Clinical Simulation in Medicine

Clinical Simulation in Medicine

For all Examinations in Cardiology, Critical Care, Anesthesia and Pulmonary Medicine

Editor-in-Chief

Poonam Malhotra Kapoor
MD DNB MNAMS FIACTA (Hony) FTEE (Hony) FISCU (Hony)

Professor
Department of Cardiac Anesthesia
Cardiothoracic Center (CTC)
All India Institute of Medical Sciences
Ansari Nagar, New Delhi, India

Chief-Editor
Annals of Cardiac Anesthesia

President
Extracorporeal Membrane Oxygenation (ECMO) Society of India

Secretary
Society of Cardiac Anesthesia (SCA)
New Delhi and NCR
The Simulation Society
Secretary and Chairperson Academics
The Simulation Society (TSS)

Section Editors

Navin C Nanda
Yatin Mehta
HK Chopra
KK Kapur

Forewords

MC Misra
Balram Airan

Under the aegis of
THE SIMULATION SOCIETY

The Health Sciences Publisher

New Delhi | London | Philadelphia | Panama

Jaypee Brothers Medical Publishers (P) Ltd.

Headquarters
Jaypee Brothers Medical Publishers (P) Ltd.
4838/24, Ansari Road, Daryaganj
New Delhi 110 002, India
Phone: +91-11-43574357
Fax: +91-11-43574314
E-mail: jaypee@jaypeebrothers.com

Overseas Offices

J.P. Medical Ltd.
83, Victoria Street, London,
SW1H 0HW (UK)
Phone: +44-20 3170 8910
Fax: +44(0) 20 3008 6180
E-mail: info@jpmedpub.com

Jaypee-Highlights Medical Publishers Inc.
City of Knowledge, Building 235, 2nd floor
Clayton, Panama City, Panama
Phone: +1 507-301-0496
Fax: +1 507-301-0499
E-mail: cservice@jphmedical.com

Jaypee Medical Inc.
325, Chestnut Street
Suite 412, Philadelphia, PA 19106, USA
Phone: +1 267-519-9789
E-mail: support@jpmedus.com

Jaypee Brothers Medical Publishers (P) Ltd.
17/1-B, Babar Road, Block-B
Shaymali, Mohammadpur
Dhaka-1207, Bangladesh
Mobile: +08801912003485
E-mail: jaypeedhaka@gmail.com

Jaypee Brothers Medical Publishers (P) Ltd.
Bhotahity, Kathmandu, Nepal
Phone: +977-9741283608
E-mail: kathmandu@jaypeebrothers.com

Website: www.jaypeebrothers.com
Website: www.jaypeedigital.com

Clinical Simulation in Medicine (For all Examinations in Cardiology, Critical Care, Anesthesia and Pulmonary Medicine)

First Edition: **2017**

ISBN: 978-93-5152-563-9

Printed at Replika Press Pvt. Ltd.

Dedicated to

My father and family

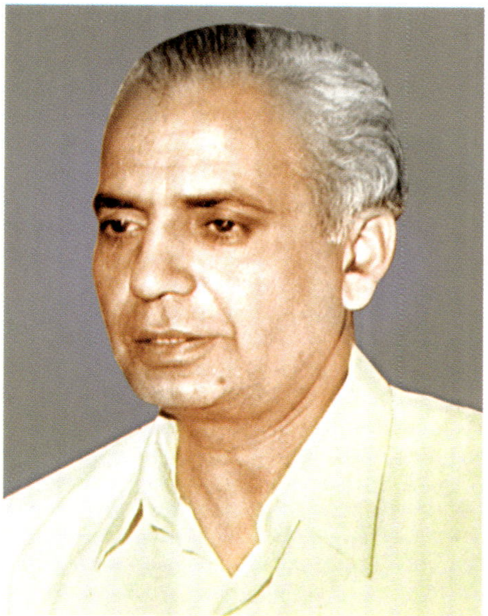

Dr KK Malhotra
(4.7.1929–4.1.2011)

My father is a never-ending song in my heart—of comfort, happiness and well-being. I may sometimes forget the words but I always remember the tune.

My mentor, guide and inspiration in life
An extraordinary physician and human being with boundless affection, witty, hardworking and godly qualities who five years after he's gone, still inspires me to read and write. He is my bridge and a good luck charm.

—Poonam Malhotra Kapoor

CONTRIBUTORS

Amit Gupta
Professor of Surgery
Division of Trauma Surgery
and Critical Care
Jai Prakash Narayan Apex Trauma Center
All India Institute of Medical Sciences
New Delhi, India

Anant Mohan
Professor
Department of Pulmonary Medicine
and Sleep Disorders
All India Institute of Medical Sciences
New Delhi, India

Arindam Choudhury
Assistant Professor
Cardiac Anesthesia
Cardiothoracic Center
All India Institute of Medical Sciences
New Delhi, India

Arun Kumar
Research Scholar
Coagulation Testing
Vijayashree Diagnostics
Bengaluru, Karnataka, India

Bishnu Panigrahi
Group Head
Medical Strategy and Operations
Fortis Healthcare Ltd, India

BS Sethi
Senior Resident
Cardiac Anesthesia
Cardiothoracic Center
All India Institute of Medical Sciences
New Delhi, India

D Bhattacharya
Consultant, Chest Physician
Department of Pulmonary
Critical Care and Sleep Medicine
Safdarjung Hospital
New Delhi, India

Dattatreya Prabhakumar
Consultant
Cardiac Anesthetist
Fortis Workhardt Hospital
Bengaluru, Karnataka, India

Dharmesh Agarwal
Senior Consultant
Cardiac Anesthesiologist and Pain
Specialist
Apollo Hospital
Bengaluru, Karnataka, India

Dhruv Bibra
Consultant
Spine and Pain Medicine
Delhi Pain Management Center
New Delhi, India

Geethanjali Ramachandra
Senior Consultant
Pediatric Intensivist
Rainbow Children's Hospital
Bengaluru, Karnataka, India

GP Dureja
Chief Consultant
Spine and Pain Medicine
Delhi Pain Management Center
New Delhi, India

HK Chopra
Chairman
National CSI Affairs
President, Cardiological Society
of India, 2015
President, World Wellness Foundation,
World Heart Academy, and
Indian Academy of
Echocardiography, 2017
American Heart Association: Courtry Head
Formerly Editor, Indian Heart Journal
and JIAE
Chief Cardiologist, Moolchand Medcity
New Delhi, India

JC Suri
Head
Department of Pulmonary
Critical Care and Sleep Medicine
Safdarjung Hospital
New Delhi, India

Jitin Narula
Associate Consultant
Department of Cardiac Anesthesiology
Max Superspecialty Hospital
Patparganj, New Delhi, India

Kalpana Irpachi
Senior Resident
Cardiac Anesthesia
Cardiothoracic Center
All India Institute of Medical Sciences
New Delhi, India

Kamal Ahuja
Consultant
Division of Cardiovascular Disease
University of Alabama at Birmingham
Birmingham, Alabama, USA

Kanchi Muralidhar
Director (Academic)
Senior Consultant and Professor
Anesthesia and Intensive Care
Narayana Hrudyalaya Hospital
Bengaluru, Karnataka, India

Karan Madan
Assistant Professor
Department of Pulmonary Medicine
and Sleep Disorders
All India Institute of Medical Sciences
New Delhi, India
Executive Member
The Simulation Society

KK Kapur
Sr Consultant and Co-director
Noninvasive Cardiology
Indraprastha Apollo Hospital
New Delhi, India

Klaus Gorlinger
Medical Director and
Former Head, Anesthesia
University of Duisburg-Essen
Germany

Kumar Belani
Professor of Medicine
Department of Anesthesiology
University of Minnesota Health
Minneapolis, MN 55455, USA

Mahesh Vakamudi
Senior Consultant and Head
Anesthesiology and Critical Care
Sri Ramachandra Medical Center
Chennai, Tamil Nadu, India

Manju Mani
Chief Consultant
Cardiac Anesthesiology
Director, Quality
Saket City Hospital
New Delhi, India

Marisa Joson
Consultant
Division of Cardiovascular Disease
University of Alabama at Birmingham
Birmingham, Alabama, USA

Mayadhar Barik
Research Scholar
Biomarker and Genetic Testing
AIIMS, New Delhi, India

Munveer Thind
Consultant
Division of Cardiovascular Disease
University of Alabama at Birmingham
Birmingham, Alabama, USA

Naga Sai Shravan Turaga
Consultant
Division of Cardiovascular Disease
University of Alabama at Birmingham
Birmingham, Alabama, USA

Naman Shastri
Chief Cardiac Anesthesiologist
and Intensivist
SAL Hospital
Ahmedabad, Gujarat, India
Treasurer and Chief Advisor
The Simulation Society

Naveen Garg
Consultant
Department of Cardiology
Indraprastha Apollo Hospital
New Delhi, India

Navin C Nanda
Distinguished Professor of Medicine
and Cardiovascular Disease
Section Head of Electrocardiography
Director of the Clinical Echocardiography
Fellowship Program
UAB School of Medicine
Birmingham, Alabama, USA

Poonam Malhotra Kapoor
Professor
Department of Cardiac Anesthesia
Cardiothoracic Center (CTC)
All India Institute of Medical Sciences
Ansari Nagar, New Delhi, India
Chief-Editor
Annals of Cardiac Anesthesia
President
Extracorporeal Membrane Oxygenation
(ECMO) Society of India
Secretary
Society of Cardiac Anesthesia (SCA)
New Delhi and NCR
The Simulation Society
Secretary and Chairperson Academics
The Simulation Society

Pranay Oza
ECMO Specialist and Intensivist
Riddhivinayak Critical Care
and Cardiac Center
Mumbai, Maharashtra, India

Praveen Kalligudd
Consultant
Cardiac Anesthetist
Fortis Workhardt Hospital
Bengaluru, Karnataka, India

Priyanka Saxena
Senior Resident
Department of Clinical Hematology
Institute of Liver and Biliary
Sciences (ILBS)
New Delhi, India

R Gopinath
Head
Department of Anesthesiology
Nizam's Institute of Medical Sciences
Hyderabad, Telangana, India

Raghu B
Consultant
Anesthesia and Critical Care
Narayana Hrudyalaya Hospitals
Bengaluru, Karnataka, India

Rajiv Juneja
Director
Institute of Critical Care and
Anesthesiology
Medanta—The Medicity
Gurgaon, Haryana, India
President
SCA—Delhi and NCR

Rakesh Garg
Assistant Professor
Department of Anesthesiology
Intensive Care Pain and Palliative Care
Dr BRAIRCH: All India Institute of
Medical Sciences
Ansari Nagar, New Delhi, India

Rakesh Gupta
Director and Chief Cardiologist
Echo and Color Doppler Center
JROP Institute of Echocardiography
Ultrasound and Vascular Doppler, India

Rakshay Shetty
Lead Pediatric Intensivist
24 Bed Tertiary Care PICU
Rainbow Children's Hospital
Bengaluru, Karnataka, India
Section Editor, Cardiology
Annals of Cardiac Anesthesia (ACA)

Randeep Guleria
Professor and Head
Department of Pulmonary Medicine
and Sleep Disorders
All India Institute of Medical Sciences
New Delhi, India
Vice President
The Simulation Society

Richie Jain
Attending Consultant
Department of Cardiac Anesthesiology
Medanta—The Medicity
Gurgaon, Haryana, India

Rohan Magoon
Senior Resident
Department of Cardiac Anesthesia
CN Center
All India Institute of Medical Sciences
New Delhi, India

S Mohan
Senior Consultant
Liver Transplant Anesthesia
Global Hospital
Hyderabad, Telangana, India

Sameer Srivastava
Head
Department of Noninvasive Cardiology
Fortis Escorts Heart Institute
New Delhi, India
Principal Coordinator
Postgraduate Diploma in Clinical
Cardiology, Program at FEHI
New Delhi, India
Section Editor, Cardiology
Annals of Cardiac Anesthesia

Sameer Taneja
Senior Resident
Cardiac Anesthesia
Cardiothoracic Center
All India Institute of Medical Sciences
New Delhi, India

Sanjay Goel
Senior Consultant
Cardiac Anesthesia
Max Super Specialty Hospital
Saket, New Delhi, India

Sanjeev Bhoi
Additional Professor and In-charge
Department of Emergency Medicine
Jai Prakash Narayan Apex Trauma Center
All India Institute of Medical Sciences
New Delhi, India

Sanketh Hiremath
Research Scholar
Coagulation Testing
Vijayashree Diagnostics
Bengaluru, Karnataka, India

Sarvesh Pal Singh
Assistant Professor
Department of CTVS
Cardiothoracic Center
All India Institute of Medical Sciences
New Delhi, India

Saurabh Gaba
Consultant
Division of Cardiovascular Disease
University of Alabama at Birmingham
Birmingham, Alabama, USA

Serkan Bulur
Consultant
Division of Cardiovascular Disease
University of Alabama at Birmingham
Birmingham, Alabama, USA

SN Das
Additional Professor
Cardiac Anesthesia
Cardiothoracic Center
All India Institute of Medical Sciences
New Delhi, India

Sujatha Thyagarajan
Consultant PICU/ER
Rainbow Children's Hospital
Bengaluru, Karnataka, India

Sunit Singhi
Head
Department of Pediatric Medicine
Postgraduate Institute of Medical
Education and Research
Chandigarh, India

Surabh Gaba
Consultant
Division of Cardiovascular Disease
University of Alabama at Birmingham
Birmingham, Alabama, USA

Suruchi Hasija
Assistant Professor
Cardiac Anesthesia
Cardiothoracic Center
All India Institute of Medical Sciences
New Delhi, India

TA Patil
Consultant
Cardiac Anesthetist
Fortis Workhardt Hospital
Bengaluru, Karnataka, India

Ujjwal Chowdhury
Professor
Department of CTVS
Cardiothoracic Center
All India Institute of Medical Sciences
New Delhi, India

Vandana Bhardwaj
Senior Resident
Cardiac Anesthesia
Cardiothoracic Center
All India Institute of Medical Sciences
New Delhi, India

Venkat Goyal
ECMO Specialist and Cardiologist
Riddhivinayak Critical Care
and Cardiac Center
Mumbai, Maharashtra, India
President Elect
The South and West Asia Chapter of
Extracorporeal Life Support Organization
(SWAC-ELSO)

Vilash Hiremath
Research Scholar
Coagulation Testing
Vijayashree Diagnostics
Bengaluru, Karnataka, India

Viswas Malik
Additional Professor
Cardiac Anesthesia
Cardiothoracic Center
All India Institute of Medical Sciences
New Delhi, India

Yatin Mehta
Chairman
Institute of Critical Care and
Anesthesiology
Medanta—The Medicity
Gurgaon, Haryana, India
Chancellor, Indian College of Cardiac
Anesthesia
National President
The Simulation Society
Advisor
Annals of Cardiac Anesthesia
Former President
Society of Cardiac Anesthesia
Delhi and NCR Branch
President
Critical Care Society of India

FOREWORD

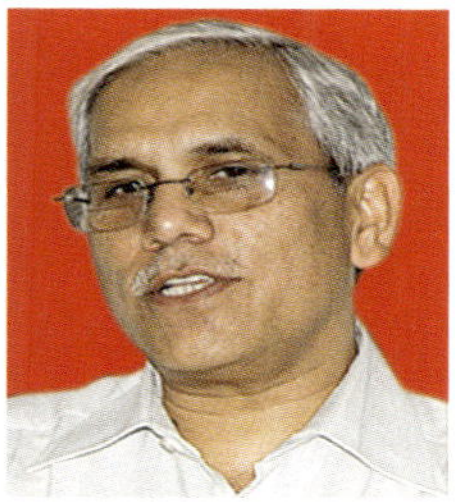

Medical simulation is a branch of simulation technology related to education and training in medical fields of various industries. It can involve simulated human patients, educational documents with detailed simulated animations, casualty assessment in homeland security and military situations, and emergency response. Its main purpose is to train medical professionals to reduce accidents during surgery, prescription, and general, clinical practice.

This book *Clinical Simulation in Medicine* edited by Dr Poonam Malhotra Kapoor and other stalwarts in academic teaching is a handbook for individuals working in or preparing to work in simulation and for academic and service organizations that are using simulation or are planning to use simulation. It provides the knowledge needed to become a simulation professional and generates information on how to best use that knowledge to effectively use simulation in their organizations for day-to-day procedures. Evidence-based and pragmatic, this book raises awareness of the knowledge and expertise required to utilize simulation strategies.

A true benefit of simulation can be harvested when the simulation models are fully integrated into the routine fabric of health care delivery and academics. Health professionals embarking on a career teaching simulation are embracing a world of innovation in which both teachers and students can develop their healthcare skills more rapidly and promote better patients' outcomes. This is the first practice manual to assist healthcare simulation educators in India and internationally in preparing for certification in this rapidly emerging field.

Healthcare decision makers need reliable tools to support them in decision making for adapting policies to help cutting costs or reducing waiting time, and to provide visualization which allows them to rehearse innovative ideas before they are implemented. The tools should facilitate an evidence-based and informed decision-making environment. Simulation models, especially with transparency into their structure and underlying variables, which can be easily understood and trusted by decision makers, are a helpful tool in decision support, communication and discussion of ideas and policies, and analysis of scenarios.

The book is a guide and reference to the latest technology, operations and opportunities presented by clinical simulation in the field of bronchoscopy and the difficult airway, trauma and basic life support, echocardiography, hemodynamic monitoring and latest trends in monitoring the bleeding surgical patients in point-of-care testing. It shows how to develop and make efficient use of resources, and provides hands-on information to those tasked with setting up and delivering simulation facilities for medical, clinical and related purposes, and the development and delivery of simulation-based education programs.

All in all, the *Clinical Simulation in Medicine* is a very important entry into what I would consider the "examination preparation" category of cardiac critical skills for the fellows and students in the subject. The chapters are well illustrated, and most have an extensive number of topics that they may need to review in greater depth. With expert contributors and sound editing, the book would be a valuable addition to the library of anesthesiologists, surgeons, pulmonologists, pediatric intensivists, and cardiologists interested in a text covering the breadth of topics related to clinical medicine.

"The eyes do not see what the mind does not know" is very true about clinical medicine. As a result, a simple aortic stenosis may be missed. This first-of-its-kind book on the subject of clinical medicine has brought together different contributors from various branches of medicine. There is a great need for a book of this type and the author's present work goes a long way in fulfilling this need.

I wish the contributors, all success in their venture.

MC Misra
Director
All India Institute of Medical Sciences
Ansari Nagar, New Delhi, India

FOREWORD

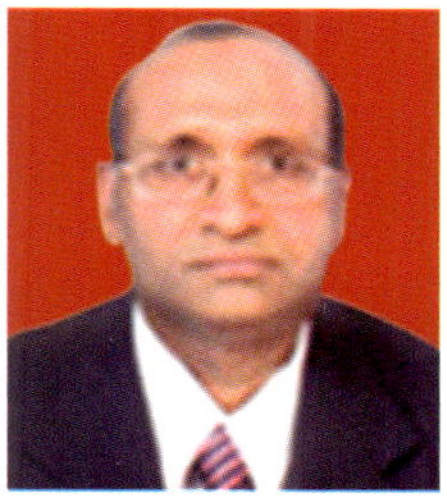

The book promotes the value of simulation in healthcare and its associated outcomes while clarifying the operational requirements of successful simulations, featuring numerous contributions from international and national experts, consultants and specialists in clinical medicine in simulation.

The use of simulation to gain and maintain skills in healthcare has become critical to the delivery of the curricula in medical schools, nursing schools, residency programs, and hospital-based practice. Specialty boards, such as the American Board of Anesthesiology, now require simulation training as part of the maintenance of certification. This trend is fast catching up in medical simulation.

Medical simulation is a relatively new science that is achieving respectability among healthcare educators worldwide. Simulation and skills centers have become established to integrate simulation into mainstream education in all medical, nursing, and paramedical fields. Borrowing from the experience and methodologies of industries that are using simulation, medical educators are grappling with the problem of rapidly acquiring the skills and techniques required to implement simulation programs into established curricula. This book assists both novice and experienced workers in the field to learn from established practitioners in medical simulation. Simulation has been used to enhance the educational experience in a diverse range of fields; therefore, a wide variety of disciplines are represented.

The book begins with a section on the logistics of establishing a simulation and its role in the medical field and hospitals. Different sections deal with simulation in transthoracic and transesophageal echocardiography, hemodynamic monitoring, ECMO and many of miscellaneous diseases, such as advanced cardiovascular life support (ACLS), basic life support (BLS), and airway management that is required to equip a stand-alone or institution-based center. The features, strengths, and weaknesses of training devices are presented to help the readers find the appropriate simulator to fulfill their training requirements.

The book will continue to vibrate you from the beginning to the end and going through the book is a pleasure. The contributors of the book are unmatched in their pediatric perioperative TEE skills who have excelled in their fields.

I am sure the book will find a permanent place on the desk of all clinicians interested in simulation. I congratulate Dr Poonam Malhotra Kapoor and her team for this wonderful endeavor and wish the book and her great success.

Balram Airan
Professor and Head
Department of Cardiothoracic and Vascular Surgery (CTVS)
Dean, Academic, AIIMS
Chief, Cardiac Center
All India Institute of Medical Sciences (AIIMS)
Ansari Nagar, New Delhi, India

PREFACE

Medical textbooks, continuing education programs and reference sources all provide the knowledge base needed for competent medical practice. This book presents the rest of what we need to know to be an outstanding clinician—that is practicing your clinical skills on simulators. *Clinical Simulation in Medicine* goes beyond basic routine teachings. It helps the clinicians improve patients' outcomes with simulation-based learning to enhance practitioners' skills, clinical competence and interdisciplinary collaboration. To advance the field of healthcare simulation, this book provides a platform for every clinician in improving and reforming education amongst the health professionals, in a more robust way!

Today, clinicians, hunting for the answers to questions can find more timely information online and they can find it faster than searching the index and then the numbered pages of a heavy book!! But, how do you practice your clinical skills? The physician participants in this book have discovered better and in some cases, incredibly effective ways to learn the clinical skills over the years by simulating them first, without weakening the conventional system and in most cases, learning and teaching it on the simulators to clear their concepts better! Research studies have proven their success!

The path to mastery and improved performance involves practice and experience. This is true if you are an athlete or a helicopter pilot, but not as a practicing clinician, on a live patient! For education and professional development in the medical field, simulation has provided practice and experiential learning opportunities for years. In my experience of teaching at AIIMS, simulation is the most essential to educate medical professionals.

Any individuals, societies or organizations discussed in this book are mentioned without malice. To the best of my knowledge, this book reports the truth, not with the intent to harm, but to inform to the best of my ability as a scholar who has devoted much time and is passionate about using simulation for academic teaching.

I am grateful to all my section editors, contributors and readers for their constant interest and expert help with this manuscript.

This book collaborates physicians from different fields, first time together with one aim—"Academic teaching and learning different clinical subjects with medical simulation". Most of my thanks go to my teachers, students and family members—my first readers and key critics.

This is lucid text, explained simply by all of us in the words of Einstein, the Great—"If you cannot explain it simply enough, then you do not understand it well enough".

Poonam Malhotra Kapoor

ACKNOWLEDGMENTS

I am highly indebted to acknowledge the contributors of this book and deeply appreciate their cooperation. I am also grateful to my AIIMS colleagues for facilitating the preparation of this manuscript and using simulation ardently in teaching our students. My gratitude also goes to the assistance offered by Mr Sandeep Balyan, Mr Pradeep and Mr Sachin my efficient office staff. My son, Pranav Kapoor helped me with images in this book and I feel proud of his talent. My husband and son I remain most indebted to for bearing my long absence from home while I was preparing this first-of-its-kind book together in *Clinical Simulation in Medicine*. My parents and three lovely sisters are my constant source of inspiration. I thank them for their continuous support and patience. God bless each one of the above-mentioned supporters into formulating this book, especially the "students of cardiac critical care science".

Writing and illustrating are part of a book, yet never the whole and my special thanks are due to Shri Jitendar P Vij (Group Chairman), Mr Ankit Vij (Group President), Mr Tarun Duneja (Director–Publishing), Mrs Samina Khan (Executive Assistant to Director Publishing), and whole production team of M/s Jaypee Brothers Medical Publishers (P) Ltd, New Delhi, India, for their cooperation in formulating this book.

CONTENTS

SECTION 1: Introduction to Simulation in Medicine

SECTION 2: Simulation in Transthoracic Echocardiography

SECTION 5: Simulation for Hemodynamic Monitoring

SECTION 6: Transesophageal Echocardiography in the Cardiac Intensive Care Unit

SECTION 7: Pediatric Simulation

SECTION 8: Simulation for ECMO and Pain Medicine

SECTION 9: Simulation, Cardiac Critical Care and Resources

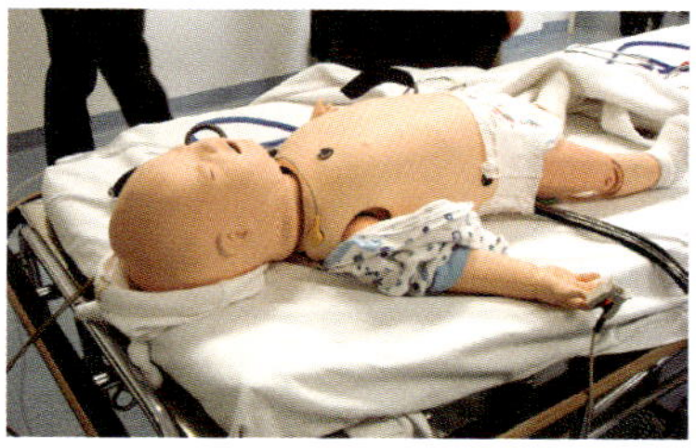

Section 1

Introduction to Simulation in Medicine

Section Outline

- What is Simulation?
- Role of Simulation in Medicine

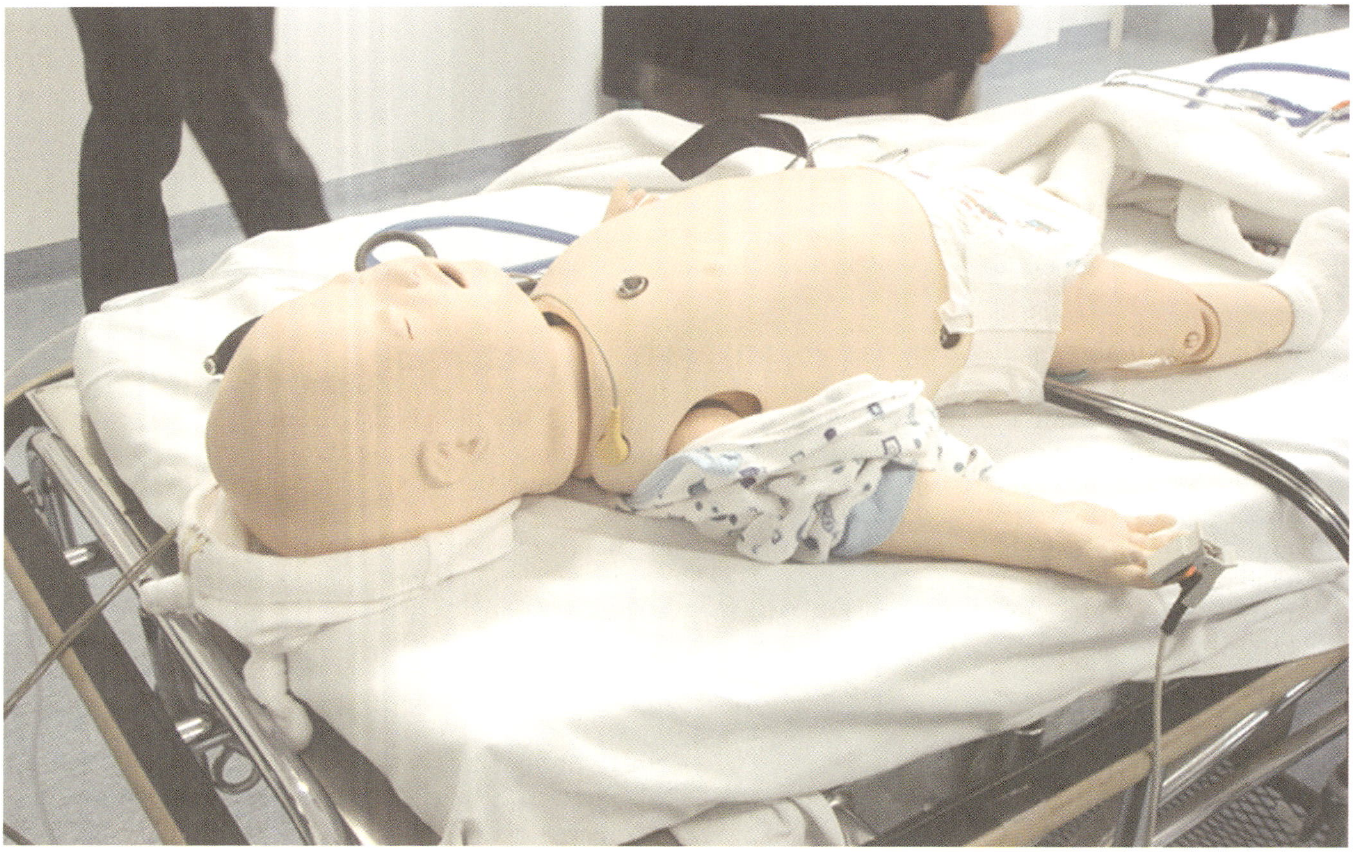

Chapter 1

What is Simulation?

Poonam Malhotra Kapoor, Yatin Mehta

Chapter Outline

- Simulation in Various Medical Fields
- Advantages of Simulation Learning
- Freedom to Error and Learn from Mistakes
- Learning can be Customized
- Simulation Provides Detailed Feedback and Evaluation
- Simulation in Health Care
- To Summarize about Simulation in Education
- Objectives of Simulation
- Activities of the Simulation Society
- Modern Medical Simulation
- Advantages of Mannequin-based Computer Simulators
- Transesophageal Echocardiography Simulation
- Importance of Transesophageal Echocardiography Simulation

INTRODUCTION

One of the most important steps in curriculum development is the introduction of simulation-based medical teaching and learning. Simulation is a generic term that refers to an artificial representation of a real world process to achieve educational goals through experiential learning. Simulation based medical education is defined as any educational activity that utilizes simulation aides to replicate clinical scenarios. Although medical simulation is relatively new, simulation has been used for a long time in other high risk professions such as aviation. Medical simulation allows the acquisition of clinical skills through deliberate practice rather than an apprentice style of learning. Simulation tools serve as an alternative to real patients. A trainee can make mistakes and learn from them without the fear of harming the patient. There are different types and classification of simulators and their cost vary according to the degree of their resemblance to the reality, or 'fidelity'. Simulation-based learning is expensive. However, it is cost-effective if utilized properly. Medical simulation has been found to enhance clinical competence at the undergraduate and postgraduate levels. It has also been found to have many advantages that can improve patient safety and reduce health care costs through the improvement of the medical provider's competencies. The objective of this narrative review article is to highlight the importance of simulation as a new teaching method in undergraduate and postgraduate education.

Simulation technology (**Figure 1**) has been used successfully to advance medical training, especially in

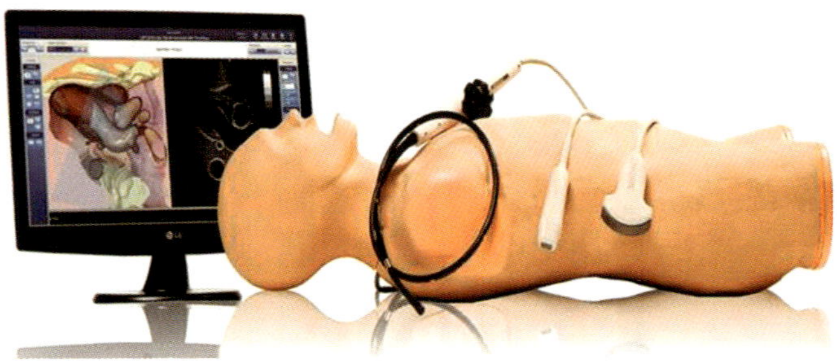

Figure 1 Simulation mannequin

the last 10 years.[1] Recently, the emphasis has been on scenarios when the skill involved is critical to patient safety and/or the number of procedures required to achieve proficiency is impractical.[2,3] Simulation technology can be complemented with parallel three-dimensional (3D) models that improve the spatial perception of the procedure (reality-enhanced simulators) or with devices that allow visual feedback and kinesthetic interactions between an operator and the simulator (haptic technology).

DEFINITION

The dictionary meaning of simulation is "the representation of the behavior or characteristics of one system through the use of another system, especially using a computer". One can learn in a particular zone of development by what vygotsky called the "Lure to learn" **(Figure 2)**. Particular zones of development can be referred to as the domain where people are acting a particular scenario. For a simulation procedure (SP), it would be within the constraints of a simulated patient examining room. For a construction scene, the constraints will be at work site. Being able to successfully improvise within the particular zone of learning and engaging with the other members of the interaction will allow a fluid dynamic in interaction.

Medical simulation is a branch of simulation technology related to education and training in medical fields of various industries. It can involve simulated human patients, educational documents with detailed simulated animations, casualty assessment in homeland security and military situations, and emergency response. Its main purpose is to train medical professionals to reduce accidents during surgery, prescription, and general practice. However, it now has been extended in its use for training students

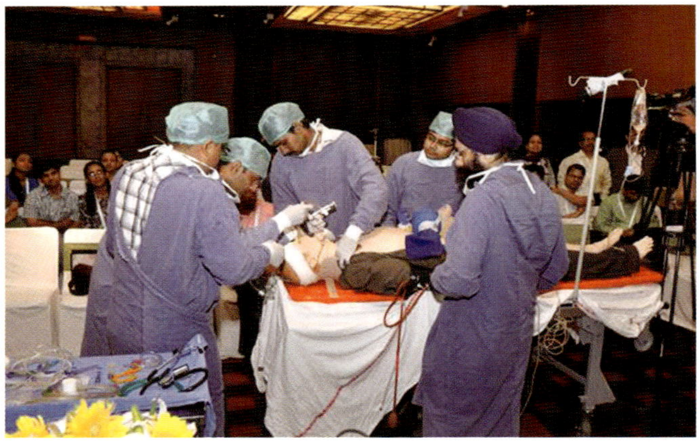

Figure 2 Simulation mannequin for teaching and learning

in anatomy and physiology during their clinical training as allied health professionals. These professions include nursing, sonography, pharmacy assistants and physical therapy. Advances in technology are advancing geometrically and a McGraw Hill textbook, Medical Simulation, by VanCura and Bisset interfaces the simulator technology with any medically related course of study.

Many medical professionals are skeptical about simulation, saying that medicine, surgery, and general healing skills are too complex to simulate accurately. But technological advances in the past two decades have made it possible to simulate practices from yearly family doctor visits to complex operations such as heart surgery.

SIMULATION IN VARIOUS MEDICAL FIELDS

The utility of simulation is widely recognized and becoming a greater part of medical education across fields. Each major specialty in medicine has worked to shape and optimize the use of simulation in ways that not only address common medical challenges but also specifically address competencies unique to a given specialty. To better understand simulation as a changing entity across medical fields, we briefly survey key components of the use of simulation in each of five major medical specialties outside neurosurgery: anesthesiology, emergency medicine, surgery, obstetrics and pediatrics.

The nature of certain medical fields in which spontaneous emergent intervention is required (e.g. anesthesiology, surgery and emergency medicine) is such that learning opportunities in critical cases may be sporadic and somewhat limited given the rapidity with which intervention must be implemented. Unacceptable consequences may occur should care be delayed or errors take place during training.

Procedural simulation has been demonstrated to improve clinical implementation of advanced cardiac life support protocols.[4] Therefore, given the often high-acuity environments of anesthesiology, simulations have provided a natural supplement to clinical anesthesia training, with 70% of medical schools using some form of simulation for teaching.[5]

KEY POINTS

- Simulation has a rich history in medical fields; it is particularly useful in fields that carry high risk and cost in the event of errors.
- Medical and surgical education is constantly being pushed to meet the demands of the public and society for excellent results with minimal morbidity and mortality.
- Cardiological surgery, because of its high-risk and complex procedures that affect quality and quantity of life, may augment traditional training with multimodality didactic tools.

ADVANTAGES OF SIMULATION LEARNING

Simulation Learning Provides the Following Opportunities

Learning in healthcare is too frequently in an apprenticeship model. In many disciplines, as opportunities to learn and practice come along, it is hoped that learners encounter enough situations to insure that they become competent. This is ultimately a haphazard way to learn, and puts learners and patients at a disadvantage. Simulation offers scheduled, valuable learning experiences that are difficult to obtain in real life. Learners address hands-on and thinking skills, including knowledge-in-action, procedures, decision making, and effective communication. Critical team work behaviors such as managing high workload, trapping errors, and coordinating under stress can be taught and practiced **(Figure 3)**. Training runs the gamut from preventive care to invasive surgery. Because any clinical situation can be portrayed at will, these learning opportunities can be scheduled at convenient times and locations and repeated as often as necessary.

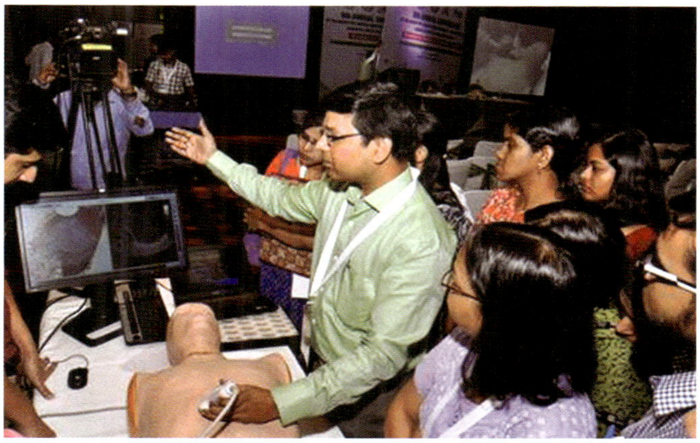

Figure 3 A trainee receiving instruction on anatomical correlation with echocardiographic images using a TEE simulator

Simulation offers scheduled, valuable learning experiences that is difficult to obtain in real life.

FREEDOM TO ERROR AND LEARN FROM MISTAKES

Working in a simulated environment allows learners to make mistakes without the need for intervention by experts to stop patient harm. By seeing the outcome of their mistakes, learners gain powerful insight into the consequences of their actions and the need to **"get it right"**.

LEARNING CAN BE CUSTOMIZED

Simulation can accommodate a range of learners from novices to experts. Beginners can gain confidence and "muscle memory" for tasks that then allow them to focus on the more demanding parts of care. Experts can better master the continuously growing array of new technologies from minimally invasive surgery and catheter-based therapies to robotics without putting the first groups of patients at undue risk. Some complex procedures and rare diseases simply do not present enough opportunities for practice, even to established clinicians. Examples include treating a severe allergic reaction or heart attack in an outpatient clinic setting, or handling a case of malignant hyperthermia in the operating room. This is a gap that simulation training methods can help fill **(Figure 4)**.

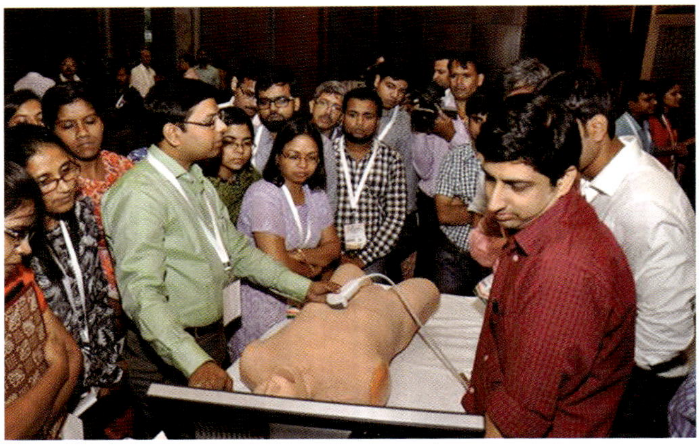

Figure 4 Simulation teaching is easy to teach and easy to learn

SIMULATION PROVIDES DETAILED FEEDBACK AND EVALUATION

Real events and the pace of actual healthcare operations do not allow for the best review and learning about why things took place, or how to improve performance. Controlled simulations can be immediately followed by videotape-supported or after-action reviews that richly detail what happened. Advanced surgical and task simulators gather much data about what the learner is actually doing. These performance maps and logs provide a solid and necessary feedback mechanism to learners and help instructors target necessary improvements.

SIMULATION IN HEALTH CARE

Health care simulation is coming of age, and has begun to share much with established methods in aviation, spaceflight, nuclear power, shipping and the military. The rapid advance of computer science, bioengineering, and design has met demands from all stakeholders for safer, more effective and efficient ethical healthcare. When the stakes are high and real settings do not lend themselves to artificial handling for other purposes, simulation methods will find applications.

TO SUMMARIZE ABOUT SIMULATION IN EDUCATION

- Simulation-based education (SBE) is a rapidly developing method of supplementing and enhancing the clinical education of medical students.
- Clinical situations are simulated for teaching and learning purposes, creating opportunities for deliberate practice of new skills without involving real patients.

  Experts can better master the continuously growing array of new technologies from minimally invasive surgery and catheter-based therapies to robotics without putting the first groups of patients at undue risk.
- Simulation takes many forms, from simple skills training models to computerized full-body mannequins, so that the needs of learners at each stage of their education can be targeted.
- Emerging evidence supports the value of simulation as an educational technique; to be effective it needs to be integrated into the curriculum in a way that promotes transfer of the skills learnt in clinical practice.
- Currently, SBE initiatives in India are fragmented and depend on local enthusiasts; Health Workforce Australia is driving initiatives to develop a more coordinated national approach to optimize the benefits of simulation.

OBJECTIVES OF SIMULATION

- To develop standards of practice regarding the key applications of simulation including education, research and patient care.
- To foster a network of professionals working within the simulation field.
- To advocate for continued development and availability of simulation-based modalities for key applications including education, research and patient care.
- To form affiliations with societies and groups having common goals in relation to simulation and safety and quality in health care.
- To promote the professional development of individuals working in the simulation field.
- To advise on legislation related to the use of simulation in health care.
- To be recognized as the official representative of these groups in the national and international scenarios.

ACTIVITIES OF THE SIMULATION SOCIETY

The Simulation Society (TSS) from India formulated in August 2014 by, the authors of this chapter conducts workshop on simulation regularly. Simulation in cardiac critical care is in the curriculum of medical education which is essential to promote technical skills in clinical practice.

- Conducting conferences, seminars and workshops including the SimHealth conference.
- Sponsoring student scholarships.
- Contributing to the development of Indian and international standards of simulation.
- Liaising with international simulation organizations.
- Encouraging research.
- Information dissemination via newsletters and the website.
- Running a college and a journal to enhance simulation based education and learning in medical sciences.
- Providing certification courses and fellowship examinations in simulation based teaching in medicine and cardiac critical care on a regular basis.

MODERN MEDICAL SIMULATION

The American Board of Emergency Medicine employs the use of medical simulation technology in order to accurately judge students by using "patient scenarios" during oral board examinations.[6] However, these forms of simulation are a far cry from high fidelity models that have surfaced since the 1990s **(Figure 5)**.[7]

Due to the fact that computer simulation technology is still relatively new relative to flight and military simulators, there is still much research to be done about the best way to approach medical training through simulation. That said, successful strides are being made in terms of medical education and training. A thorough amount of studies has shown that students engaged in medical simulation training have overall higher scores and retention rates than those trained through traditional means.

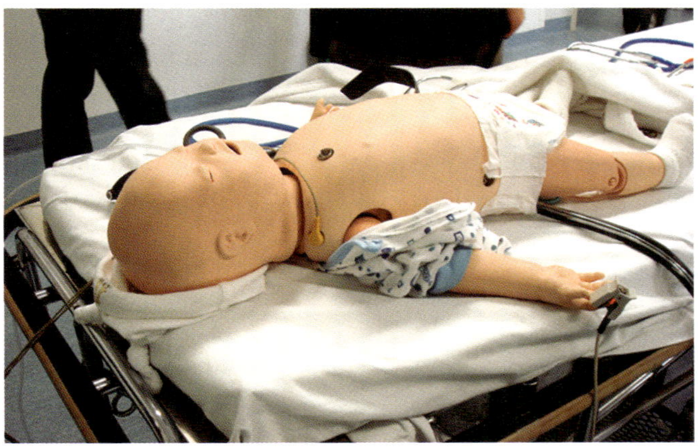

Figure 5 High fidelity simulator for teaching and training

The Council of Residency Directors (CORD) has established the following recommendations for simulation.

Students engaged in medical simulation training have overall higher scores and retention rates than those trained through traditional means.

- Simulation is a useful tool for training residents and in ascertaining competency. The core competencies most conducive to simulation-based training are patient care, interpersonal skills, and systems based practice.
- It is appropriate for performance assessment but there is a scarcity of evidence that supports the validity of simulation in the use for promotion or certification.
- There is a need for standardization and definition in using simulation to evaluate performance.
- Scenarios and tools should also be formatted and standardized such that simulation educators can use the data and count on it for reproducibility, reliability and validity **(Figures 6A and B)**.

ADVANTAGES OF MANNEQUIN-BASED COMPUTER SIMULATORS

- Students can refine and apply their skills in realistic health care situations
- Learning tailored to the educational needs of students
- Allows unlimited creation of situations that might be too dangerous or expensive to perform live
- Allows students repeated practice of procedures to reach proficiency
- Allows adherence to standard guidelines by reinforcement
- Allows evaluation of individual or group performance
- Scenarios can be halted at any time to allow for discussion of management strategies
- No issues of patient safety or confidentiality.

TRANSESOPHAGEAL ECHOCARDIOGRAPHY SIMULATION

A perfect example of high fidelity simulation.

Transesophageal echocardiography (TEE) is a widely-used technique in the cardiovascular

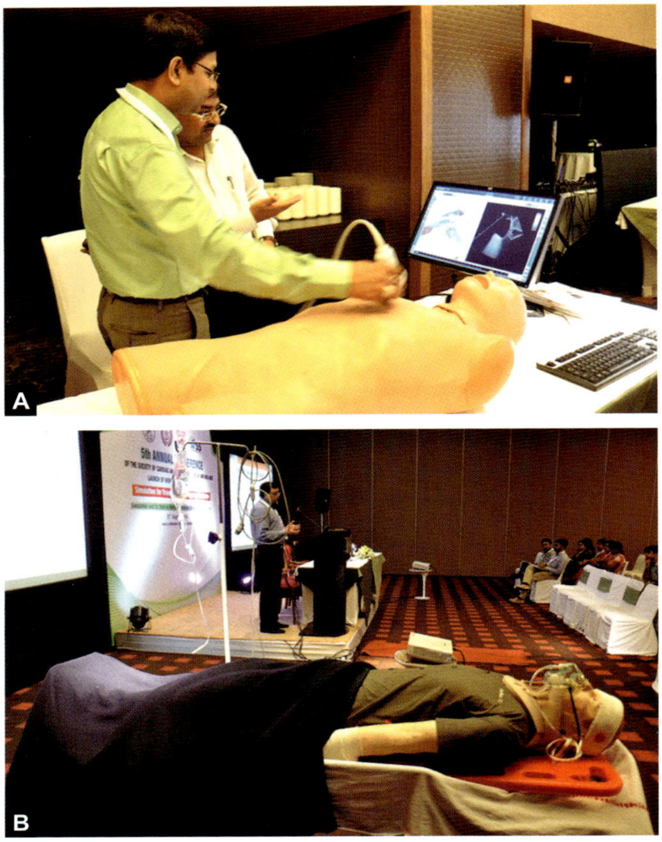

Figures 6A and B The teaching macrosimulation for one to one learning as "hands on experience"

assessment of patients undergoing complex surgery or those that are critically ill.

It is recognized as an important element that impacts surgical technique, especially in patients undergoing mitral valve surgery **(Figure 7)**.[8,9] Image acquisition and interpretation using TEE can also be subject to variability depending on experience and skill of the operator. The National Board of Echocardiography and the Society of Cardiovascular Anesthesiologists (SCA) have therefore established training guidelines that define expectations of competency in TEE during the training period for perioperative physicians.[10] Acquiring minimal proficiency in perioperative TEE can also be challenging for trainees and teaching faculty, as the number of cases required learn TEE is considerable as is the time for acquiring the cognitive skills through didactic education.[10]

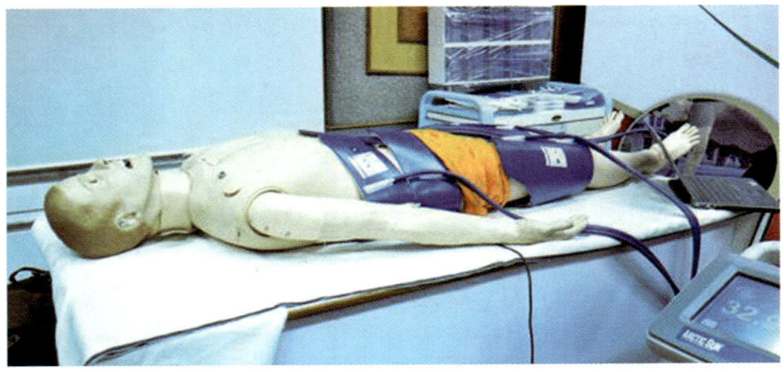

Figure 7 Mannequin for TEE simulation in echocardiography

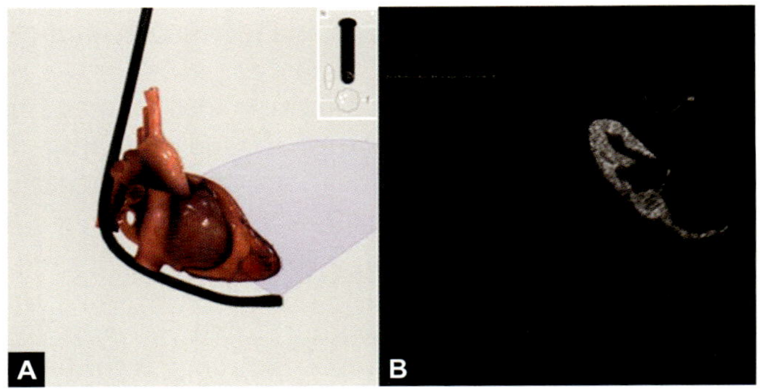

Figures 8A and B (A) An image from the TEE simulator showing the location of the TEE probe in close proximity to the heart with the intervening structures removed to better demonstrate the relationship. (B) The panel on the right simultaneously displays the echocardiographic correlate

A TEE simulator is capable of displaying two images—one that shows a three-dimensional representation of cardiac anatomy, while the other shows the simultaneous echo correlate **(Figures 8A and B)**. The location of the TEE probe with the esophagus removed is an added advantage that helps the user visually with anatomical relationships. The manipulation of the echocardiographic scan plane can be accomplished using a keyboard or a connected mannequin.

IMPORTANCE OF TRANSESOPHAGEAL ECHOCARDIOGRAPHY SIMULATION

This technology can also be used by trainees in several disciplines such as anesthesiology, cardiology, cardiac surgery and critical care to improve proficiency in basic TEE image acquisition and interpretation. At the present time, exposure to intraoperative TEE is challenging for trainees outside the operating room environment

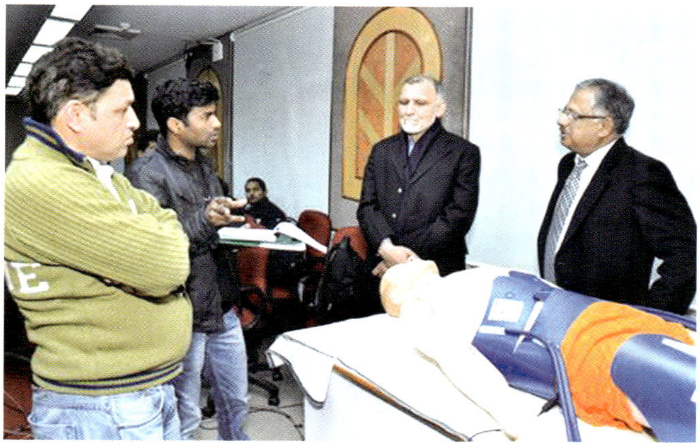

Figure 9 The simulation for TEE is challenging for trainee's outside the operating room environment

(Figure 9). The development of cardiac pathology will greatly help trainees develop the interpretative skills in areas either too complex or infrequent in occurrence to permit enough time for education in the clinical environment. This technology can be used for helping physicians maintain competency in situations where clinical case volume may be insufficient to support current competency requirements.

Significance of Simulation Training

The availability of reality-enhanced TEE simulation is a significant departure from traditional training models that rely on a combination of didactics and real time clinical teaching. While more 'real world' in application, the challenges of simultaneous clinical management may place additional burden on educators in the operating room. Simulation in TEE provides a more controlled environment in which to assess the efficacy of this training methodology over conventional approaches while also providing objective data to justify its routine use.

Limitations of Simulation Training

Simulation technology is expensive and TEE simulators are not immune to this phenomenon. A TEE simulator can cost from US$ 22,000 up to US$100,000. Maintenance expenses add to the overall cost of a simulator. A simulator also needs to be placed in a dedicated training area and this cost should also be accounted for. Other echo modalities such as M-mode, spectral Doppler and color flow are challenging to reproduce and are not currently available. Similarly simulation of transducer functions, such as gain, compression and depth are not available. Simulation of pathologic states is the next frontier in TEE simulation when the touch of a button can produce mitral valve prolapse, aortic stenosis, or a regional wall motion abnormality.

CONCLUSION

Simulation patients are the issues, learning gaps, and needs that are required to improve simulation patient education. Simulation based education are requiring for the concept of virtual humans, embodied conversational agents, fundamentals of acting, clinical play, virtual humans, and future immersive technologies. A fresh look is needed into looking at standardized patient education. Improvization is essential in simulation in which there is a need to show and simulation can get us to a better level of quality when educating these essential medical role players.

REFERENCES

1. Cooper JB, Taqueti VR. A brief history of the development of mannequin simulators for clinical education and training. Postgrad Med J. 2008;84:563-70.
2. Ziv A, Wolpe PR, Small SD, Glick S. Simulation-based medical education: An ethical imperative. Acad Med. 2003;78:783-8.
3. Ziv A, Wolpe PR, Small SD, Glick S. Simulation-based medical education: An ethical imperative. Simul Healthc. 2006;1:252-6.
4. Nishisaki A, Keren R, Nadkarni V. Does simulation improve patient safety? Selfefficacy, competence, operational performance, and patient safety. Anesthesiol Clin. 2007;25(2):225-36.
5. Morgan PJ, Cleave-Hogg D. A worldwide survey of the use of simulation in anesthesia. Can J Anaesth. 2002;49(7):659-62.
6. Chakravarthy B. Academic resident. Medical simulation in EM training and beyond. Edited by the SAEMGME Committee.
7. Ahmed K, Jawad M, Abboudi M, Gavazzi A, Darzi A, Athanasiou T, et al. Effectiveness of procedural simulation in urology: A systematic review. J Urol. 2011 May 13. PMID 21571338.
8. Practice guidelines for perioperative transesophageal echocardiography. A report by the american society of anesthesiologists and the society of cardiovascular

CHAPTER 1

anesthesiologists task force on transesophageal echocardiography. Anesthesiology. 1996;84:986-1006.
9. Cheitlin MD, Armstrong WF, Aurigemma GP, Beller GA, Bierman FZ, Davis JL, et al. ACC/AHA/ASE 2003 guideline update for the clinical application of echocardiography: Summary article. A report of the American College of Cardiology/American Heart Association task force on practice guidelines (ACC/AHA/ASE committee to update the 1997 guidelines for the clinical application of echocardiography). J Am Soc Echocardiogr. 2003;16:1091-110.
10. Cahalan MK, Abel M, Goldman M, Pearlman A, Sears-Rogan P, Russell I, et al. American Society of Echocardiography and Society of Cardiovascular Anesthesiologists task force guidelines for training in perioperative echocardiography. Anesth Analg. 2002;94:1384-8.

Chapter 2

Role of Simulation in Medicine

Poonam Malhotra Kapoor, Bishnu Panigrahi

Chapter Outline

- Simulation
- Levels of Simulation
- True Benefit of Simulation
- Smarter Simulation Modes Now Available
- Importance of Simulation
- Decision Support
- Training and Quality
- Complexity
- Process Improvement
- User Acceptance
- Healthcare Processes
- Conclusion: Modules Provide Dynamic Effects
- Greater Insight
- Wider Applicability
- A Flexible Tool
- Healthcare Simulation Challenges
- Simulation Makes the Learner "Higher Up on the Learning Curve"
- Clinical Simulation: Role and Significance in Student Training
- Utility of Simulation in Medical Education

SIMULATION

Creation of a artificial scenario for a real life technique in a virtual, mechanical, graphic or computerized version or on a mannequin for the training or testing of that technique. This is done to enhance learning and teaching through hands on repeated practice and feedback, without any harm caused to the patient.

Objectives of Clinical Simulation[1]

- Promotion of modern training methods, self-training and team work **(Figure 1)**
- Acquirement of practical abilities and competences
- Individualization of student training

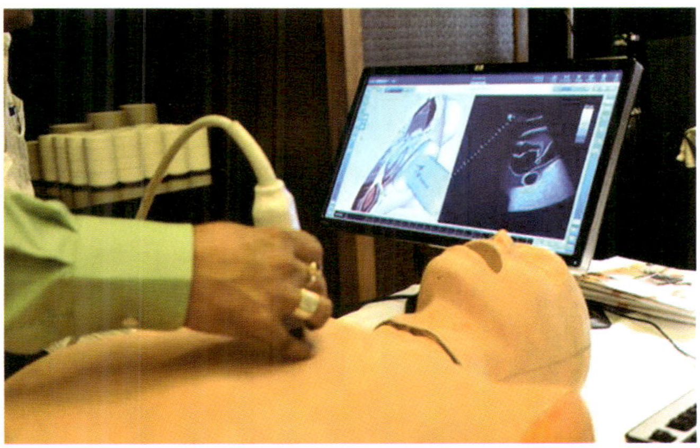

Figure 1 Simulation promotes training

- Increase of practical efficiency
- Increased security for the patient.

LEVELS OF SIMULATION

The level to which simulation modeling is applied depends on the maturity of a facility or process.

- *Macro-level simulation:* It is used for high-level strategic planning and concept development, such as determining room capacity in facility planning.
- *Micro-level simulation:* It is used to analyze processes such as patient flow or process/technology tradeoffs.

TRUE BENEFIT OF SIMULATION

A true benefit of simulation can be harvested when the simulation models are fully integrated into the routine fabric of healthcare delivery, i.e. the existing information system applications which support the daily operation of the healthcare provider.[2] Essentially, the vision is not to treat simulation as a tool for conducting a one-time set of experiments when a major change is planned, but make the simulation models run in parallel to other applications as a routine part of the everyday work environment. With this approach, healthcare efficiency becomes an ongoing objective and the future may require even tougher demands. Furthermore, with the rapidly changing variables of the healthcare system (technology, finance, policy, service demands, market, etc.), healthcare efficiency is becoming more of a moving target that needs to be periodically retargeted and re-addressed. Emerging from past skeptics and resistance toward simulation, today healthcare is showing more maturity and the necessity for simulation to play a significant role in solving healthcare challenges. Moreover, the current economic situation, policy shift, and the environment in which healthcare is delivered are ripe for institutionalization of simulation as a standard tool supporting the steering, management, and control of healthcare delivery.

SMARTER SIMULATION MODES NOW AVAILABLE

Virtual actors are getting 'smarter'. The full power of fuzzy logic, continuous variability, deictic context, and conversational logic being combined with advances in human social, behavioral and cultural (HSBC) research has resulted in virtual humans with emotive behavior, personality traits and motive—they are beginning to appear to have perception and cognition **(Figures 2A and B)**.

While scripted actors have served in the past, the advanced research herein points to a new generation of virtual actors that are demonstrating some elements of artificial intelligence, though they certainly cannot pass the Turing Test yet. While there are varying definitions of multimedia, it can be generally defined as "extending

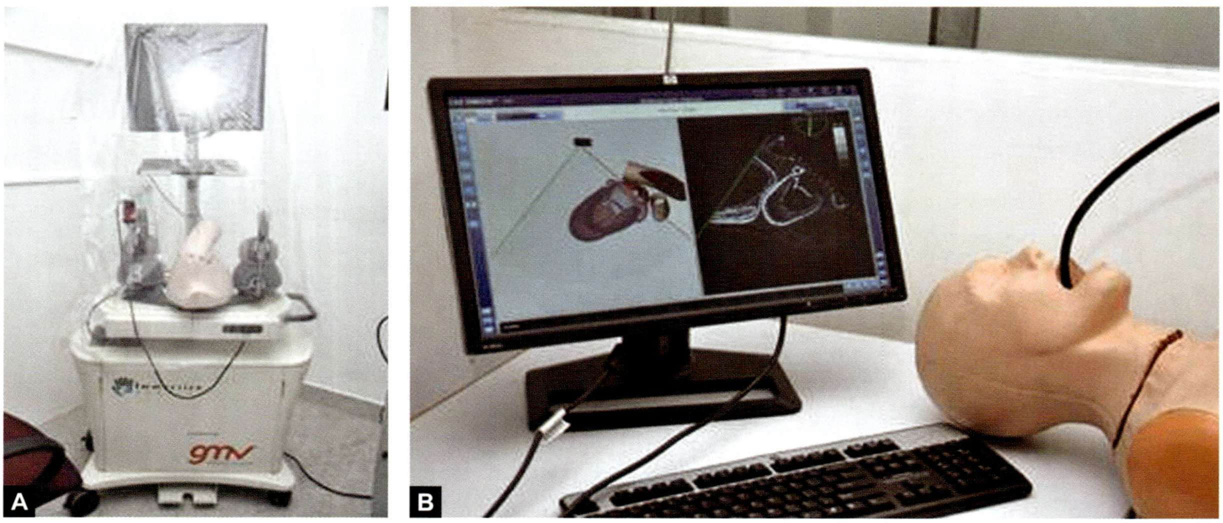

Figures 2A and B CAE Viamedix simulator for transesophageal echocardiography (TEE) learning for beginners and advanced cases, incorporating all comprehensive TEE views and 80 different TEE pathologies

training beyond pure text using a combination of several potential media types such as graphics, animations, video, auditory, and photographs".[3] "Indeed, technological advances continue to produce new media types that can be used in multimedia based training and educational venues".[3] In Conkey's case, the experiment uses an integrated multimedia training tool for comparison of a machinima interface vs. prerecorded skills when learning soft skills. An electronic educational system should assist the user in achieving a mastery of skills that are needed to complete a task on job. Training fidelity is essential in providing a robust educational solution. This solution should provide the user with an experience that are immersive and provides retention of a learning task.

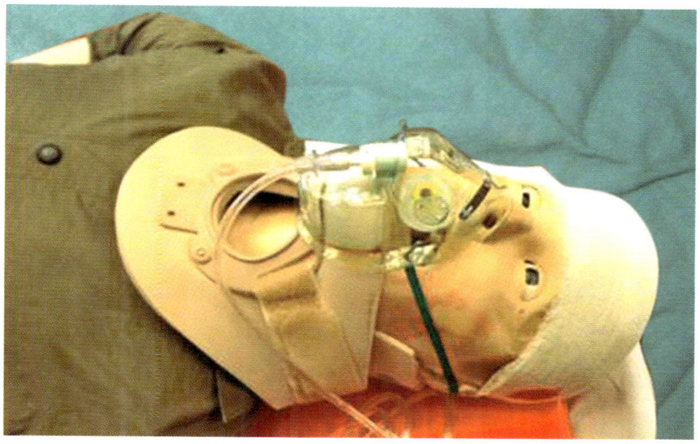

Figure 4 The upper head and neck part of SimMan 3G to recognize different parts and learn to anatomy of the upper airway

IMPORTANCE OF SIMULATION

Information Technology Alignment Development of national electronic health record (EHR) systems has created unprecedented opportunity for healthcare systems around the world to transition to electronic health practice (eHealth) and to benefit economically from it **(Figure 3)**. The path for harvesting the benefits of eHealth lies through designing innovative healthcare processes and redesigning existing practices to cope with the changes resulting from the adoption of the new technology. The work by Hillestad et al.[4] estimates potential savings and costs of electronic medical record (EMR) in the US, which finds that effective implementation of EMR (interoperable with other systems) could eventually save more than $81 billion annually. This saving is merely achieved by improving healthcare efficiency and safety. However, the author[4] recognizes that this is unlikely to be realized without related changes to the healthcare system. Thus, the simulation application in redesigning existing healthcare business processes and IT alignment is a critical scientific potential to explore **(Figures 4 and 5)**.

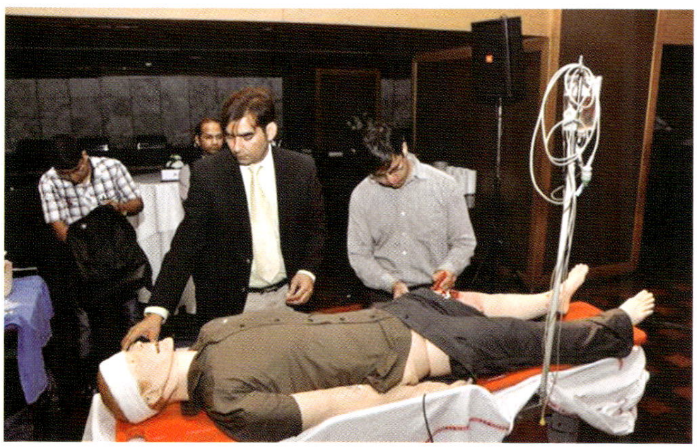

Figure 3 Learning on simulation is a teamwork which works well economically

DECISION SUPPORT

Healthcare decision makers need reliable tools to support them in decision making for adapting policies to help cutting costs or reducing waiting time, and to provide visualization which allows them to rehearse innovative ideas before they are implemented. The tools should facilitate an evidence-based and informed decision making environment. Simulation models, especially with transparency into their structure and underlying variables, which can be easily understood and trusted by decision makers, are a helpful tool in decision support, communication and discussion of ideas and polices, and analysis of scenarios.

TRAINING AND QUALITY

Adequate training of clinicians has direct impact on the quality of service. It will reduce errors and promote the adoption of best practices. Training of healthcare staff (clinicians, administrators and managers) is costly, time consuming, and assumes commitments and dedication that are usually not embraced because of time constraints. Simulation can successfully enhance and

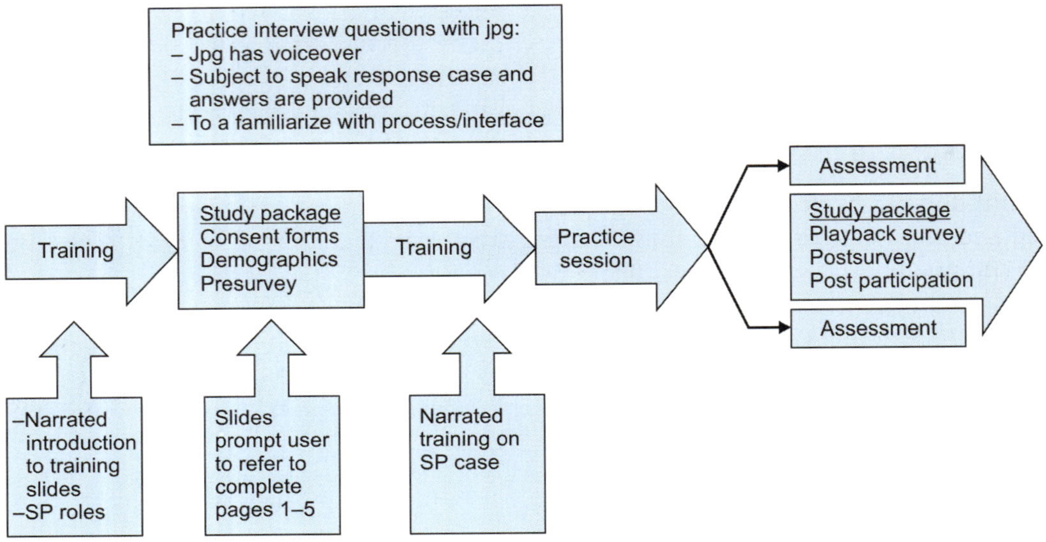

Figure 5 The SimMan 3G simulator for upper airway simulation learning

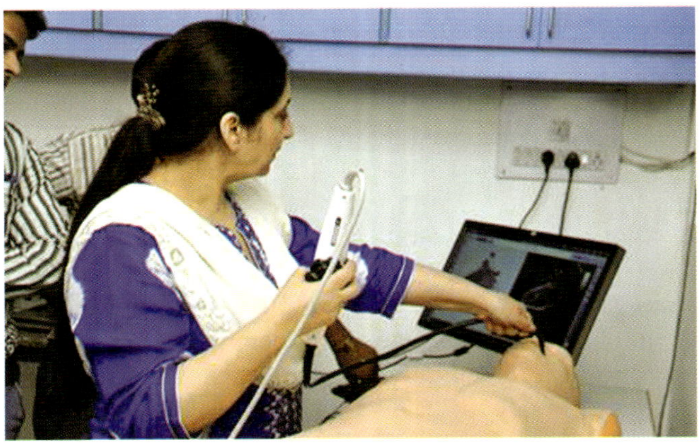

Figure 6 Training and quality in TEE enhanced by good views which are clear and have two interfaces, the section of the heart cut at that plane and structures studied at that level

improve clinicians' expertise, accomplish acquaintance with new procedures and processes, and prevent errors that are caused by the lack of training and hands-on experience **(Figure 6)**.

COMPLEXITY

The complexity of healthcare processes is growing exponentially, with various services like laboratories being outsourced, multiplication of specialties, and extreme mobility of patients resulting from competition in the free market. Modern hospitals are complex systems of distributed subsystems with intricate healthcare processes, human interactions, and interorganizational workflows. For example, citizens easily can plan a different healthcare service based on less waiting time, prominent quality, or many other factors that lead them beyond their local, regional or even national borders. This makes healthcare processes more interconnected and more complex, and simulation can be a way of tackling such complexity. Thus, the complexity of healthcare systems makes simulation a potential tool for healthcare analysts.[5]

PROCESS IMPROVEMENT

In majority of healthcare simulation projects, where efficiency is the goal, the reduction of patient waiting time seems to be the main target. Both waiting for the service date and waiting while receiving service are important indicators of efficiency. Essentially, waiting time is the root cause of many problems healthcare is facing. Increased waiting time affects patient's perception of the quality, requires more space (waiting area), long waiting time for the service causes many no-shows and cancellation, and so on.[6] If one was to conduct root-cause analysis of healthcare operational problems, patient waiting time would certainly appear in the root of many issues. Apart from application potentials, healthcare simulation as a whole is facing a myriad of interesting scientific challenges, which open up a fascinating research domain for simulation researchers and practitioners.

USER ACCEPTANCE

There is no doubt that the healthcare industry is now more prepared and ready to embrace simulation with all its capacity and potential. They are now fully aware of the values and the benefits simulation may yield to improve their operational and management processes.

However, simulation is still a highly technical and sophisticated tool for common user comprehension, which triggers user resistance. User resistance is a major barrier to a successful simulation implementation in healthcare. This barrier exists in concert with the fact that simulation, especially detailed simulation, requires tremendous effort and time. These challenges require theoretical breakthrough. While expedition of simulation can be improved through innovative approaches such as development of different libraries, reuse of models, rich graphical interactive development environments, the reconciliation of users and the technicality of simulation models is still a least studied research field.[7]

HEALTHCARE PROCESSES

Organizational and workflow complexity of the modern healthcare system is huge and extensive. Modern hospitals have a large number of interacting units consisting of specialized and acute units, third-party facilities, external labs, interhospital transfers. This complex collaboration and interaction contributes to a complex interorganizational workflow and even a complex business model. The challenge of a simulation model is capturing this complexity of interorganizational flow in a systematic and manageable manner. Models should adhere to certain qualities such as hierarchical representation, granularity, multiple views, etc. While rich in representation, at the same time, models should be still an easy means of communication and understanding among stakeholders, including those with no or moderate technical knowledge.

CONCLUSION: MODULES PROVIDE DYNAMIC EFFECTS

Models can often be run in 'simulation' time to analyze dynamic effects. For example, if we change arrival rates and available resources during a time period what are the effects on throughput, queues (both queue size and time in queue) and what are the cost implications? Using time-based analysis, we can also determine whether resources are under-used at certain times of the day and over stretched at other times. Another benefit of simulation models is that often they are more flexible and easier to understand than mathematical models.

GREATER INSIGHT

The outputs of this model have provided a greater insight into the interaction of arrival rates throughout the day and impact of resource levels on queues and service throughput. Findings then allowed resources to be optimized to maximize efficiency.

WIDER APPLICABILITY

An example of the wide applicability of simulation is shown here by a recent case study at a large UK National Health Service trust. Simulation modeling was used to study patient based nursing time on decentralized wards versus centralized wards. The simulation modelled specific key service factors as 'interruptions' that took nurses away from patients.

The study illustrated that patients in decentralized wards had an average of approximately 80% of the total nursing time available compared to approximately a 30% in centralized wards. Decentralized wards also showed less variability compared to centralized wards due to queuing effects. In addition, this application demonstrates that simulation modelling can identify opportunities to improve not only operational performance but also quality of care.

A FLEXIBLE TOOL

Simulation can also be used as a multilevel tool modelling a range of activities such as:

- *Whole system modeling:* Achieving the right balance between hospital, community and primary care
- *Subsystems modeling:* The recent National Audit Office report on trauma care recommended formal transfer systems to provide more appropriate complex or specialist care as required for trauma patients. Simulation can help to model the rebalancing of care between major trauma centers and local hospitals.

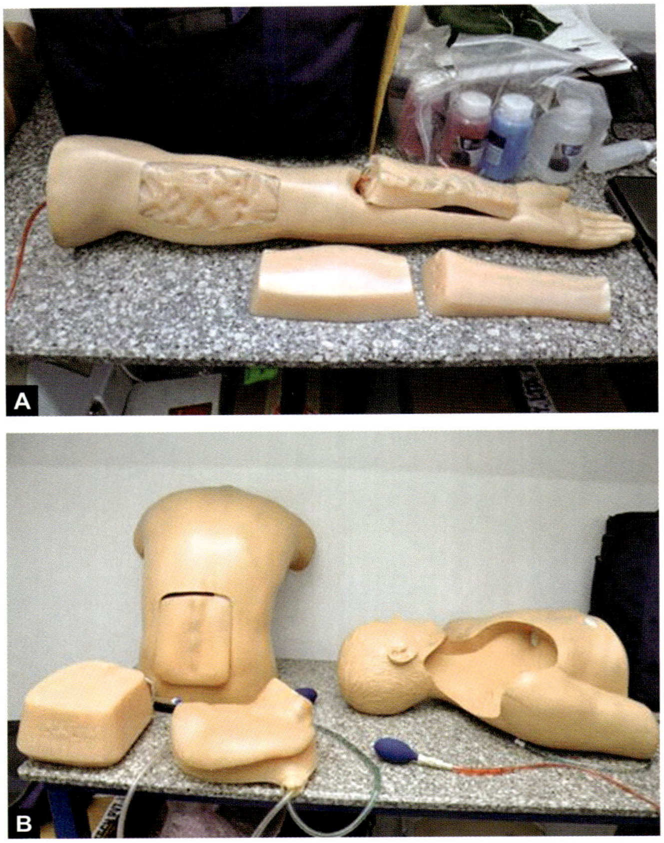

Figures 7A and B (A) Phantom limbs for studying anatomy of lower limbs and anatomical sites for pain relief. (B) Flexible tool of head, neck and thorax by DSS for teaching landmarks on different sites

- *Specific process modeling:* With increased competitive intensity in healthcare systems, successful providers will be those who fully understand the operating economics of high technology services and the risk of stranded capacity. In areas such as imaging, simulation can be used to optimize patient schedules for increased productivity and efficiency.

Simulation modeling is a powerful tool—if used properly and with a full understanding of the services and processes which are being modeled. It is not a black box but enables testing of scenarios to aid decision making **(Figures 7A and B)**.

HEALTHCARE SIMULATION CHALLENGES

From what we discussed so far, it becomes evident that healthcare is a multidisciplinary, complex field. As such, the main challenge of healthcare simulation is a theoretical breakthrough that should focus on multimethods (methods for formal and informal representation), multiparadigms (discrete event simulation paradigm, continuous paradigm, agent based paradigm), and multidisciplines (organization, information, technology, policy, etc). Although diligent research has been conducted in relation to multiplicity of theories and paradigms, the current practice of simulation, in many aspects, is single-method, single-paradigm, and single-discipline minded.

The main objective and premise of multiparadigm modeling and simulation is based on the idea of delivering a solution tool and theoretical framework allowing multilevel abstraction for the targeted domain and multiperspective view of the domain problem.

SIMULATION MAKES THE LEARNER "HIGHER UP ON THE LEARNING CURVE"

Simulated mannequins, on the other hand, provide a number of advantages—which help solve some of the limitations above. And given the current difficulties with the 80 hours workweek (potentially soon to be even less hours) that lessens the time available for the learners, the increasing cost of space, salaries, and time, having a virtual actor residing on a computer, available at any time (and from any place over the internet) without any substantive additional cost above the initial investment, provides a substantial cost and efficiency benefit. In addition, a library of virtual patients with multiple variations of the presentation of a disease type, in many different cultures and for both sexes, increases the richness of the experience of the learner **(Figure 8)**.

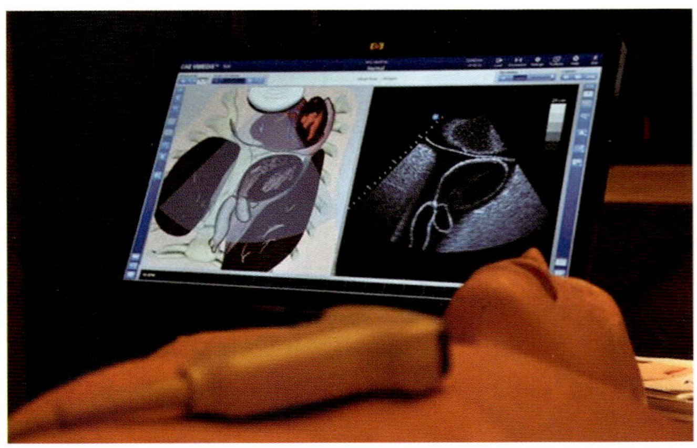

Figure 8 The clarity of 2D and 3D structures, makes learning echocardiography on the simulator, easier

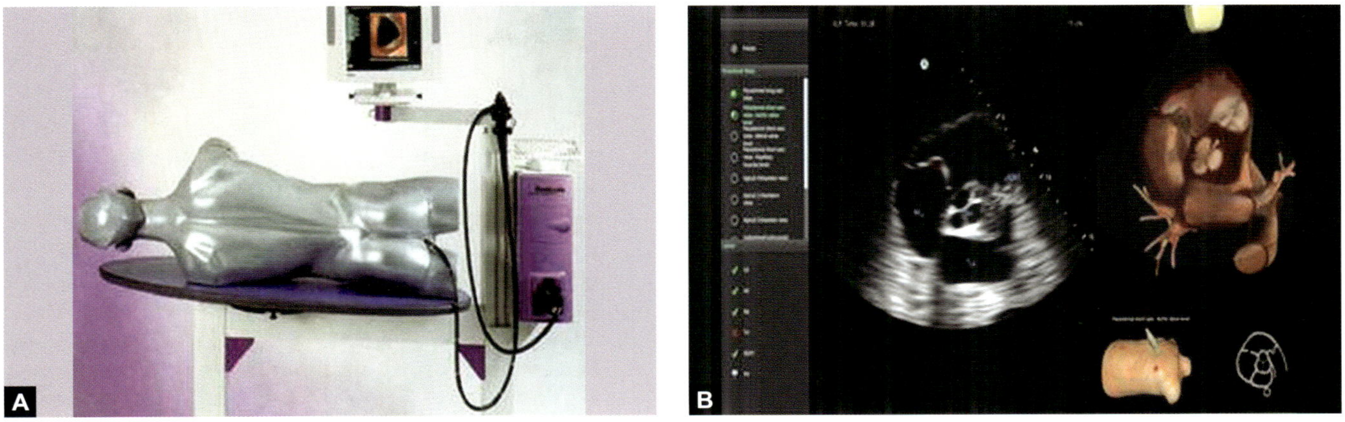

Figures 9A and B Clinical validation, features and benefits of Gastrointestinal Mentor

CLINICAL SIMULATION: ROLE AND SIGNIFICANCE IN STUDENT TRAINING

The aim of simulation is to train students—future doctors, in order to facilitate the integration in modern medical environment, taking in to account the fact that medical education by clinical simulation is an active method of formation, through the accumulation and implementation of knowledge, in the framework of a practice very close to the real one.

For an integrated context of presentation of clinical simulation we will associate the theoretical considerations with the experience of application and implementation of this method/learning strategy in an account of the experience with the students of the faculty of medicine in the University of Medicine and pharmacy "Gr. T. Popa" Iasi.

The implementation of clinical simulation with the interactive simulators Human Patient Simulator (HPS) and GI mentor as an applicable system for the analysis and evaluation of the practical individual ability, and the supervision of their development during the module of student training, in order to gain competences and efficiency **(Figures 9A and B)**.

Purpose of Training and Assessment

- Initial assessment of fundamental abilities (aptitude)
- Basic skills and established procedures
- New procedures (residents, students and established surgeons)
- Maintenance of certification
- Retraining (or re-entry training) of skills after absence from performing surgery
- Remediation

UTILITY OF SIMULATION IN MEDICAL EDUCATION

Simulation in medical education serves several purposes, including procedure planning, visual-spatial learning, skill acquisition, and minimizing errors that occur during the early phases of training. Simulation training has the possibility, if implemented correctly, to maximize a surgical resident's training in the setting of reduced resident work hours and increasingly complex procedures. There has been wide support from both surgical program directors and residents for the implementation of simulation in the curricula.[8,9] However, there is concern regarding lack of evidence for its efficacy. Reznick and colleagues[10,11] at the University of Toronto introduced in the mid-1990s the objective structured assessment of technical skills, an assessment tool that they validated. Briefly, for any given task, use of the objective structured assessment of technical skills allows an evaluator to assess the trainee's skill using both a task-specific checklist and a global rating scale.

In determining the value and effectiveness of simulation training, outcomes must be assessed at different levels. In a review of simulation education, Griswold et al[12] referenced a system by which to measure simulation outcomes (T1, T2, T3, Tvalue). At the T1 research level, simulation outcomes are measured in a laboratory setting. At the T2 level, transfer of skills acquired from simulation training is measured by clinical performance outcomes. T3 level studies assess patient safety. Finally, Tvalue studies measure the costsaving benefits of simulation training. In this review, we focus primarily on the T1 and T2 levels to demonstrate the value of simulation in a resident's medical education.

CONCLUSION

By producing results that have had positive impact on cost savings and the quality of care, simulation modeling is becoming widely recognized as a valuable application in the healthcare industry. Prior to the introduction of simulation modeling, healthcare administrators relied on rough estimates and guidelines from previous projects in order to make planning and investment decisions. Today, however, simulation modeling enables administrators to make more accurate decisions based on detailed discrete-event analyses that accommodate more variations and complexities than traditional spreadsheet analyses. Simulation modeling also presents physical movement not available in traditional analysis. This dynamic animation allows the simulation concept to be easily presented, providing decision makers with a better understanding of the variations and complexities involved in the model. As healthcare simulation embarks on tackling major challenges, it might be worthwhile to adapt the experience of traditional fields. For example, study of healthcare processes from the perspective or analogy of engineering processes, manufacturing processes, will benefit the future of healthcare simulation by brining engineering knowledge into the field. We briefly discussed areas, where theoretical breakthrough and developments are needed to make simulation a holistic methodology for accurately and adequately conducting analysis and studying healthcare processes and dealing with their underlying complexity.

REFERENCES

1. Bradley C. The role of high fidelity clinical simulation in teaching and learning in the health professions. Higher Education Research Network Journal. 2011;4:33-42.
2. Gaba DM. The future vision of simulation in health care. Quality and Safety in Health Care. 2004;13:i2-i10.
3. Conkey C. Machinima Technology: Serious Games Lite. Paper presented at the Interservice/Industry Training, Simulation, and Education Conference 2009, Orlando, Fl; 2009.
4. Hillestad R. Can electronic medical record systems transform health care? Potential health benefits, savings, and costs. Health Affairs. 2005;24(5):1103-17.
5. Lowery JC. Introduction to simulation in health care. In Proceedings of the 28th Conference on Winter Simulation (Coronado, California, United States; 1996).
6. Eilers GM. Improving patient satisfaction with waiting time. Journal of American College Health. 2004;53(1):41-8.
7. McGaghie WC, Issenberg SB, Petrusa ER, Scalese RJ. A critical review of simulation based medical education research: 2003–2009 Medical Education. 2010;44(1):50-63.
8. El Ahmadieh TY, EL Tecle NE, Aoun SG, Yip BK, Ganju A, Bendok BR. How can simulation thrive as an educational tool? Just ask the residents. Neurosurgery. 2012;71(6):N18-N19.
9. Ganju A, Aoun SG, Daou MR, et al. The role of simulation in neurosurgical education: a survey of 99 United States neurosurgery program directors [published online ahead of print November 24, 2012]. World Neurosurg. doi:10.1016/j.wneu. 2012.11.066. Accessed: May 01, 2013 [PMID: 23182732].
10. Martin JA, Regehr G, Reznick R, et al. Objective structured assessment of technical skill (OSATS) for surgical residents. Br J Surg. 1997;84(2):273-8.
11. Faulkner H, Regehr G, Martin J, Reznick R. Validation of an objective structured assessment of technical skill for surgical residents. AcadMed. 1996;71(12):1363-5.
12. Griswold S, Ponnuru S, Nishisaki A, et al. The emerging role of simulation education to achieve patient safety: translating deliberate practice and debriefing to save lives. Pediatr Clin North Am. 2012;59(6):1329-40.

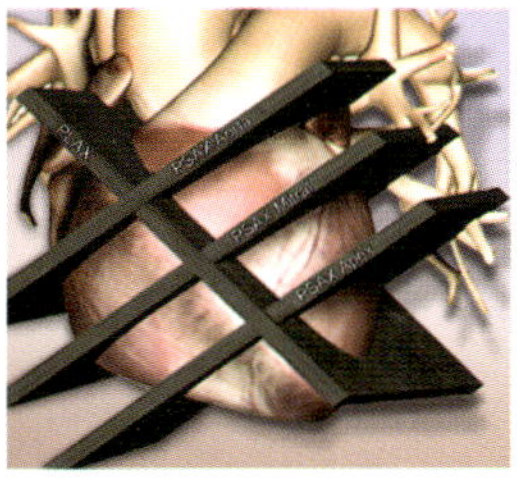

Section 2

Simulation in Transthoracic Echocardiography

Section Outline

- Simulation for Transthoracic Echocardiography for Echo Views
- Understanding Echocardiographic Assessment of Left Ventricular Systolic and Diastolic Function for Simulation Training
- Simulation for Transthoracic Echocardiography of Mitral Valve
- Simulation for Transthoracic Echocardiography of Aortic Valve
- Use of Simulation for Transthoracic Echocardiography in Ischemic Heart Disease

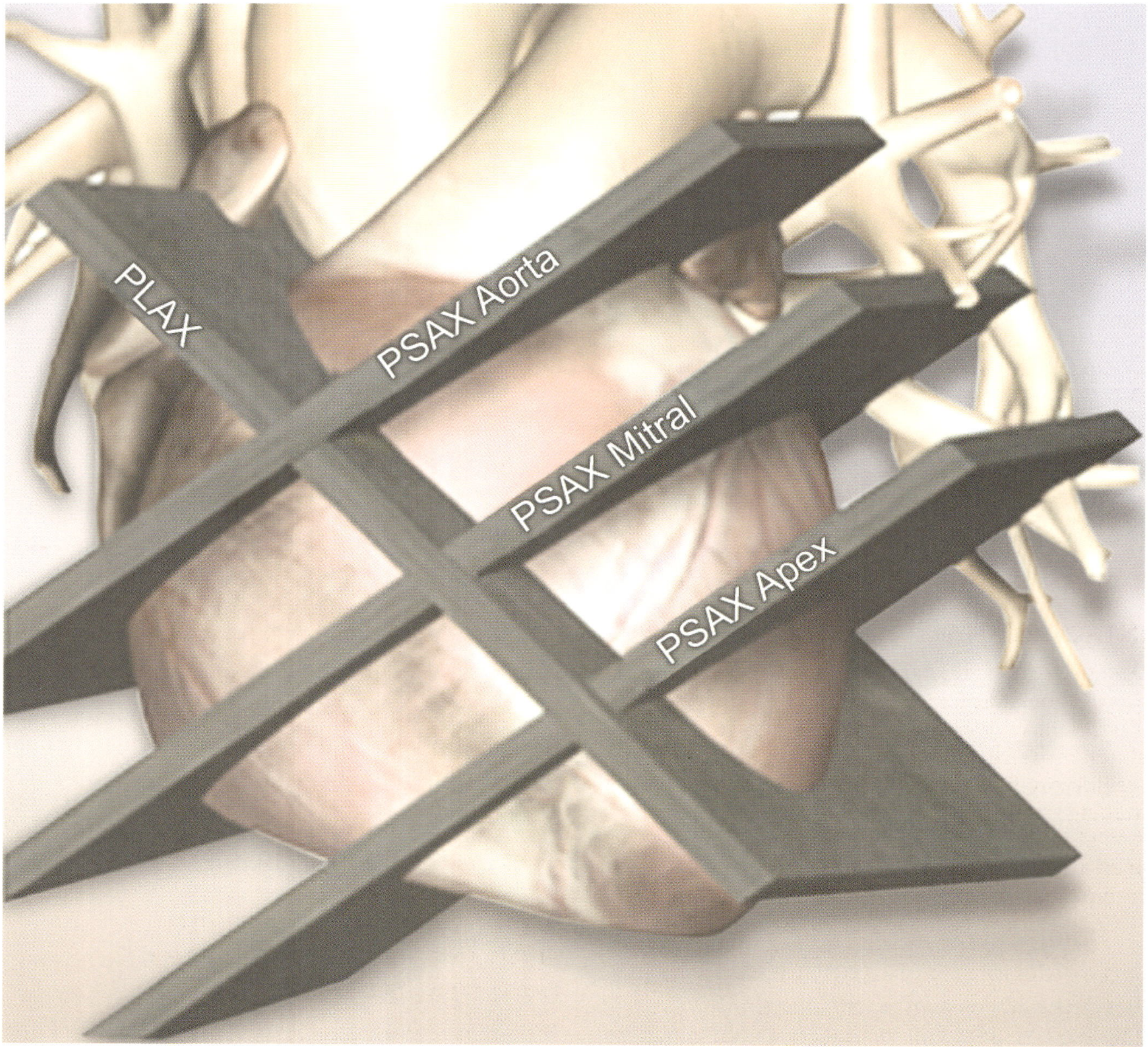
PLAX
PSAX Aorta
PSAX Mitral
PSAX Apex

Chapter 3

Simulation for Transthoracic Echocardiography for Echo Views

KK Kapur

Chapter Outline

- Acquisition of Various 2D Echocardiographic Planes on Mannequin
- Several Variations of Long Axis Projection
- Short Axis Projection
- Apical Views (Coronal Section)
- Subcostal Planes
- Suprasternal Views
- Right Parasternal View

INTRODUCTION

Over the last several decades, there has been introduction of simulators for teaching, training and acquisition of skills in various fields of medical sciences. These simulators are mannequin based, which simulate real life situations and have been approved for use in training and evaluation in several medical and surgical disciplines. Only recently, these mannequins have been used for training technologist, physician and cardiologists in echocardiography both transthoracic (TTE) and Transesophageal (TEE).[1]

As in any field of human activity the acquisition of skills and expertise in echocardiography requires repetitive and constant practice. Hitherto these skills have been acquired on volunteers or actual patients. However, owing to time constraints and ethical issues, the traditional training programs are being replaced by patient-simulators. These simulators facilitates in acquisition of necessary the following:

- Various echocardiography imaging planes
- Interpretation and evaluation of these images
- Diagnosis of various cardiac pathologies based on this interpretation.

Several common and as well as rare cardiac pathologies are depicted using computer based video programs integrated into the plastic mannequins.

ACQUISITION OF VARIOUS 2D ECHOCARDIOGRAPHIC PLANES ON MANNEQUIN

The simulated human heart can be viewed just as a real time heart in three basic projections:

1. Longitudinal (Sagittal) section

2. Transverse or cross-section
3. Coronal section.

Several echocardiographic planes are then obtained from these basic sections **(Figure 1)**.

Parasternal long axis (PLAX) in this plane the heart is cut in the long axis (sagittal) section between the right shoulder and left hip with the index mark on the simulated ultrasonic probe at the 10 o'clock position. The probe itself is placed in the left 3rd or 4th intercostal space parasternally. The orientation is anteroposterior and superoinferior **(Figures 2A and B)**.

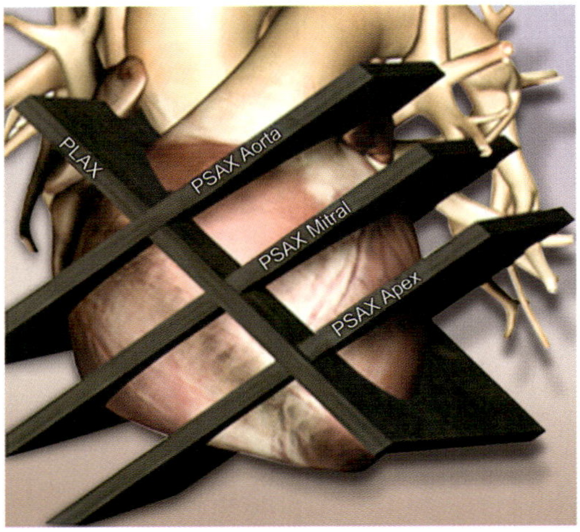

Figure 1 Various tomographic planes of the heart that are used in transthoracic echocardiography

SEVERAL VARIATIONS OF LONG AXIS PROJECTION

Several variations of long axis projection are available:

- *High PLAX*: In which the probe is placed one intercostal space higher and allows visualization of a larger segment of ascending aorta **(Figures 3A and B)**.
- *Low PLAX*: In which the probe is placed one intercostal space lower and allows visualization of more distal segments of LV (**Figures 4A and B**).
- *RV-inflow view*: It is obtained by a medial and inferior tilt from standard PLAX position and allows visualization of RA, RV and coronary sinus CS, and entry of IVC **(Figures 5A and B)**.
- *Mitral Pulmonic Plane*: It is obtained by superior and lateral tilt from standard PLAX and allows visualization of RV outflow, PV, PA and MV **(Figure 6)**.

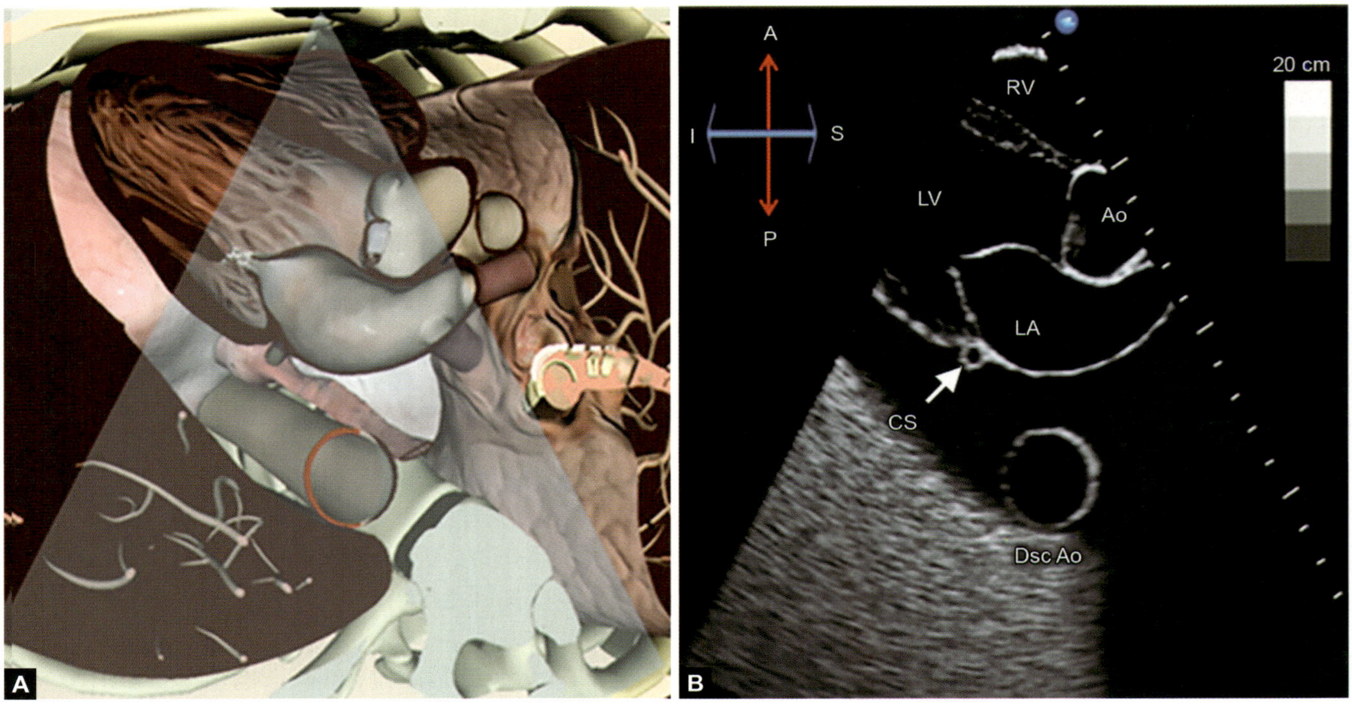

Figures 2A and B Parasternal long axis standard view at left 4th parasternal ICS, showing RV lying anteriorly and LA posteriorly. Coronary sinus (CS) is seen adjacent to LA and descending aorta (Dsc Ao) little more posteriorly. Ascending aorta is superior and LV cavity inferiorly placed
Abbreviations: ICS, intercostal space; RV, right ventricle; LA, left atrium; LV, left ventricle; Ao, aorta

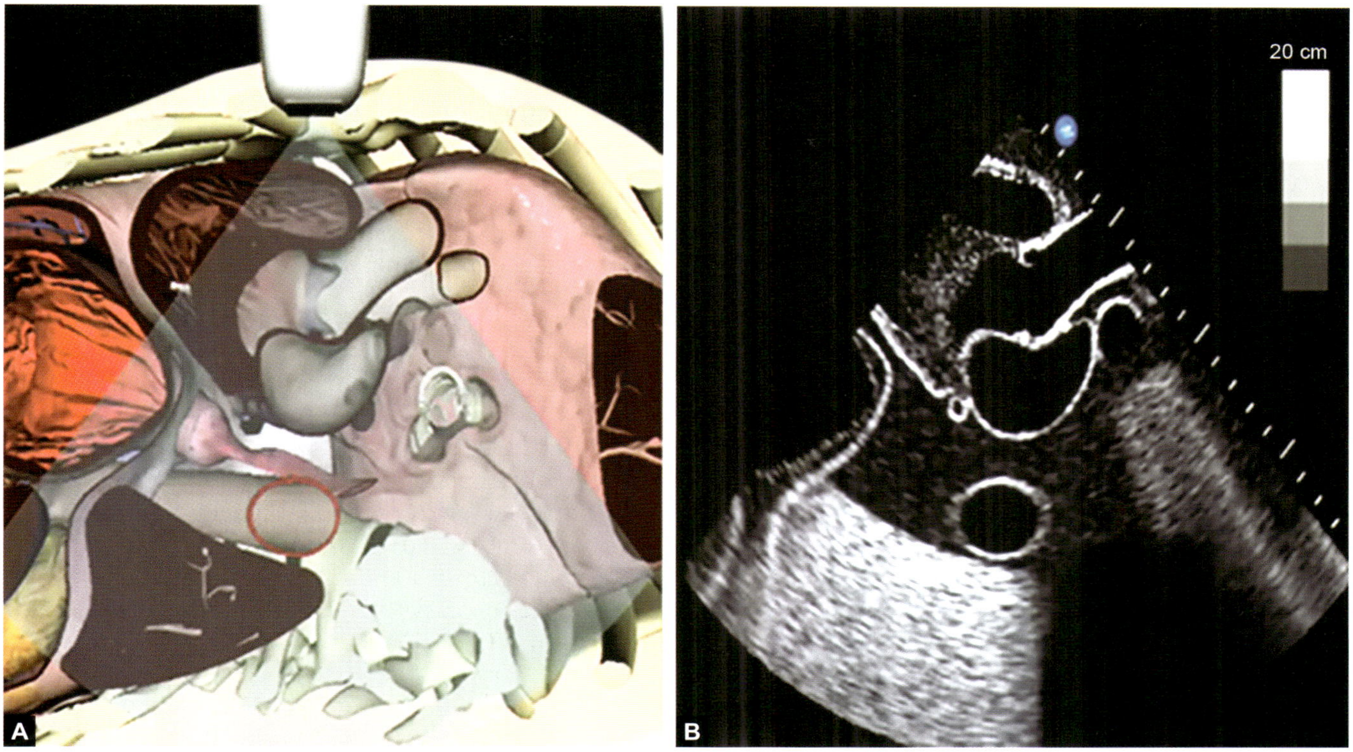

Figures 3A and B Long segment of ascending aorta can be visualized in this view by placing probe one ICS higher
Abbreviation: ICS, intercosta space

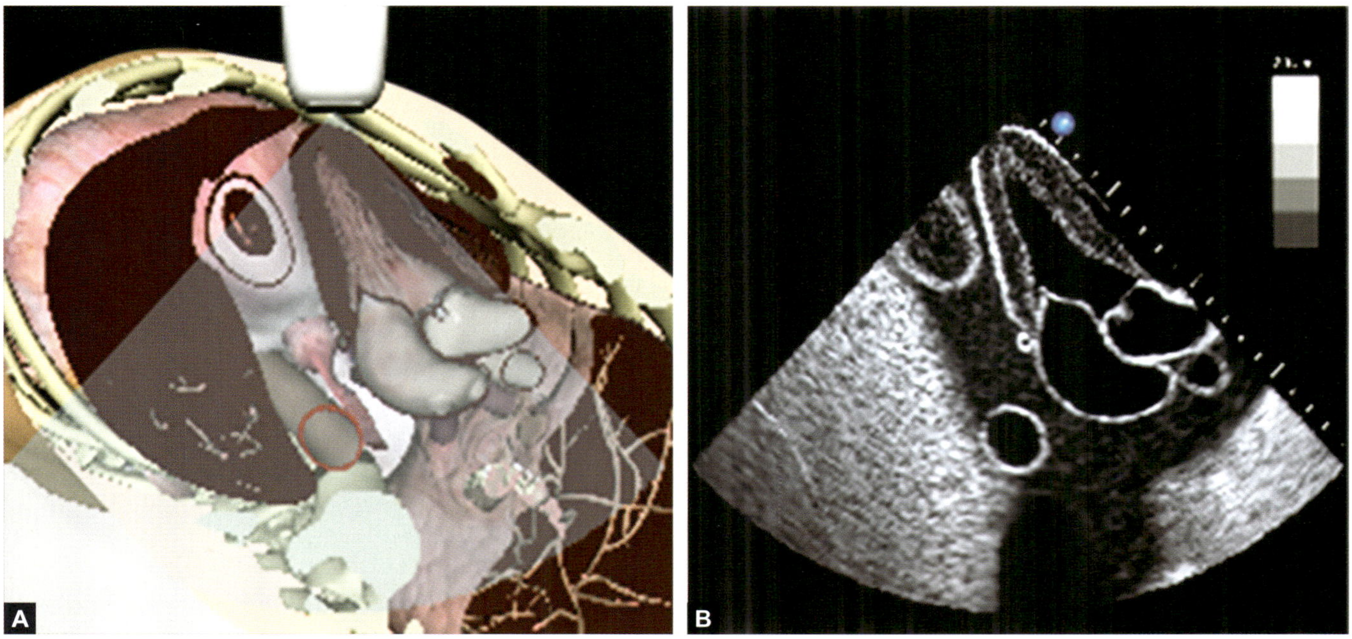

Figures 4A and B Low PLAX view at one ICS lower of standard view shows cistal part of LV and 3 Chambers namely LA, LV and aorta
Abbreviations: ICS, intercostal space; LV, left ventricle; LA, le-t atrium; PLAX, parasternal long axis

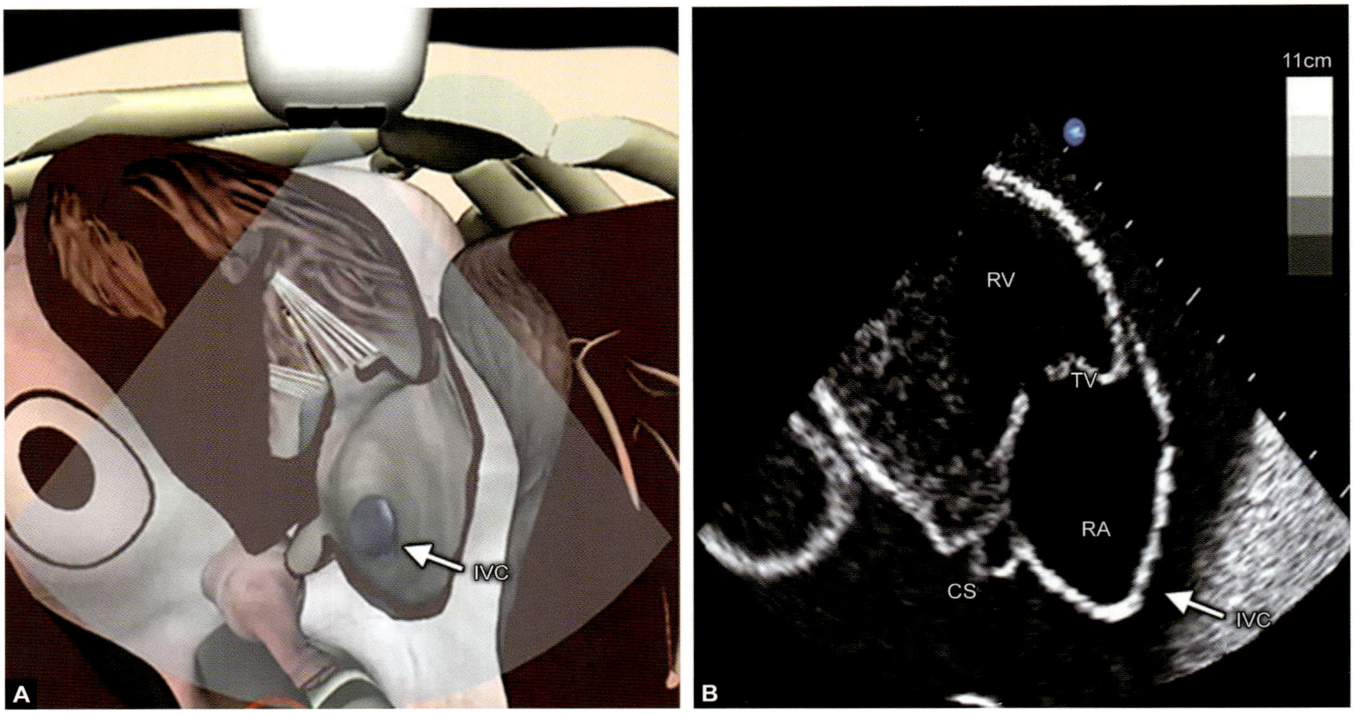

Figures 5A and B RV inflow view depicts CS opening in RV and IVC opening (not clearly seen) and TV
Abbreviations: RV, right ventricle; CS, costal space; IVC, inferior vena cava; RA, right atrium; TV, tricuspid valve

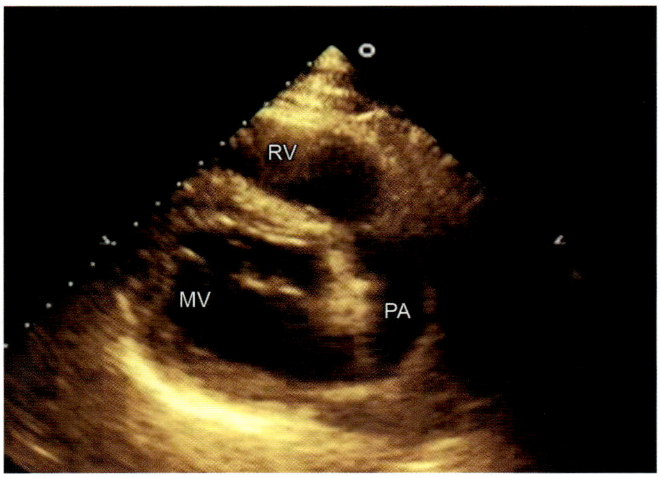

Figure 6 The MV, RV outflow and PA, the view is obtained by outward and upward angulation of probe at PLAX standard position
Abbreviations: MV, mitral valve; RV, right ventricle; PA, pulmonary artery

SHORT AXIS PROJECTION

The parasternal SAX plane is obtained by clockwise rotation of the probe from 10 o'clock to 1 o'clock position and sliding/angulating the probe inferiorly. The orientation is anteroposterior, right and left. The right sided structures (RA, RV, TV) are situated on the operator's left side while the left sided structures (PV, PA) are on right side of the operator. Several standard and nonstandard tomographic views are then obtained.

- *SAX aorto pulmonic level*: It is obtained from the standard position at the 3rd and 4th ICS. The trileaflet aortic valve is situated in the center of the image and PV is anteriorly and to the left, while the tricuspid valve is situated to the right. A slight angulation shows the origin of LMCA and LAA at 4 o'clock position **(Figures 7A and B)**.
  While a mild anterior and rightward angulation visualizes the origin of the RCA at 11 o'clock **(Figure 8)**.

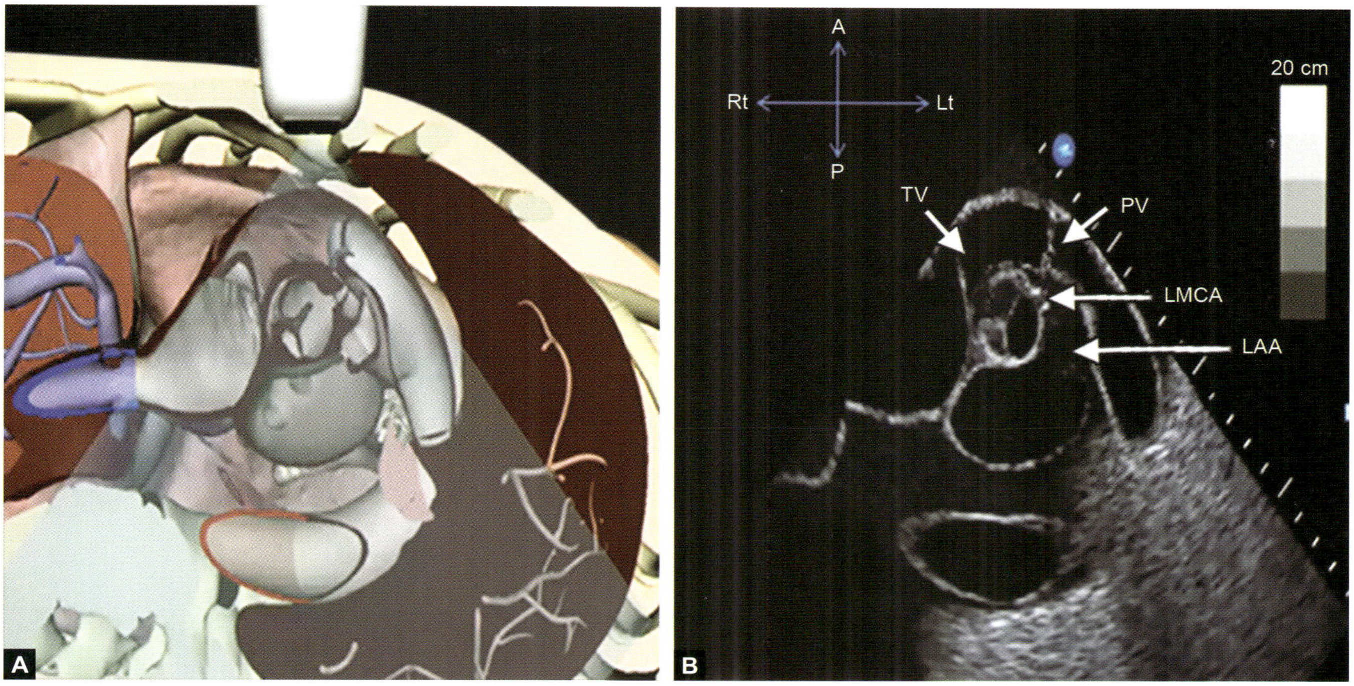

Figures 7A and B SAX at aorta level showing TV, PV and trileaflet aorta in the center. Left main coronary artery can be seen at its origin at 2 o'clock position (in this picture)
Abbreviations: AX, short axis; TV, tricuspid valve; PV, pulmonary valve; LAA, left atrial appendage

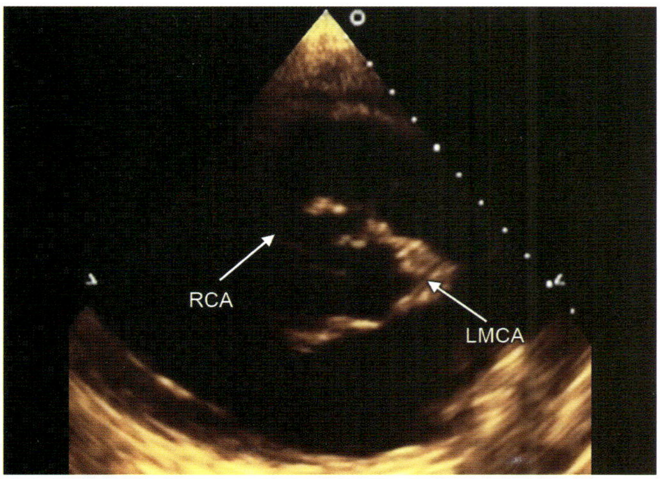

Figure 8 Echocardiographic SAX-view at aorta showing LMCA and RCA at their origin
Abbreviations: LMCA, left main coronary artery; RCA, right coronary artery

- *High SAX for PA bifurcation*: A superior and lateral angulation from the conventional SAX position or one ICS higher, allows visualization of PA bifurcation with RPA behind the ascending aorta **(Figures 9A and B)**.
- *Parasternal short axis (PSSAX) at*
  - MV level or basal level **(Figures 10A and B)**
  - Papillary muscle (Pm) or midlevel **(Figures 11A and B)**
  - LV apex or apical level **(Figures 12A and B)**

These are obtained by successive inferior angulations and/or sliding of the probe from the standard position. Thus the entire LV segments are imaged.[2] (6 segments at MV-level, 6 segments at PM level and 4 segments at apical level).

The mitral orifice can be traced at the basal short axis level and the orifice area thus computed.

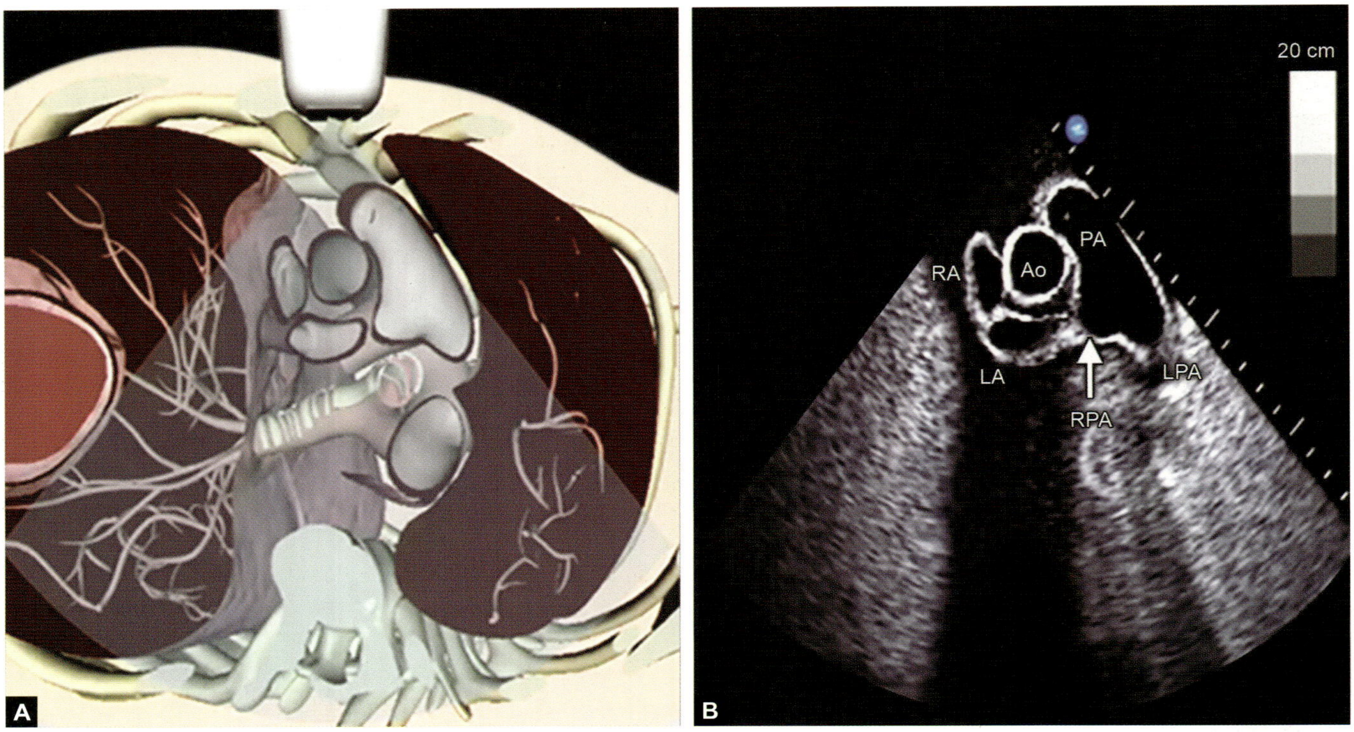

Figures 9A and B High SAX view showing bifurcating pulmonary trunk with RPA curving along the aorta whereas LPA moving away posteriorly. Pulmonary emboli are often captured at this junction

Abbreviations: RPA, right pulmonary artery; LPA; left pulmonary artery

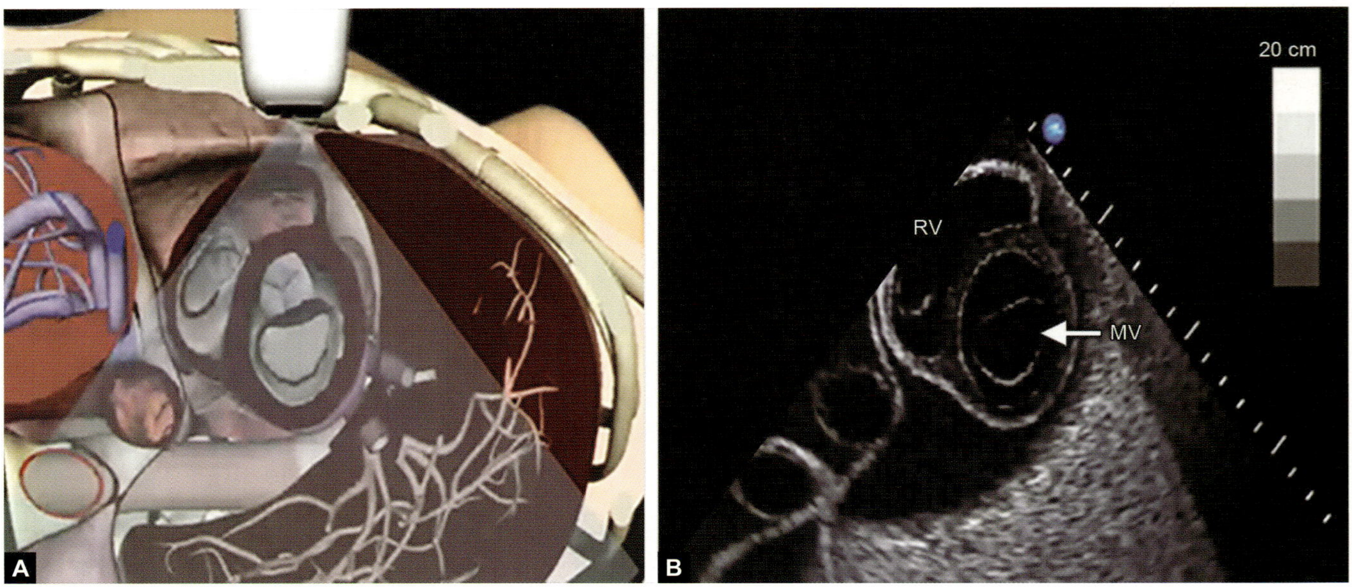

Figures 10A and B Parasternal short axis at basal level shows mitral cusps, MV orifice and interventricular septum. This view offers planimetry of MV area and deformities of cusps

Abbreviations: MV, mitral valve; RV, right ventricle

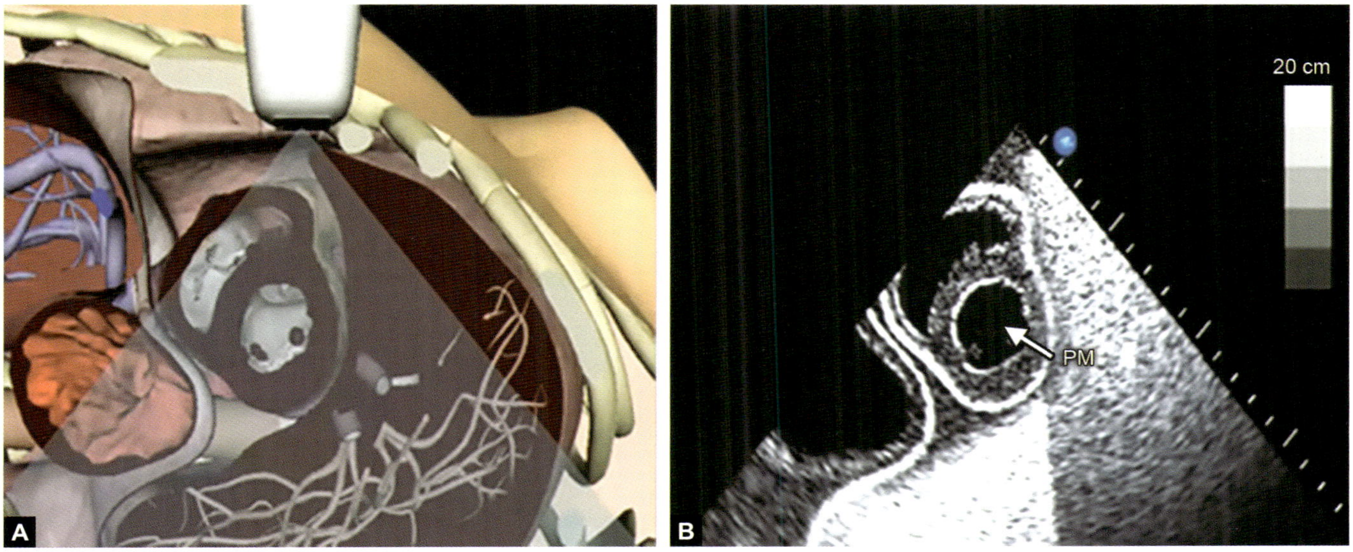

Figures 11A and B Papillary muscles (PM) can be seen as two rounded balls at 5 and 7 o'clock position of LV cavity in cross-section

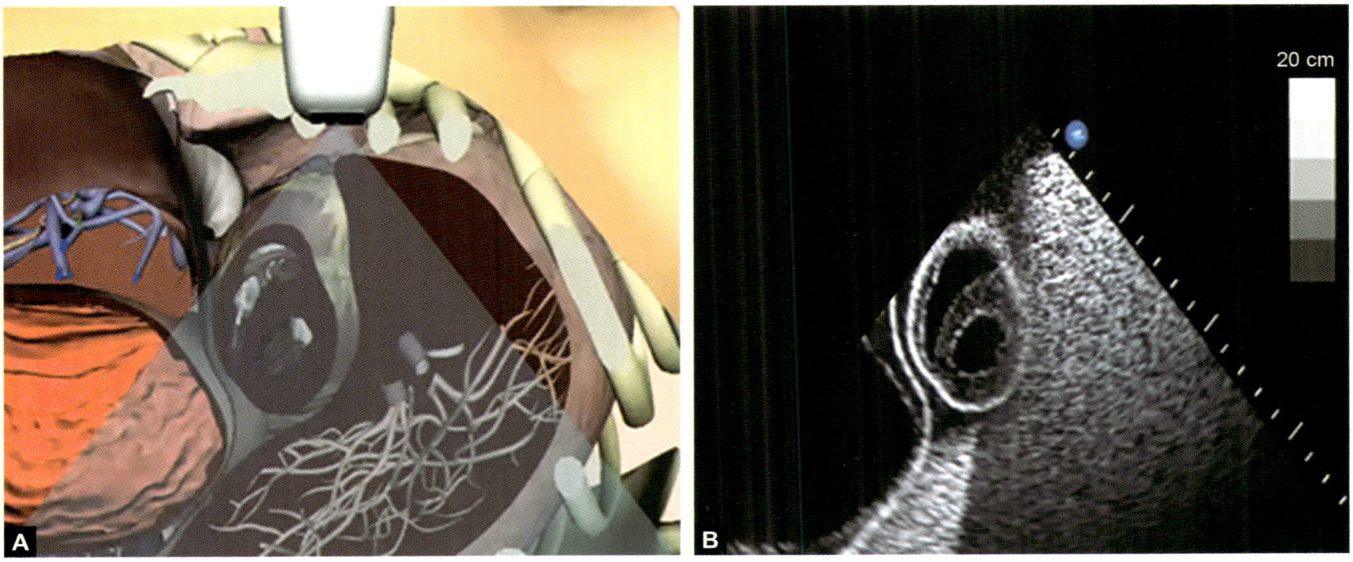

Figures 12A and B Parasternal short axis at apex shows apical segment of LV and interventricular septum. This view is important in visualizing small VSDs or clot at apex

Abbreviations: VSDs, ventral septal defect; LV, left ventricle

APICAL VIEWS (CORONAL SECTION)

The transducer is placed on the 5th ICS midclavicular line (adjusted as always by hand-eye co-ordination). The index mark is placed by clockwise rotation at the 4 o'clock position and the apical 4 chamber (4C) is obtained **(Figures 13A and B)**. The orientation is superior-inferior, right and left. This view is optimized such that the LV is in the middle of the sector and LV apex is inferior to RV apex. The image so obtained is inverted superior-inferiorly with the ventricles on top and atria below.[3]

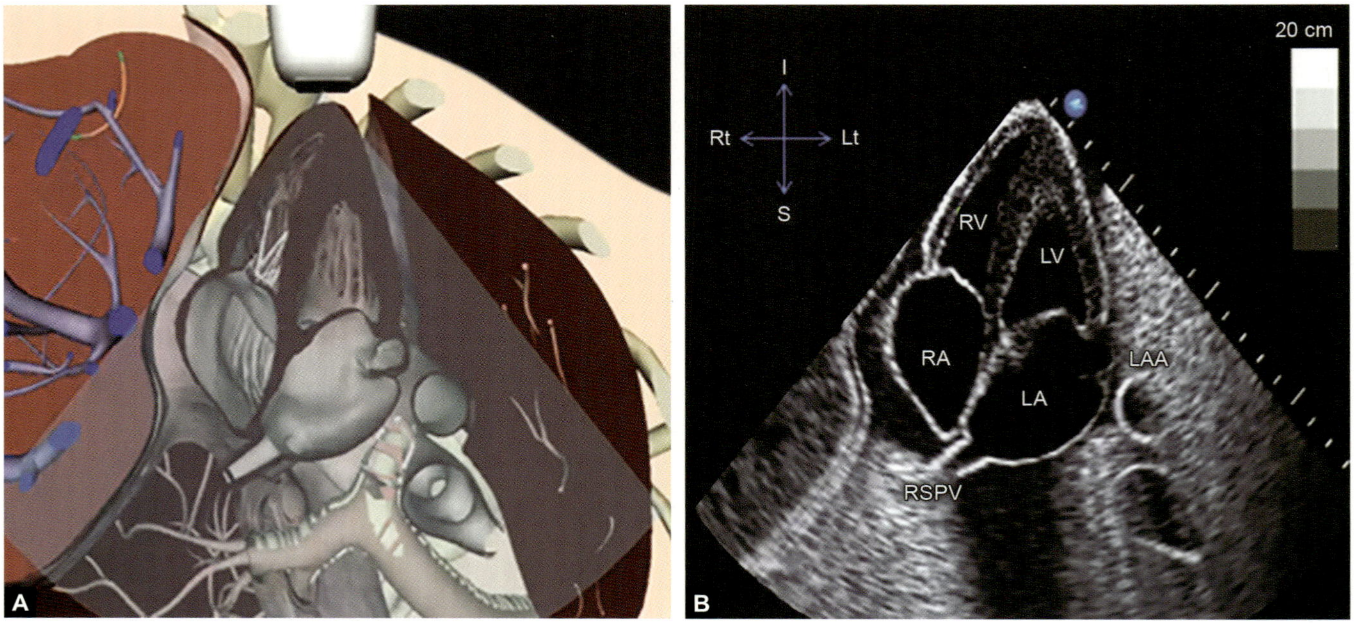

Figures 13A and B 4 chamber view at apical position shows all four chambers of the heart. It may depict LAA and RSPV also
Abbreviations: LAA, left atrial appendage; RSPV, right superior pulmonary vein; RA, right atrium; RV, right ventricle; LA, left atrium; LV, left ventricle

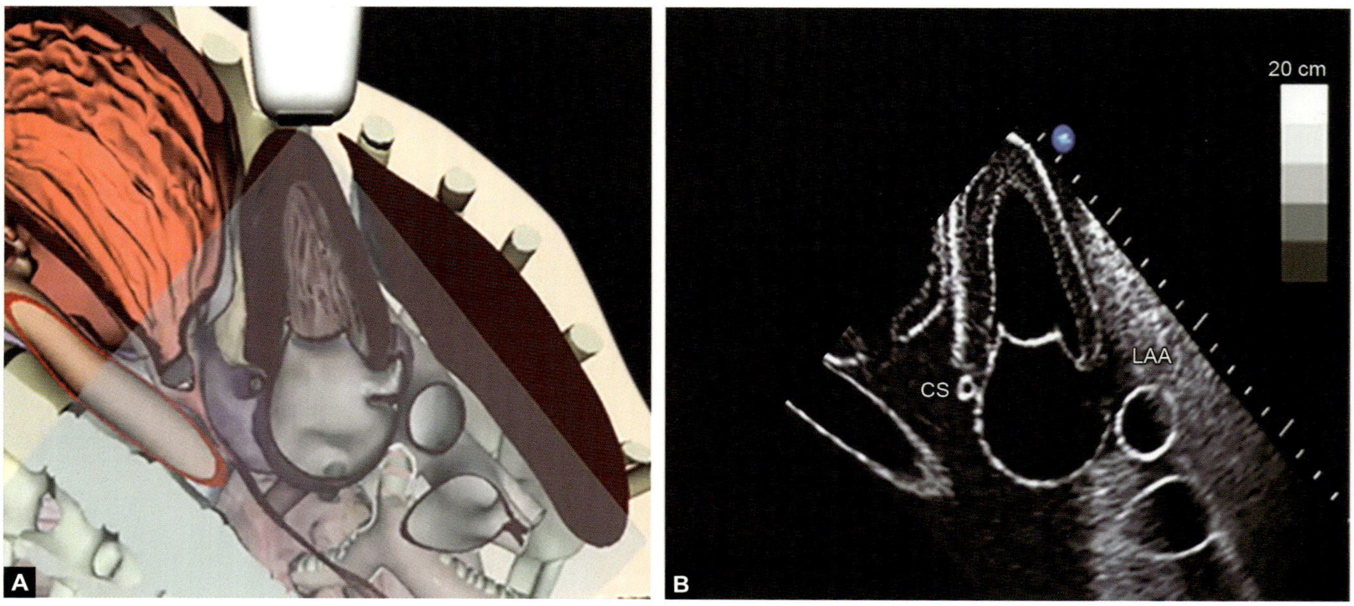

Figures 14A and B 2 chamber view shows LA and LV cavity with LAA and CS. This view portrays the LV inferior wall on left side of operator and anterior wall on right side of operator
Abbreviations: CS, costal space; LAA, left atrial appendage

The apical 2C view is obtained by counter-clockwise rotation such that the index mark is at 1o'clock position. The IVS (interventricular septum) disappears from this view and is replaced by LV inferior wall (on the left side of the operator). The diametrically opposite wall on the Rt. side is the LV anterior wall **(Figures 14A and B)**.

Apical Long Axis View

This is obtained by further counter-clockwise rotation such that the index mark pointing at the 10 o'clock position. This is also called apical 3C plane. **Figures 15A and B** and is useful view for imaging and interrogation MV and AoV. As well as visualizing the proximal, mid and distal segments of LV located in the anteroseptal and inferolateral walls.[4]

Apical 5 chamber image 3 is obtained by anterior angulation from the apical 4C placement, (index mark at the 4 o'clock position). This is an excellent view for Doppler interrogation of LVOT and aortic valve **(Figures 16A and B)**.

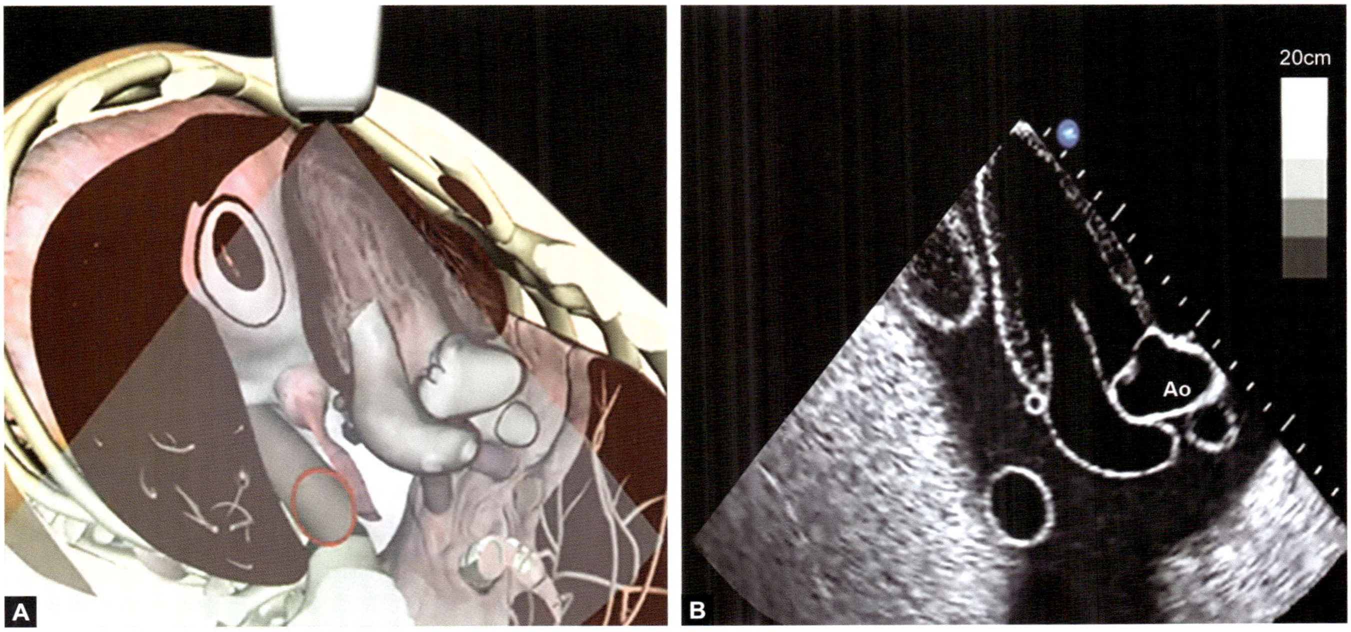

Figures 15A and B 3 chamber view at apical position shows distal segments of LV. This view is similar to low PLAX
Abbreviations: PLAX, parasternal long axis view; Ao, aorta

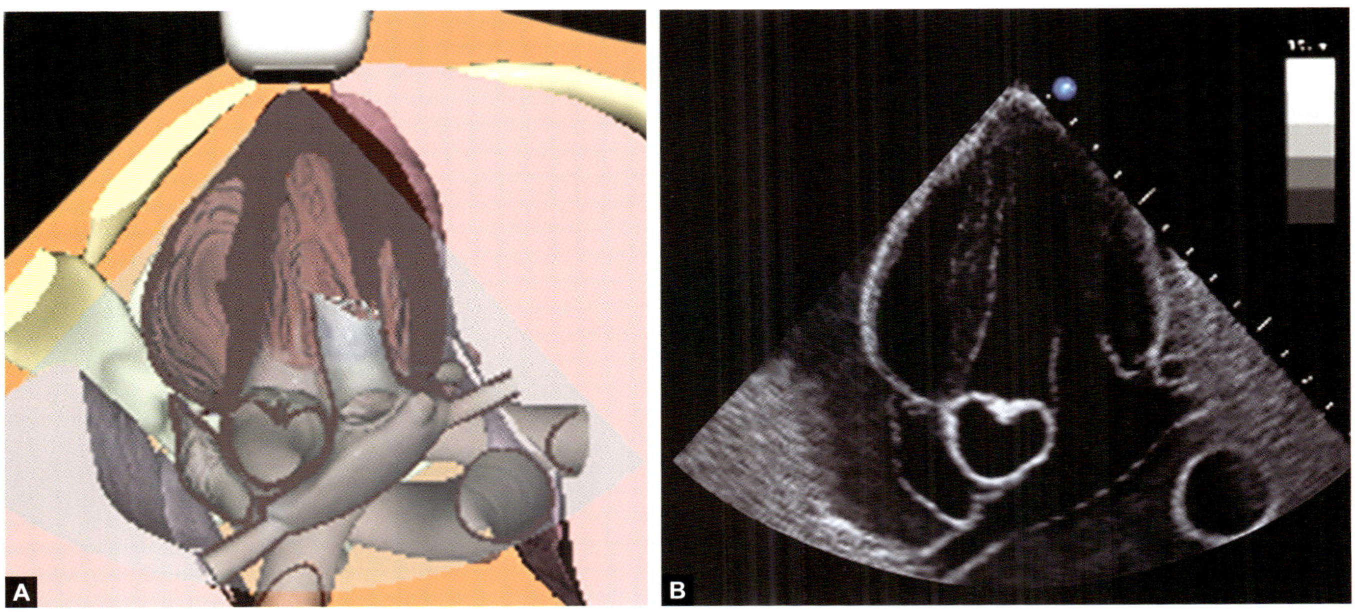

Figures 16A and B Slight upward (anterior) tilting the probe at apical position portrays 5 chambers of the heart

Unconventional variations from the apical 4C position include apical RV 2C projection (by medial angulation); the apical short axis tomographic plane with the transducer at apex as well as the RV inferobasal plane (biventricular view) **(Figures 17A and B)**. The latter plane is obtained by the combination of counter clockwise rotation and basal angulation such that the atria disappear from the imaging plane. This view is useful to evaluate the right ventricular regional function as well as to detect infero-basal VSD (postinferior MI).

The apical short axis plane is useful to differentiate LV apical clots from the artifactual apical clutter.

SUBCOSTAL PLANES

The subcostal view is also a coronal plane which is cut from side to side rather than apex to base.

This view is obtained by placing the transducer at the epigastric position and several projections can be acquired. The subcostal imaging is especially useful in patients with chronic obstructive lung diseases who usually have poor transthoracic windows as well as in pediatric patients including neonates and infants **(Figure 17C)**.

- *The 4C* view is obtained by keeping the index mark at the 4 o'clock position. This plane is extremely useful to assess the RV systolic function especially its diaphragmatic wall. It is also particularly helpful in evaluating atrial septal defect (ASD) because the interatrial septum (IAS) in this projection is at right angle to the direction of ultrasound beam while simultaneously a parallel alignment of the flow from LA to RA also occurs **(Figures 18A and B)**.

  A slight anterior angulation allows acquisition of subcostal *5C* projection **(Figures 19A and B)**.

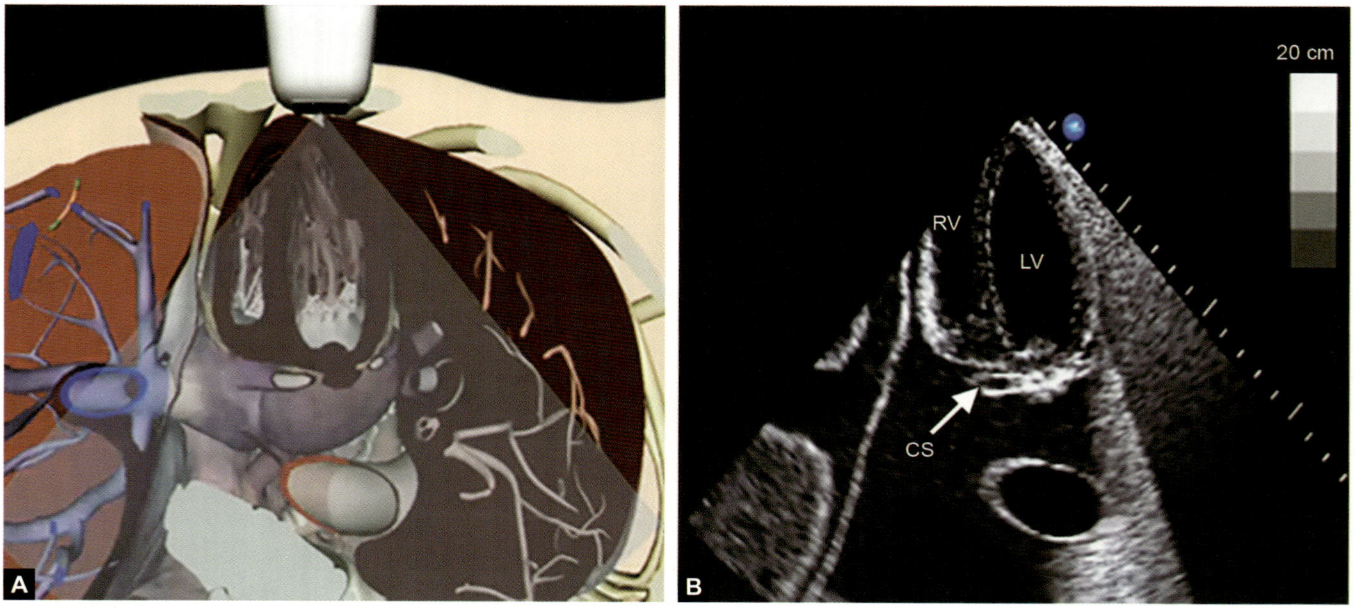

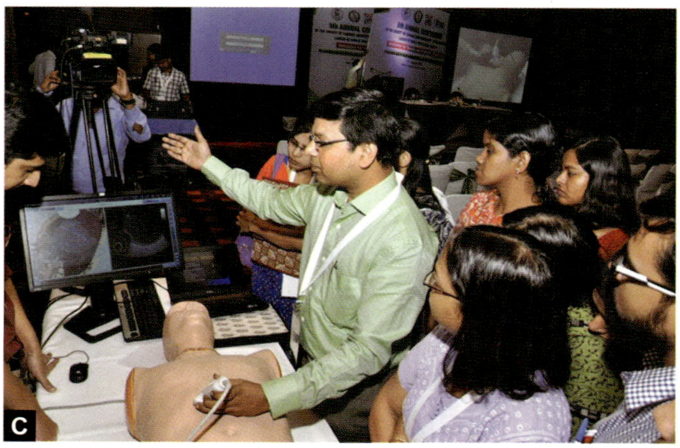

Figures 17A to C (A and B) Biventricular view by downward angulation of probe at apical position. It shows diaphragmatic wall of RV and also displays coronary sinus; (C) Transthoracic views using subcostal approach on the TTE simulator

Abbreviations: RV, right ventricle; LV, left ventricle; CS, costal space

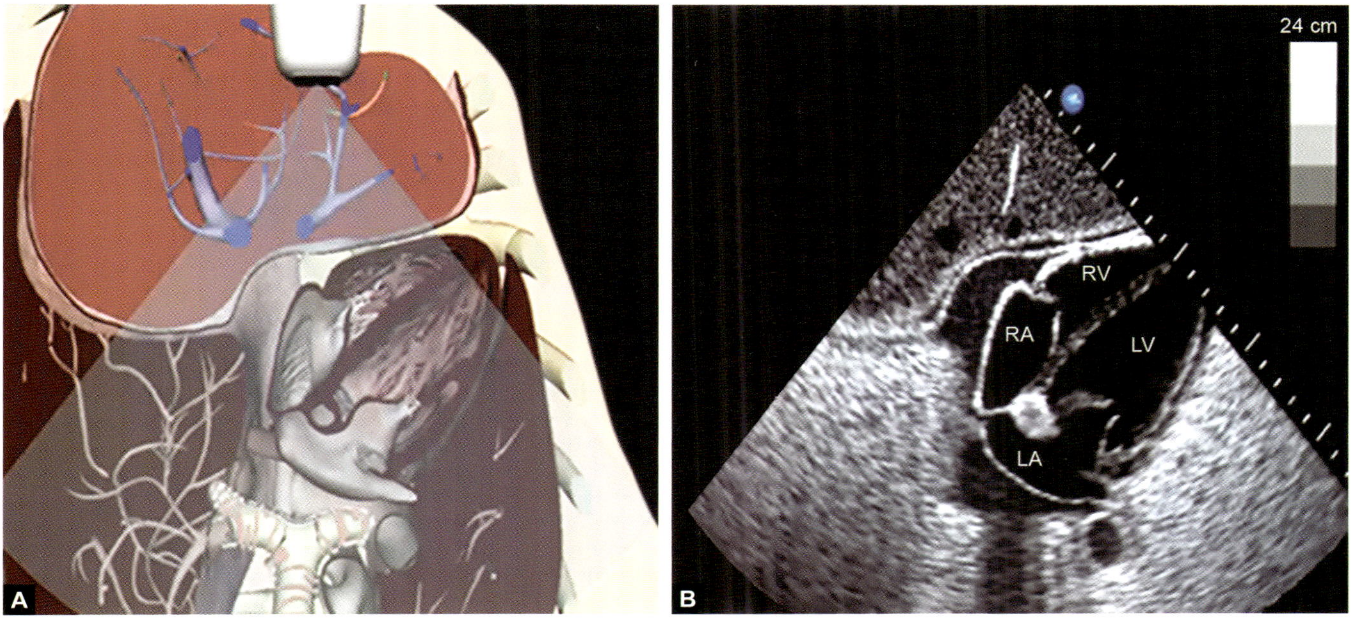

Figures 18A and B Subcostal 4C view showing all chambers of the heart
Abbreviations: LA, left atrium; LV, left ventricle; RV, right ventricle; RA, right atrium

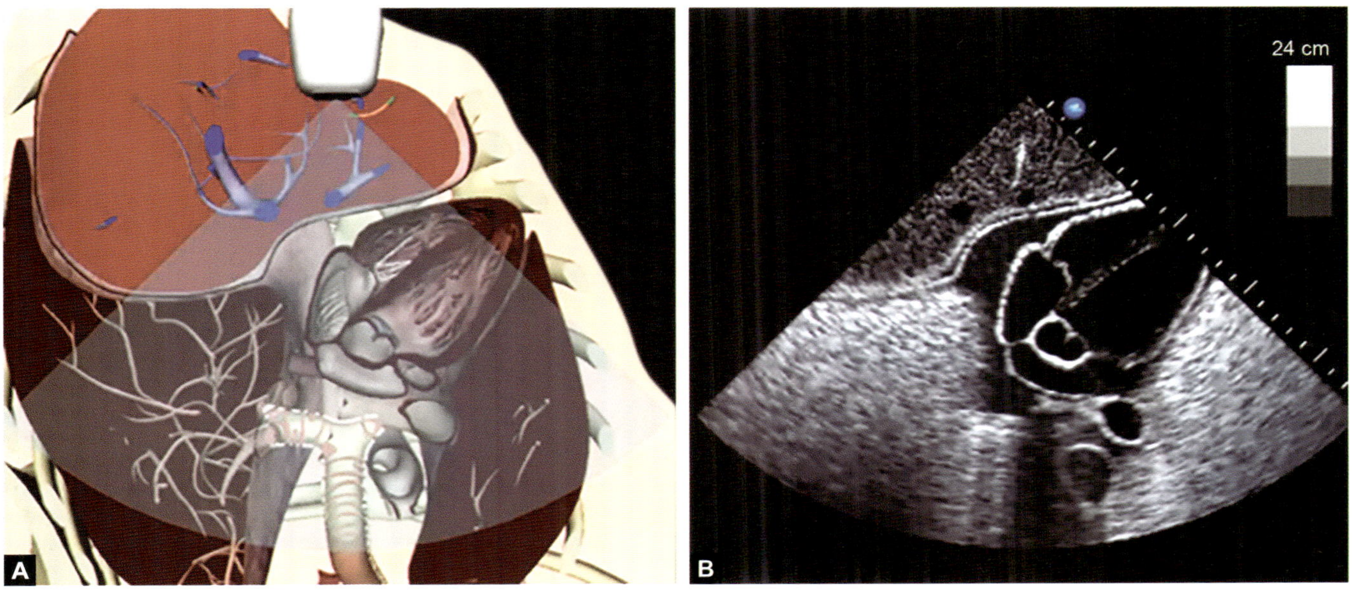

Figures 19A and B Slight angulation at subcostal plane yields 5C, showing 5 chambers of the heart

- *The subcostal SAX plane:* It is obtained by rotating the transducer counter-clockwise, with the index mark now at 1 o'clock position. Several tomographic planes can be acquired from this position including SAX at aortopulmonary position (RV inflow-apical-outflow view) as well as the SAX projections of the LV at Papillary muscle and apex **(Figures 20A and B)**.
- *Subcostal long axis*: It is obtained by rotating the transducer counter-clockwise with the index mark at

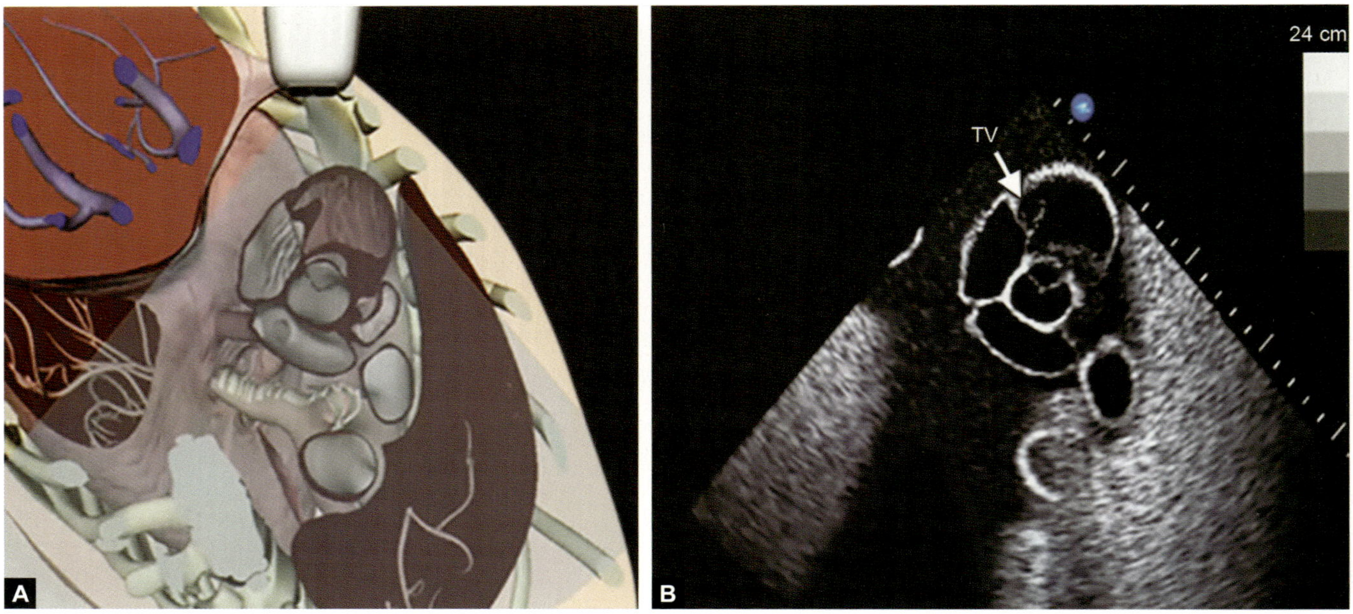

Figures 20A and B Short axis at subcostal showing aorta and RV inflow as well as outflow
Abbreviations: RV, right ventricle; TV; tricuspid valve

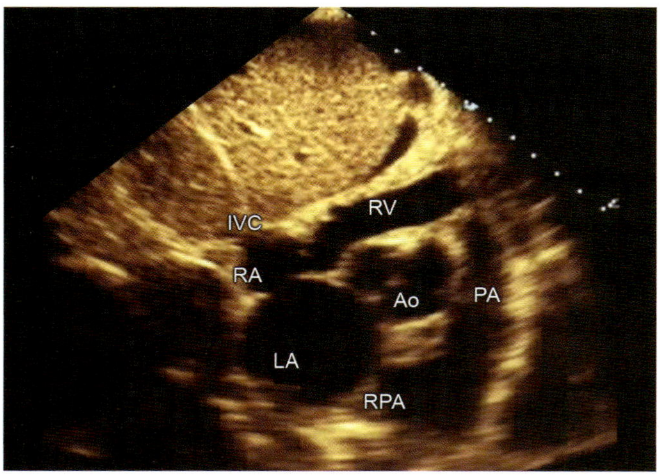

Figure 21 RV inflow-apical-outflow view
Abbreviations: LA, left atrium; Ao, aorta; RA, right atrium; PA, pulmonary artery; IVC, inferior vena cava; RPA, right pulmonary artery

10 o'clock position. This view is more easily obtained in pediatric population as well as in thin patients **(Figure 21)**.

- *Subcostal plane for IVC delineation*: It is obtained by rightward tilt of the probe with the index mark at 1 o'clock position. The drainage of the hepatic veins into the IVC as well as the ostium of the IVC guarded by the Eustachian valve can be well delineated. This view is extremely useful to evaluate the right sided filling pressures (CVP) **(Figures 22A and B)**.
- *Subcostal plane for thoracoabdominal aorta*: Is readily obtained by posterior and inferior angulation of the transducer with the index mark at 1 o'clock position. This view is extremely useful for delineating thoracoabdominal aneurysm, atherosclerotic plaques and stenosis **(Figure 23)**.

SUPRASTERNAL VIEWS

The suprasternal transducer position yields long axis and short axis cuts of the ascending aorta, aortic arch and its branches as well as the proximal descending aorta and the SVC. The main pulmonary artery/RPA is located immediately below the aortic arch and the left. Atrium is immediately below and behind the main pulmonary artery. The transducer is placed in the suprasternal notch with the index mark at 1 o'clock position and the suprasternal long axis view is thus obtained. **Figures 24A and B** long axis. This view is extremely useful to delineate ascending aortic arch aneurysms, aortic dissection as well as to profile aortic coarctation. In the pediatric population this view also facilitates accurate delineation of PA anatomy in patients with congenital heart diseases **Figure 19**.

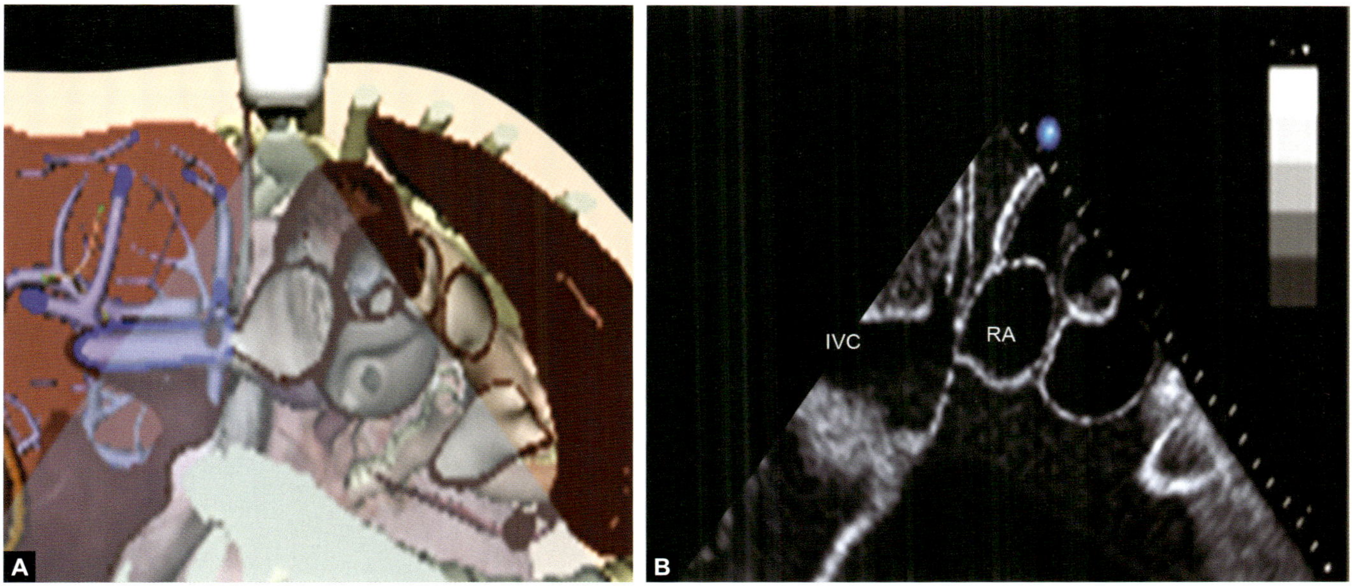

Figures 22A and B Subcostal plane showing IVC draining into RA
Abbreviations: IVC, inferior vena cava; RA, right atrium

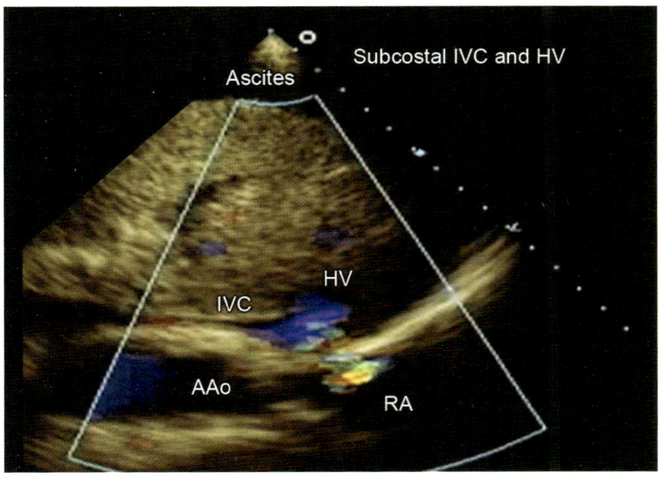

Figure 23 Colour Doppler view at subcostal level showing IVC draining into RA and hepatic veins (HV) draining into IVC
Abbreviation: AAo, ascending aorta

Suprasternal Short-axis

A slight clockwise rotation of the probe such that the index mark at 3 o'clock position and with rightward tilt facilitates the acquisition of the suprasternal short-axis (SSSAX) view with the right pulmonary artery (RPA) is seen in the long axis just behind the SVC **(Figures 25A and B)**.

A left ward tilt and a slight counter clockwise rotation from 3 o'clock to 1 o'clock position yields the suprasternal SAX with LPA over the proximal descending thoracic aorta **(Figures 26A and B)**.

RIGHT PARASTERNAL VIEW

The right sternal transducer location allows interrogation of the ascending aorta and the aortic valve in patients with aortic stenosis and helps in accurate alignment of the Doppler beam with the direction of the aortic stenosis jet. This helps in accurate computation of the pressure gradients and aortic valve area. The transducer is placed in the 2nd ICS at right sternal border with the index mark at 1 o'clock position (high right parasternal view). This transducer position also facilitates the identification of aortic dissection, aneurysm as well as pulmonary artery anatomy.

A lower transducer position at 4th or 5th ICS, helps in delineation of the atrial septum in profile with the SVC at the superior position and IVC inferior (eqivalent of Bicaval-view). The left atrium and right atrium are imaged on either side of the atrial septum and drainage of the pulmonary veins into the LA is also demonstrated (Lower right parasternal view) **(Figures 27A and B)**.

CHAPTER 3

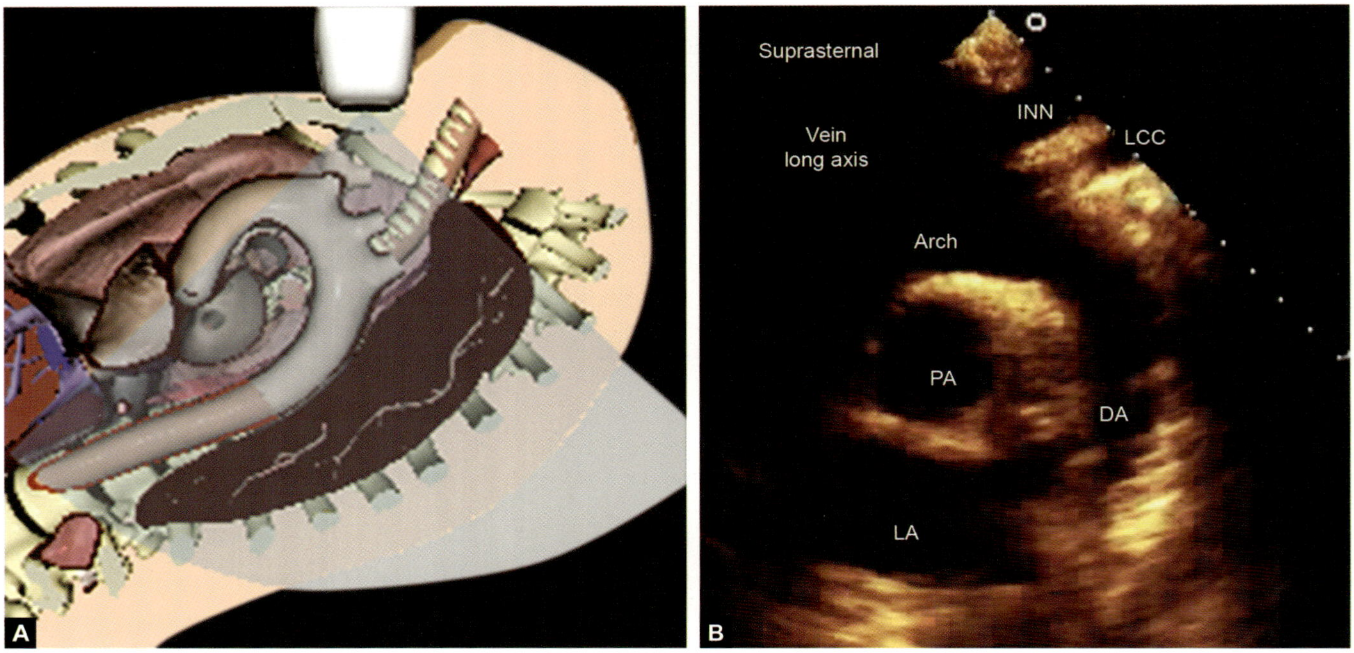

Figures 24A and B Long axis at suprasternal view showing arch of aorta with its branches and PA below it
Abbreviations: INN, innominate vein; Arch, aortic arch; PA, pulmonary artery; DA, descending aorta; LA, left atrium; LCC, left coronary cusp

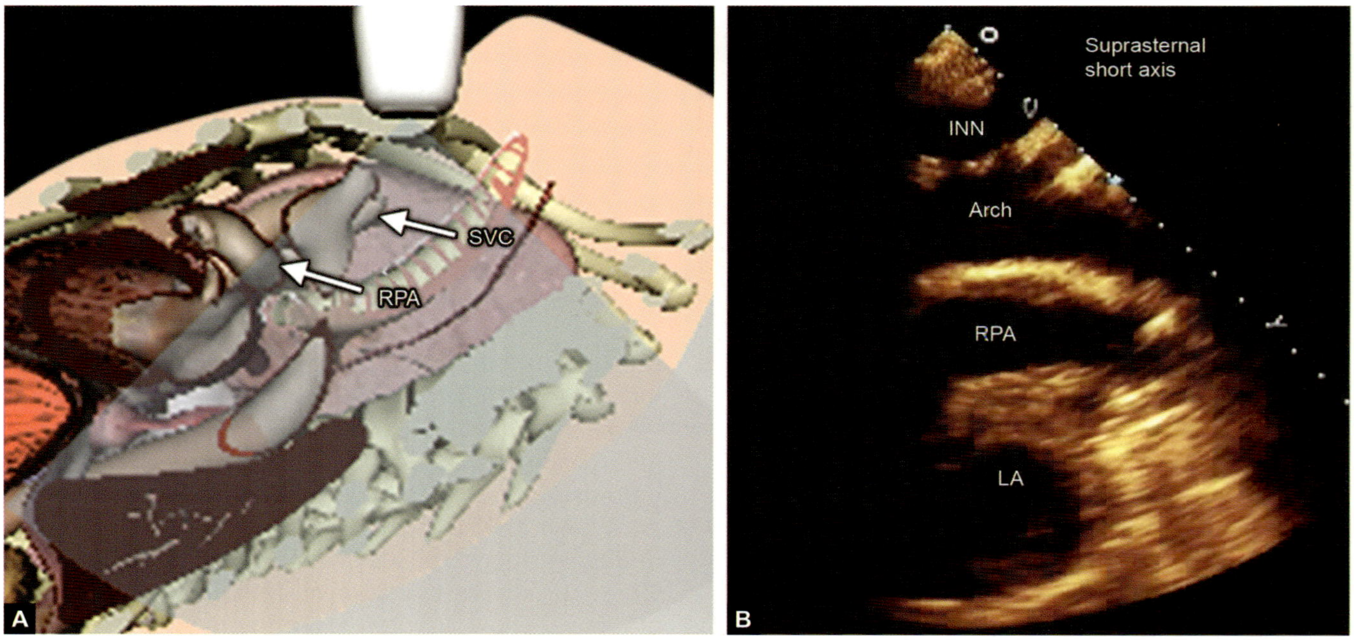

Figures 25A and B Suprasternal short axis view showing arch of aorta with SVC above and RPA below it
Abbreviations: INN, innominate vein; SVC, superior vena cava; RPA, right pulmonary artery; LA, left atrium

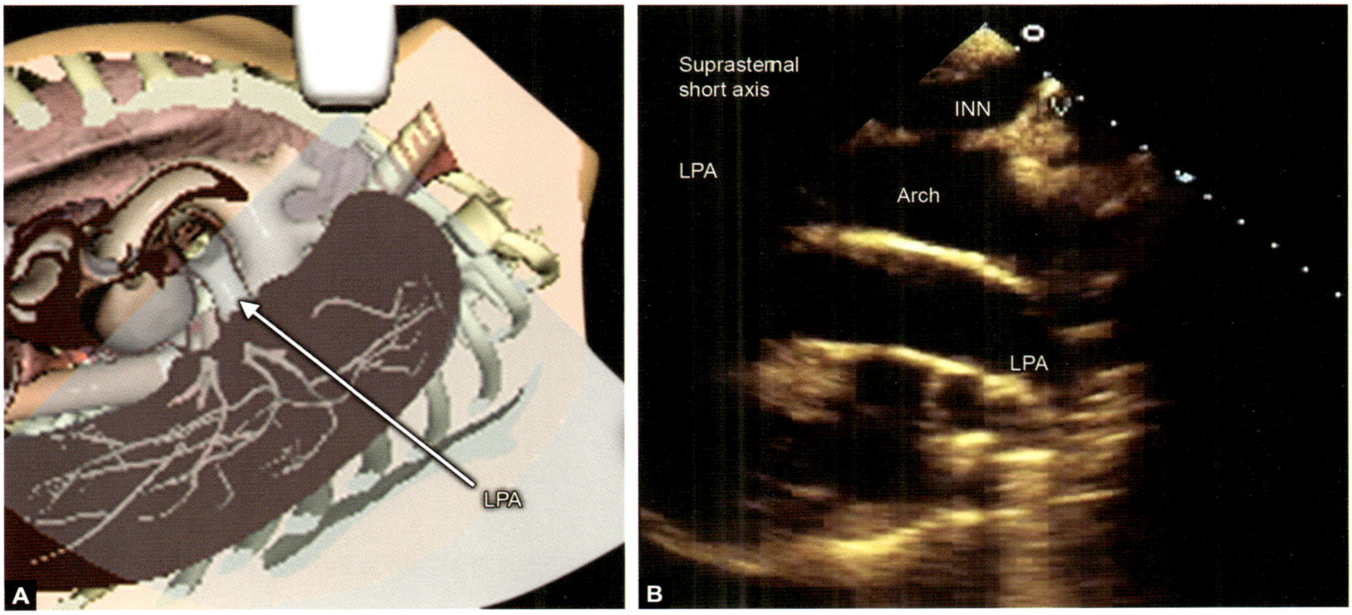

Figures 26A and B Suprasternal short axis depicting LPA over the proximal descending aorta
Abbreviation: LPA, left pulmonary artery; INN, innominate vein

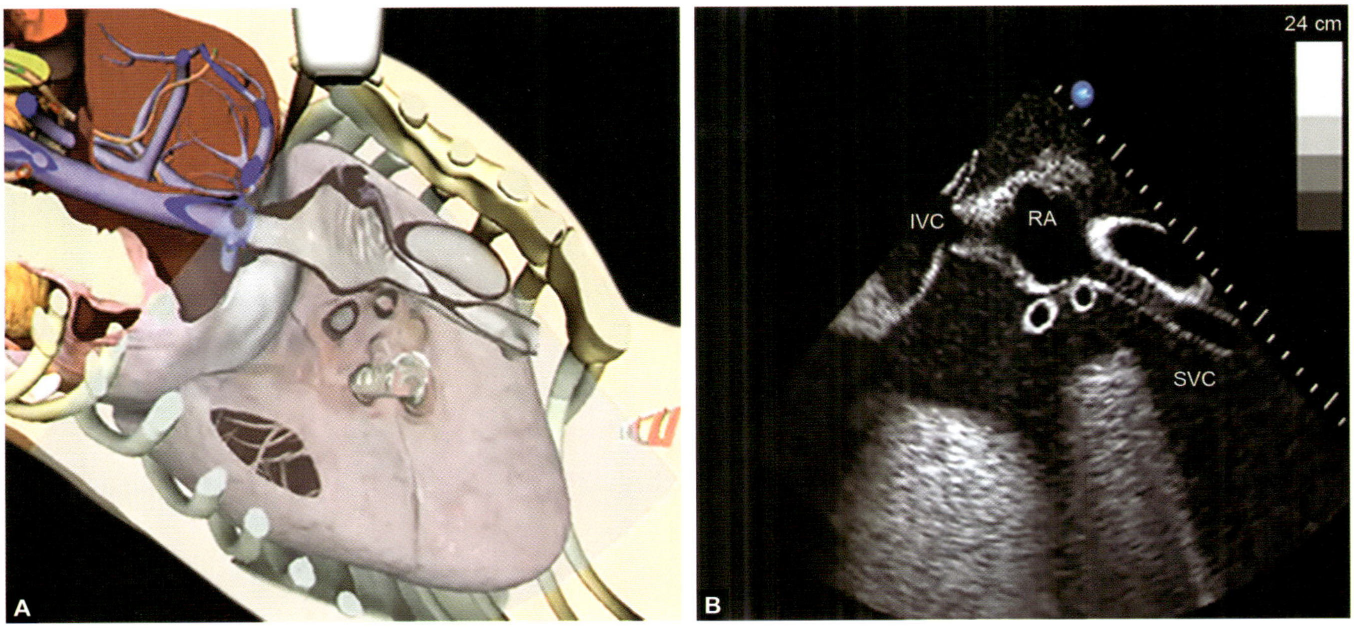

Figures 27A and B Lower right parasternal view showing IVC and SVC draining into the RA. The right pulmonary veins are just to the right-side of atrial septum
Abbreviations: IVC, inferior vena cava; SVC, superior vena cava; RA, right atrium

SUMMARY

The use of mannequin simulator for the acquisition of the transthoracic echocardiographic skills is a novel approach for training various categories of echocardiographic personnel including technologist, physicians and cardiologists. This facilitates and simulates hands-on approach without infringing on patients privacy and the work flow in the echo lab. Therefore, it is gaining in popularity and has been widely appreciated as a logical and practical approach to systematic training. However, several limitations do exists which are related to the variability of acoustic windows in real life situations as well as the inability of the simulator to provide good quality quantitative Doppler spectral data in various valvular and congenital cardiac pathologies.

REFERENCES

1. Fernando Clau-Terré, Vivek Sharma, Bernard Cholley, Nick Fletcher. Can Simulation Help to Answer the Demand for Echocardiography Education? Anesthesiology. 2014;120:32-41.
2. Paul A Roberts, Brett R Cowan, Yingmin Liu, Aaron CW Lin, Poul MF Nielsen, Andrew J Taberner, et al. Real-time aortic pulse wave velocity measurement during exercise stress testing. J Cardiovasc Magn Reson. 2015;17:86.
3. Josep Brugada, Nico Blom, Georgia Sarquella-Brugada, Carina Blomstrom-Lundqvist, John Deanfield, Jan Janousek, et al. Pharmacological and non-pharmacological therapy for arrhythmias in the pediatric population: EHRA and AEPC-Arrhythmia Working Group joint consensus statement. Europace. 2013;15:1337-82.
4. Ahmed Fathala. Myocardial Perfusion Scintigraphy: Techniques, Interpretation, Indications and Reporting. Ann Saudi Med. 2011;31(6):625-34.

Chapter 4

Understanding Echocardiographic Assessment of Left Ventricular Systolic and Diastolic Function for Simulation Training

Navin C Nanda, Munveer Thind, Saurabh Gaba, Marisa Joson, Serkan Bulur, Kamal Ahuja, Naga Sai Shravan Turaga, Sameer Srivastava

Chapter Outline

- Diastolic Function Assessment
- Conventional Two-dimensional Echocardiography
- Conventional and Color Doppler Echocardiography
- Tissue Doppler Imaging
- Two-dimensional Speckle Tracking Echocardiography and Velocity Vector Imaging
- Three-dimensional Speckle Tracking Echocardiography

DIASTOLIC FUNCTION ASSESSMENT

When a patient presents with dyspnea in spite of a documented normal systolic function, it is essential to consider diastolic dysfunction (DD) as a cause of heart failure. Diastolic heart failure (DHF) is also known as heart failure with preserved or normal left ventricular ejection fraction (LVEF). In this condition, left atrial pressures, which are equivalent to left ventricular filling pressures in the absence of mitral stenosis, are elevated causing increased pulmonary venous pressures and eventually affect the pulmonary circulation leading to dyspnea and pulmonary hypertension. Left ventricular diastolic function can be evaluated by two-dimensional transthoracic echocardiography (2DE), Doppler studies such as transmitral inflow velocities, pulmonary venous flow and flow propagation velocity, tissue Doppler imaging, pulmonary artery pressure, and with the emerging techniques of velocity vector imaging and 2D and three (3)D speckle tracking echocardiography.

CONVENTIONAL TWO-DIMENSIONAL ECHOCARDIOGRAPHY

According to current guidelines, DHF is diagnosed in the presence of the following three criteria: clinical picture consistent with heart failure, demonstration of preserved LVEF and documentation of diastolic dysfunction (DD).[1] Conventional two-dimensional echocardiography (2DE) can accurately measure LVEF and determine whether systolic dysfunction is present. Left atrial (LA) size, which is best assessed using LA volume, reflects mean pulmonary wedge pressure and is a reliable marker of chronic DD. If LA size is normal, elevated LA pressures are less likely to be present except in an acute setting where the LA may not have had time to dilate.[2] Alternatively, a dilated LA may not always be due to DD because conditions like atrial fibrillation, flutter, bradycardia, mitral valve disease, hypertension and anemia may cause significant atrial dilatation.[3] Concentric LV hypertrophy characterized by increased LV mass and relative wall thickness and remodeling, wherein LV mass is normal but relative wall thickness is increased, can be noted in DD.[4] Likewise, accurate determination of wall motion abnormalities is important as they contribute to decreased relaxation and compliance. DHF is associated with LVEF > 50% and LV mass ≥ 90 g/m² for women and ≥115 g/m² for men, LA volume index ≥34 mL/m² and abnormal wall motion.[1,2]

CONVENTIONAL AND COLOR DOPPLER ECHOCARDIOGRAPHY

Transmitral Velocities

Echocardiographic evaluation of diastolic function has been conventionally carried out by measuring the transmitral flow parameters. The mitral inflow Doppler profile provides the following indices for assessing diastolic function:

1. **E wave (early diastolic filling velocity).**
2. **A wave (late diastolic filling velocity due to atrial contraction).**
3. **E/A** (E to A ratio).
4. **DT** (deceleration time which is the time interval from the peak of E to its extrapolation to the baseline, and
5. **IVRT** (isovolumic relaxation time which is the time interval from aortic valve closure to mitral valve opening).

   DD may be present when any of the following is noted: (a) E/A < 1 or >2; (b) DT <150 ms or >220 ms or (c) **IVRT** <60 ms or >100 ms.[4]

The **peak E velocity** may be augmented by either increased LA pressure in the presence of heart disease, or by rapid LV relaxation typical of normal young adults. Hence, a high E/A may either be normal or abnormal. The transmitral flow parameters should be interpreted in the context of the loading conditions of the heart. Preload reduction decreases LA pressure and reduces the gradient between the LA and LV, leading to decreased E velocity and increased DT as it takes a longer time for the LV to fill. An increase in preload, as in severe mitral regurgitation, on the other hand, increases E velocity and reduces DT as there is increased gradient between the LA and LV pushing blood forward. In tachycardia or nonsinus rhythm, it may not be possible to acquire the biphasic E and A waves in the transmitral flow signal and evaluation of E, A and DT would be difficult.

Diastolic dysfunction can be graded according to variations in E/A ratio. In a normal heart, the LA empties rapidly into a relaxed and compliant LV resulting into a tall E wave and a shorter A wave, E > A. In Grade I DD or impaired relaxation with normal filling pressures, E < A since atrial contraction is the main contributor to LV filling. In Grade II or pseudonormalization pattern characterized by impaired relaxation and mildly elevated LV filling pressures, E > A. Finally, in Grade III or restrictive pattern with markedly elevated filling pressures and decreased deceleration time, a high E/A ratio is noted **(Figures 1 and 2)**.

The Valsalva maneuver, which by increasing intrathoracic pressure reduces cardiac preload, can be used to differentiate the normal pattern from pseudonormalization as they both present as E > A. In the presence of DD, the decreased preload with Valsalva

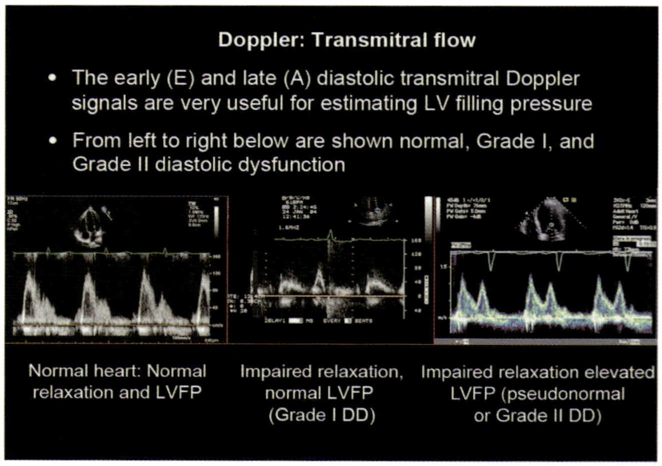

Figure 1 Transmitral diastolic inflow for the assessment of left ventricular filling pressures. (Left panel): mitral inflow in the normal heart shows early transmitral diastolic inflow greater than late transmitral diastolic inflow (E > A) due to rapid diastolic function and normal left ventricular filling pressures (LVFP); (Middle panel): in the patient with impaired LV relaxation but normal LVFP, E is lower than A, as the LV depends more on atrial kick for LV filling; this is also termed Grade I diastolic dysfunction (DD); (Right panel): in the patient with pseudonormal filling pattern, there is impaired LV relaxation but E > A, and is caused by elevated LA pressures; this is also termed Grade I diastolic dysfunction (DD). Valsalva maneuver and tissue Doppler imaging can help distinguish normal from pseudonormal filling.

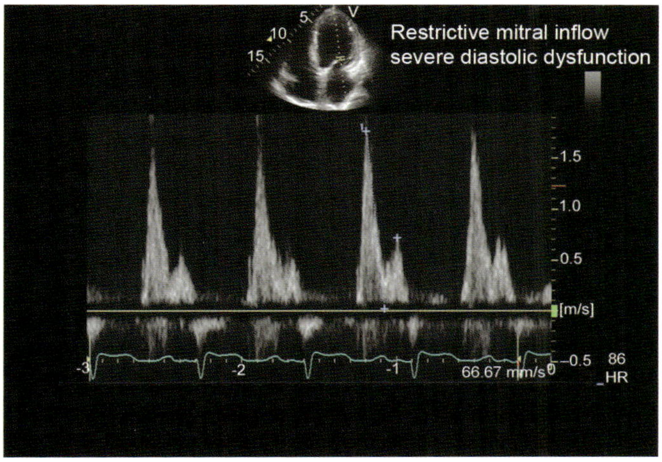

Figure 2 Restrictive transmitral filling pattern. When left ventricular (LV) filling pressures are severely elevated due to increased LV diastolic stiffness, early transmitral diastolic flow (E) has a high velocity because there is an initial high gradient between very elevated left atrial (LA) pressure and LV diastolic pressure. However, due to elevated resting LV diastolic pressures, the LA and LV pressures rapidly equilibrate, resulting in a rapid deceleration time (DT) of transmitral E. In general, in a patient with cardiac disease, restrictive filling occurs when E/A > 2 and DT < 150 milliseconds. A = late transmitral diastolic velocity.

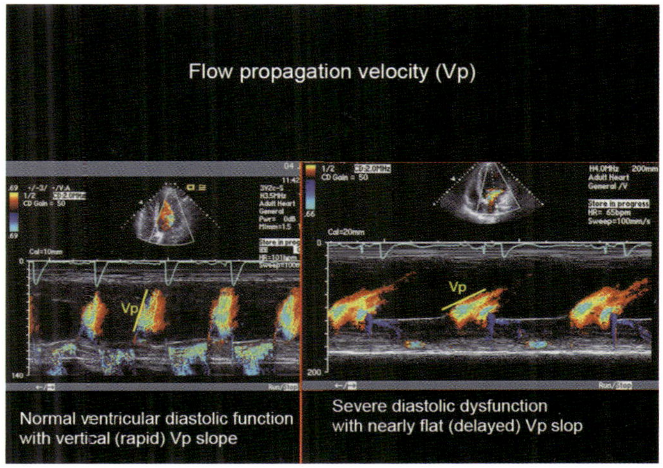

Figure 3 Color Doppler flow propagation velocity (Vp) in the assessment of left ventricular diastolic function. Placing the color Doppler sample volume from the mitral annular level to the left ventricular (LV) apex, the more rapid the LV relaxation, the faster blood travels from the mitral annular level to the LV apex, and hence the more vertical the color Doppler mitral inflow M-mode and the more rapid the Vp slope (left panel). On the other hand, the more impaired the LV relaxation, the slower it takes for blood to go from the mitral annular to the LV apex, hence a "flatter" Vp slope (right panel).

will unmask the tall E and elicit the pattern E < A. When diastolic function is normal, E > A will remain. Likewise, Valsalva maneuver can help determine whether a restrictive pattern is reversible or not. With reversibility, usually referred to as Grade IIIA DD, the pattern can change to either E < A or E > A. With irreversible restrictive pattern or Grade IIIB, the E/A ratio remain the same. [5]

In reality, Valsalva maneuver is not always a practical tool to use. Not all patients can follow the instructions and the procedure is not standardized. The innovation brought about by tissue Doppler imaging (TDI) has lessened the performance of this maneuver particularly in busy echocardiography laboratories.[4]

Flow Propagation Velocity

This modality combines color Doppler imaging and M mode using apical 4-chamber view to measure blood transit time from the mitral valve annulus to the LV apex. The early diastolic filling wave by color M mode, which appears in red color as blood flows from the mitral valve to the LV apex is identified (V_p). The slope of this early diastolic M mode is rapid and vertical with normal diastolic function. With DHF, the slope gets flatter and flatter reflecting progressively impaired relaxation. **Also, E/V_p correlates with mean LA pressure such that E/V_p >15 reasonably correlates with PCWP >15 mm Hg.**[6,7] In practice, many echo laboratories do not use this modality as many technological concerns contribute to significant inter observer variability **(Figure 3)**.[7, 8]

Pulmonary Venous Flow

Pulsed wave Doppler of the pulmonary veins is also used to evaluate for DD. In a normal heart, blood flows rapidly through the pulmonary veins into the LA and passes through the mitral valve into the LV. The Doppler signals are made up of forward systolic (S), and diastolic (D) velocities into the LA and a backward late diastolic A reversal wave (Ar) corresponding to atrial contraction. Other measurements include the duration of Ar velocity and the time difference between Ar duration and mitral A wave duration (Ar-A), systolic filling fraction and DT (deceleration time). In normal subjects, S < D (due to rapid diastolic suction in the healthy LV) and Ar < 35 ms. In grade I DD, S > D as rapid diastolic function is lost. In the setting of elevated LA pressure S < D, and in significiantly elevated LA pressure DT of D wave < 150 ms. Therefore, as with mitral inflow E/A, pulmonary

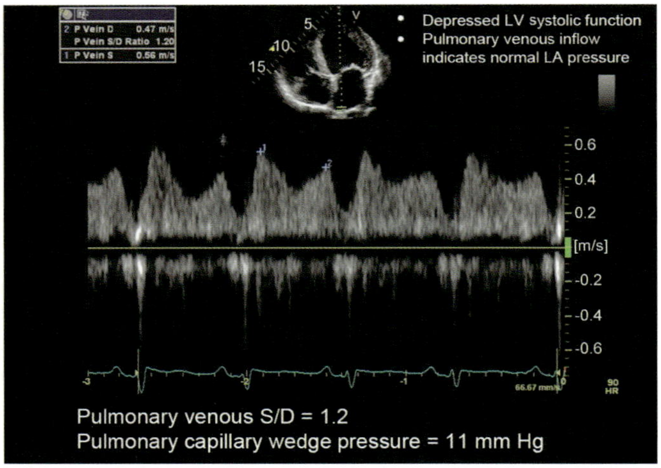

Figure 4 Pulmonary venous Doppler velocities in the assessment of left atrial pressures. In normal heart, systolic pulmonary venous (PV) flow (S) is lower than diastolic PV flow (D), as rapid left ventricular (LV) suction during diastole results in elevated PV D velocities; thus, PV S < D. In patients with impaired LV relaxation and elevated LA pressure, when the mitral valve (MV) is closed in ventricular systole, the elevated LA pressure prevents PV S flow, and therefore most flow occurs when the MV opens, resulting in S < D. Therefore, as with mitral inflow velocities, PV velocities are also prone to pseudonormal filling. In this example, there is impaired LV relaxation due to cardiomyopathy, but LA pressure is not elevated; thus, when the MV is closed (LV systole), there is unimpeded flow through the PV, and hence S > D.

venous S/D also has normal and pseudonormal patterns. Ar-A velocity duration >30 ms indicates an elevated LV end diastolic pressure. DD can also be graded using the values of the pulmonary venous flow velocities mentioned above.[9]

It is obvious that measurement of pulmonary venous flow is not always feasible, as high quality recordings suitable for measurement are not always obtainable. In contrast to mitral inflow velocities, only a small number of studies have documented the prognostic role of pulmonary venous flow **(Figure 4)**.[10-12]

Pulmonary Artery Pressure (PAP)

When there is elevated LA pressure, this pressure is transmitted back into the pulmonary veins and across the pulmonary venous-capillary bed into the pulmonary arterioles then into the pulmonary arteries leading to pulmonary arterial hypertension (PAH). In this way, PA pressure estimated by addition of right atrial (RA) pressure (by assessing inferior vena cava size and response to respiration) is a good surrogate marker of significant, and often chronic, LA pressure elevation.

It has been proven that PA systolic pressure (PASP) >35 mm Hg often characterizes advanced or significant LV DD with elevated LA pressures.[4,13] However, as with LA volume, the existence of significant PAH does not necessarily mean significant DD, as significant elevation in pulmonary vascular resistance (PVR) due to intrinsic lung disease must first be excluded. Likewise, normal PASP can be helpful in ruling out significant and long-standing LA pressure elevation, as long as a complete tricuspid regurgitation (TR) jet is obtained with correct Doppler sample volume angulation in respect of the direction of TR, and with correct RA pressure estimation. PA end-diastolic pressure, which in the absence of significant elevations in PVR can be a good estimate of mean LA pressure, can be approximated from the pulmonary artery regurgitation diastolic wave, with RA pressure then added to it as is done with PASP.[13]

TISSUE DOPPLER IMAGING

Measurement of mitral annulus velocities using TDI has been shown to be a sensitive tool to evaluate for DD since it is less dependent on cardiac loading conditions. Contraction and relaxation of myocardial segments result in long axis shift of the mitral annulus toward the quite immobile LV apex during systole and in the opposite direction in diastole. Three velocities are recorded:

a. **S′ corresponding to ventricular ejection,**
b. **E′ corresponding to early filling as in the E of transmitral Doppler.**
c. **A′ corresponding to late filling as in A wave.**[8,13,14]

Of the three velocities recorded, E′ is considered to be the most valuable for the evaluation of DD. E′ progressively decreases as relaxation becomes slower in the setting of many cardiac diseases such as dilated, restrictive and hypertrophic cardiomyopathies.[8] It is less affected by preload and remains low in patients with pseudonormalized E/A. These velocities are recorded at the septal and lateral annuli. Septal E′ is usually less than lateral E′, except in the setting of lateral wall infarction or constrictive physiology. Studies suggest that the lateral E′ is preferable if one is obtaining only a single measurement in a patient with normal LVEF, as the septal E′ has been shown to be changed by preload in patients with normal LV function, although this alteration may decrease as LV relaxation becomes more deranged. Also, the septal E′ may be affected by right ventricular DD.[15] Computing for E/E′ provides an estimate of LV filling pressure, with E/lateral E′ >12 and E/septal E′ > 15 indicating increased LV filling pressure. With regional LV dysfunction, it is advised to utilize the average value of E′ of septal and lateral annuli to better reflect LV filling pressures.[16] Tissue Doppler imaging also measures the time interval, TE-E′ which is the time interval between the QRS complex and the onset of mitral E velocity minus the time interval between the QRS and the onset of E′. In particular, IVRT/T E-E′ < 2 reasonably identifies patients with elevated LV filling pressures.[17] Diastolic dysfunction can also be graded in the same way as with transmitral Doppler velocities using the values for E′ and E/E′.[6]

Tissue Doppler imaging has the edge, against other modalities of being easy to execute and validate in clinical practice.[18] There are procedural limitations, however, such as its being angle dependent and requiring proper attention to the location of the Doppler sample volume which should be placed at the tips of the mitral leaflets for measurement of E and A. The presence of significant mitral annular calcification, surgical rings, mitral stenosis, significant mitral regurgitation, prosthetic mitral valve and constrictive pericarditis, among others affect the mitral inflow velocities rendering the application of E to E′ ratio unreliable in these settings **(Figures 5A to D)**.[19]

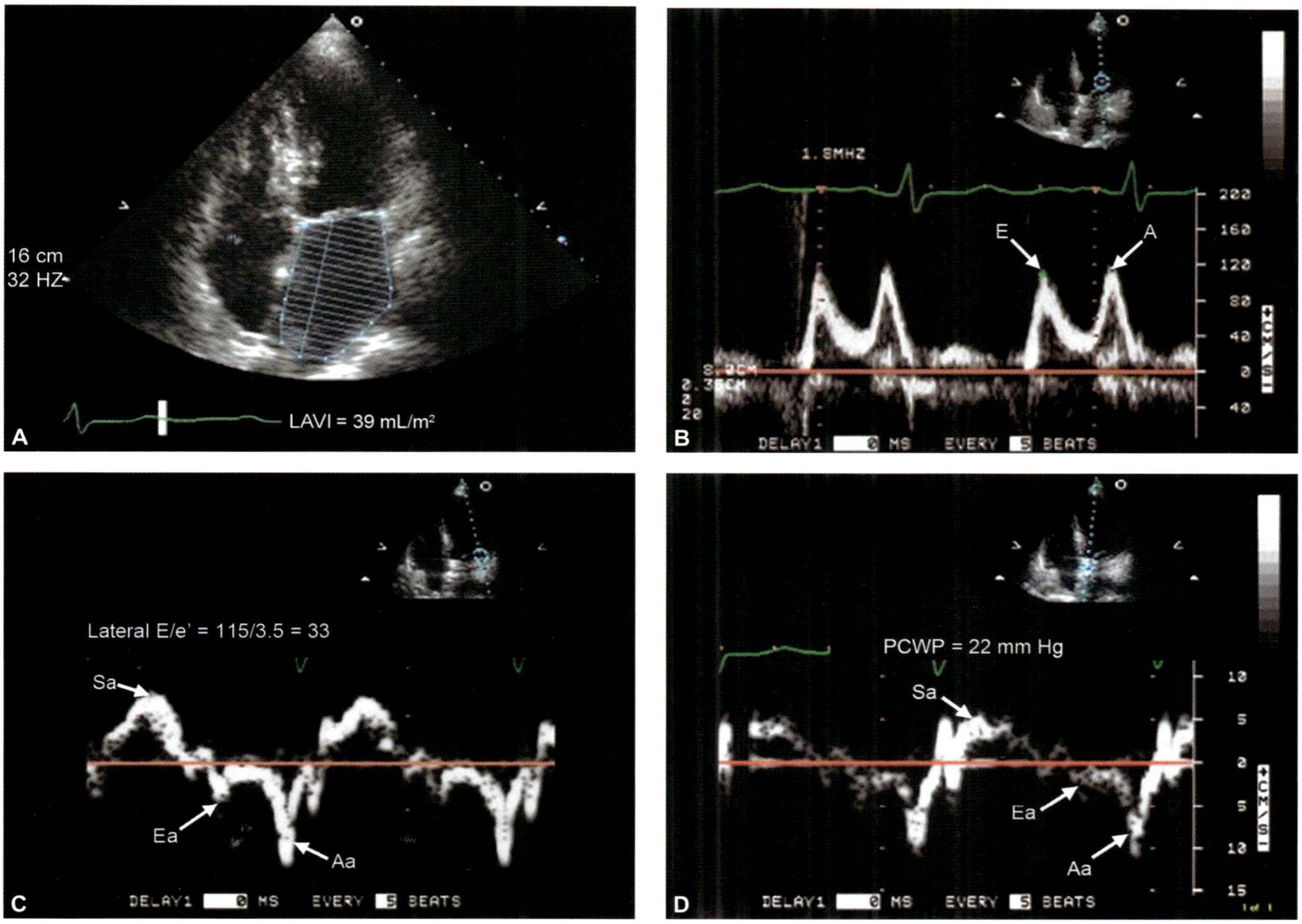

Figures 5A to D Tissue Doppler imaging for the assessment of left ventricular (LV) diastolic function. (A) An apical four-chamber view with moderate to severe dilation of the left atrium (LA) with an LA volume index of 39 mL/m^2; (B) Elevated early transmitral diastolic velocity (E) = 117 cm/s; (C) Very depressed mitral lateral annular early diastolic relaxation velocity (e') = 3.5 cm/s; (D) Very depressed septal tissue Doppler (TD) early diastolic velocity (e') = 2.5 cm/s. Therefore, E/e' septal = 47, and E/e' lateral = 33, indicating severely impaired LV relaxation with elevated LV filling pressures.
Abbreviations: LAVI, left atrial volume index; PCWP, Pulmonary capillary wedge pressure.

TWO-DIMENSIONAL SPECKLE TRACKING ECHOCARDIOGRAPHY AND VELOCITY VECTOR IMAGING

Two-dimensional speckle tracking echocardiography (2D STE) is an innovative technology of cardiac imaging that allows for calculating complex cardiac movement based on frame-to-frame tracking of ultrasonic speckles on gray scale 2D images. Speckles are small dots or groups of myocardial pixels that are routinely created by the interface of ultrasonic beams and the myocardium. Identifying and tracking these speckles all through the cardiac cycle by 2D technology provides information about myocardial muscle mechanics which can then be used to evaluate cardiac function and confirm the presence of abnormalities. Many vendors have developed algorithms for speckle tracking **(Figures 6A to C)**.[20-22]

Though TDI also provides information on myocardial velocities from which myocardial deformation (strain) can be obtained, the method is complex and requires parallel alignment of the ultrasound beam to tissue movement. On the other hand, 2D STE is angle independent since it is based on 2 DE and not on Doppler. **Table 1** compares 2D STE with TDI and presents the advantages and disadvantages of each technology.

Clinically, 2D STE has been utilized to evaluate systolic and diastolic function and a host of cardiac pathologies like ischemia, cardiomyopathy, valvular and congenital heart diseases, and the athlete's heart, among others. It is also being utilized to evaluate the effectiveness of treatment as in cardiac resynchronization therapy and the effects of chemotherapeutic drugs and stem cell therapy on the heart.[22]

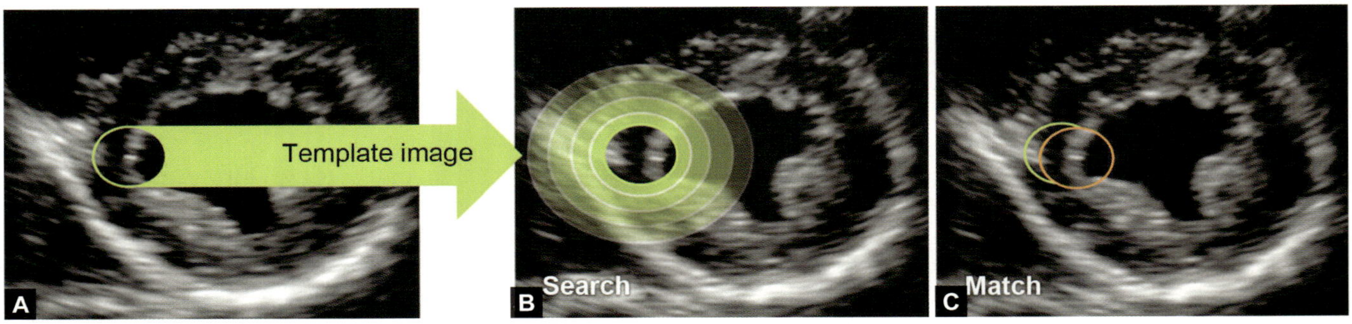

Figures 6A to C Speckle tracking imaging. Left ventricular short-axis view showing frame-by-frame tracking of a large group of pixels (denoted by a circle).
Courtesy: Toshiba Medical Systems Europe BV.

TABLE 1 Comparison of tissue Doppler imaging with speckle tracking for evaluation of strain

Tissue Doppler imaging	*Speckle tracking*
Dependent on angle of insonation	Angle independent
Can measure deformation only along one axis (axis of the transducer)	Can measure longitudinal, radial, and circumferential strain. Can also measure left ventricular twist mechanics
Movement assessed in relation to transducer	Movements assessed in relation to adjacent speckles
Higher frame rates and hence good temporal resolution	Lower frame rates and poor temporal resolution. Hence limited utility in tachycardic patients and in those with nonsinus rhythms
Limited spatial resolution	Better spatial resolution
Measures regional strain only	Both regional and global strain can be computed
Measures tissue velocity, strain is derived	Strain and strain rate can be measured directly
Influenced by translational motion	Less influenced by translational motion
Image quality less important	Relies on good image quality
Less reproducibility	Greater concordance among observers

Adapted from Biswas M, et al. Two- and three-dimensional speckle tracking echocardiography: clinical applications and future directions. Echocardiography. 2013;30(1):88-105.

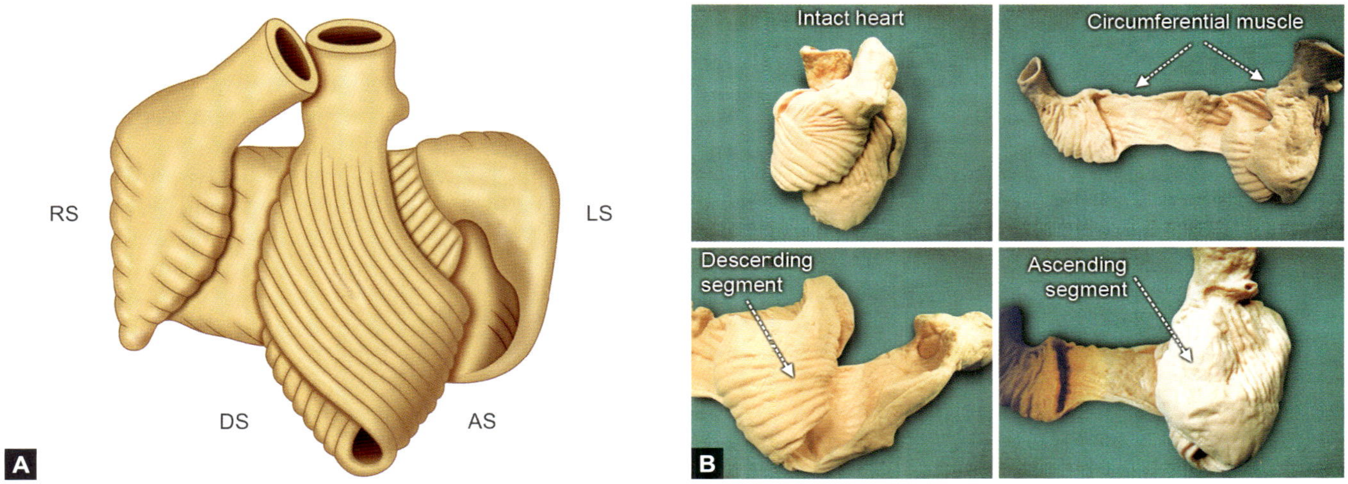

Figures 7A and B Schematic model and dissected heart model showing myocardial fiber arrangements. (A) Depicts the apical and basal loops. The apical loop consists of an outer ascending segment (AS) with oblique counterclockwise fiber orientation and an inner descending segment (DS) with fibers oriented in an oblique clockwise direction. The basal loop covers the upper two-thirds of the apical loop and its fibers are oriented in a circumferential or transverse direction. It can be considered to have two segments: right (RS) and left (LS); (B) Depicts the way the circumferential fibers of the basal loop wrap around the ascending and descending segments.
Reproduced from Buckberg G, Hoffman JI, Nanda NC, et al. Ventricular torsion and untwisting: further insights into mechanics and timing interdependence: a viewpoint. Echocardiography. 2011;28:782-804, with permission from Wiley-Blackwell.

A reasonable understanding of cardiac muscle mechanics is needed to appreciate how 2D STE works. According to the model popularized by Buckberg, et al, the heart is a helix made up of a single myocardial muscle band with fibers of different orientations folded upon itself in 3 layers. This single muscle band has 2 loops, a transverse basal loop which is the middle layer and an oblique apical loop that has two segments. The descending apical segment is the inner layer and twists clockwise while the ascending apical segment is the outer layer and twists counterclockwise. The transverse basal loop wraps around two thirds of the upper ascending and descending segments leaving the lower third of the apex and the ventricular septum free **(Figures 7A and B)**.[20,23,24]

The heart does not move in one direction but in several planes with each cardiac cycle. In systole, long axis motion is shortening from base to apex while radial, transverse and circumferential motions bring the muscle inward. There is also translational motion with the base moving anteriorly. At the same time, the heart rotates with the base moving clockwise and the apex, counterclockwise in systole. In diastole, all these movements are reversed. During the isovolumic contraction period, both the base and apex move in the counterclockwise direction while the ascending apical segment does not move. During the isovolumic relaxation period, both base and apex rotate clockwise with no contraction of the descending apical segment. If there is extended contraction of the descending segment or if contraction crosses over to diastole, (post-systolic contraction or shortening), diastolic filling will be affected because 50% of untwisting motion of the heart or relaxation occurs at this time.[24]

Based on the above movements of the myocardial muscle, parameters of strain (myocardial deformation), strain rate (rate of deformation), and rotational mechanics of rotation, twist and torsion are measured by 2D STE and become useful clinically. 2D STE can also measure these parameters in the other chambers of the heart but are less well investigated.

Strain refers to the percentage thickening or deformation of the cardiac muscles during the cardiac cycle and 2D STE measures 4 types of strain:

1. **Radial strain** (using short axis views).
2. **Transversal strain** (using apical views) that measure thickening of the wall during inward motion and is assigned a positive (+) sign **(Figures 8 and 9)**.
3. **Longitudinal strain** measures the percentage decrease in length as the base predominantly moves toward the apex and is expressed as a negative (–) sign **(Figure 10)**.

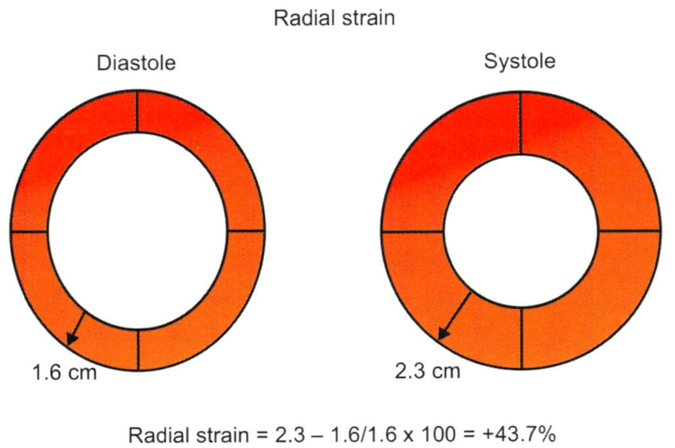

Figure 8 Radial strain shows radial thickening of the myocardium during systole. In the end-diastolic frame on the left, the myocardial thickness is 1.6 cm and increases to 2.3 cm in end systole as depicted on the right; hence, the radial strain will be +43.7%.
Courtesy: Toshiba Medical Systems Europe BV.

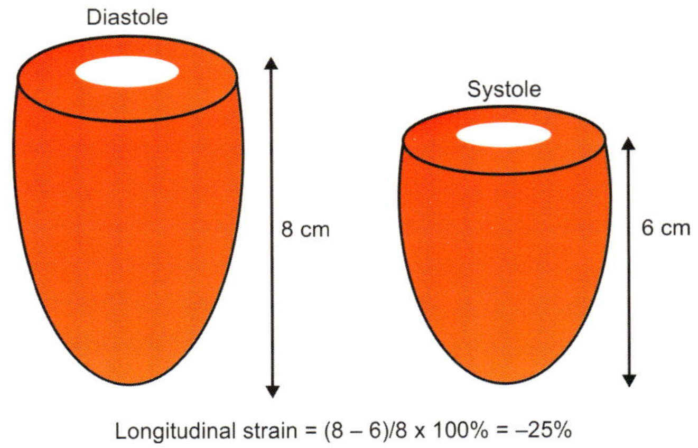

Figure 10 Longitudinal strain shows shortening of ventricular length during systole. The figure on the left denotes end diastole and the one on the right depicts end systole. Note the downward descent of the mitral annulus toward the apex in systole. There is a reduction in length by 2 cm, which is a 25% decrease. As there is a decrease in the longitudinal length, it will be denoted by a negative (–) sign; hence the longitudinal strain will be –25%.

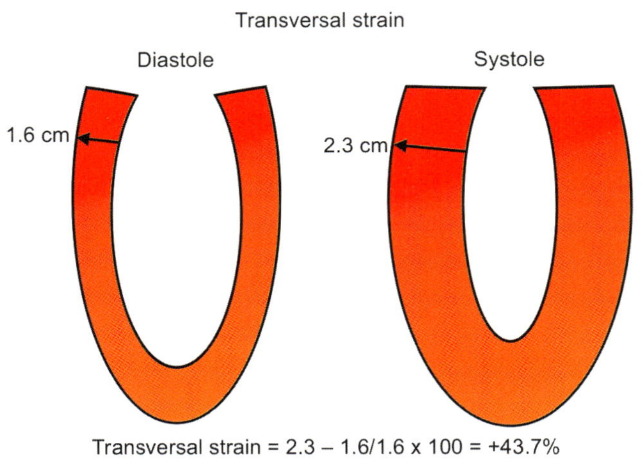

Figure 9 Transversal strain: The calculations are similar to radial strain, except that the measurements are done using apical views.

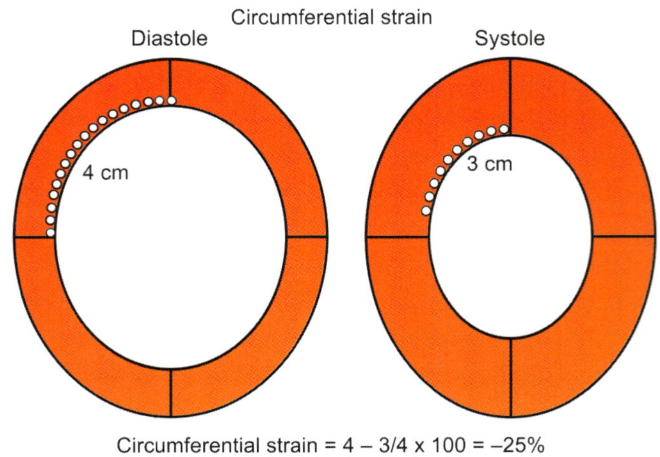

Figure 11 Circumferential strain. This refers to the change in the circumference of each segment as denoted by the dotted yellow line in the figure. There is a 25% reduction in the circumferential length in end-systole from the baseline end-diastole; hence the circumferential strain will be –25%.
Courtesy: Toshiba Medical Systems Europe BV.

4. Circumferential strain measures the change in length along the circular or circumferential perimeter and is assigned a negative (–) sign **(Figure 11)**.

All these strain parameters can be measured individually for each myocardial segment or can be averaged for all the segments to provide global strain. Strain rate is the rate of change of thickness or deformation of the myocardium.

The time from the start of the QRS complex (end diastole) to the time when peak strain occurs (at end systole, end of T wave) coincides with minimum LV volume. Measuring the time difference when peak strain occurs for each muscle segment is also clinically useful as it gives information on dyssynchrony of muscle

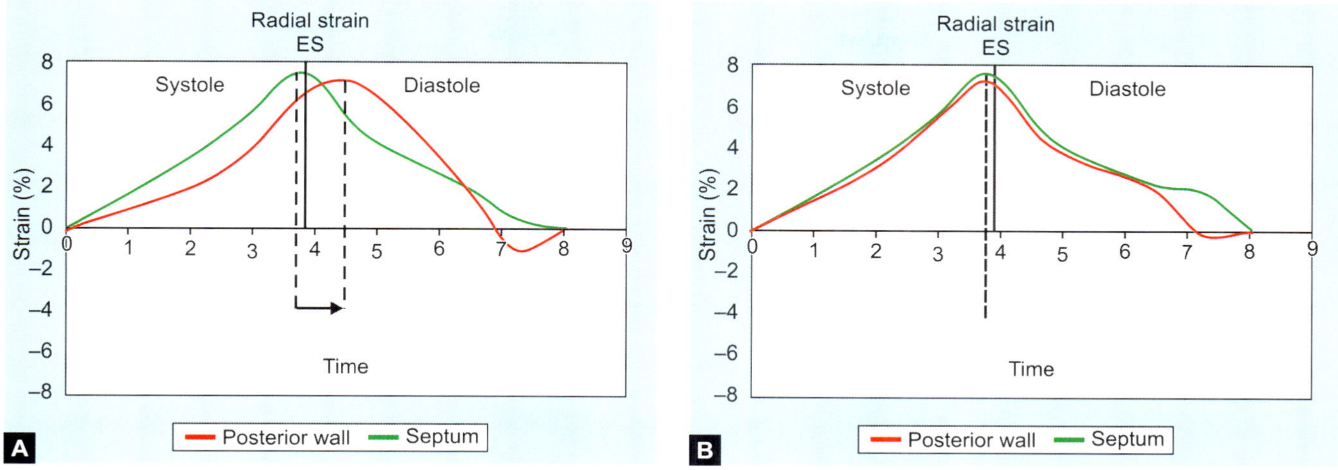

Figures 12A and B Dyssynchronous left ventricular contraction depicted by radial strain. Note the time difference between peak strain of the posterior wall and ventricular septum denoted by the yellow arrow. The peak strain or contraction of the posterior wall is much delayed in comparison with the septum (A). The goal of resynchronization therapy is to get the peak strains (contractions) as close as possible to each other as depicted in (B).
Abbreviation: ES, end-systole.

contraction, as occurs with left bundle branch block. Recognizing this condition, appropriate management such as biventricular pacing can be provided **(Figures 12A and B)**.

For rotational mechanics, the following parameters are measured by 2D STE:

1. Rotation, which is the rotation around a designated long axis line drawn from apex to base through the middle of the LV cavity with clockwise movement given a negative (-) value and counterclockwise, a positive (+) value.
2. Twist measures the algebraic difference between the apex and base rotation.
3. Torsion is twist normalized to the length of the LV cavity. Both twist and torsion can be computed for between any two segments of the myocardium. Likewise, the rate and total duration of rotation can also be calculated **(Figure 13)**.[20]

Some 2D STE applications present tracking results as velocity vectors and this technique is called Velocity Vector Imaging. Each arrow or vector expresses the direction and magnitude of myocardial movement during each cardiac cycle. The vectors are compared along a tracked contour placed over the echo view of the heart **(Figures 14 and 15)**.

Myocardial strain data obtained from 2D STE compare positively with hemodynamics, tissue Doppler, tagged MRI and sonomicrometry studies. Normal values for both strain and rotational mechanics have been published.[20] **Tables 2 and 3** show these values.

Strain and rotational parameters have been described in many cardiac conditions attesting to the clinical usefulness of this technology. **Table 4** presents such a list which is large and may be quite overwhelming. The following general principles should make for a better appreciation of these findings and the tremendous utility of this modality.[20, 25]

- The subendocardial longitudinal fibers are deemed the most susceptible in many disease processes manifested as early deterioration of longitudinal strain and next by radial and circumferential strains.
- Decrease in radial or transversal and circumferential strains are considered more conclusive than wall motion abnormalities in the assessment of ischemic heart disease because the latter are subjectively assessed, and as such are prone to greater interobserver variability.
- Abnormalities of the pericardium lead to aberration of circumferential strain first.
- The hyperactive rotational motion during systole acts as a compensatory process early in the disease causing diastolic dysfunction.
- Untwisting during the post ejection isovolumic interval (isovolumic relaxation period) is hampered early in DD.
- As the diseases become more severe, all the parameters may become further abnormal.

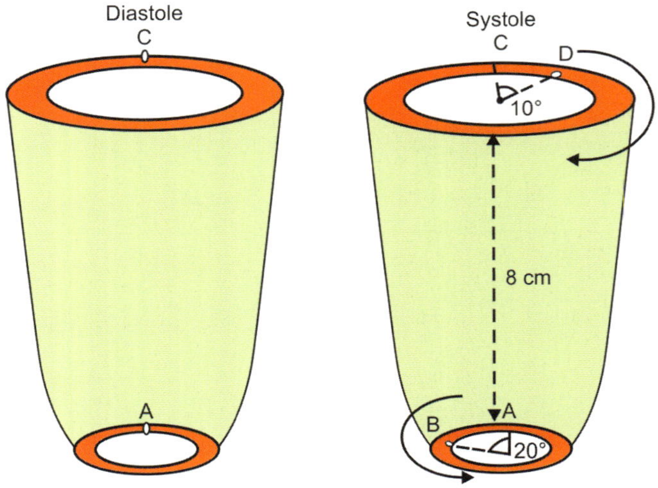

Figure 13 Differential rotational movements of left ventricular apex and the base. In the normal individual, the apex rotates more than the base. By convention, counterclockwise motion is assigned a positive (+) sign and clockwise motion a negative (–) sign. In the above example, the apex rotates 20° in counterclockwise direction from end diastole (point A) to end systole (point B); hence the rotation of the apex will be +20°. As the base rotates at the same time 10° clockwise from point C to D, the rotation of the base will be –10°. "Twist" is calculated as the algebraic difference in the rotation of the apex and base; in other words, how far apart a point in the apex and base move from each other. In the above example, the twist will be apex rotation (20°) minus base rotation (–10°), that is, 20 – (–10) = +30°. Twist can be calculated for any point in the myocardium compared to a reference basal point. "Torsion" is a way of adjusting for the distance of a point of interest from the reference point in the base, as it is expected that the twist will be higher for the segments farther away from the base. Torsion = twist/the distance from the base or distance between any two points that are evaluated. In the above example, the torsion, calculated between apex and base, would be 30/8 = 3.75°/cm. As would be expected, the middle portion of the left ventricle would not show any rotation.

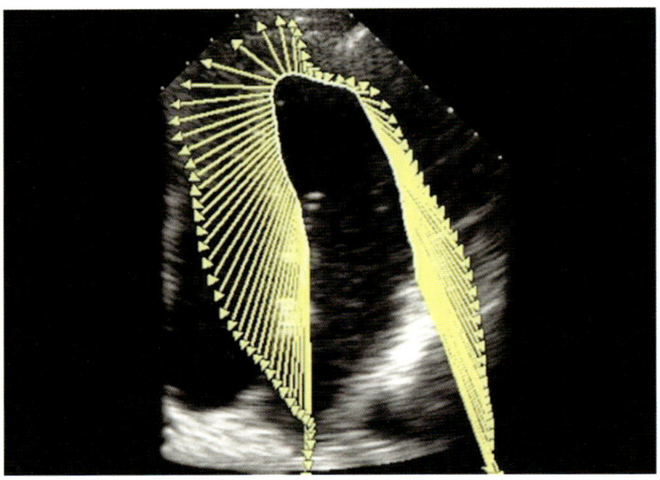

Figure 14 Velocity vector imaging. Apical four-chamber view: the direction of the arrows indicates the direction of the movement of the left ventricular myocardium, and the length of the arrows indicates the velocity of such movement.

2D STE is particularly useful in differentiating the athlete's heart from hypertrophic cardiomyopathy which both present with LV hypertrophy and normal systolic function. **Table 5** shows how these two conditions differ from each other by 2D STE and other parameters.[20]

THREE-DIMENSIONAL SPECKLE TRACKING ECHOCARDIOGRAPHY

The addition of 3D technology has expanded the scope of STE. It eliminates the inherent limitation of 2DE such as out of plane motion when only a thin slice of the myocardium can be imaged whereas a bigger pyramidal volume can be analyzed with 3D STE. One apical volume acquired in a 4-chamber view alone may be enough for the evaluation of all segments and chambers. Real-time acquisition of the motion of

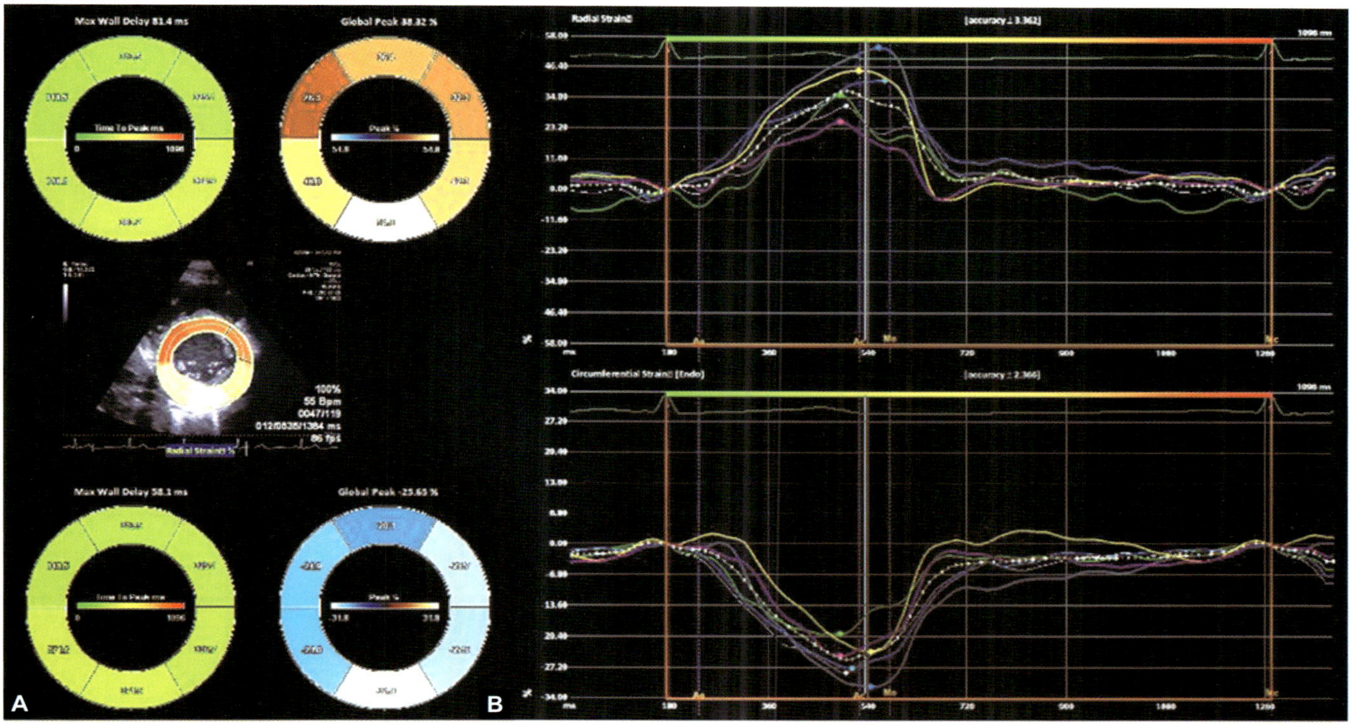

Figures 15A and B Radial and circumferential strain (A) and longitudinal strain rate; (B) From different segments using velocity vector imaging. The left panel also depicts global peak strain and maximum wall delay.
Courtesy: Siemens ultrasound.

Table 2 Mean percentage strain values by left ventricular region in normal adults

Longitudinal strain	Apical septal 21 ± 4	Mid septal 19 ± 4	Basal septal 17 ± 4	Apical lateral 21 ± 7	Mid lateral 19 ± 6	Basal lateral 19 ± 6
Circumferential strain	Anterior 24 ± 6	Lateral 22 ± 7	Posterior 21 ± 7	Inferior 22 ± 6	Septal 24 ± 6	Anteroseptal 26 ± 11
Radial strain	Anterior 39 ± 16	Lateral 37 ± 8	Posterior 37 ± 17	Inferior 37 ± 17	Septal 37 ± 19	Anteroseptal 39 ± 15

Source: Hurlburt HM, Aurigemma GP, Hill JC. Direct ultrasound measurement of longitudinal, circumferential, and radial strain using 2-dimensional strain imaging in normal adults. Echocardiography. 2007;24:723-31.

Table 3 Normal rotation and torsion in young adults

Peak apical rotation (°)	10.1 ± 1.9
Peak apical rotation rate (°/s)	61.6 ± 25.3
Peak basal rotation (°)	4.9 ± 2.0
Peak basal rotation rate (°/s)	44.2 ± 17.8

Source: Takahashi K, Al Naami G, Thompson R. Normal rotational, torsion and untwisting data in children, adolescents and young adults. J Am Soc Echocardiogr. 2010;23:286-93.

basal and apical segments is possible by 3D STE while with 2D STE; information is gathered from 2 short axis views taken at 2 different time points which would be altered by different heart rates and thus, results in unreliable determination of rotational parameters. A joint assessment of longitudinal and circumferential strains, termed area strain, can also be performed with 3D while this is not possible with 2D **(Figures 16A and B)**.[25-27]

TABLE 4 Clinical conditions where two-dimensional speckle tracking is useful

1. Myocardial ischemia	Reduction in strain by 2D STE more objective and accurate than the traditional visual method of assessing WMA
	Longitudinal, radial, and circumferential strain reduced in ischemic areas in coronary artery disease
	Postsystolic thickening (deformation), detected by radial strain correlates with the severity of ischemia
2. Myocardial infarction	2D STE successful in differentiating transmural from subendocardial infarction by showing lower circumferential strain in the former
	Reduced subendocardial LV twist also noted in patients with ST-segment elevated myocardial infarction
	Decreased LV torsion and segmental longitudinal strain predicts progressive
	LV dilatation after myocardial infarction
3. Myocardial viability	Strain measurements by 2D STE more objective and accurate than visual WMA for assessment of myocardial viability during low-dose dobutamine stress echocardiography. 2D STE differentiates active contraction from passive motion due to tethering
4. Heart failure with normal LVEF	Reduced and delayed LV untwisting—at rest and exercise
5. Cardiac resynchronization therapy (CRT)	Combining longitudinal strain from TDI velocity with 2D STE radial strain may help in predicting response to CRT
	Longitudinal strain delay index (calculated from the difference between peak and end-systolic strain) of >25% predicts response to CRT (sensitivity 95%, specificity 83%)
	Speckle tracking and resynchronization (STAR) study showed that radial and transversal strain were better than longitudinal and circumferential strain in predicting LVEF response and long-term survival after CRT
	Lack of dyssynchrony before CRT by 2D STE radial strain associated with death or hospitalization for heart failure
6. Stress cardiomyopathy	Impaired longitudinal strain noted particularly in apical and midventricular segments
7. Restrictive cardiomyopathy	Impaired longitudinal deformation and twist mechanics are noted
8. Constrictive pericarditis	Impaired LV circumferential deformation and torsion
9. Detection of rejection and coronary stenosis in heart transplant patients	Sudden reduction of ≥15% in global radial strain associated with acute rejection
	Decrease in strain and strain rate at rest and with dobutamine stress echo also useful to detect significant coronary stenosis
10. Early detection of chemotherapy-induced cardiotoxicity	Reduction in radial strain may occur before reduction in LVEF and associated with histologic changes
11. Detection of subclinical diseases/ early myocardial involvement	Reduction in strain may occur before changes in LVEF in systemic hypertension, diabetes mellitus, systemic sclerosis, amyloidosis, Duchenne's muscular dystrophy, and Kawasaki syndrome
12. Valvular heart disease	Decreased radial, circumferential, and longitudinal strain in patients with severe aortic stenosis and normal LVEF. Long-term follow-up after valve replacement showed significant improvement with no change in EF
	Reduced preoperative 2D STE longitudinal strain in the ventricular septum (apical four-chamber view) predicts a postoperative LVEF decrease of ≥10% in patients with chronic severe mitral regurgitation
13. Congenital heart disease	Atrial septal defect—basal clockwise rotation during systole is reduced
	Tetralogy of Fallot—right ventricular global longitudinal strain and strain rate is decreased significantly

Abbreviations: 2D, two-dimensional; EF, ejection fraction; LV, left ventricle; LVEF, left ventricular ejection fraction; TDI, tissue Doppler imaging; STE, speckle tracking echocardiography; WMA, wall motion abnormalities.

Source: Biswas M, et al. Two- and three-dimensional speckle tracking echocardiography: clinical applications and future directions. Echocardiography. 2013;30(1):88-105.

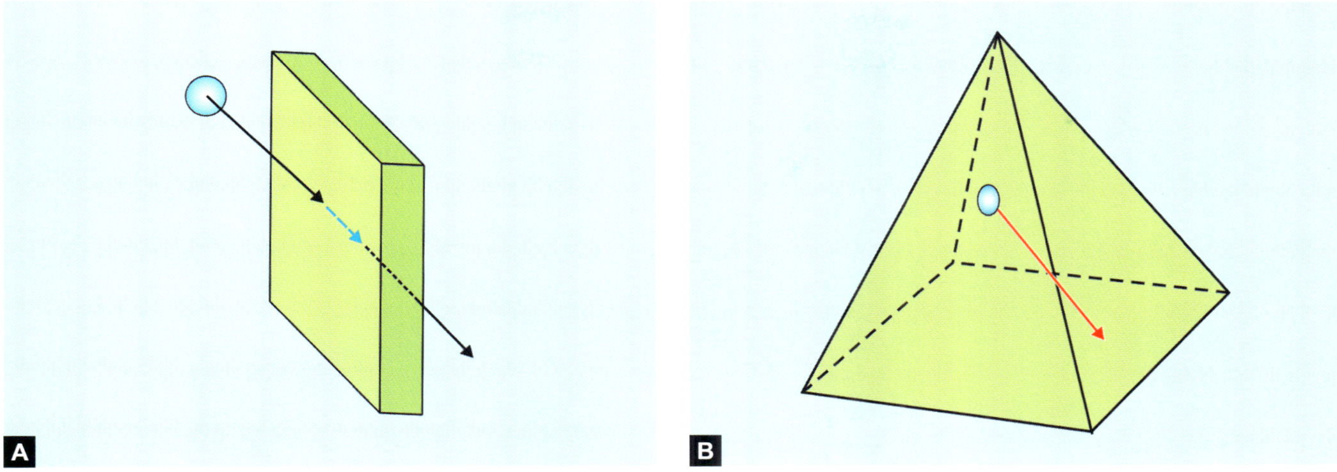

Figures 16A and B Advantage of three-dimensional speckle tracking echocardiography over the two-dimensional (2D) technique. (A) As 2D echocardiography represents only a thin slice through the cardiac structures, it is easy for the speckle particle to move out of the scanning plane as the heart moves, making it difficult or impossible to track the same speckle during the cardiac cycle; (B) On the other hand, with the three-dimensional (3D) technique, a much larger pyramidal-shaped section is obtained, making it more difficult for the speckle particle to move out of the 3D data set.
Courtesy: Toshiba Medical Systems Europe BV.

TABLE 5 Differentiation of athlete's heart from hypertrophic cardiomyopathy using speckle tracking

Athlete's heart	*Hypertrophic cardiomyopathy*
Normal longitudinal and other types of strain	Decreased longitudinal strain
Increased LV EDV	Decreased LV EDV
Decreases after deconditioning for 3 months	No change with deconditioning
Increased LV twist	Delayed LV untwisting
Increased early LA strain rate	Reduced LA strain and strain rate
No postsystolic thickening	Postsystolic thickening present

Abbreviations: EDV, end-diastolic volume; LA, left atrium; LV, left ventricle.
Reproduced with permission from Biswas M, et al. Two- and three-dimensional speckle tracking echocardiography: clinical applications and future directions. Echocardiography. 2013;30(1):88-105.

SUMMARY

A patient with dyspnea and normal LV systolic function may either have diastolic heart failure or a non cardiac cause of dyspnea. When the transmitral flow pattern is normal, this may reflect either normal diastolic function, or pseudonormal filling pattern, which does reflect significant DD. Thus, multiple echo-Doppler parameters (LV mass, LA volume, TDI, pulmonary veins and pulmonary artery pressures) must be integrated to establish if heart failure is present or not.

There is a need to reconcile all clinical information with the echocardiographic findings and learn the same on simulation **(Figures 17 to 19)**. A small LA often excludes a diagnosis of DHF, as long as echocardiography is performed prior to diuresis or BP lowering in a patient presenting with dyspnea. Concentric LVH or remodeling and wall motion abnormalities are clues that underlying DD may be present. A young, healthy patient, on the other hand, may have E > A, but this pattern likely reflects

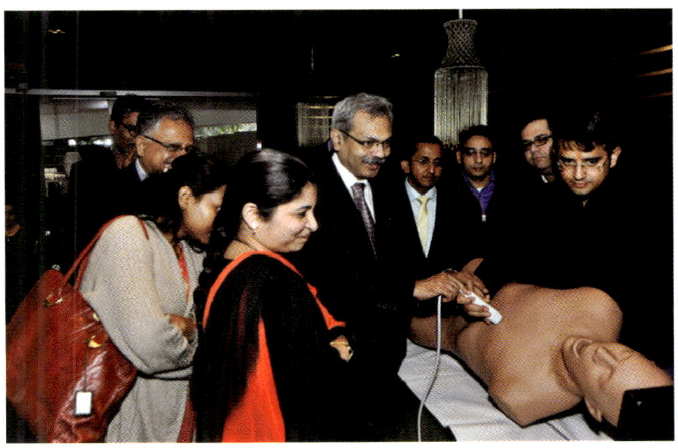

Figure 17 The transthoracic echo probe simulator position to learn left ventricular diastolic function

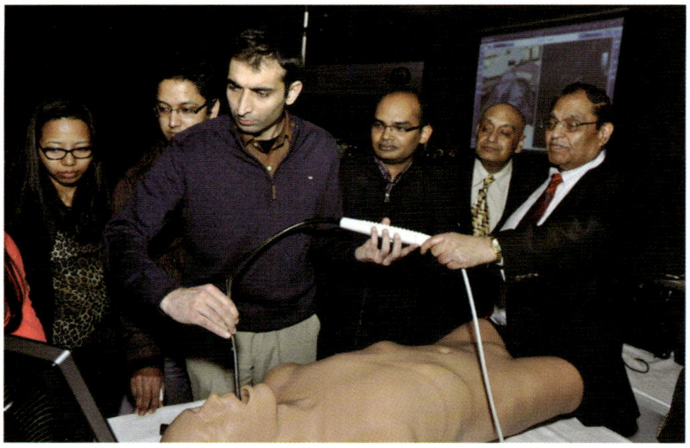

Figure 18 Holding the probe in the right manner is essential for preventing probe related complications. Practice on simulator is best

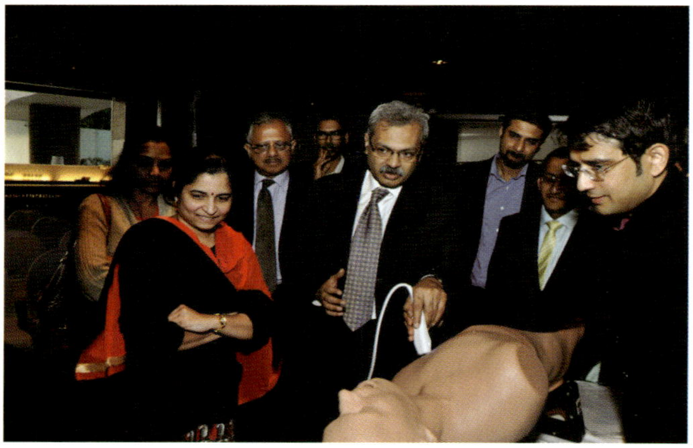

Figure 19 The exact position of the transesophageal echocardiography probe on the simulator is learnt best in experienced hands.

Flow chart 1 An integrated approach to the assessment of left ventricular diastolic function: normal LV ejection fraction. As recommended in the current guidelines, use of multiple echo Doppler parameters results in a more accurate assessment of left ventricular (LV) diastolic function than using any single echo Doppler parameter in isolation. In the patient with normal LV ejection fraction (EF), it is reasonable to start with early transmitral diastolic velocity/tissue Doppler early diastolic velocity (E/e'), as it can be difficult to discern whether a patient with preserved LVEF has impaired or normal LV relaxation. Following E/e', other echo Doppler variables are added to result in an accurate assessment of LV diastolic function.

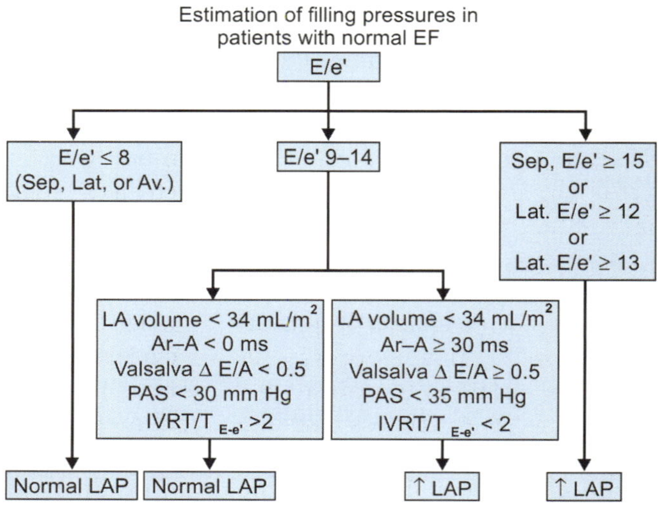

Reproduced with permission from Nagueh SF, Appleton CP, Gillebert TC, et al. Recommendations for the evaluation of left ventricular diastolic function by echocardiography. J Am Soc Echocardiogr. 2009;22(2):107-33.

Flow chart 2 Practical approach to grading diastolic dysfunction

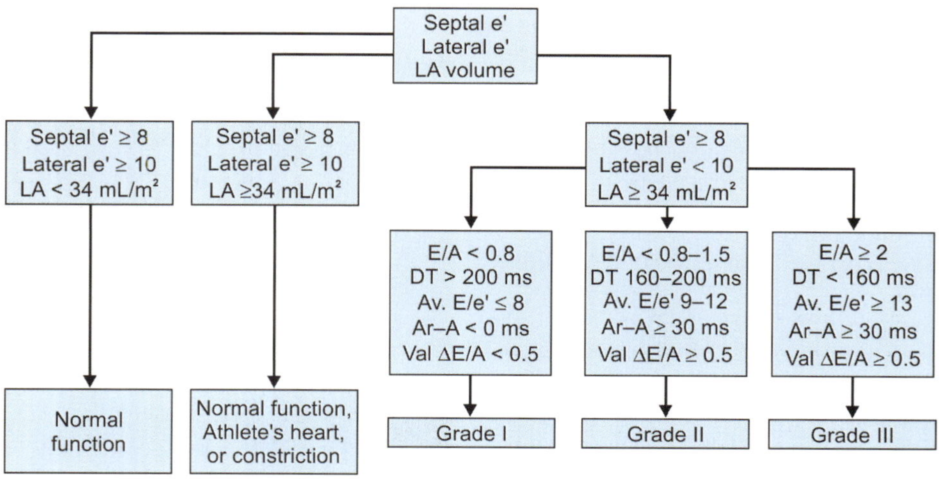

Abbreviations: Av, average; LA, left atrium; Val, Valsalva.

Source: Nagueh SF, Appleton CP, Gillebert TC, et al. Recommendations for the evaluation of left ventricular diastolic function by echocardiography. J Am Soc Echocardiogr. 2009;22(2):107-33.

normal diastolic function. When the transmitral flow shows E<A, impaired relaxation with normal LA pressures (grade I DD) is usually present. With a normal or pseudo normal pattern, proceeding to TDI and measuring E′ velocity to calculate E/e′ often distinguishes normal from pseudonormal filling pattern. Valsalva maneuver may also be used to distinguish normal from pseudonormal filling; however, TDI is often more practical and reliable. Other echo-Doppler variables can be used additionally if the results are still indeterminate. **Flow chart 1** provides an algorithm for the estimation of LV filling pressures in patients with normal estimate filling pressure.[4]

In a patient with low LVEF, diastolic dysfunction is almost always present. One does not need to do an elaborate evaluation of diastolic function but the goal is to approximate LV filling pressures which has a direct bearing for prognosis and treatment.

A scheme on how to grade diastolic dysfunction is presented in **Flow chart 2.**[4] Increasing severity of DD relates to poor prognosis in spite of normal LVEF.

Transmitral flow Doppler remains central to the diagnosis of DD in the presence of normal LVEF, in combination with the less load dependent modality of TDI. They are more practical and reliable to use than pulmonary venous flow, flow propagation velocity or the Valsalva maneuver. The emergence of 2D and 3D STE add incremental value to the definite assessment of many cardiac conditions with both preserved and poor LVEF, decreasing errors in the evaluation of DHF.[28]

REFERENCES

1. Paulus WJ, Tschöpe C, Sanderson JE, et al. How to diagnose diastolic heart failure: a consensus statement on the diagnosis of heart failure with normal left ventricular ejection fraction by the Heart Failure and Echocardiography Associations of the European Society of Cardiology. Eur Heart J. 2007;28(20):2539-50.
2. Dokainish H, Zoghbi WA, Lakkis NM, et al. Incremental predictive power of B-type natriuretic peptide and tissue Doppler echocardiography in the prognosis of patients with congestive heart failure. J Am Coll Cardiol. 2005;45(8):1223-6.
3. Abhayaratna WP, Seward JB, Appleton CP, et al. Left atrial size: physiologic determinants and clinical applications. J Am Coll Cardiol. 2006;47(12):2357-63.
4. Nagueh SF, Appleton CP, Gillebert TC, et al. Recommendations for the evaluation of left ventricular diastolic function by echocardiography. J Am Soc Echocardiogr. 2009;22(2):107-33.
5. Oh JK, Hatle L, Tajik AJ, et al. Diastolic heart failure can be diagnosed by comprehensive two-dimensional and Doppler echocardiography. J Am Coll Cardiol. 2006;47(3):500-6.
6. Garcia MJ, Ares MA, Asher C, et al. An index of early left ventricular filling that combined with pulsed Doppler peak E velocity may estimate capillary wedge pressure. J Am Coll Cardiol. 1997;29(2):448-54.
7. Rivas-Gotz C, Manolios M, TV, et al. Impact of left ventricular ejection fraction on estimation of left ventricular filling pressures using tissue Doppler and flow propagation velocity. Am J Cardiol. 2003;91(6):780-4.
8. Mottram PM, Marwick TH. Assessment of diastolic function: what the general cardiologist needs to know. Heart. 2005;91:681-95.
9. Appleton CP, Galloway JM, Gonzalez MS, et al. Estimation of left ventricular filling pressures using two-dimensional and Doppler echocardiography in adult patients with cardiac disease. Additional value of analyzing left atrial size, left atrial ejection fraction and the difference in duration of pulmonary venous and mitral flow velocity at atrial contraction. J Am Coll Cardiol. 1993;22(7):1972-82.
10. Poulsen SH, Jensen SE, Gotzsche O, Egstrup K. Evaluation and prognostic significance of left ventricular diastolic function assessed by Doppler echocardiography in the early phase of a first acute myocardial infarction. Eur Heart J. 1997;18:1882-9.
11. Dini F, Michelassi C, Micheli G, Rovai D. Prognostic value of pulmonary venous flow Doppler signal in left ventricular dysfunction: contribution of the difference in duration of pulmonary venous and mitral flow at atrial contraction. J Am Coll Cardiol. 2000;36:1295-302.
12. Dini FL, Dell'Anna R, Micheli A, Michaelassi C, Rovai D. Impact of blunted pulmonary venous flow on the outcome of patients with left ventricular systolic dysfunction secondary to either ischemic or idiopathic dilated cardiomyopathy. Am J Cardiol. 2000;85:1455-60.
13. Dokainish H. How to assess diastolic function. In: Nanda NC (Ed). Comprehensive Textbook of Echocardiography. (1st edn) New Delhi, India. Jaypee Brothers Medical Publishers Pvt Ltd. 2014;2:pp.1124-33.
14. Nagueh SF, Middleton KJ, Kopelen HA, Zoghbi WA, Quinones MA. Doppler tissue imaging: a non-invasive technique for evaluation of left ventricular relaxation and estimation of filling pressures. J Am Coll Cardiol. 1997;30:1527-33.
15. Firstenberg MS, Greenberg NL, Main ML, et al. Determinants of diastolic myocardial tissue Doppler velocities: influences of relaxation and preload. J Appl Physiol. 2001;90:299-307.
16. Rivas-Gotz C, Manolios M, Thohan V, Nagueh SF. Impact of left ventricular ejection fraction on estimation of left ventricular filling pressures using tissue

Doppler and flow propagation velocity. Am J Cardiol. 2003;91:780-4.
17. Rivas-Gotz C, Khoury DS, Manolios M, Rao L, Kopelen HA, Nagueh SF. Time interval between onset of mitral inflow and onset of early diastolic velocity by tissue Doppler: a novel index of left ventricular relaxation: experimental studies and clinical application. J Am Coll Cardiol. 2003;42:1463-70.
18. Ommen SR, Nishimura RA, Appleton et al. Clinical utility of Doppler echocardiography and tissue Doppler imaging in the estimation of left ventricular filling pressures: a comparative simultaneous Doppler catheterization study. Circulation. 2000;102:1788-94.
19. Diwan A, McCulloch M, Lawrie GM, Reardon MJ, Nagueh SF. Doppler estimation of left ventricular filling pressures in patients with mitral valve disease. Circulation. 2005;111:3281-9.
20. Biswas, M, Sudhakar S, Nanda NC, Buckberg G, Pradhan M, Roomi AU, Gorissen W, Houle H. Two- and Three-Dimensional Speckle Tracking Echocardiography: Clinical Applications and Future Directions. Echocardiography. 2013;30:88-105.
21. Dandel M, Hetzer R. Echocardiographic strain and strain rate imaging–clinical applications. Int J Cardiol. 2009;132:11-24.
22. Dokainish H, Sengupta R, Pillai M, et al. Usefulness of new diastolic strain and strain rate indexes for the estimation of left ventricular filling pressure. Am J Cardiol. 2008;101:1504-9.
23. Torrent-Guasp F, Buckberg GD, Clemente C, et al. The structure and function of the helical heart and its buttress wrapping. I. The normal macroscopic structure of the heart. Semin Thorac Cardiovasc Surg. 2001;13:301-19.
24. Buckberg G, Hoffman JI, Nanda NC, et al. Ventricular torsion and untwisting: Further insights into mechanics and timing interdependence: A viewpoint. Echocardiography. 2011;28:782-804.
25. Padmanabhan S, Singh S, Nanda NC. Speckle tracking echocardiography: Clinical usefulness. In: Nanda NC (Ed). Comprehensive Textbook of Echocardiography. (1st edn). New Delhi, India. Jaypee Brothers Medical Publishers Pvt Ltd. 2014;1:pp.360-79.
26. Saito K, Okura H, Watanabe N, et al. Comprehensive evaluation of left ventricular strain using speckle tracking of echocardiography in normal adults: Comparison of three-dimensional and two-dimensional approaches. J Am Soc Echocardiogr. 2009;22:1025-30.
27. Wen HL, Liang ZS, Zhao YF, et al. Feasibility of detecting early left ventricular systolic dysfunction using global area strain: A novel index derived from three-dimensional speckle-tracking echocardiography. Eur J Echocardiogr. 2011;12:910-6.
28. Gorrisen W, Nanda NC. Speckle tracking acquisition: Basics and practical tips. In: Nanda NC (Ed). Comprehensive Textbook of Echocardiography (1st edn). New Delhi, India. Jaypee Brothers Medical Publishers Pvt Ltd. 2014;1:pp.87-98.

Chapter 5

Simulation for Transthoracic Echocardiography of Mitral Valve

KK Kapur

Chapter Outline

- Anatomy of Mitral Valve
- Criteria for Mitral Stenosis
- Mitral Regurgitation
- Criteria for Mitral Regurgitation
- Mitral Valve Prolapse
- Utility of Transthoracic Echocardiography for Mitral Valve
- Fast Interactive Simulations of Mitral Valve Repair

ANATOMY OF MITRAL VALVE

Mitral valve apparatus consists of the mitral annulus, mitral leaflets, chordae, tendinae, papillary muscles and the underlying left ventricular wall. The mitral annulus is complex structure and part of the fibrous trigon **(Figures 1A to D)**. It can be measured anteroposteriorly in the parasternal long axis view (PSLAX) and mediolateraly in apical 4C view.

Mitral leaflets: There are two mitral leaflets, anterior also called the septal leaflet is the larger of the two, while the posterior (mural) leaflet is smaller. The posterior leaflet is divided into three scallops which are numbered P1, P2 and P3 from lateral to medial (most lateral is P1 and most medial is P3). The anterior mitral leaflet is not divided into scallops however, the corresponding segments on the anterior mitral leaflet (AML) are numbered A1, A2 and A3 from lateral to medial.

Chordae tendineae: There are primary, secondary and tertiary chordae, they connect the mitral leaflets to the papillary muscles **(Figure 2)**.

Papillary muscles: There are two papillary muscles anterolateral and posteromedial; more appropriately called lateral and medial respectively. The lateral papillary muscle has dual blood supply (LAD and LCx) while the medial papillary muscle has the single blood supply from the right coronary artery (RCA).

During systole MV coaptation occurs, which extends to a variable length of mitral leaflet tissue and is called zona coapta (ZC) (usually 5–8 mm).

Simulator mannequin teaching and training for mitral valve (MV) pathologies. The use of the mannequin and simulator coupled to the various MV pathologies has been found to facilitate and accelerate the learning curve.

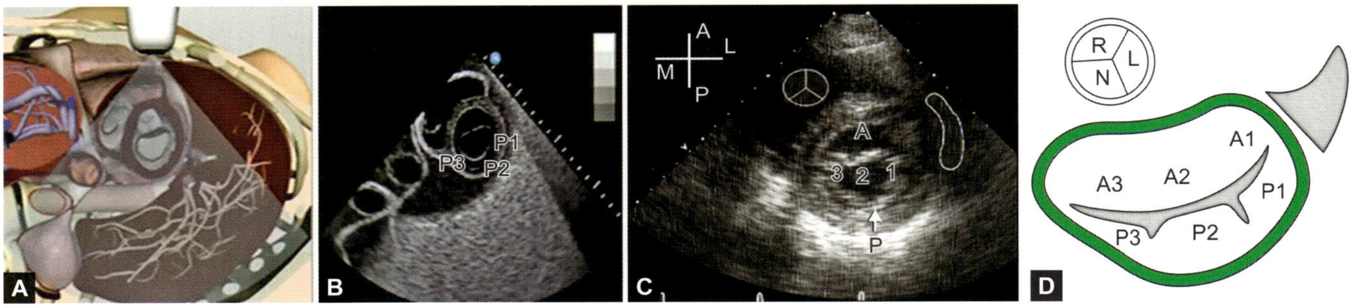

Figures 1A to D Depicting the mitral valve anatomy in parasternal short axis view illustrating various scallops on posterior leaflet
Abbreviations: P1, P2, P3, posterior mitral leaflet scallops; A1, A2, A3, lateral, central and medial scallops of anterior mitral value leaflet; A, anterior; P, posterior

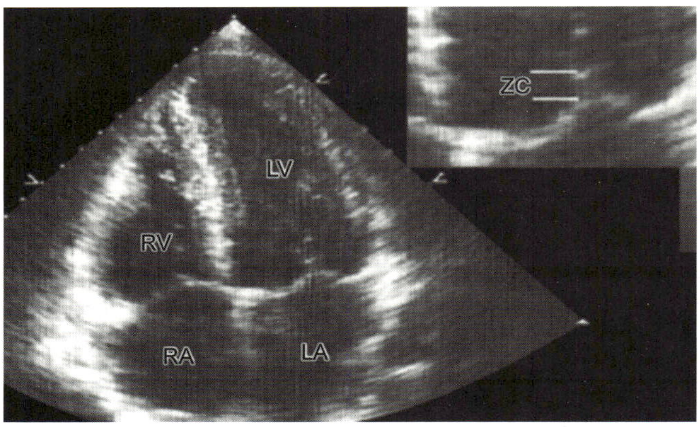

Figure 2 The zona coapta (ZC) of mitral valve leaflets
Abbreviations: LV, left ventricle; RV, right ventricle; RA, right atrium; LA, left atrium

The various 2D and color Doppler echocardiograms of different cardiac pathologies are compiled in a systematic manner. The operator manipulates the probe in various transducer positions and angulations and images the various cardiac pathologies which have been incorporated in the computer software of the computer software. Most of the MV pathologies included in this chapter are based on our experience with the mannequin simulator. Hemodynamic consequences of mitral valve disease are MS, MR and MS + MR.

Mitral Stenosis

In mitral stenosis (MS), there is commissural fusion leading to narrowing the mitral orifice. The most common etiology is rheumatic however, the congenital mitral stenosis in pediatric population and calcific mitral stenosis in the elderly population is not uncommon.

Rheumatic Heart Disease

Rheumatic heart disease (RHD) is characterized by leaflet doming and varying degrees of thickening and calcification. The posterior mitral leaflet moves with the anterior leaflet (paradoxical movement) or it may be severely restricted. A normal progressive multifocal leukoencephalopathy (PML) motion excludes a rheumatic etiology.

The various methods for computation of MV area are plainemetry, Doppler pressure half time and continuity equation.

CRITERIA FOR MITRAL STENOSIS

Valve area (cm^2)	1.5–2.5 mild, 1.0–1.5 moderate, <1.0 severe
Peak gradient (mm Hg)	<10 mild 10–20 moderate >20 severe
Mean gradient (mm Hg)	<5 mild 5–10 moderate >10 severe

MITRAL REGURGITATION

The RHD is the most common cause of mitral regurgitation (MR) in the under developed or in developing countries. It is characterized by varying degrees of thickening, calcification and fibrosis which eventually leads to noncoaptation. The fibrotic process causing the retraction of mitral leaflets and loss of leaflet tissue. The mitral annulus is usually large. Besides RHD, the other various causes of MR includes myxomatous

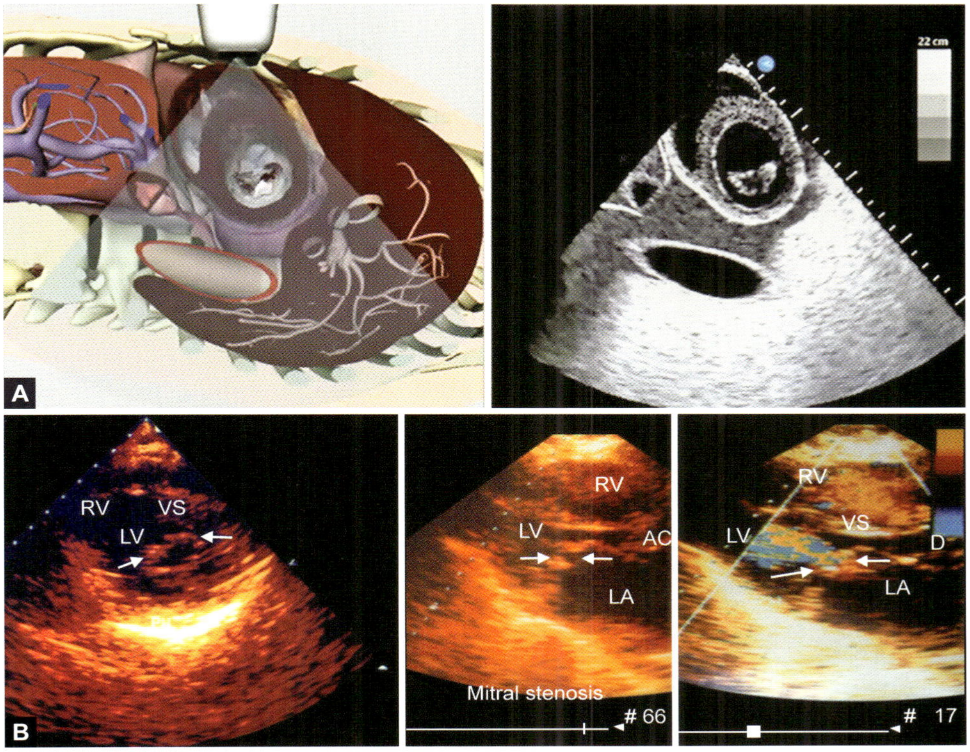

Figures 3A and B Mitral orifice in short axis (A) and doming seen in long-axis along with the turbulent color jet (B)
Abbreviations: RV, right ventricular; LV, left ventricular; VS, ventricular septum; AC, anterior commissure; D, doming; LA, left atrium

MV disease leading to mitral valve prolapse (MVP) and or flail leaflet due to chordal rupture. Mitral valve endocarditis, dilated and hypertrophic cardiomyopathy are other common causes of MR. The pathophysiological mechanism of MR is well described by Carpentier, who described three basic mechanisms; type-1 includes normal leaflet motion (annular dilatation, perforation), type-2: excessive leaflet motion (MVP, Flail-leaflet), type-3: restrictive MV motion. The type-3 MR can be further divided into restricted diastolic and systolic (3a, e.g. RHD) and only systolic restriction (3b), e.g. ischemic MR in CAD, or DCMP **(Figures 3A and B)**. The severity of MR is assessed by the area of the regurgitation jet either absolute or in proportion to the left atrial area (LAA) with the Nyquist limit kept at 45–50 cm/s in any of the standard or nonstandard view. Other methods include the vena contracta (VC) method, PISA method and spectral Doppler computation of regurgitant volumes **(Figures 4A to C)**.

CRITERIA FOR MITRAL REGURGITATION

Jet area absolute (cm^2)	<4 mild, 4–8 moderate, >8 severe	
Jet area relative to LA area	<20% mild, 20–40% moderate, >40% severe	
Vena contracta (mm)	<3 mild, 3–6 moderate, >6 severe	
PISA-ROA (cm^2)	<0.2 mild, 0.2–0.4 moderate, >0.4 severe	In ischemic MR ROA of >0.2 is severe
Spectral Doppler	Regurgitant volume >60 mL or regurgitant fraction >60% is severe	

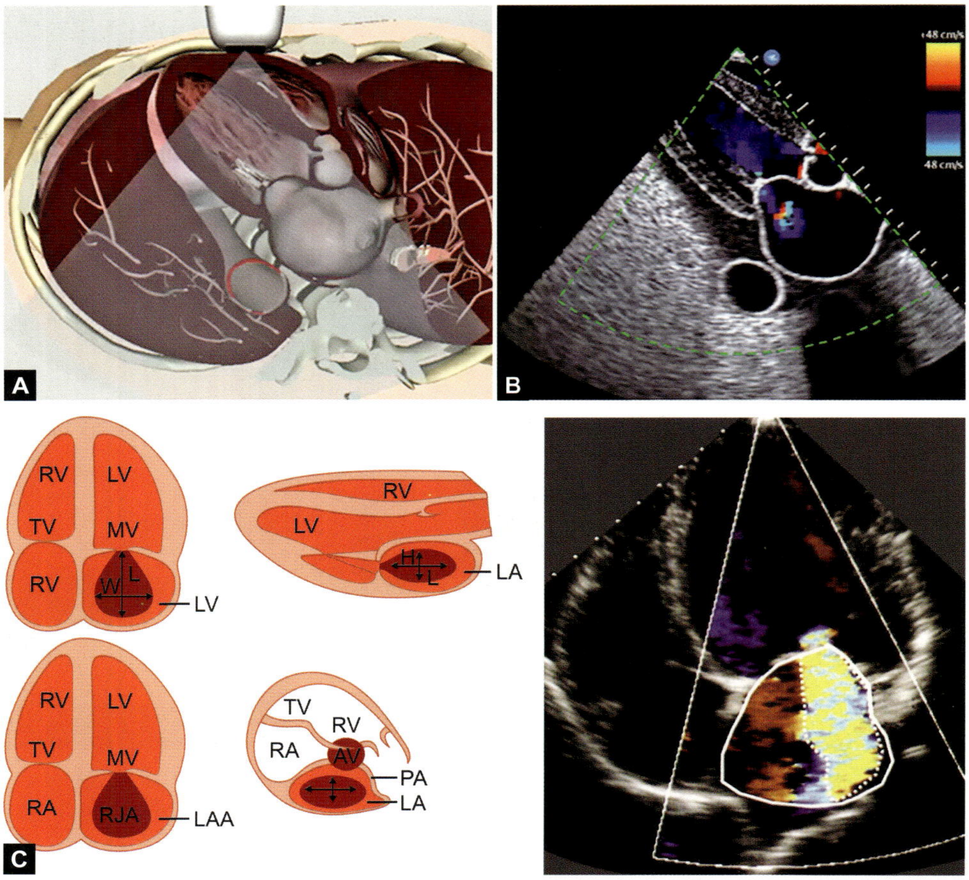

Figures 4A to C (A) Simulator showing MR in RHD on simulator; (B) Quantifying the severity of MR by area method; (C) MR in apical 4C view

Abbreviations: RV, right ventricle; TV, tricuspid valve; LV, left ventricle; MV, mitral valve; RJA, right jugular artery; LA, left atrium; PA, pulmonary artery; RA, right atrium; LAA, left atrial area

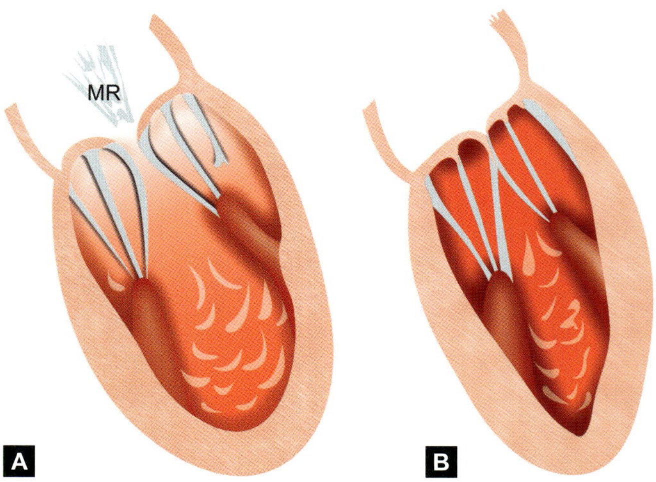

Figures 5A and B Acute ischaemic MR with mitral annular dilatation

Acute ischemic MR (IMR) is caused by acute and chronic ischemia or infarction. Acute IMR is either due to acute myocardial infraction; rupture of the papillary muscle, acute ischemic myocardial dysfunction or due to acute ischemia/rupture of papillary muscle (Carpentier type-2) chronic IMR is due to tethering (Carpentier type 3b) of the mitral leaflets caused by either dilatation of the LV cavity and/or infarction of the LV wall. This usually associated with mitral annular dilatation (Carpentier type-1) **(Figures 5A and B)**.

MITRAL VALVE PROLAPSE

The mitral valve prolapse (MVP) is characterized by deposition of myxomatous tissue into the mitral leaflets causing them to be thickened, redundant and displaced

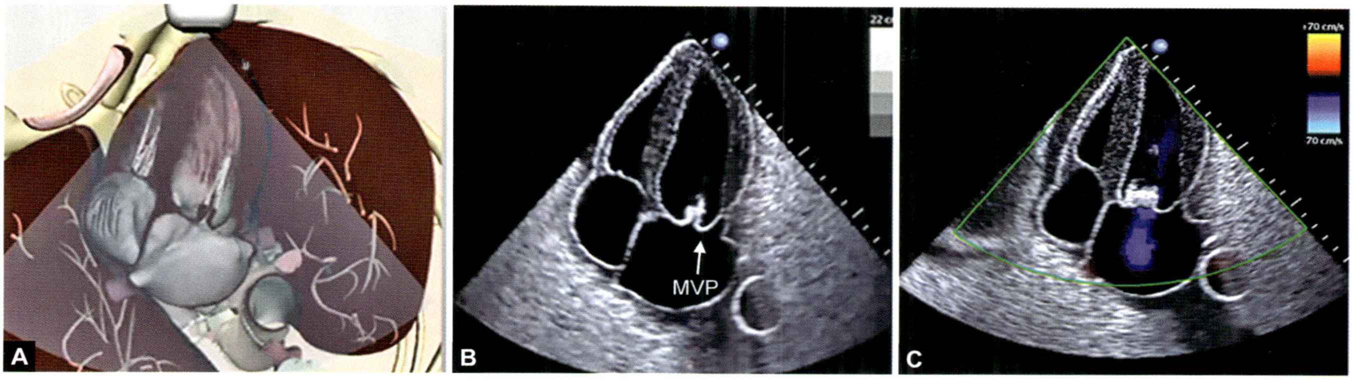

Figures 6A to C Simulator picture shows the MV prolapsing into LA and MR due to noncoaptation
Abbreviations: MVP, mitral valve prolapse

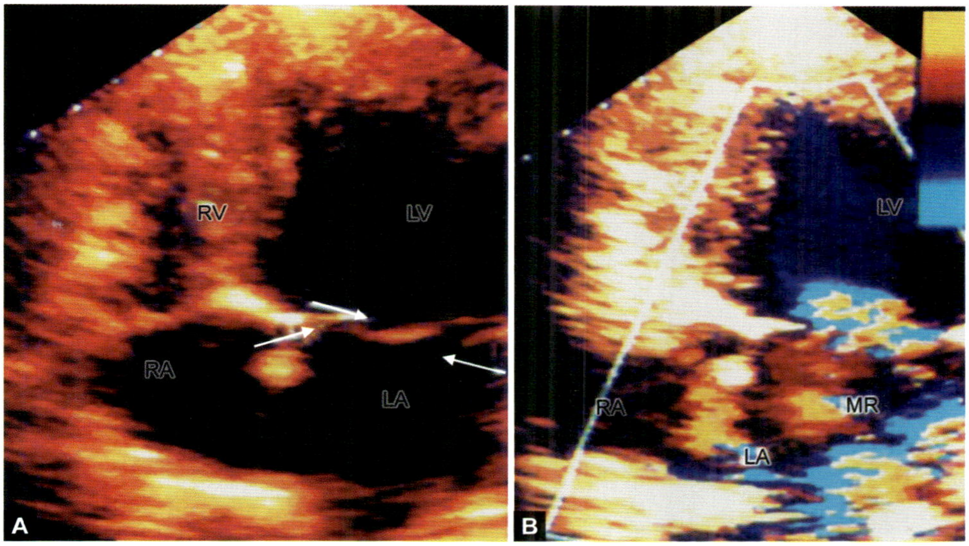

Figures 7A and B 2D apical 4C echocardiographic view shows prolapsed mitral valve and MR in colored Doppler
Abbreviations: RV, right ventricle; LV, left ventricle; RA, right atrium; LA, left atrium; MR, mitral regurgitation

into the left atrium into the systole. Additionally the chordae tendinae are elongated and mitral annulus shoes varying degrees of enlargement. The mismatch between the mitral leaflets and mitral annulus size causes protrusion into the left atrium (LA). Varying degrees of MR associated depending on the degree of noncoaptation of redundant leaflets and/or associated chordal rupture **(Figures 6 and 7)**. Rupture of the primary chordae usually leads severe MR. The MR jet is eccentric and is in the direction opposite to the flail or prolapsed leaflet.

UTILITY OF TRANSTHORACIC ECHOCARDIOGRAPHY FOR MITRAL VALVE

The clinical utility of focused transthoracic echocardiography (TTE) is increasingly recognized in perioperative medicine. However, its use is limited among anesthesiologists because of a lack of training. The most efficient training methods have not been determined. We hypothesized that simulation-based TTE training would be more effective than traditional lecture-based methods for teaching basic TTE skills to the anesthesiology residents.

A proposed alternative to real-time patient-based learning is simulation-based training that allows anesthesiologists to learn complex concepts and procedures.[1-5] Recently, a TTE simulation tool has become available (Heartworks, Inventive Medical Ltd, London, UK). Simulation allows interactive TTE learning using a virtual 3-dimensional model of the heart and may aid in the acquisition of the cognitive and technical skills needed to perform TTE.[1] The ability to link probe manipulation, cardiac anatomy, and echocardiographic images using a simulator has been shown to be an effective model for training anesthesiology residents in transesophageal echocardiography **(Figures 8A and B)**.[3]

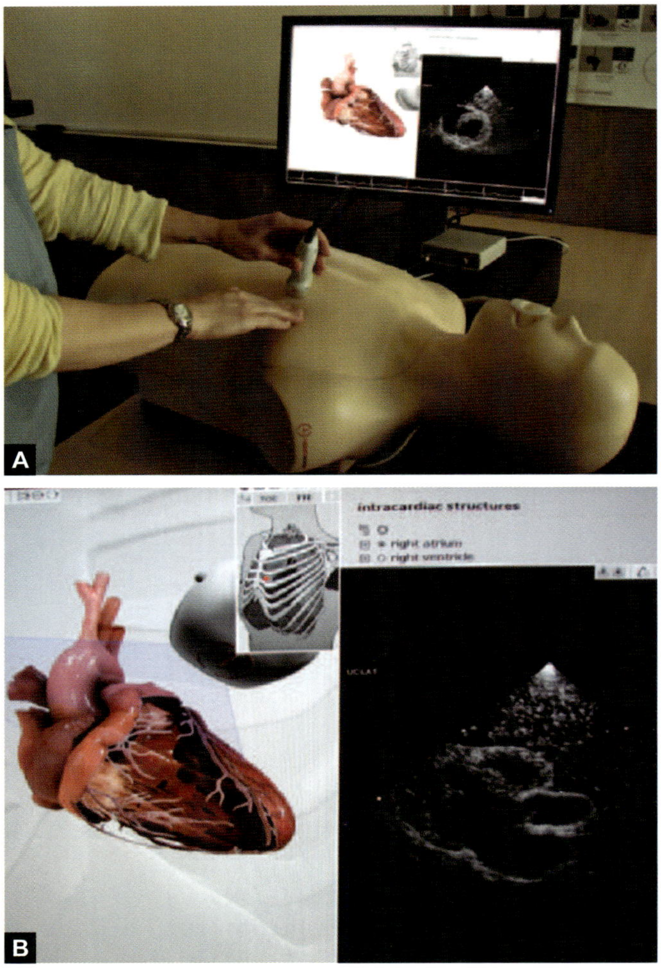

Figures 8A and B Sample views of transthoracic echocardiography simulator showing probe manipulation, 3-dimensional simulated cardiac anatomy, and echoanatomic image correlation

Simulation-based TTE training would be more effective than traditional teaching methods, and that the educational benefits of TTE simulation compared to traditional didactics would be sustained with subsequent addition of volunteer subject training in both groups. The goal of this prospective randomized study was to examine the use of simulation in teaching basic principles of echocardiography and TTE skills of image acquisition and anatomy recognition to anesthesiology residents.

FAST INTERACTIVE SIMULATIONS OF MITRAL VALVE REPAIR

A healthy mitral valve ensures the one-way flow of oxygenated blood from the left atrium to the left ventricle. Mitral regurgitation is a potentially serious condition in which oxygenated blood flows backwards across the valve, reducing cardiac efficiency and often necessitating surgical intervention.

Simulation of Tissue Mechanics

While finite element models are the standard for mechanical membrane simulations, they are an order of magnitude slower than models based on mass-spring approximations. As shown by Hammer,[6] these mass-spring models result in a minimal loss of accuracy for mitral leaflet tissue. Therefore, the system uses a bilinear mass-spring model of leaflet tissue with a critical strain of 25% to approximate a more complex Fung-elastic constitutive law **(*see* Figures 3A and B)**. Chordae tendineae are treated as linear-elastic cylindrical rods with a 1 mm diameter supporting only uniaxial tension. Finally, Dirichlet boundary conditions are provided by the vertices located on the fibrous mitral annulus and papillary muscles.

Simulation of Pressurization

Simulation of dynamic blood flow in the heart is infeasible in a clinical planning system as it typically requires days of simulation time for each model. Therefore, we assess valve competency under a static peak-systolic pressure as this provides the greatest mechanical challenge to the valve and therefore, the greatest potential for regurgitation. It also approximates a common intraoperative test for assessing valve competency.

CONCLUSION

The increased practice and knowledge integration from simulation leads to improved focused TTE skills among anesthesiology residents compared to traditional teaching methods. This may translate into more efficient TTE education and better clinical diagnosis; however, the impact of these short-term educational approaches on longer-term retention and actual clinical application warrants further investigation.

REFERENCES

1. Matyal R, Bose R, Warraich H, Shahul S, Ratcliff S, Panzica P, et al. Transthoracic echocardiographic simulator: normal and the abnormal. J Cardiothoracic Vasc Anesth. 2011;25:177-81.
2. Sinz E. Simulation based education for cardiac, thoracic, and vascular anesthesiology. Semin Cardiothorac Vasc Anesth. 2005;9:291-307.
3. Bose R, Matyal R, Warraich H, Summers J, Subramaniam B, Mitchell J, et al. Utility of a transesophageal echocardiographic simulator as a teaching tool. J Cardiothorac Vasc Anesth. 2011;25:212-5.
4. Sturm LP, Windsor JA, Cosman PH, Cregan P, Hewett PJ, Maddern GJ. A systematic review of skills transfer after surgical simulation training. Ann Surg. 2008;248:166-79.
5. Good ML. Patient simulation for training basic and advanced clinical skills. Med Educ. 2003;37(Suppl 1): 14-21.
6. Hammer P. Simulating heart valve mechanical behavior for planning surgical repair. Dissertation. Tufts University, 2011.

Chapter 6

Simulation for Transthoracic Echocardiography for Aortic Valve

KK Kapur, Naveen Garg

Chapter Outline

- Brief Anatomy
- Aortic Stenosis
- Etiology of Aortic Stenosis
- Criteria for Aortic Stenosis
- Aortic Regurgitation
- Aortic Valve Implantation
- Infective Endocarditis (IE): Aortic Valve

BRIEF ANATOMY

Aortic valve is a trileaflet valve which is thickened at its tips (Arantius) and allows a complete seal, while closing to avoid any backflow into the left ventricular cavity, by overlapping neighboring leaflets by 2–3 mm.

Sinuses of Valsalva are outpouching's behind the aortic cusps when the valve is open. The sinuses support the aortic leaflets superiorly. The sinuses provide a reservoir for diastolic blood flow to the coronary vessels right coronary artery arises from the right anterior sinus while the left coronary artery arises from the left posterior sinus **(Figure 1)**.[1] The right posterior sinus does not give rise to coronary artery and is called non-coronary sinus.

The fibrous annulus supports the aortic cusp and is continuous with the mitral annulus as well as the mitral aortic intervalvular ridge.

Hemodynamic affections of aortic valve include aortic stenosis (AS), aortic regurgitation (AR) or both.

AORTIC STENOSIS

Severe aortic stenosis (AS) has an extremely adverse prognosis for symptomatic patients not eligible for the standard surgical aortic valve replacement (SAVR).[2] Transcatheter aortic valve replacement (TAVR) has been emerged as a new minimally invasive treatment for such high-risk patients. In the case of the Edwards Sapien® valve, the procedure consists of the delivery of a balloon-expandable stented tissue valve to the site of the native pathological valve via transfemoral or transapical catheterization. We hypothesize that the presence of large deposits of calcium *in situ* is a significant cause of intra- and postprocedural complications. Hence, the simulation of the deployment in patient-specific

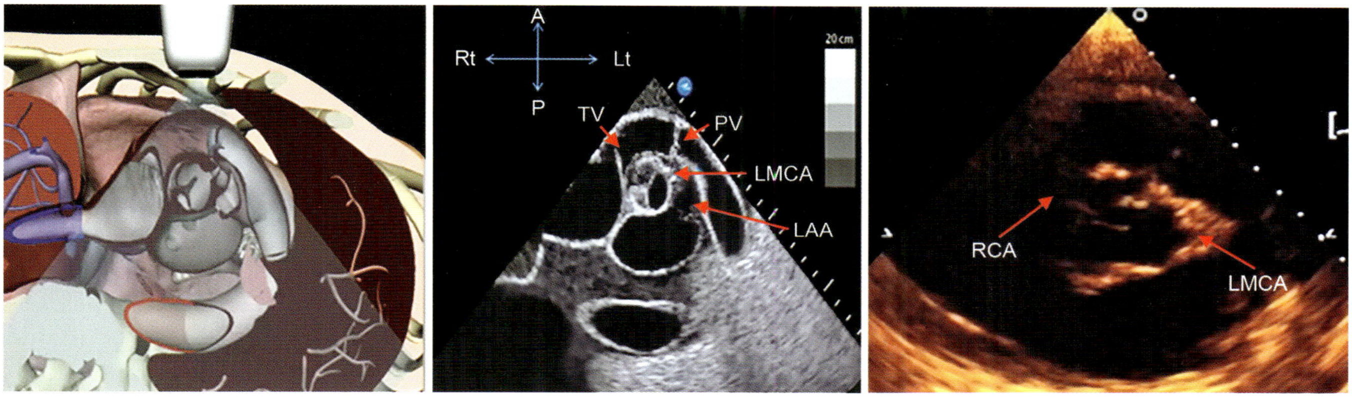

Figure 1 Aortic valve on mannequin in parasternal short axis view (PSSAX), it is being trileaflet and left main coronary artery (LMCA) is originating from left posterior sinus. RCA is shown in similar echocardiographic view being arising from right anterior sinus

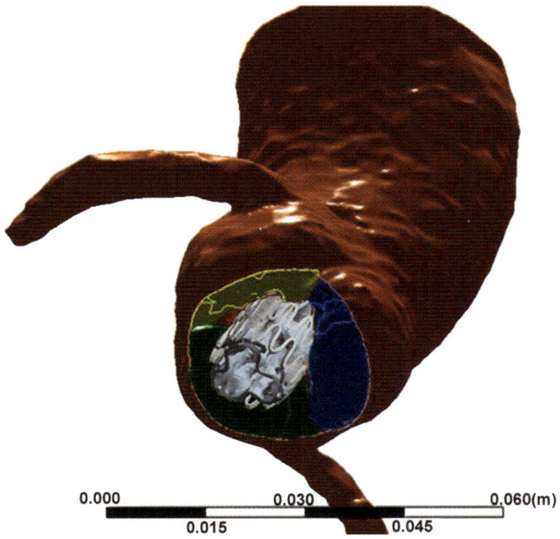

Figure 2 FE model of a patient-specific aortic root and SAPIEN® valve in midway position before deployment

aortic root (AR) models encompassing the patient's pathophysiological features may both represent a valuable procedural planning tool and lead to improved design of TAVR device **(Figure 2)**.

Indications of TTE in Aortic Stenosis

Class 1

- To confirm presence and severity of AS.
- Assessment of left ventricular size, function.
- Re-evaluation in mild/moderate aortic stenosis on symptom change.
- Re-evaluation for LV size/function in asymptomatic severe AS.

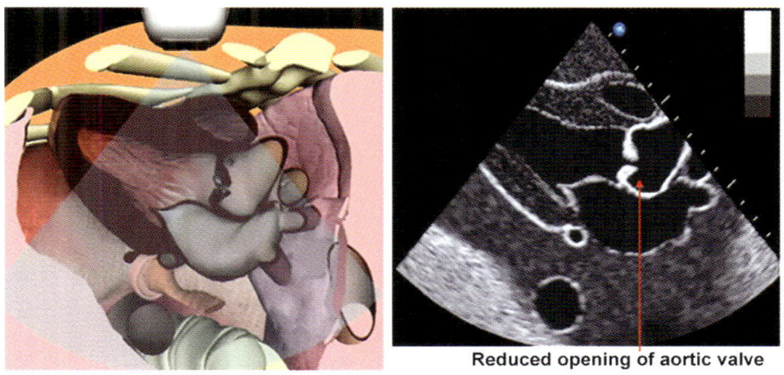

Figure 3 Simulated parasternal long axis view (PLAX) view of aortic stenosis, depicting the reduced opening of the aortic valve

ETIOLOGY OF AORTIC STENOSIS

The etiology of aortic valve stenosis may be congenital (unicuspid, bicuspid or trileaflet aortic valve with unequal cusps), rheumatic aortic valve stenosis or sclerodegenerative aortic stenosis **(Figure 3)**.[3] However, other pathologies causing LVOT obstruction may mimic AS includes subaortic membrane, hypertrophic cardiomyopathy and supravalvular stenosis. The aortic stenosis jet is usually eccentric and therefore a multiple imaging planes are required for parallel Doppler interrogation. Usually apical 5C, right parasternal and high left parasternal imaging planes are utilized for optimal alignment of the Doppler beam to the direction of AS jet **(Figure 4)**.

CRITERIA FOR AORTIC STENOSIS

In asymptomatic patients with severe AS, a closely monitored treadmill stress echo can be performed to objectively to evaluate exercise capacity and to observe for any improvement in the calculated aortic valve

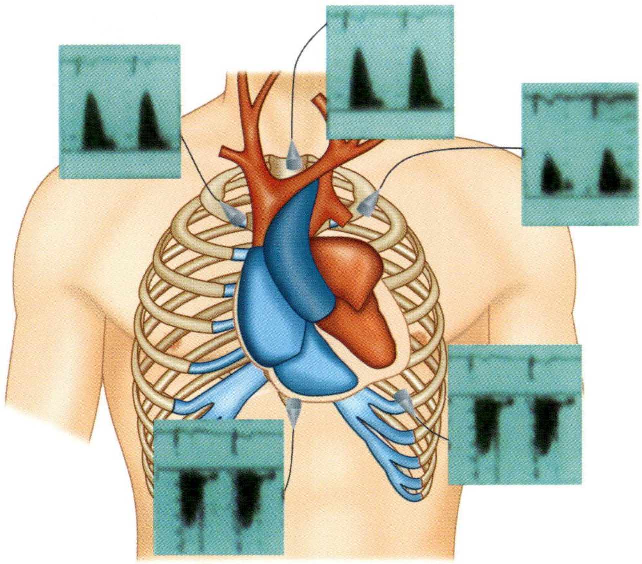

Figure 4 Proper alignment to AS jet for better Doppler study

TABLE 1 Quantification of aortic stenosis severity

Aortic valve area (cm^2)	>1.5 mild 1–1.5 moderate 0.75–1 moderately severe <0.75 severe
Peak gradient (mm Hg*)	20–40 mild 40-60 moderate >60 severe
Mean gradient (mm Hg*)	<20 mild 20–40 moderate >40 severe
*at average heart rates 70–100/min and average cardiac-output	

area.[4] In patients with significant LV dysfunction and AS, a markedly low AVA is sometime observed together with low transvalvular gradient. This "low gradient" aortic stenosis can be appropriately categorized into critical versus non-critical using dobutamine infusion to increase cardiac output in an attempt to increase the aortic valve opening **(Table 1)**.

Bicuspid Valve

Bicuspid aortic valve is one of the most common cardiac abnormalities occurring in 1% of the population. It can result in AS, AR or combined AS and AR. Usually, the AS is initially mild and progressively increases over several years **(Figures 5A and B)**.

The bicuspid aortic valve is also prone to infective endocarditis. A classical bicuspid valve has two aortic sinuses. However, several variations of the bicuspid aortic valve occur including an incomplete cusp called raphe. This variant usually has three aortic sinuses. The commissural plane dividing the cusps could be horizontal, oblique or vertical. An "acquired" bicuspid valve sometime results from inflammatory (rheumatic) or calcific fusion of two adjacent cusps; thus giving an appearance similar to congenital bicuspid valve.

AORTIC REGURGITATION

Aortic regurgitation may be the cause of diseases affecting the aorta-like dilatation, aortic dissection etc., or may be due to pathologies of the leaflets-like congenital bicuspid valves, calcifications, myxomatous, rheumatic or infective endocarditis. AR causes volume overload in LV that leads to its progressive dilatation and could lead to systolic dysfunction **(Figures 6A and B)**.

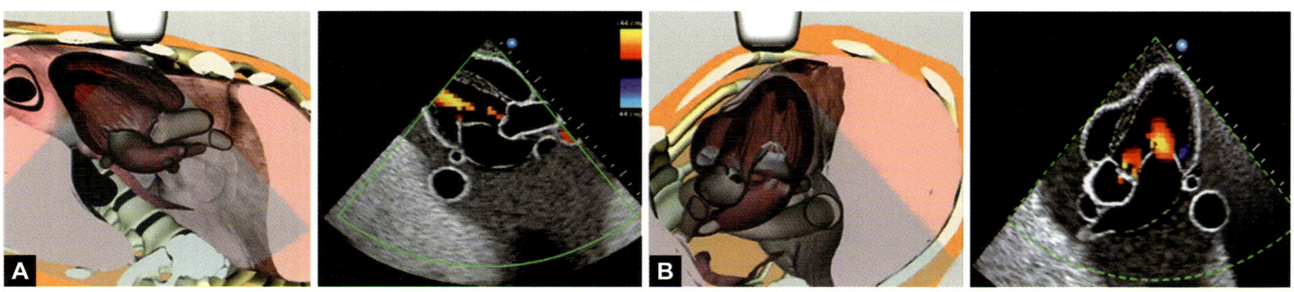

Figures 5A and B AR on simulator in different views of aortic valve. (A) Parasternal long axis view (PSLAX); (B) Apical 5-chamber view

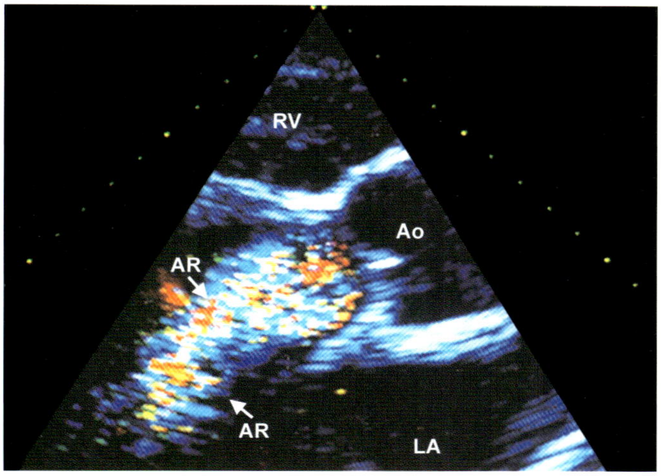

Figure 6A Echocardiographic picture showing torrential AR in PSPLAX- view
Abbreviations: RV, right ventricle; AR, aortic root; LA, left atrium; Ao, aorta

Indications of TTE in Aortic Regurgitation

- To confirm presence and severity AR **(Table 2)**.
- Assessment of jet ventricular size, function.
- Re-evaluation in mild/moderate AR on symptom change.
- Assessment of regurgitation and severity of aortic dilatation in patients with enlarged aortic root.

TABLE 2 Aortic regurgitation severity

1. Jet width proportional to LVOT width (%)	<25 mild 25–66 moderate >66 severe
2. Vena contracta (mm)	< 2 mild, 3–6 moderate, >7 severe
3. PISA- ROA (cm^2)	<0.1 mild 0.1–0.3 moderate >0.3 severe
4. Regurgitant fraction (%)	<30 mild 30–50 moderate >50 severe
5. Regurgitant volume (mL)	<30 mild 30–60 moderate >60 severe
6. Pressure half time (msec)	>350 mild 250–350 moderate <250 severe
7. A pan-diastolic back flow in descending aorta using supra-sternal view, indicates more than moderate regurgitation.	

AORTIC VALVE IMPLANTATION

Mentice aortic valve implantation is designed for interventional cardiologists and cardiac/cardiothoracic surgeons who wish to start training on transcatheter aortic valve implantation/replacement (TAVI/TAVR) **(Figure 7)**. The module allows for safe and cost-effective training, either for individual instruction or as part of a hospital quality improvement or change-of-process program **(Figure 7)**.

This module assumes familiarity with preoperative CT imaging, echocardiography and extensive experience with endovascular intervention and cardiac catheterization. Both balloon-expandable and self-expandable valve types are supported, which facilitates a discussion on pros and cons, as well as to understand the differences in deployment technique. The stepwise approach, where each step of the procedure is carried

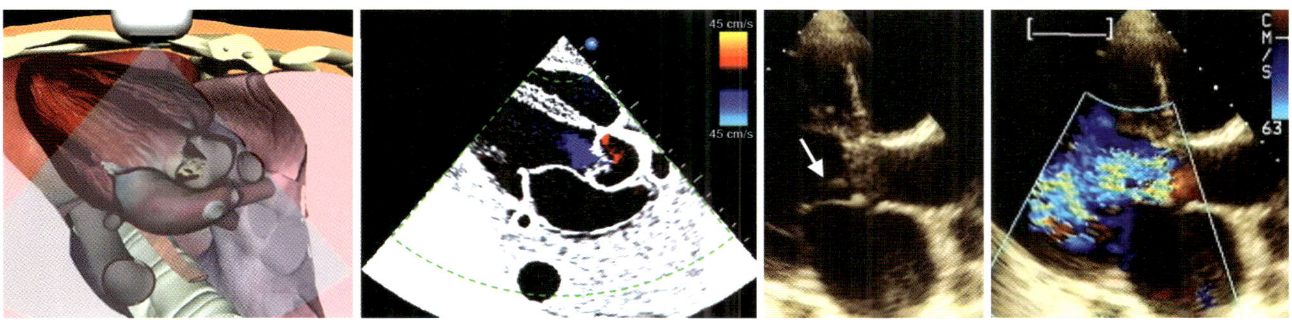

Figure 6B Aortic regurgitation jet on the simulator and as well as echocardiographic PLAX view depicting aortic valvular vegetation (arrow) with torrential AR

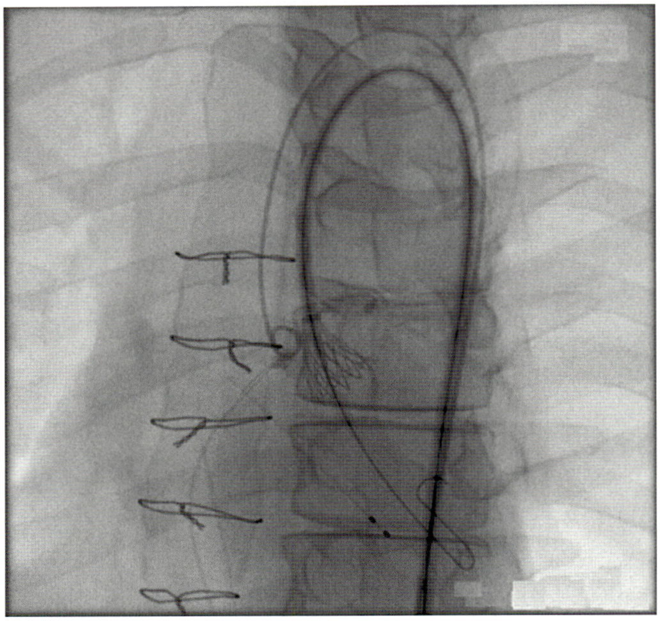

Figure 7 The module allows for safe and cost-effective training

out in a safe-simulated environment, prepares the trainee to meet unexpected events in the operating room. Together with a VIST®-C extension, the module can be run with bifemoral access to further enhance training realism.[5]

An ideal platform for:

- Teaching patient selection and preoperative planning
- Training of TAVI/TAVR in a stepwise approach
- Managing and minimizing radiation dose exposure
- Training of required technical and manipulation skills
- Review, validation and amendment of the procedure plan.

Aortic valve implantation is designed for understanding and learning the critical steps involved in the complex high-risk procedure of transcatheter aortic valve implantation/replacement (TAVI/TAVR).

INFECTIVE ENDOCARDITIS (IE): AORTIC VALVE

Infective endocarditis involving the AV occurs either on a pre-existing rheumatic or bicuspid aortic valve disease. However, a normal valve infective endocarditis is also fairly common. The echocardiographic hallmark of infective endocarditis is a mobile oscillating nodular, linear or shaggy echo density on the involving either one or more aortic valve cusps. Varying grades of AR are usually seen in such patients. Sub-acute or chronic complications include ring or annular abscess, pseudo-aneurysm of the ascending aorta, aorta to LA/RV fistula and flail aortic leaflets **(Figure 8)**. Transthoracic echocardiography has sensitivity and specificity of 65–70% in detecting vegetation. If a strong clinical suspicion for IE exists in a patient with a negative TTE study, TEE should be suggested, which has a much higher predictive accuracy (more than 90%).

Pathology of Simulator for Aortic Valve

HeartWorks pathology modules for both TTE and TEE imaging have been created to facilitate the echocardiographic evaluation of patients with structural and hemodynamic disturbances.

This module includes:

- Mechanical aortic valve
- Aortic stenosis and mitral stenosis Doppler.

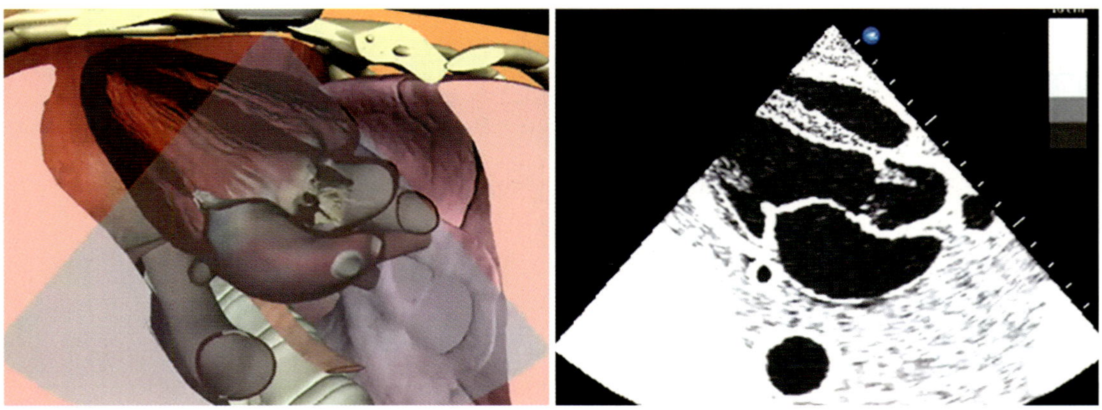

Figure 8 Aortic valve vegetation's (Shaggy, fluffy echo densities) on simulated images

Mechanical Aortic Valve

This model demonstrates a bileaflet mechanical aortic valve prosthesis **(Figure 9)**. The Doppler profile permits **(Figure 10)** detailed evaluation of prosthetic function while the characteristics of the left ventricle and aorta reflect the underlying native pathology ventricular hypertrophy and poststenotic dilation of the ascending aorta.

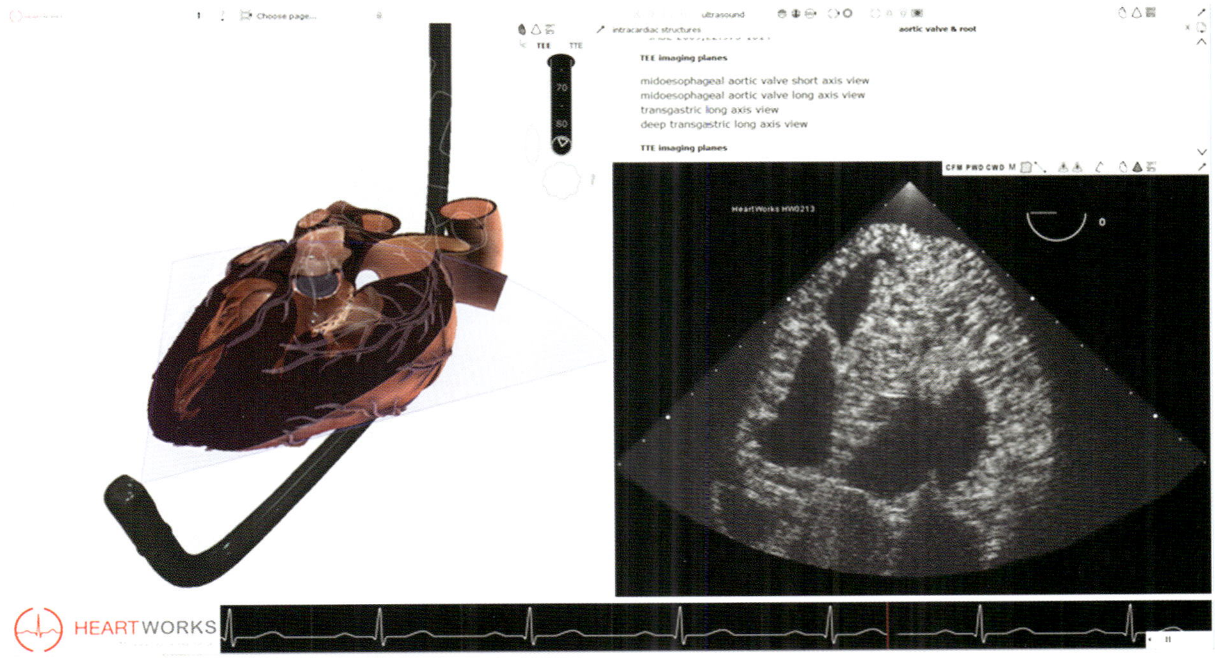

Figure 9 TEE image of mechanical aortic valve

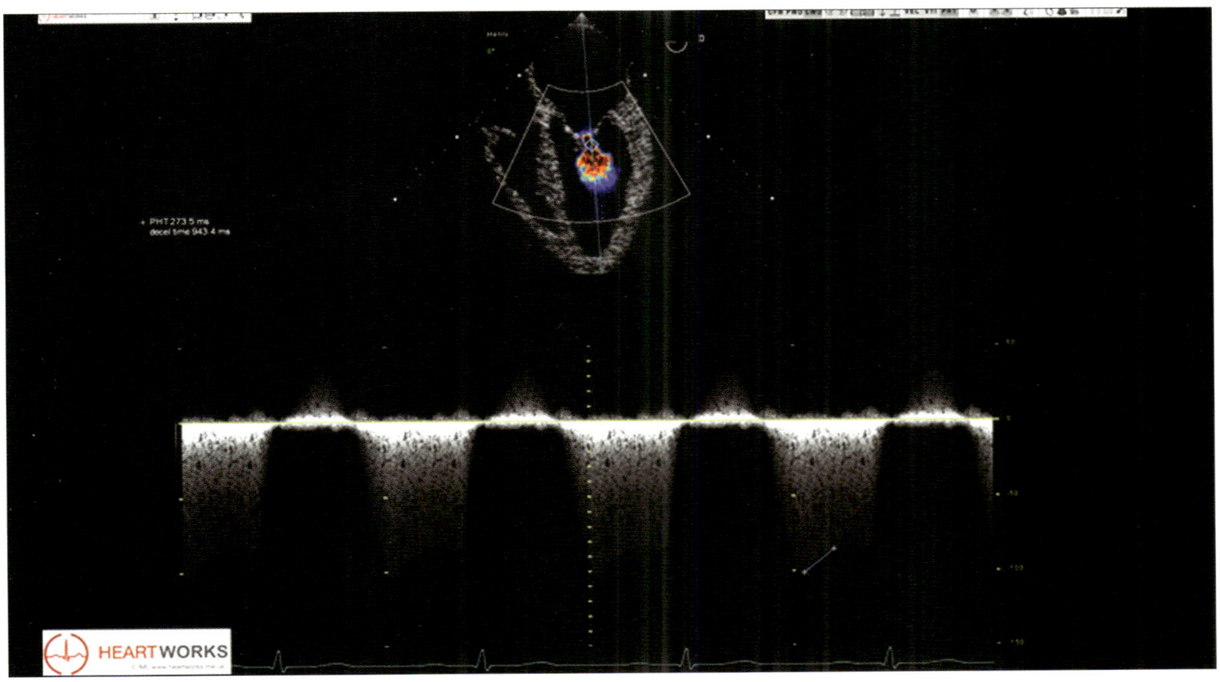

Figure 10 TEE image of mitral stenosis with Doppler

Aortic Stenosis and Mitral Stenosis Doppler

Flow velocity has been added to the existing aortic stenosis and mitral stenosis models (Pathology Module 2). Spectral and color flow Doppler displays demonstrate characteristic appearances with stenotic flow.

CONCLUSION

Accurate patient-specific AR models including the vessel wall thickness and calcification deposits represent a useful tool to guide TAVR and to help in preventing the migration of the valve during the deployment procedure. Also, optimizing the positioning of the valve during deployment, as well as alternative approaches to TAVR valves tailored to patient's specific pathology, e.g. polymeric valves, may offer better procedural outcome.

REFERENCES

1. Joshi SD, Joshi SS, Athavale SA. Origins of the coronary arteries and their significance. Clinics (Sao Paulo). 2010;65(1):79-84.
2. Lannaccone A, Marwick TH. Cost effectiveness of transcatheter aortic valve replacement compared with medical management or surgery for patients with aortic stenosis. Appl Health Econ Health Policy. 2015;13(1):29-45.
3. Siu SC, Silversides CK. Bicuspid aortic valve disease. J Am Coll Cardiol. 2010;55(25):2789-800.
4. Maganti K, Rigolin VH, Sarano ME, Bonow RO. Valvular heart disease: diagnosis and management. Mayo Clin Proc. 2010;85(5): 483-500.
5. Stout KK, Verrier ED. Valvular heart disease: changing concepts in disease management: acute valvular regurgitation. Circulation. 2009;119:3232-41.

Chapter 7

Use of Simulation for Transthoracic Echocardiography in Ischemic Heart Disease

Rakesh Gupta, Navin C Nanda, HK Chopra

Chapter Outline

INTRODUCTION

Coronary heart disease (CHD) is a common cardiovascular disease and the leading cause of death in western countries.[1] The early diagnosis and post-treatment assessment of CHD are clinically significant. Transthoracic echocardiogram provides important diagnostic and prognostic information for CHD because of its lack of invasiveness, simple examination technique, and ability to provide ample anatomical and hemodynamic information. Abnormal segmental ventricular wall motion is a sensitive and specific indicator for myocardial ischemia **(Figure 1)**. To facilitate data exchange among various imaging modalities, including ultrasonography, radionuclide imaging, MRI, and CT, the American Heart Association (AHA) has suggested a myocardial segmentation method that divides the myocardium into 17 segments.

In contrast to other imaging modalities, Transthoracic echocardiography (TTE) suggests the presence of an occluded coronary artery by detecting the abnormal motion of the ventricular wall.[2]

TRANSTHORACIC ECHOCARDIOGRAPHY AND ANESTHESIOLOGISTS

The TTE is a noninvasive and readily available diagnostic technique that is seeing increased perioperative use by anesthesiologist. A focused, goal-directed examination can be performed in less than 10 minutes, has been shown to alter patient management, and may improve outcomes. A prospective observational study demonstrated that a focused TTE performed by anesthesiologist resulted in alterations in management for 84% of the patients and the results correlated with cardiologists' formal results in 90% of cases.[3] In the hands of a trained anesthesiologist, clinical information may be obtained quickly when sufficient time is lacking to obtain a formal TTE examination.

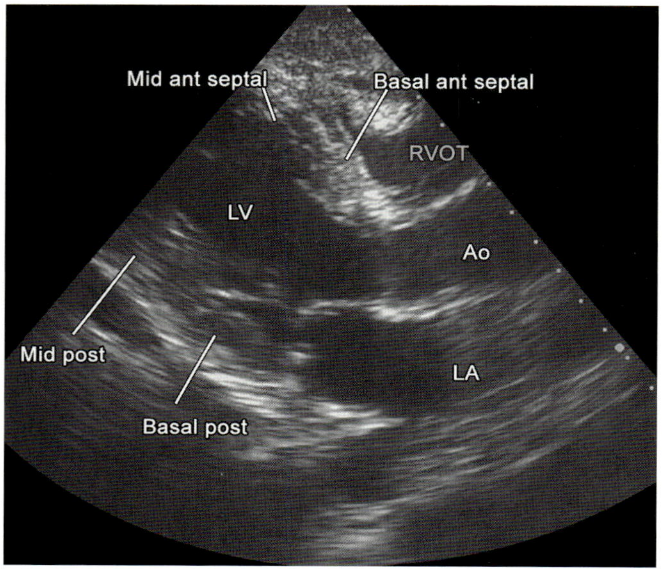

Figure 1 Regional wall motion abnormalities in coronary artery disease
Abbreviations: LA, left atrium, Ao, aorta; LV, left ventricle, RVOT, right ventricular outflow tract

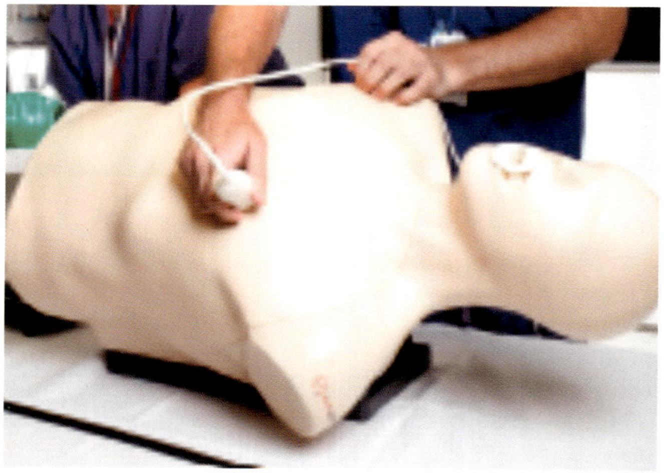

Figure 2 Transthoracic echocardiography simulator

Simulation allows interactive TTE learning using a virtual 3-dimensional model of the heart and may aid in the acquisition of the cognitive and technical skills needed to perform TTE **(Figure 2)**. The ability to link probe manipulation, cardiac anatomy, and echocardiographic images using a simulator has been shown to be an effective model for training anesthesiology residents in transesophageal echocardiography. A proposed alternative to real-time patient-based learning is simulation-based training that allows anesthesiologists to learn complex concepts and procedures.

This module allows real-time simulated TTE imaging of the virtual heart using a manikin. The life size manikin torso has soft skin with accurate, palpable anatomical landmarks to aid positioning of the handheld ultrasound probe. The screen display allows the user to identify the position of the probe on the virtual chest as well as to see the orientation of the ultrasound plane. The anatomy display includes a representation of the chest wall, ribs, sternum, and spine as well as great vessels, lungs, pericardium, diaphragm, and liver. These structures are displayed in the ultrasound view with realistic effects on cardiac imaging **(Figure 3)**.

As the learner scans the mannequin, the high-resolution monitor displays a realistic simulated ultrasound image beside a real-time 3D graphic representation of the anatomy, including surrounding structures and organs **(Figure 4)**. The 3D anatomy feature can be toggled on or off, or it can be customized to adapt to the learner's level of knowledge and ultrasound imaging skill. This augmented reality feature improves understanding of how the heart works and speeds the path to proficiency in obtaining ultrasound images. As a learner progresses, the instructor may turn off the 360° anatomical image and transform the echo simulator into an ultrasound imaging system that more closely resembles what a resident would find in a clinical setting.

Three-dimensional (3D) echocardiography is able to provide intuitive recognition of cardiac structures from

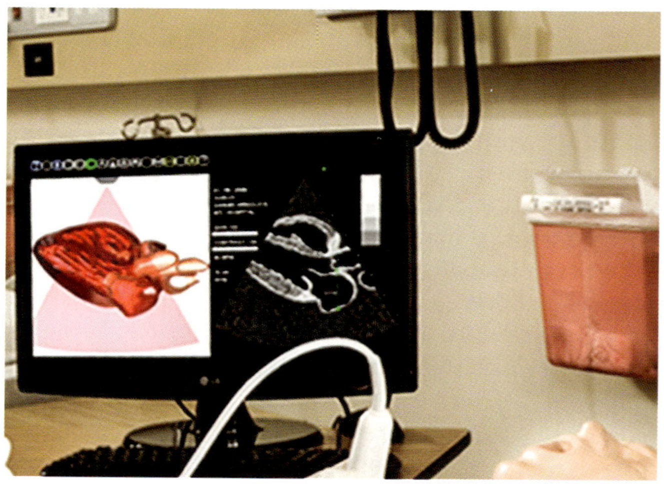

Figure 3 Real-time echo simulation with augmented reality

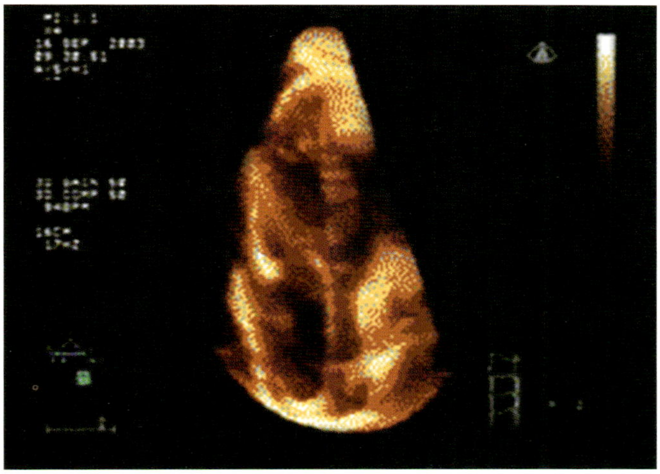

Figure 4 3D echocardiography

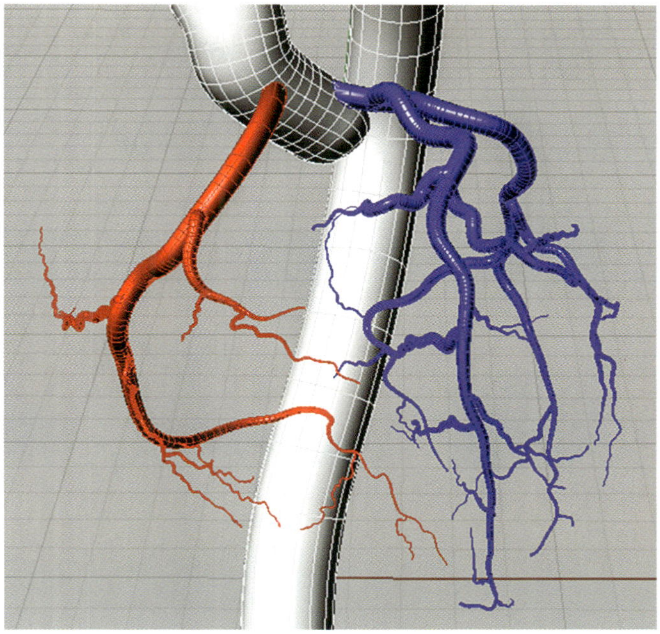

Figure 5 Establishment of 3D visible models of the coronary arteries

any spatial point of view and may provide complete information about absolute heart chamber volumes and functions. Although there are still limitations to the currently available 3D ultrasound methods due to its relatively low image quality and low time resolution, this method would be one of the ultimate goals of cardiac imaging. In light of the recent development of real-time 3D transesophageal echocardiography (TEE), this new imaging method may become a clinical standard within a few years. The coronary arteries are the first pair of branches originating from the ascending aorta and provide the primary supply of blood to the heart. The trunk of the left coronary artery originates from the left coronary sinus. The left coronary artery passes between the pulmonary artery and left auricle and bifurcates into the anterior descending branch and the left circumflex branch. The anterior descending branch divides into the left arterial cone, the right ventricular anterior branch, the left ventricular anterior branch, the anterior septal artery, and the diagonal branch. The left circumflex branch divides into the left ventricular anterior branch, the marginal branch, the left atrial branch, and the left ventricular posterior branch. The right coronary artery originates from the anterior aortic sinus; its branches include the right arterial cone, the right ventricular anterior branch, the right marginal branch, the right ventricular posterior branch, the right atrial branch, the atrioventricular nodal artery, the posterior descending branch, and the left atrial posterior branch. Three-dimensional visualizations of the coronary arteries are challenging because of the large number of thin branches from these vessels, which have a highly variable anatomy. The application of the latest ultrasound technology, in particular the 2nd harmonic, has opened new roads in ultrasound coronary evaluation. By applying anatomical knowledge and the newest technical applications it is now-a-days possible to propose a complete coronary evaluation of the left anterior descending artery and of a part of the posterior descending coronary artery in clinical practice **(Figure 5)**.

Left anterior descending (LAD) coronary anatomy was the first artery investigated with ultrasound by transesophageal and transthoracic approach. This vessel is visible by using ultrasound from proximal to distal tract and following key anatomical structures through the delivery of an ultrasound beam in an off-axis approach starting from the classical apical approach **(Figure 6)**.

Proximal LAD: The left atrial appendage and pulmonary artery represent the key reference points in detecting the proximal left anterior descending coronary tract.

Intermediate LAD: The septal perforans branches represent the key references obtainable by angulating the probe slightly lower (3, 5–5 MHz in 2nd) and maintaining the focus on the anterior interventricular sulcus.[4]

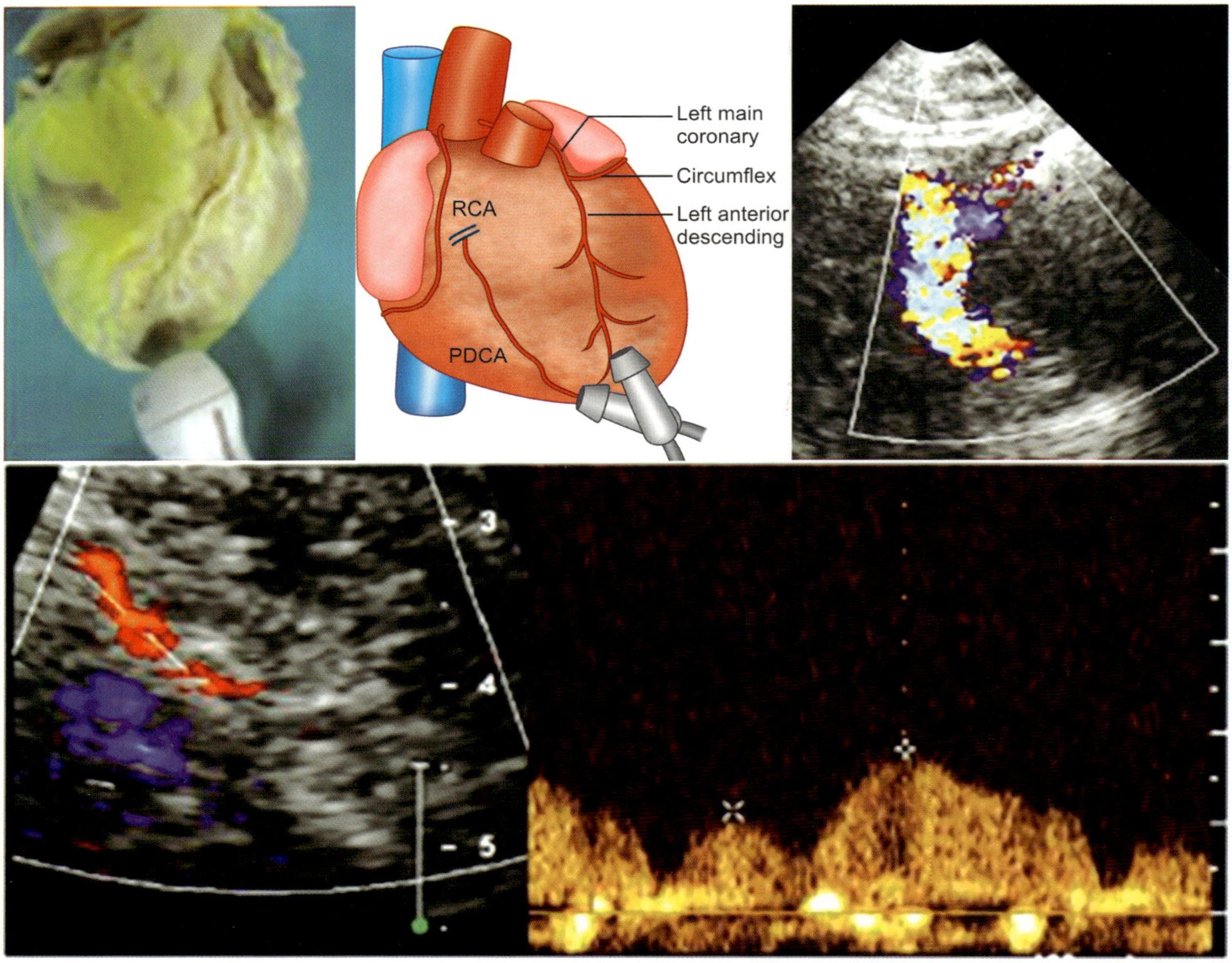

Figure 6 Represents an artist's drawing illustrating transducer beam orientations to the left anterior descending coronary artery (LAD) and to posterior descending coronary arteries with the corresponding echocardiographic images of the mid-distal tract of LAD pulse-wave flow and posterior descending coronary artery (PDCA)
Abbreviation: RCA, right coronary artery

Distal LAD tract: this can be highlighted by investigating the lower part of interventricular anterior sulcus near the apex under color Doppler guidance and adopting growing delivery frequencies (5–7 MHz in 2nd harmonic). By subsequently applying Pulse Doppler inside the coronary vessel, we may obtain the coronary spectrum and therefore quantify it. For the distal left posterior coronary artery we must address the ultrasound beam in a counter clockwise direction, and, always under color Doppler guidance, focus the ultrasound beam on the posterior descending coronary sulcus. By applying the latest technology, it is nowadays possible to investigate LAD in 98% of patients and posterior descending coronary artery (PDCA) in 60–70% of patients.[4]

LEFT VENTRICULAR VOLUMES AND LEFT VENTRICULAR EJECTION FRACTIONS

Absolute LV volumes and their dynamic changes during cardiac cycles are indispensable and fundamental indices for assessing LV function in any cardiac disease.

Three-dimensional echocardiographic methods provide unique capabilities for determining absolute.

LV volumes, stroke volumes and ejection fractions (EF). Magnetic resonance imaging (MRI) is often employed as an independent gold standard to validate the accuracy of 3D echocardiography for determining LV volumes and EF.

Absolute LV volumes and their dynamic changes during cardiac cycles are indispensable and fundamental indices for assessing LV function in any cardiac disease. Three-dimensional echocardiographic methods provide unique capabilities for determining absolute LV volumes, stroke volumes, and ejection fractions (EF).

SPECTRAL DOPPLER

Spectral Doppler is using to identify the coronary arteries in the midesophageal aortic valve views. Either of the following two 2D TEE views can be used **(Figures 7A and B)**:

- Midesophageal aortic valve short axis view
- Midesophageal aortic valve long axis view.

To identify the left main (LMCA) or the proximal anterior descending coronary artery, withdraw the probe from the midesophageal aortic valve short axis view. To aid in identification of the LMCA, apply color Doppler over the left sinus of Valsalva. The right coronary artery (RCMA) is less accessible but maybe visualized within the midesophageal aortic valve short or long axis views adjacent to the right sinus of Valsalva.

To assess flow in a coronary artery, place the pulsed wave (PW) sample volume within the artery.

A normal coronary artery spectral Doppler trace has two peaks: the systolic (S) and diastolic (D) wave. Both waves are seen below the baseline as the direction of blood flow is away from the transducer **(Figure 7A to D** and **Table 1)**.

- The D wave is larger than the S wave.
- Maximum velocity of blood in coronary arteries measured using PW Doppler.

TABLE 1 S and D wave velocities in coronary arteries on spectral Doppler

Coronary Artery	*D wave maximum velocity*	*S wave maximum velocity*
Left main	71 ± 19 cm/sec	36 ± 11 cm/sec
Right main	39 ± 12 cm/sec	25 ± 8 cm/sec

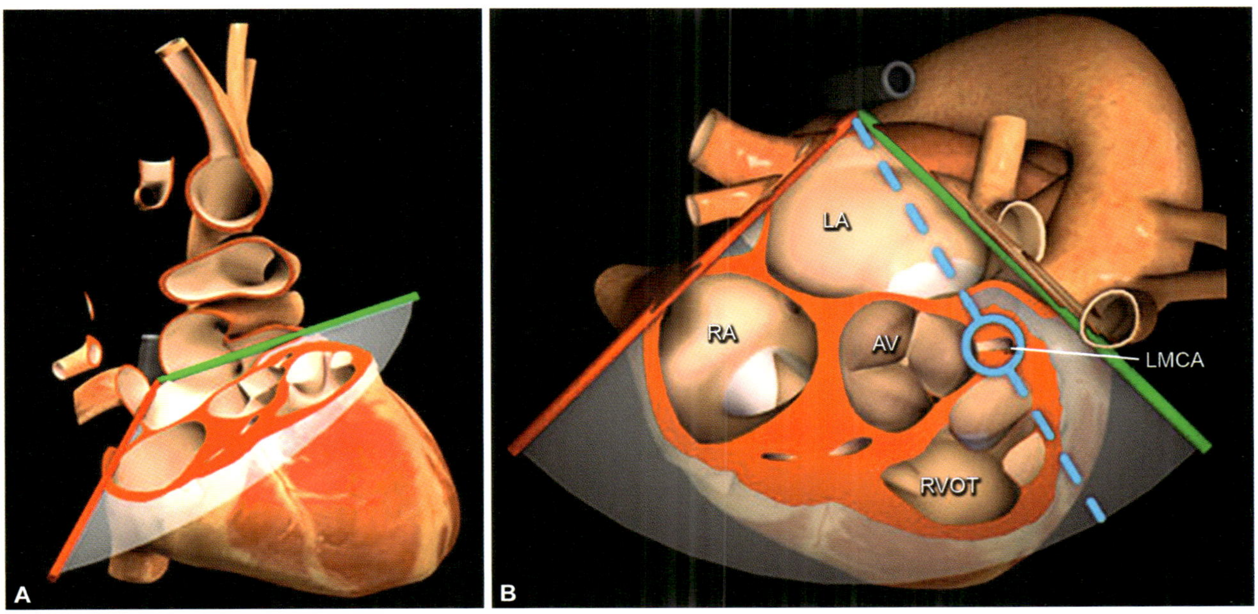

Figures 7A and B Three-dimensional heart model shown in cross-section to highlight the position of the TEE plane in the mid esophageal aortic valve short axis view. (A) Anterior view of the heart with TEE plane. (B) Superior view of the heart and TEE plane. The blue dotted line represents the orientation of the pulsed wave cursor and the blue circle indicates the position of the sample box in the left main coronary artery.

Abbreviations: AV, aortic valve; LA, left atrium; LMCA, left main coronary artery; RA, right atrium; RVOT, right ventricular outflow tract

CHAPTER 7

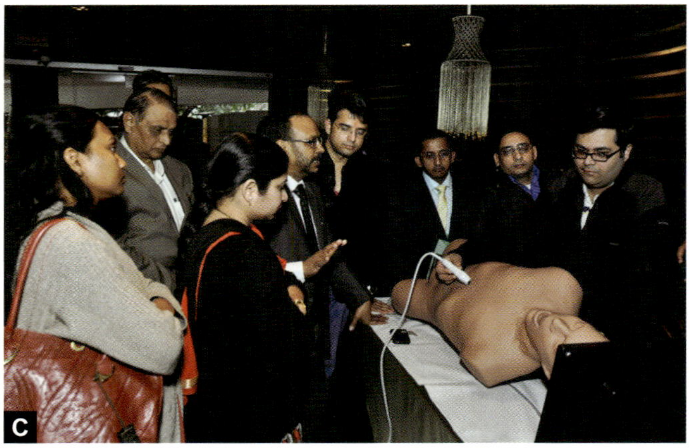

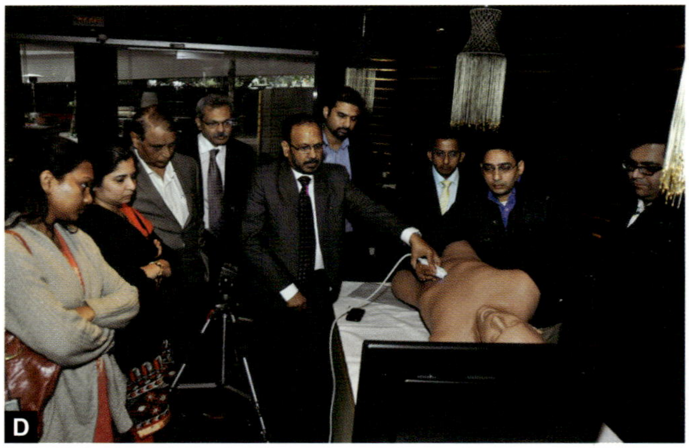

Figures 7C and D (C) Hands on TEE, probe positions to learn, transthoracic fastest; (D) A slight left lateral position and slight pressure of probe depth can be done to view the heart chambers

Simulation for Planning Services for Patients with Coronary Artery Disease

Simulation models were developed in Pascal to predict the resource use and costs arising from the treatment of patients with coronary artery disease in Indian Hospital. Results from the simulations indicated that number of cardiology beds was inadequate, causing a bottleneck in the system. There was predicted to be an overall increase in demand for treatment causing costs to rise initially, but then, unless more beds were made available, to level off. The software, which was designed to be of general application to health problems, includes facilities for the scheduling of operating theaters and the combined modelling of demands made by different groups of acute and chronic patients.[5]

The use of Simulation to Evaluate the Cost-effectiveness of Interventions

A discrete event simulation of patients with coronary heart disease (CHD) models CHD events from the first diagnosis of angina, myocardial infarction or unstable angina to death. The data have been derived mainly from published sources and databases. Using life years saved as the output, sensitivity analysis of the key parameters show how the model responds to different data assumptions.

The scenarios examined include the following:

- Changes in the availability of angiograms, angioplasties and bypass surgery
- Changes in the provision and take-up of secondary prevention
- Improvements in ambulance times
- Increase in the availability and timeliness of thrombolysis
- More widespread provision of cardiac rehabilitation.
- The presentation will show the implications of applying quality of life indicators to the years of life saved. A further model, developed at the London School of Hygiene and Tropical Medicine and concerned with the prevention of coronary heart disease, has been linked to the treatment model described above. The implications of prevention strategies, such as lowering blood pressure in high risk patients, on the need for treatment will be explored.[6]

LIMITATIONS OF TRANSTHORACIC ECHOCARDIOGRAPHY TRAINING

Limitations residents were post-tested on 1 volunteer subject with good transthoracic windows to provide consistency of imaging windows across the groups. The ability of residents, to obtain images over a large range of patients of differing body habitus or in clinical scenarios. Although the simulation group outperformed the control group in the short-term, it is unclear if this superiority will persist. Although the financial obligation of a TTE simulator is currently significant, teaching anesthesia residents TTE on volunteer subjects is time consuming and logistically difficult because of operating room commitments. Because the second training session involved volunteer subjects, a smaller subset of residents was enrolled. Although this is a limitation study and an aim to improve in future studies, it does highlight the benefit of simulation over traditional patient examination-based teaching.

CONCLUSION

Increased practice and knowledge integration from simulation leads to improved focused TTE skills among anesthesiologists compared to traditional teaching methods. This may translate into more efficient TTE education and better clinical diagnosis; however, the impact of these short-term educational approaches on longer-term retention and actual clinical application warrants further investigation.

REFERENCES

1. Thomas A. Gaziano, Asaf Bitton, Shuchi Anand, Shafika Abrahams-Gessel, Adrianna Murphy. Growing Epidemic of Coronary Heart Disease in Low- and Middle-Income Countries. Curr Probl Cardiol. Author manuscript; available in PMC 2011 February 1.
2. Zhong C, Guo Y, Huang H, Tan L, Wu Y, Wang W. Three-dimensional reconstruction of coronary arteries and its application in localization of coronary artery segments corresponding to myocardial segments identified by transthoracic echocardiography. Comput Math Methods Med. (2013). 2013:783-939.
3. Eltzschig HK, Rosenberger P, Löffler M, Fox JA, Aranki SF, Shernan SK. Impact of intraoperative transesophageal echocardiography on surgical decisions in 12,566 patients undergoing cardiac surgery. Ann Thorac Surg. 2008;85(3):845-52.
4. Rigo F, Murer B, Ossena G, Favaretto E. Transthoracic echocardiographic imaging of coronary arteries: tips, traps, and pitfalls. Cardiovasc Ultrasound. 2008;6:7.
5. Davies R, et al. Simulation for planning services for patients with coronary artery disease. 1994;72(2): Issue 2, 323-32.
6. Davies R, Cooper K, Roderick P, Raftery J. The evaluation of disease prevention and treatment using simulation models. European Journal of OR. 2003;150(1):53-66.

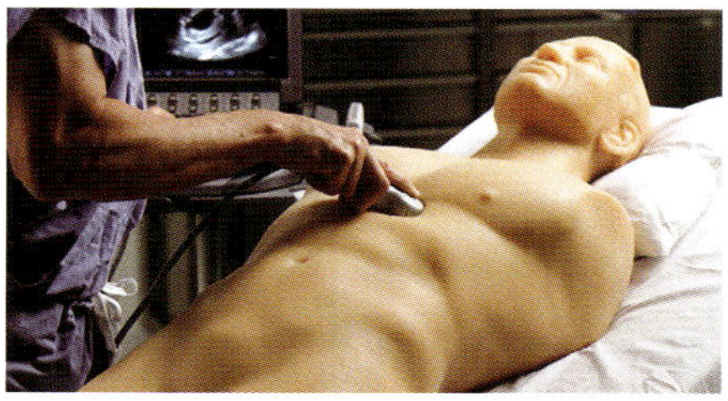

Section 3

Simulation in Transesophageal Echocardiography

Section Outline

- Importance of Simulation in Transesophageal Echocardiography Learning
- Simulation for Two-dimensional and Three-dimensional Transesophageal Echocardiography Views
- Simulation for Transesophageal Echocardiography of Mitral Valve
- Transesophageal Echocardiography in Intensive Care Unit
- Simulation for Transesophageal Echocardiography of Tricuspid and Pulmonary Valves
- Transesophageal Echocardiography Simulation for Left Ventricular Systolic Function
- Evaluation of Aorta by Simulated Transesophageal Echocardiography
- Evaluation of Aortic Valve by Simulated Transesophageal Echocardiography
- Simulation for Transesophageal Echocardiography for Aortic Valve Stenosis

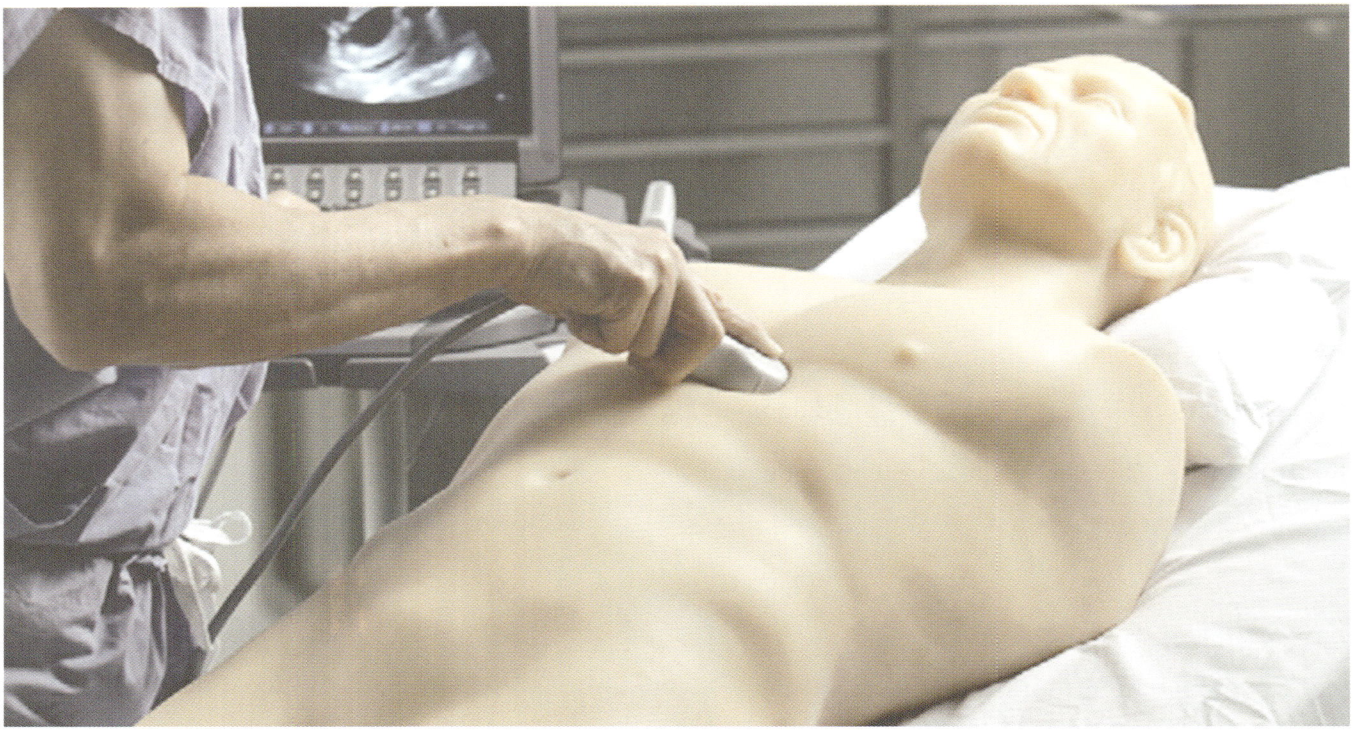

Chapter 8

Importance of Simulation in Transesophageal Echocardiography Learning

Poonam Malhotra Kapoor, Rajiv Juneja

Chapter Outline

- Measurement of Transesophageal Echocardiography Learning by Simulation
- Advantages of Simulators: Fearless and Without Distractions
- Some Simulation Pathologies of Transesophageal Echocardiography
- Different Types of Transesophageal Echocardiography and Transthoracic Echocardiography Simulators

INTRODUCTION

The role of simulation has grown exponentially in recent literature[1] as it provides an efficient method to teach complicated technical skills in a controlled environment. This rapid expansion is evident in its application to transesophageal echocardiography (TEE), where proficiency has traditionally been gained by repeated bedside examinations. While kinematic metrics data of probe motion can show the utility of simulation by improvement of movement efficiency, this technology may also be used to assess accuracy of the images acquired as an endpoint.

The role of transesophageal echocardiography (TEE) simulation in cardiac sciences residents learning is unknown **(Figures 1 and 2)**. Standard TEE training at the authors' institution though it begins in the first year itself, a resident does not get formal training in TEE until he/she is in the 2nd year of the DM cardiac anesthesia course occurs during the second of 3 clinical years. Residents spend 2 months in the TEE laboratory learning through hands-on experience on real patients and also on a daily basis in the operating room. The addition of TEE simulation to this experience may improve proficiency, speed up learning, and increase the residents comfort with TEE.

MEASUREMENT OF TRANSESOPHAGEAL ECHOCARDIOGRAPHY LEARNING BY SIMULATION

It is feasible to measure TEE position accuracy as an endpoint in the learning of TEE by simulation. It may

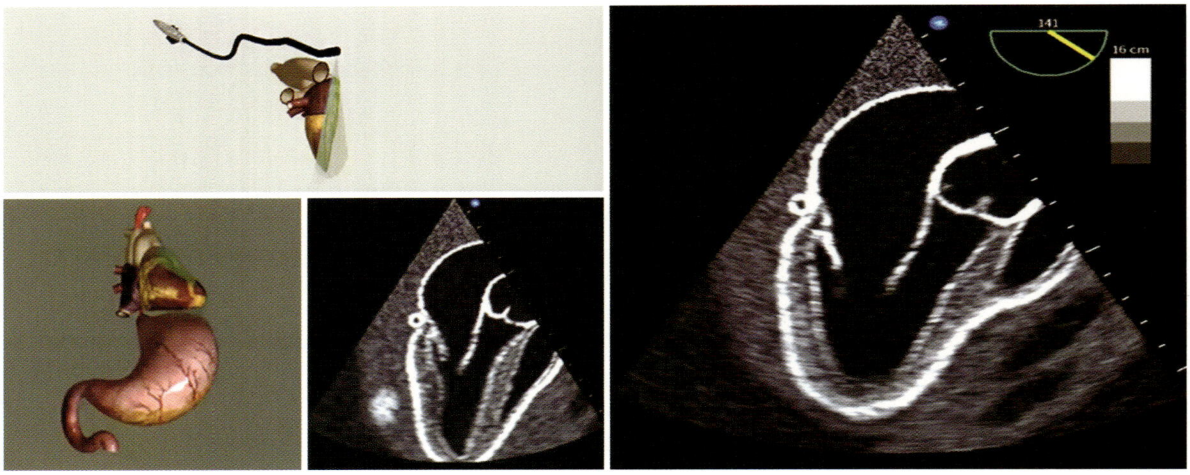

Figure 1 Cross-sectional TEE views on a simulator

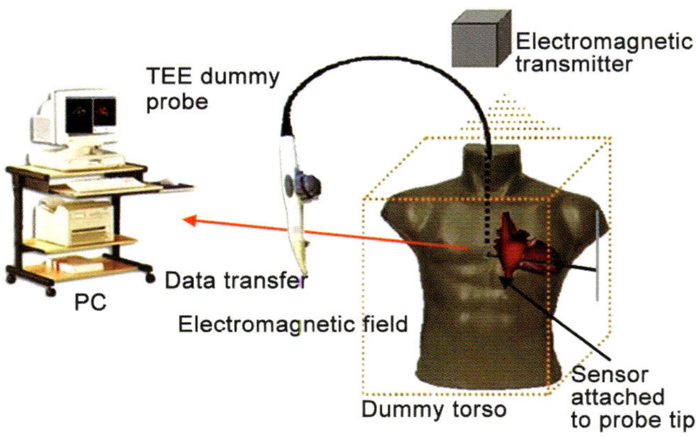

Figure 2 Parts of a TEE simulator

be used as a marker to measure the level of acquired proficiency, as a study done by Ham Kin et al,[2] to compare the efficiency of simulator based learning with standard TEE learning techniques, has shown that there are improvements in accuracy over the course of 4 weeks in residents when simulation based learning is involved. However, despite this improvement, they were still shown to be significantly less accurate when compared to experts. In this era of competency based medical education, the ability to quantify proficiency as a marker of progress of learning becomes very important.[3] TEE metrics accuracy provides an objective measurement to quantify the level and learning in a TEE curriculum. *The advantage of TEE simulation is that trainees can tailor their course according to their own timetable and needs. Difficult procedures can be trained without setting patients at risk.*

Transesophageal Echocardiography simulation is an effective tool in teaching psychomotor skills and learning views to novice echocardiographers ***(Figures 3 to 8)****.*

High-fidelity TEE simulators which have been there in the market for 2D TEE learning are an effective training adjunct for the acquisition of basic TEE psychomotor skills. It has been shown that there is no difference in improvement between the different modalities of instruction.[4] Further research will examine the need for a faculty resource for a curriculum in which a simulator is used as an adjunct.

The role of simulator training in TEE should be well defined, by the institution/association practicing TEE and using the simulation technique to enhance the academic TEE learning of its trainees. It is well known that TEE simulator learning is better than textbook learning or learning TEE skills listening to conference lectures, but it is not yet shown that TEE simulation is a better teaching tool than actual learning clinically on the patients, where the abnormal cardiac pathology is in front of the eyes and does not have to be virtually created. Authentic, comparative studies between two modes of learning are needed in handling of the probe and understanding of its manipulations to learn spatial orientation of the pathologies of the cardiac chambers. *So, simulation is excellent with the TEE probe as the patient is not needed and neither is sedation/anesthesia.*

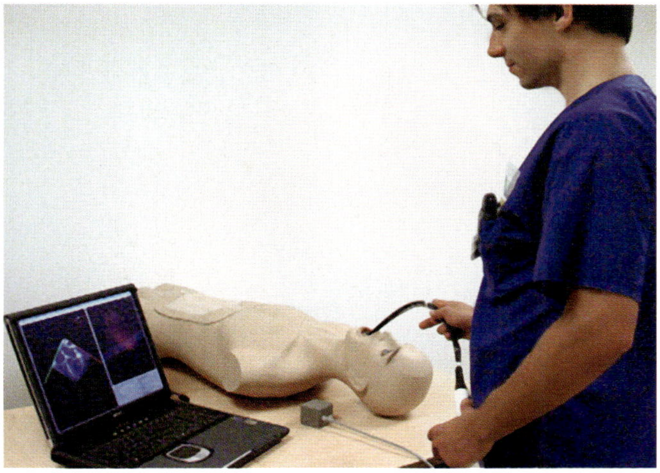

Figure 3 The EchoCom simulation system consists of a full-sized mannequin, transthoracic/transesophageal echocardiographic probe, and EchoCom software installed on a computer

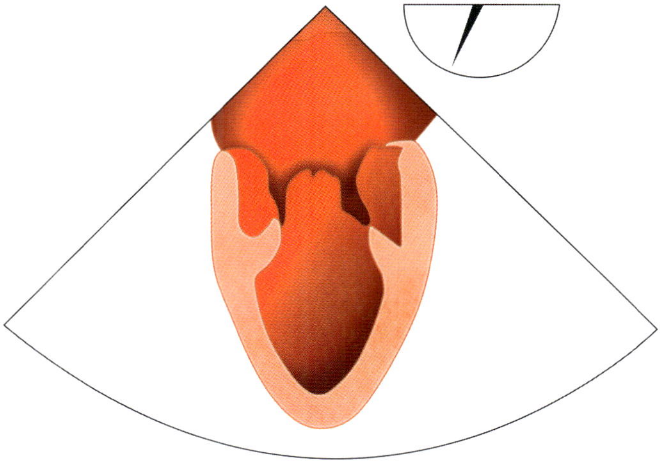

Figure 6 Midesophageal bicommissural view

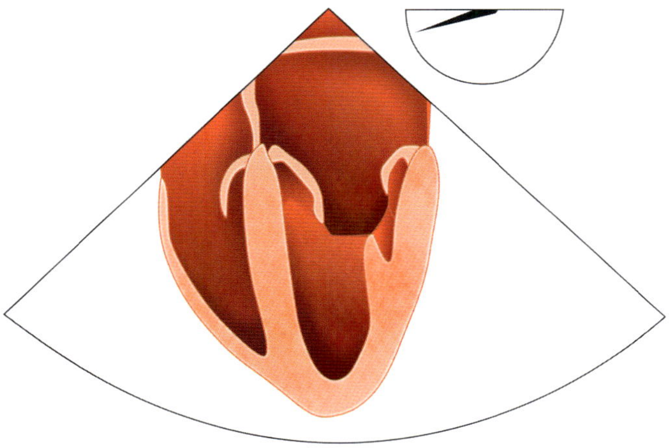

Figure 4 Midesophageal four chamber view

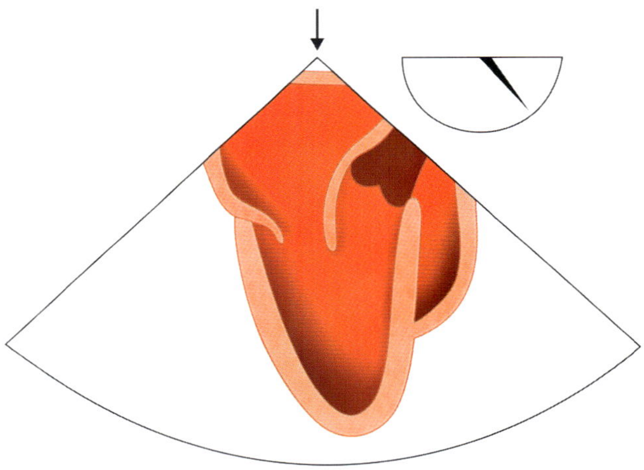

Figure 7 Midesophageal long axis view

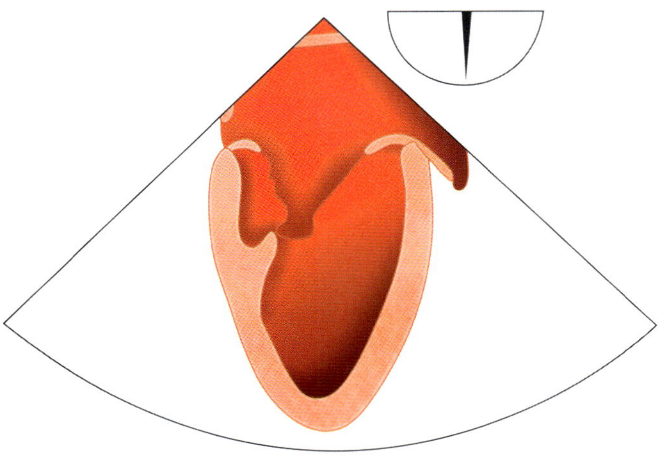

Figure 5 Midesophageal two chamber view

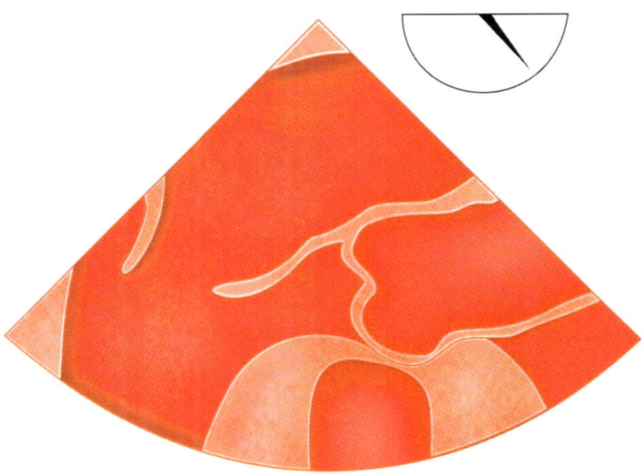

Figure 8 Midesophageal aortic valve long axis view

ADVANTAGES OF SIMULATORS: FEARLESS AND WITHOUT DISTRACTIONS

In the mannequin-based TEE simulators, the trainee is encouraged in learning the foundations of TEE probe manipulations and "knobology" which are a must to acquire and indepth knowledge of standard images, without the fear of moving the TEE probe in the esophagus of a patient who has been heparinised and is getting ready bypass. So simulator based TEE learning can be done in a fearless environment, without worrying about the rise or fall of the patient's blood pressure or saturation. There is no distraction to learning TEE on a simulator.

An advantage of the simulator is that adjustment of standard views is not learned simply by memorizing probe depth or degree of image plane rotation, but by understanding what happens when the image plane and probe are manipulated. It should be easier for the novice to transfer this knowledge to previously unknown views, although this has not been proved **(Figures 9 to 13)**. Also, for basic perioperative transesophageal echocardiography (TEE) the midoesophageal and transgastral views are the most important. The number of available 3D data sets and the quality of the data we used for the evaluation were limited due to the stepwise rotational acquisition mode. Also, they were obtained by transthoracic scanning and the structures that are in the far field in TTE with lower resolution are therefore in the near field in TOE and vice versa.

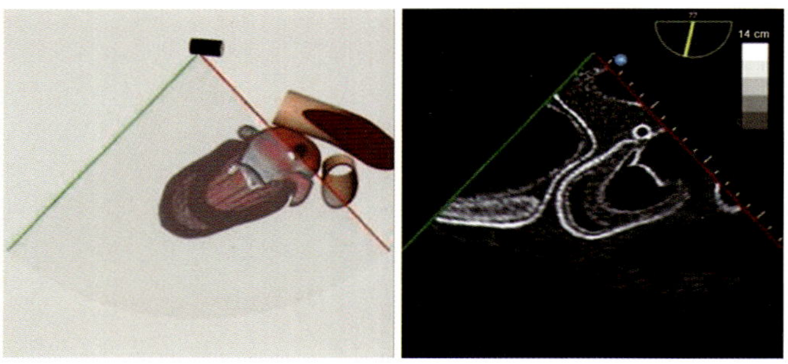

Figure 9 Transesophageal echocardiography midesophageal bicommissural view for mitral stenosis

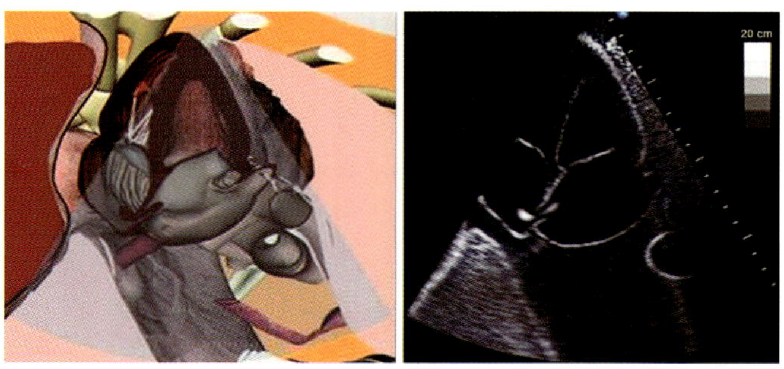

Figure 10 Deep transgastral transesophageal echocardiography view to show left ventricle hypertrophy

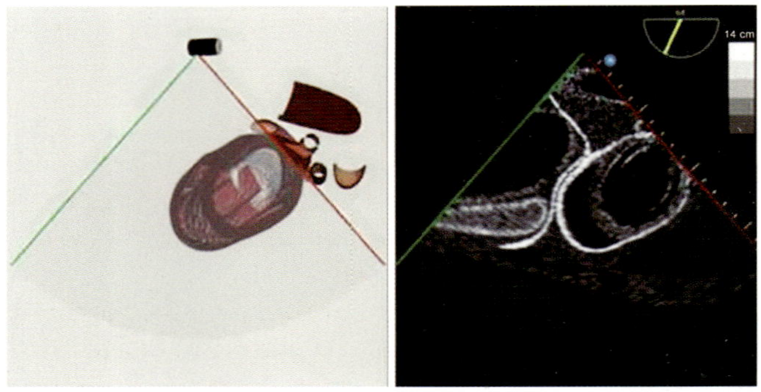

Figure 11 The transgastral basal valve view to show mitral regurgitation

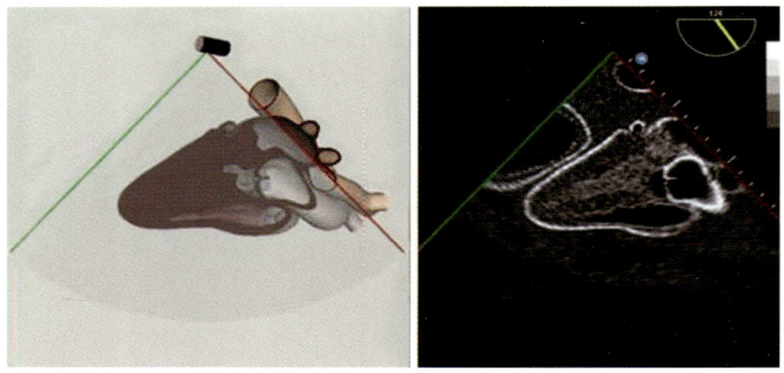

Figure 12 Transesophageal echocardiography left atrial appendage view to show left atrial appendage thrombus

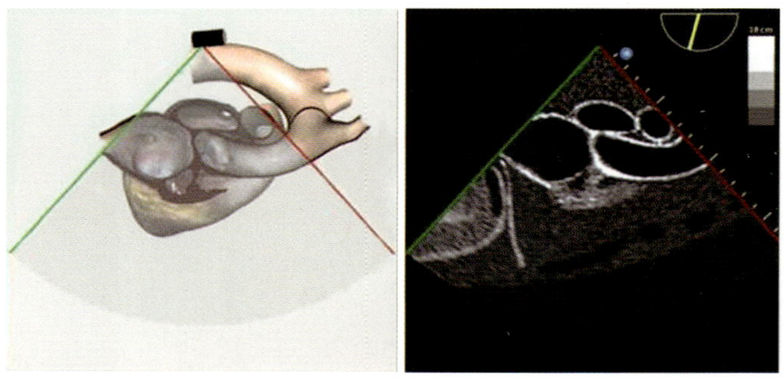

Figure 13 Transesophageal echocardiography midesophageal right ventricular outflow view

SOME SIMULATION PATHOLOGIES OF TRANSESOPHAGEAL ECHOCARDIOGRAPHY

At the present time, exposure to intraoperative TEE is challenging for trainees outside the operating room environment. The development of cardiac pathology will greatly help trainees develop the interpretative skills in areas either too complex or infrequent in occurrence to permit enough time for education in the clinical environment. This technology can be used for helping anesthetists maintain competency in situations where clinical case volume may be insufficient to support current competency requirements. Different TEE views are useful in reaching a pathology diagnosis. This is where expertise is needed. Some of the views easy to learn on the simulator are shown in **Figures 9 to 13**.

DIFFERENT TYPES OF TRANSESOPHAGEAL ECHOCARDIOGRAPHY AND TRANSTHORACIC ECHOCARDIOGRAPHY SIMULATORS

Different types of transesophageal echocardiography and transthoracic echocardiography simulators are known.

EchoCom Simulator

The EchoCom (Leipzig, Germany) simulation group was the first to publish on the use of augmented reality in the training of echocardiographic simulation. Augmented reality is based on a virtual 3D beating-heart model, which is registered spatially with actual 3D echocardiographic datasets **(Figure 14)**.[5]

Advantages/disadvantages of EchoCom: The EchoCom system has the advantage of using real TTE/TEE data, which appear more realistic. There also is the potential to incorporate different pathologic states and "normal" data. However, owing to the methodology of image acquisition, certain views, such as the upper esophageal views and imaging of the descending thoracic aorta, are not possible.[6] The ultrasound datasets used initially for image display were low-resolution images, but the simulator interface is undergoing constant upgrade. EchoCom is a prototype product and is not available commercially. It is used for local educational projects and for continuing medical education symposia for training.

Vimedix Simulator

This simulator also is based on the principle of augmented reality as described previously, but the echocardiographic images are not actual ultrasound datasets but rendered images **(Figures 15 to 18)**.

Advantages/disadvantages of Vimedix: This is a robust system with features, especially the metrics system, that make it particularly attractive for training institutions. The current simulator version does not have optimal transgastric, aortic valve short-axis, and coronary sinus images. The augmented reality model is a work in

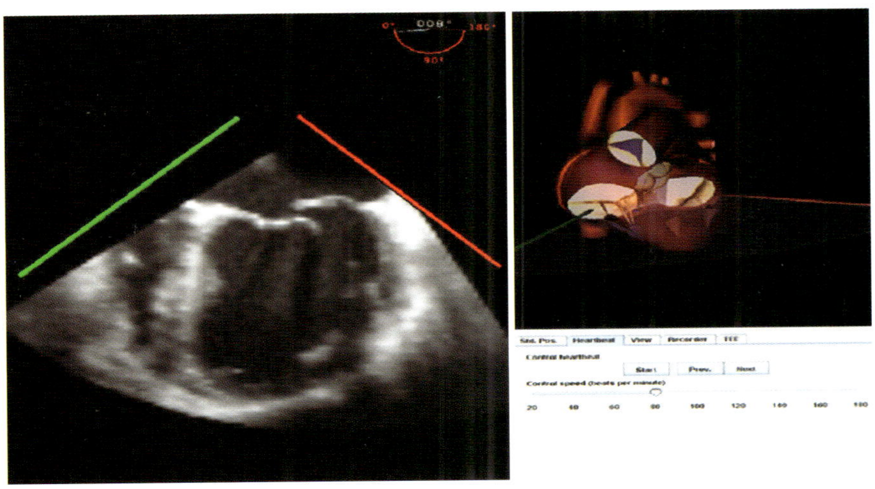

Figure 14 The computer interface of an EchoCom transesophageal echocardiogram, showing a virtual heart model and a superimposed scan plane depicting the virtual slice, which is linked to an actual transesophageal echocardiographic dataset

CHAPTER 8

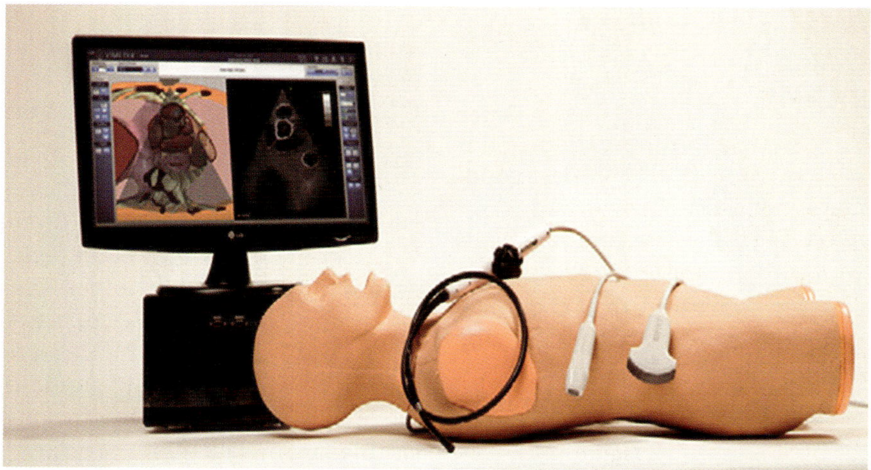

Figure 15 The Vimedix simulation system consists of a full-sized mannequin, transthoracic echocardiographic, transesophageal echocardiographic, abdominal scanning probes, and a dedicated computer

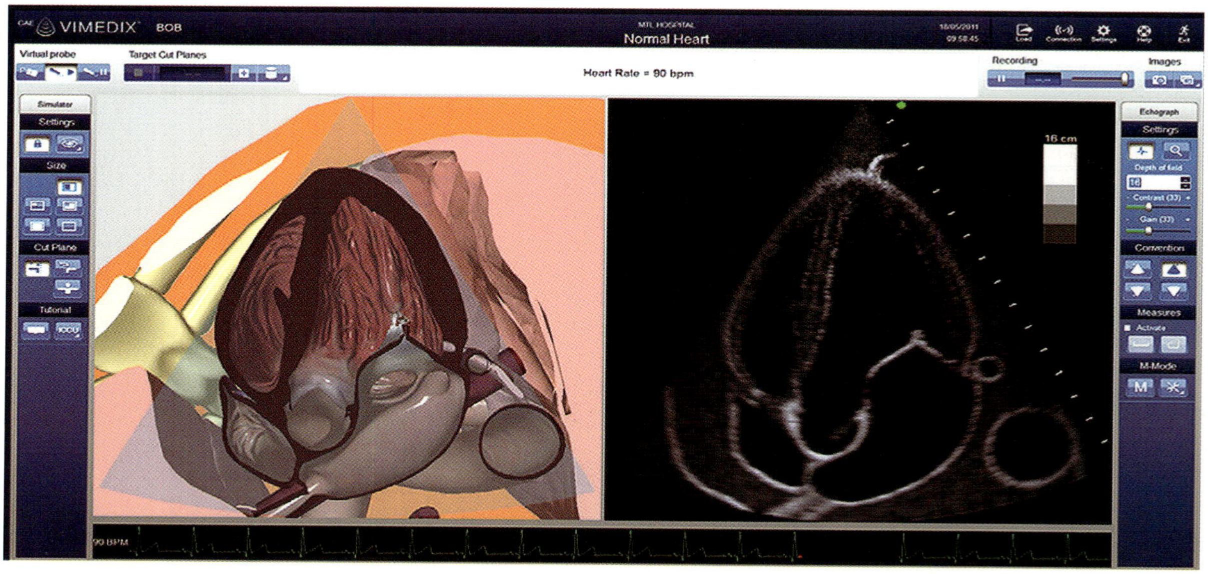

Figure 16 The computer interface and image display of the Vimedix simulation system showing a display option: an augmented reality heart model with a superimposed virtual scan plane (left) and the corresponding rendered 2-dimensional transesophageal echocardiographic image on the other

progress and, depending on the software revision, the quality of the augmented reality heart model can vary, with improvements in the quality over time. E-learning opportunity is not available in this simulator.

The CAE healthcare has developed an interactive multimedia-based curriculum, available on their Web site (*http://www.caeiccu.com*). After subscription, users have access to tutorials on echocardiography and general ultrasonography, image acquisition and interpretation, and self-testing resources. The CAE-ICCU e-learning curriculum has been endorsed by the Canadian Critical Care Society, the American College of Chest Physicians, and the American Medical Association.

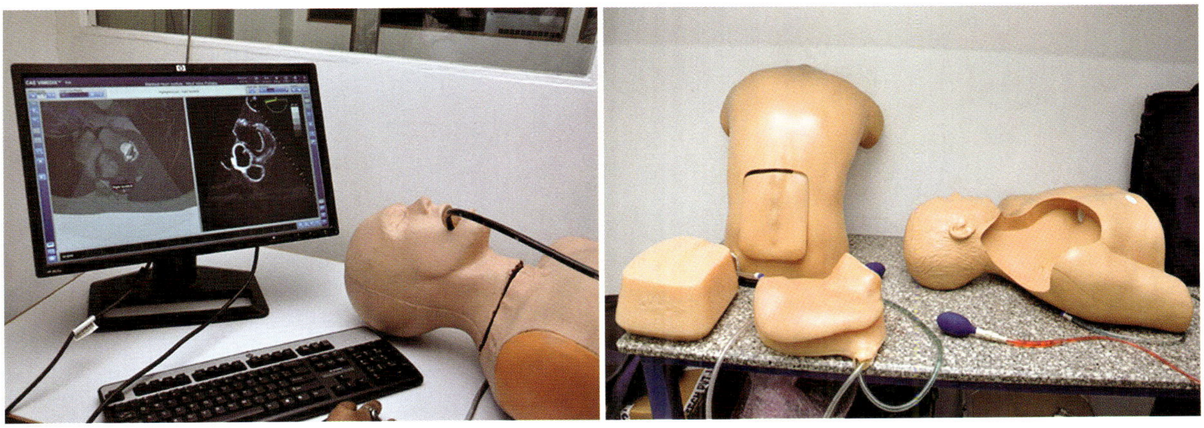

Figure 17 Vimedix simulator mannequin

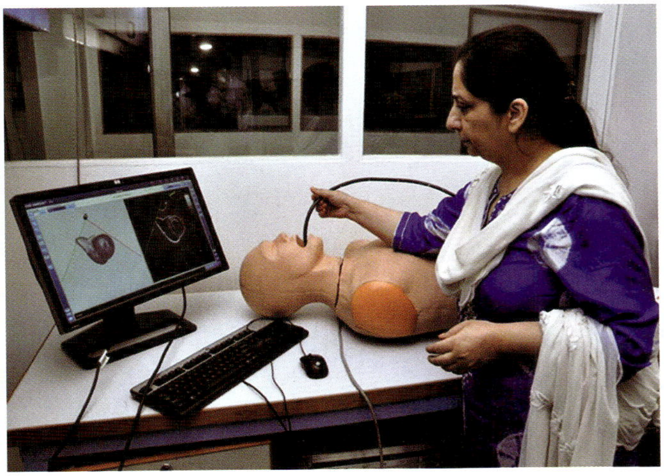

Figure 18 The simulation system consists of a full-sized mannequin, transthoracic/transesophageal echocardiographic probes, and a dedicated computer

Heartworks Simulator (Figure 19)

The system is based on an anatomically correct solid augmented reality model of the heart and ascending aorta and arch. It is offered in a range of options, from laptop-based software alone to a mannequin-based system with TEE and TTE probes. The mannequin simulation package includes a life-sized, latex-free, fiberglass, and rubber-torso mannequin and removable TTE or TEE probes with authentic control buttons.

Advantages/disadvantages of Heartworks: The repertoire of disease states is very limited in this simulator. It is a good teaching tool for normal cardiac anatomy and normal TEE and TTE examinations.[7] The ability to highlight specific intracardiac structures and add descriptive text is a useful teaching feature.

Blue Phantom Simulator (Figure 20)

The simulator is a life-sized mannequin with an articulating head and jaw, anatomically correct nonbeating model of the heart made of a composite material and suspended in the thoracic cavity, accurate anatomic landmarks, and thoracic viscera.

Advantages/disadvantages of blue fhantom simulator: Because it consists of a mannequin and an actual structural model of the heart, any of the commercially available transducers (TEE/TTE) and machines can be used to practice image acquisition skills. The heart model is static and the entire learning experience is limited to probe handling, manipulation, and image orientation.[7] E-learning opportunity is not available in this simulator.

SUMMARY

Transesophageal echocardiography is a user dependent imaging modality **(Figure 21)**. Proper steering of the probe, spatial orientation and knowledge of potential pathologies play a pivotal role. Simulator training cannot replace traditional learning methods in the learning process but can address the main obstacles in the learning process.

One of the main problems when learning TEE is the orientation in space. It can be challenging, even for echocardiographers having experience in TTE, to

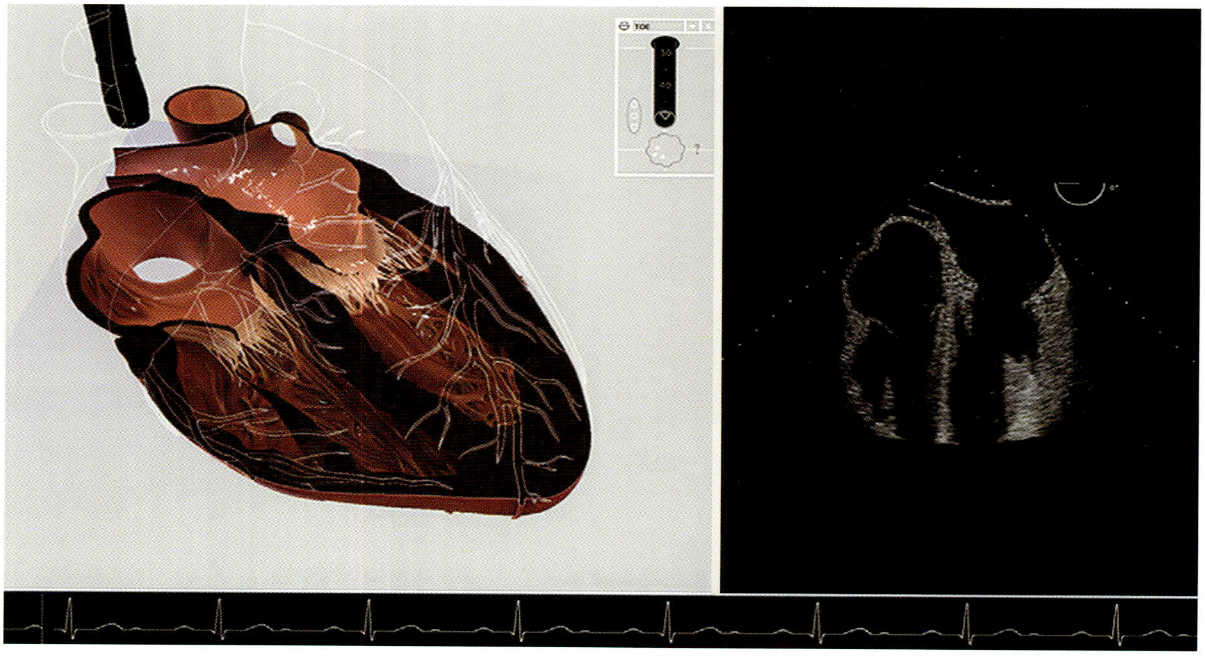

Figure 19 Computer interface of the Heartworks simulation system showing a virtual heart model and scan plane (left) and the rendered echocardiographic image (right)

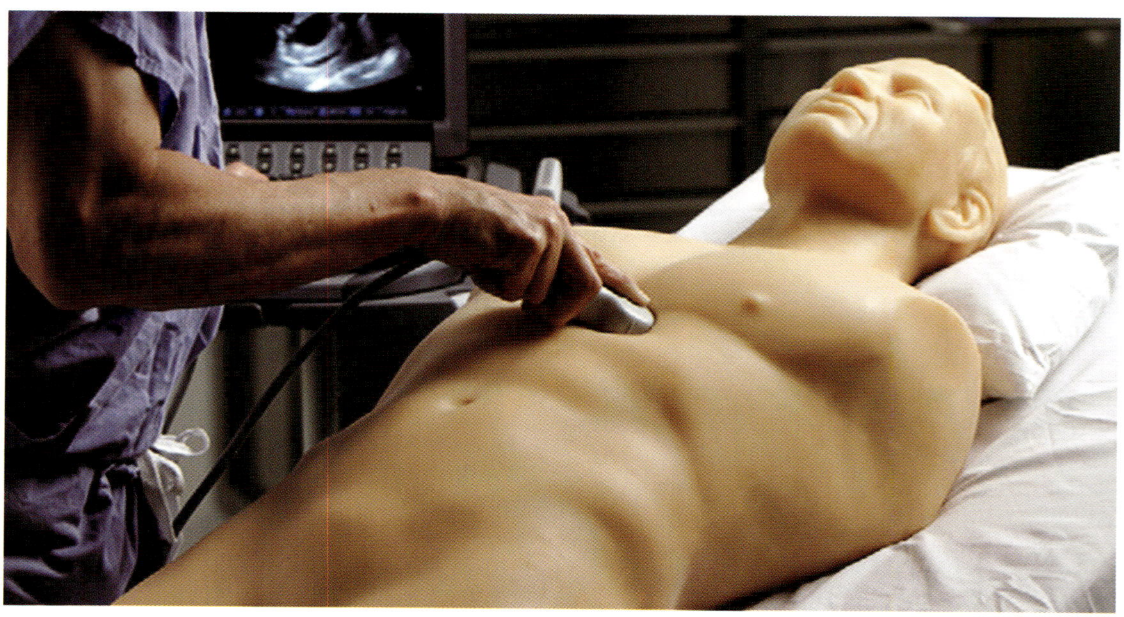

Figure 20 The blue phantom simulation system is a life-sized mannequin with a nonbeating actual model of the heart created with composite materials and suspended in the thoracic cavity of the mannequin. Because it is based on an actual heart model, the simulator can be used with any functioning ultrasound system

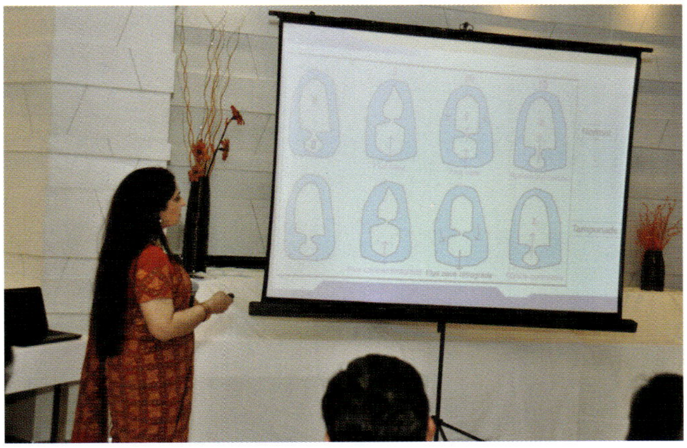

Figure 21 Computer based simulation for transesophageal echocardiography learning makes students learn grasp faster

imagine a 3D heart model seen and then cut in 2D from the esophagus, as in TEE. Experience in TTE is however helpful. It has been addressed in the recent guidelines of the European Association of Echocardiography (EAE), recommending 75 TEE examinations for users having a basic level of experience in TTE and 125 TEE examinations for those without experience in TTE and wanting to receive EAE accreditation to perform TEE independently.[8]

REFERENCES

1. Shakil O, Mahmood F, Matyal R. Simulation in echocardiography: an ever-expanding frontier. J Cardiothorac Vasc Anesth. 2012;26(3):476-85.
2. Kim H, Matyal R, Mahmood F, et al. 1653632 - Measurement of accuracy in transesophageal echocardiography by simulation. *http://www.cas.ca/English/Page/Files/812_1653632.pdf*
3. Naik VN, Wong AK, Hamstra SJ. Review article: leading the future: guiding two predominant paradigm shifts in medical education through scholarship. Can J Anaesth. 2012;59(2):213-23.
4. Sohmer B, Hudson C, Hudson J, et al. Transesophageal echocardiography simulation is an effective tool in teaching psychomotor skills to novice echocardiographers. Can J Anaesth. 2014;61(3):235-41.
5. Weidenbach M, Wick C, Pieper S, et al. Augmented reality simulator for training in two-dimensional echocardiography. Comput Biomed Res. 2000;33:11-22.
6. Weidenbach M, Drachsler H, Wild F, et al. EchoComTEE—A simulator for transesophageal echocardiography. J Anesth. 2007;62:347-53.
7. Matyal R, Bose R, Warraich H, et al. Transthoracic echocardiographic simulator: Normal and the abnormal. J Cardiothorac Vasc Anesth. 2011;25:177-81.
8. Kempny A, Piórkowski A, et al. CT2TEE—a novel, internet-based simulator of transesophageal echocardiography in congenital heart disease. Kardiologia Polska. 2010;68:3.

Chapter 9

Simulation for Two-dimensional and Three-dimensional Transesophageal Echocardiography Views

Poonam Malhotra Kapoor, Kalpana Irpachi, Sarvesh Pal Singh, SN Das, Viswas Malik, Suruchi Hasija

Chapter Outline

- Terminology of Transesophageal Echocardiography Probe Manipulation
- Multiplane Probe Angle (0°–180°)
- Midesophageal Four-chamber View
- Midesophageal Two-chamber View
- Midesophageal Mitral Commissural View
- Midesophageal Long-axis View
- Midesophageal Aortic Valve: Long-axis View
- Midesophageal Aortic Valve: Short-axis View
- Midesophageal Bicaval View
- Midesophageal Descending Aorta: Long-axis View
- Midesophageal Descending Aorta: Short-axis View
- Midesophageal Ascending Aorta: Long-axis View
- Midesophageal Ascending Aorta: Short-axis View
- Midesophageal Left Atrial Appendage View
- Midesophageal Modified Bicaval View
- Midesophageal Right Ventricular Inflow-outflow View
- Lower Esophageal Coronary Sinus View
- Transgastric Modified Hepatic Vein View
- Transgastric Two-chamber View
- Transgastric Apical: Short-axis View
- Transgastric Basal: Long-axis View
- Transgastric Basal: Short-axis View
- Transgastric Midpapillary: Short-axis View
- Transgastric Right Ventricular Inflow-outflow View
- Transgastric Right Ventricular Inflow View
- Transgastric Basal Right Ventricular Outflow View
- Deep Transgastric: Long-axis View
- Upper Esophageal Aortic Arch: Long-axis View
- Upper Esophageal Aortic Arch: Short-axis View

INTRODUCTION

Transesophageal echocardiography (TEE) has the unique advantage of portability, high resolution images of normal or abnormal cardiovascular anatomy and function, easy to perform, low risk of complication and stepwise approach is best.

The 28 basic two-dimensional (2D) and three-dimensional (3D) TEE views as described by the Society of Cardiovascular Anesthesiologists (SCA) and American Society of Echocardiography (ASE) are diagrammed here. Conveniently the views are grouped together by the structures being interrogated **(Figures 1 to 6)**:

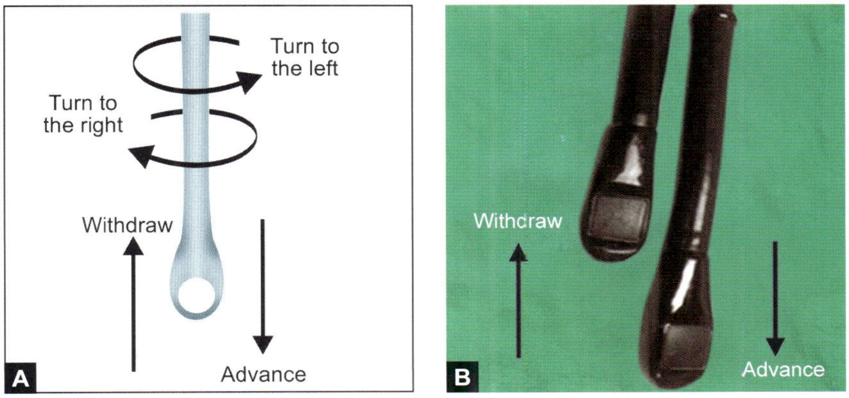

Figures 1A and B Terminology of TEE probe manipulation

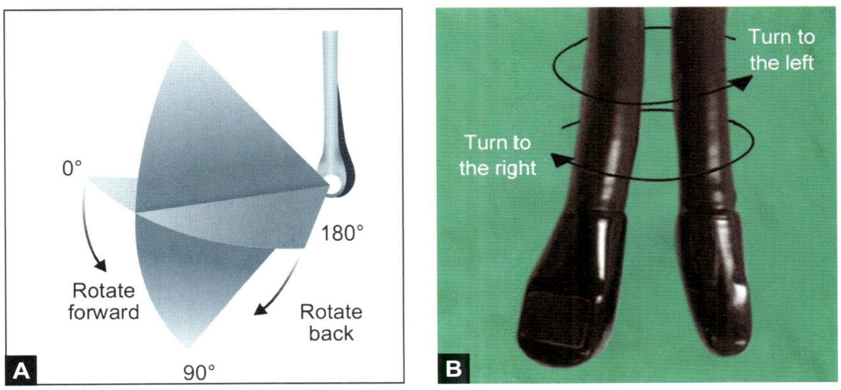

Figures 2A and B Advance, withdraw, pushing or pulling of the TEE probe

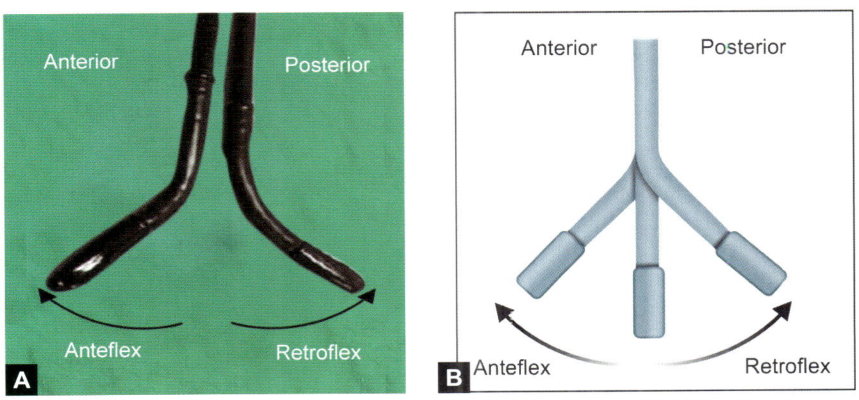

Figures 3A and B Anteflex, retroflex: anteflex is flexing the tip of the TEE probe anteriorly by turning the large control wheel clockwise. Retroflex is flexing the tip of the TEE probe posteriorly by turning the large wheel anticlockwise

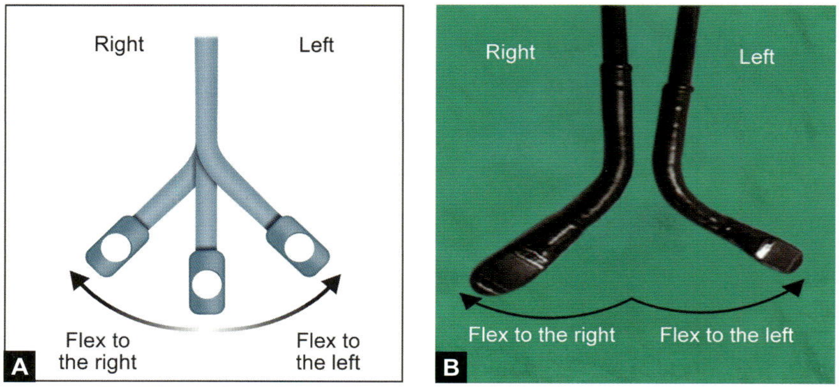

Figures 4A and B Flex to right, flex to left: flexing the tip of the TEE probe with the small control wheel to the patient's right or left. The probe flexion to the right and left may not be necessary and should be avoided to minimize trauma to the esophagus

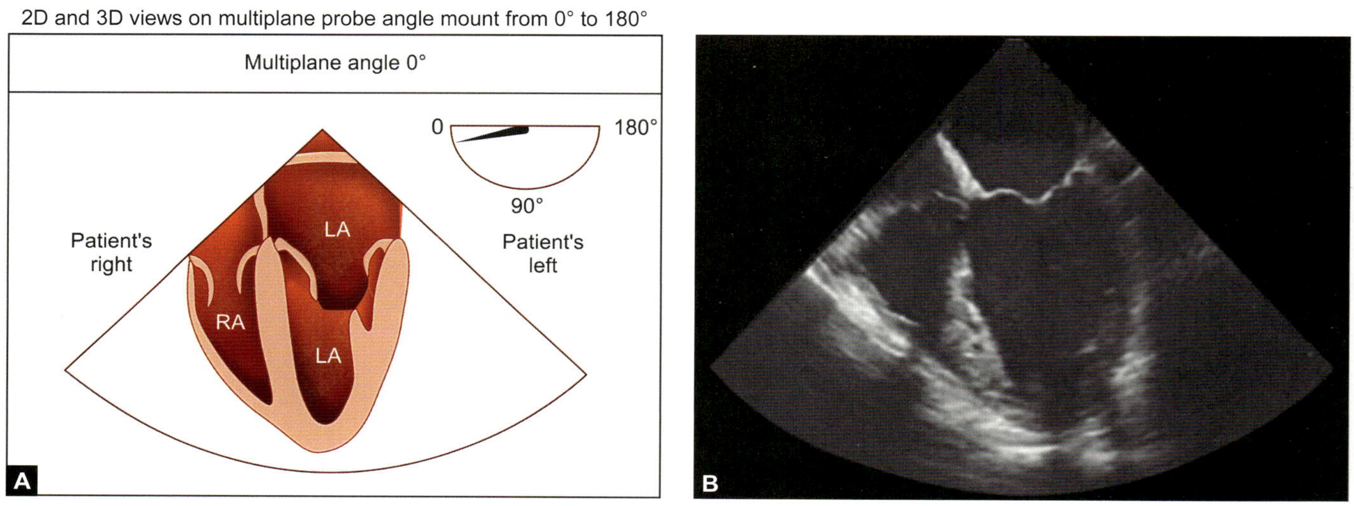

Figures 5A and B At a multiplane angle of 0 degree, the patient's right sided structures will be displayed on the left of the image display
Abbreviations: LA, left atrium; RV, right ventricle; LV, left ventricle

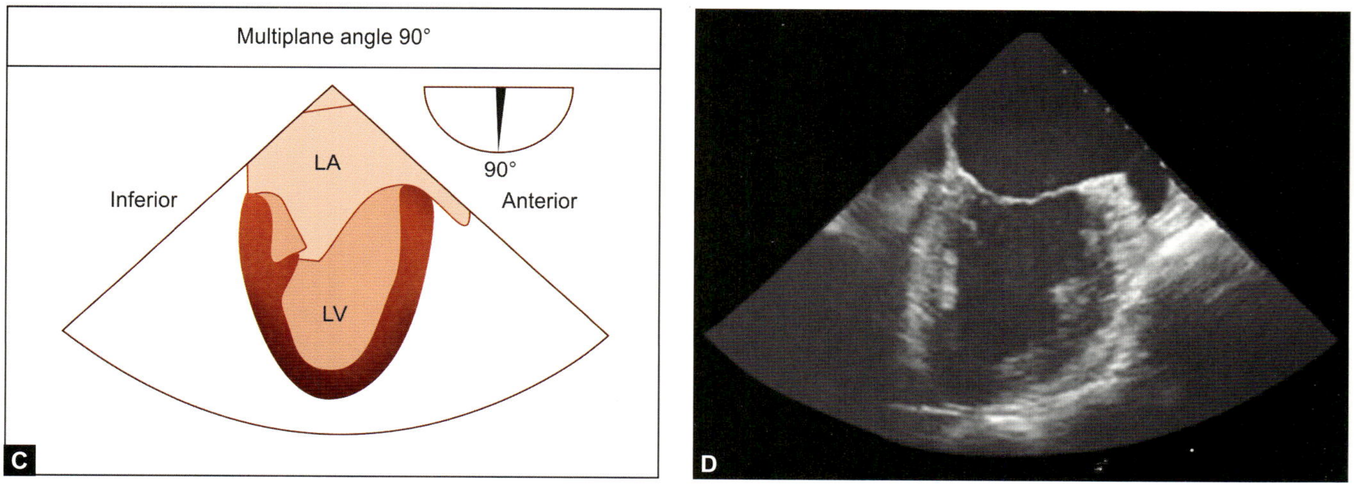

Figures 5C and D By rotating the multiplane angle forward to 90 degrees left side of the image d splay shows posterior structure
Abbreviations: LA, left atrium; LV, left ventricle

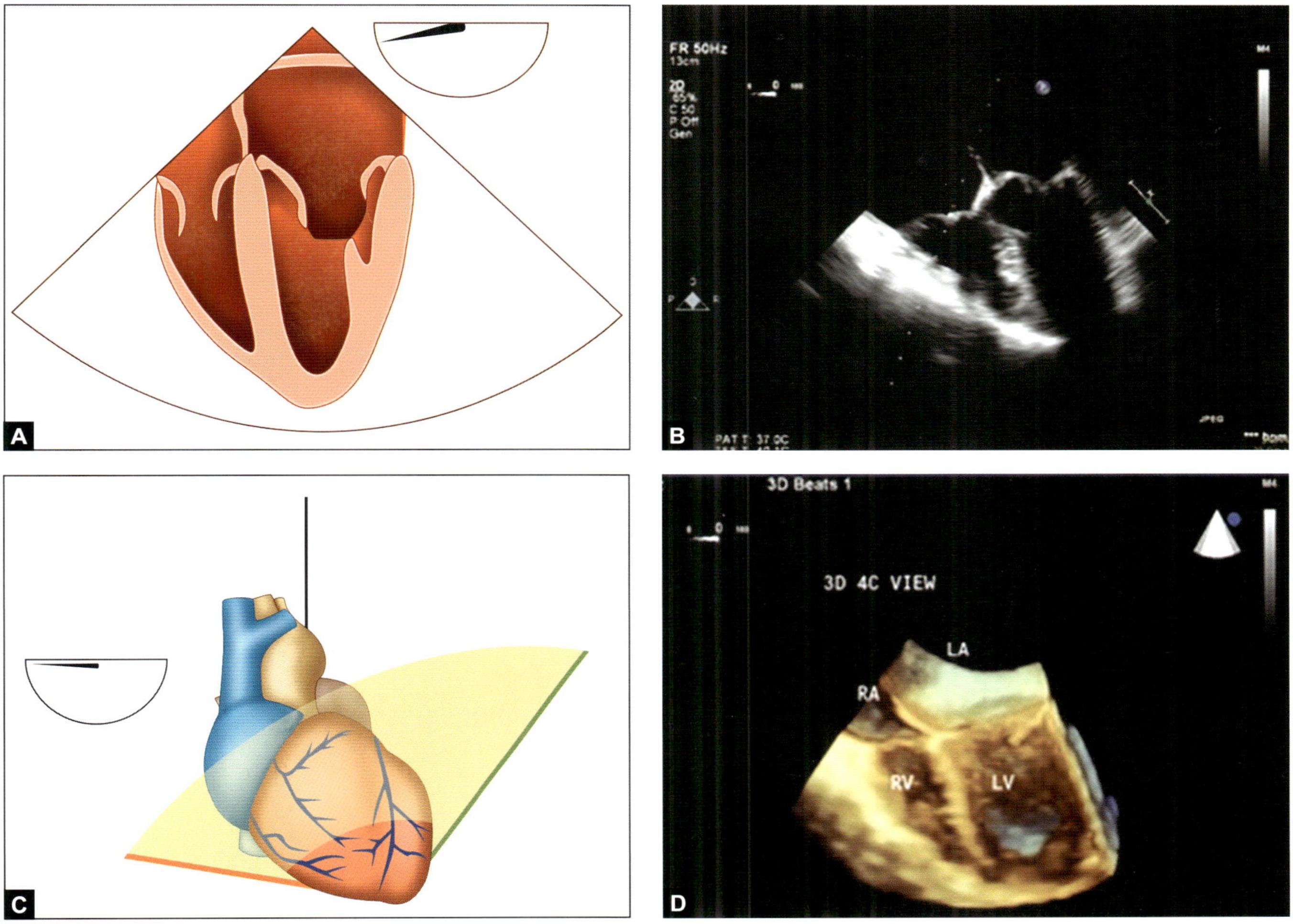

Figures 6A to D Midesophageal four-chamber view

TERMINOLOGY OF TRANSESOPHAGEAL ECHOCARDIOGRAPHY PROBE MANIPULATION

Advance, withdraw: Pushing or pulling the tip of the TEE probe.

Turn to right, turn to left (also referred to as clockwise and anticlockwise): Rotating the anterior aspect of the TEE probe to the right or left of the patient.

Anteflex, retroflex: Anteflex is flexing the tip of the TEE probe anteriorly by turning the large control wheel clockwise. retroflex is flexing the tip of the TEE probe posteriorly by turning the large wheel anticlockwise.

Flex to right, flex to left: Flexing the tip of the TEE probe with the small control wheel to the patient's right or left. the probe flexion to the right and left may not be necessary and should be avoided to minimize trauma to the esophagus.

MULTIPLANE PROBE ANGLE (0°–180°)

At a multiplane angle of 0°, the patient's right sided structures will be displayed on the left of the image display.

By rotating the multiplane angle foreward to 90° left side of the image display shows posterior structure.

MIDESOPHAGEAL FOUR-CHAMBER VIEW

The midesophageal (ME) 4C view is obtained by positioning the probe in the midesophagus behind the left atrium (LA). The imaging plane is directed through the LA, center of the mitral valve (MV) and left ventricular (LV) apex. A snapshot of the heart shows all four chambers [(LA, right atrium (RA), LV, right ventricle (RV), two valves (MV, tricuspid valve TV), the septa (interatrial septum IAS, interventricular septum IVS) and the inferoseptal (IS) and lateral (L) LV walls.

- *Multiplane angle range:*
  - 0 ~ 20°
  - *Sector depth:* ~ 12–14 cm
- *Anatomy imaged:*
  - Left ventricle and atrium
  - Right ventricle and atrium
  - Mitral and tricuspid valves
  - Interatrial and interventricular septum
- *Clinical utility:*
  - *Ventricle function:* Global and regional
  - *Intracardiac chamber masses:* Thrombus, tumor, air, foreign bodies
  - *Mitral and tricuspid valve evaluation:* Pathology, pathophysiology
  - Congenital or acquired interatrial and ventral septal defects
  - Hypertrophic obstructive cardiomyopathy evaluation.

MIDESOPHAGEAL TWO-CHAMBER VIEW (FIGURES 7A TO D)

The ME 2C view is obtained by increasing the omniplane angle to 90° from the ME 4C (0°) or ME mitral commissural (45–60°) views. The right atrium (RA) and right ventricle (RV) are eliminated from the

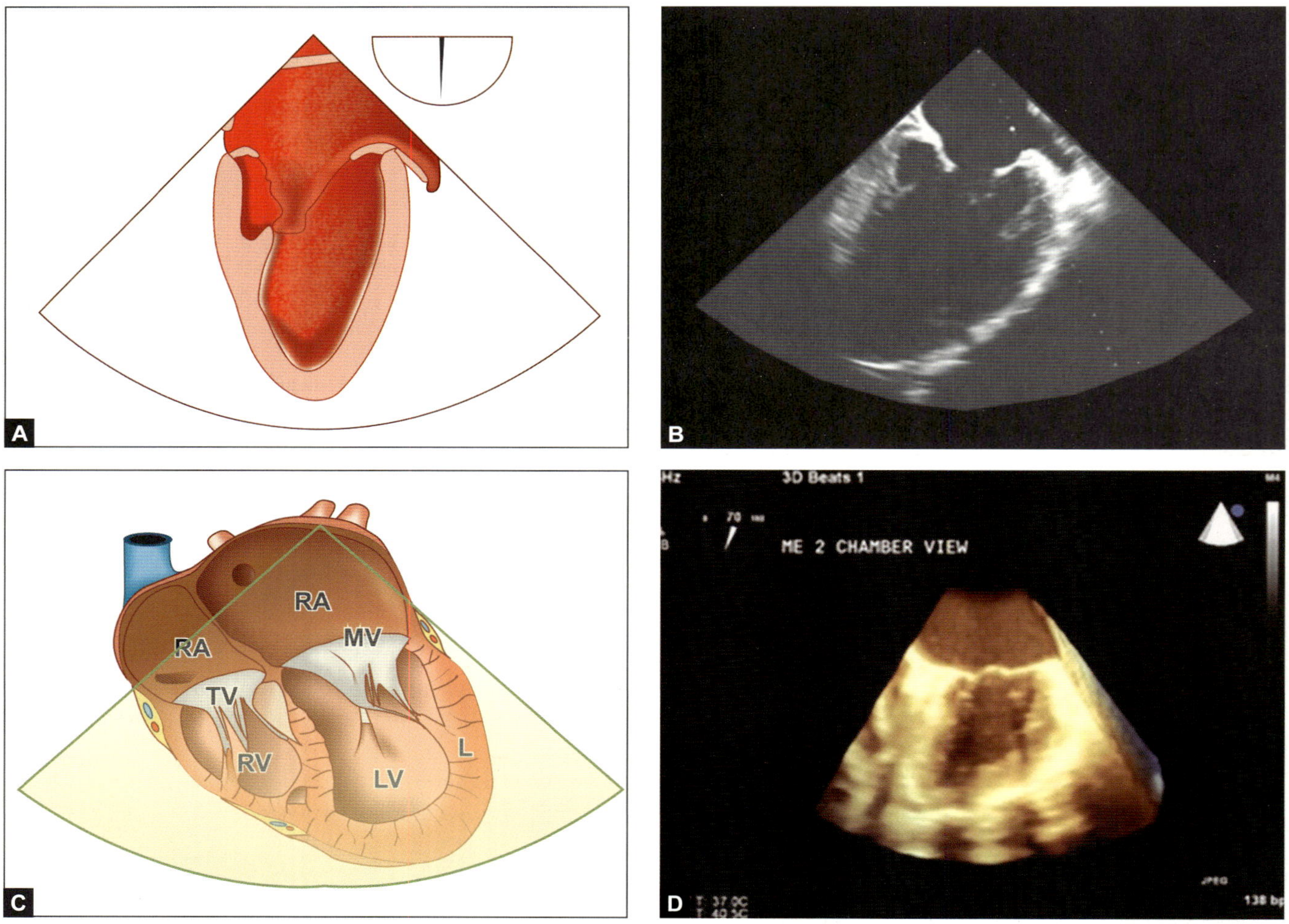

Figures 7A to D Midesophageal two-chamber view
Abbreviations: RA, right atrium; LA, left atrium; TV, tricuspid valve; MV, mitral valve; LV, left ventricle; RV, right ventricle; L, lateral

display. This view is orthogonal to the ME 4C view. The image is displayed with the cephalad part (anterior wall) below the left atrial appendage (LAA) to the right and the caudad part (inferior wall) to the left.

- *Multiplane angle range:*
  - 80–100°
  - *Sector depth:* ~ 12–14 cm
- *Anatomy imaged left ventricle, atrium, and atrial appendage:*
  - Mitral valve
  - *Left pulmonary veins:* Turning probe to left
  - Coronary sinus (short-axis or long-axis by turning probe tip to left)
- *Clinical utility:*
  - *Left ventricle function:* Global and regional
  - *Left ventricle and atrial masses:* Thrombus, tumor, air; foreign bodies
  - *Mitral valve evaluation:* Pathology, pathophysiology
  - Ventricular diastolic evaluation via transmitral and pulmonary vein Doppler flow profile analysis
  - *Coronary sinus evaluation:* Coronary sinus catheter placement; dilation secondary to persistent left superior vena cava.

MIDESOPHAGEAL MITRAL COMMISSURAL VIEW (FIGURES 8A TO D)

In the ME mitral commissural (MC) view, the scanning plane is now orientated at 45°–70° imaging through the left atrium (LA), center of the mitral valve (MV) and left ventricular (LV) apex. The P3 scallop (left), P1 scallops (right) and AMVL (usually A2) is in the middle forming

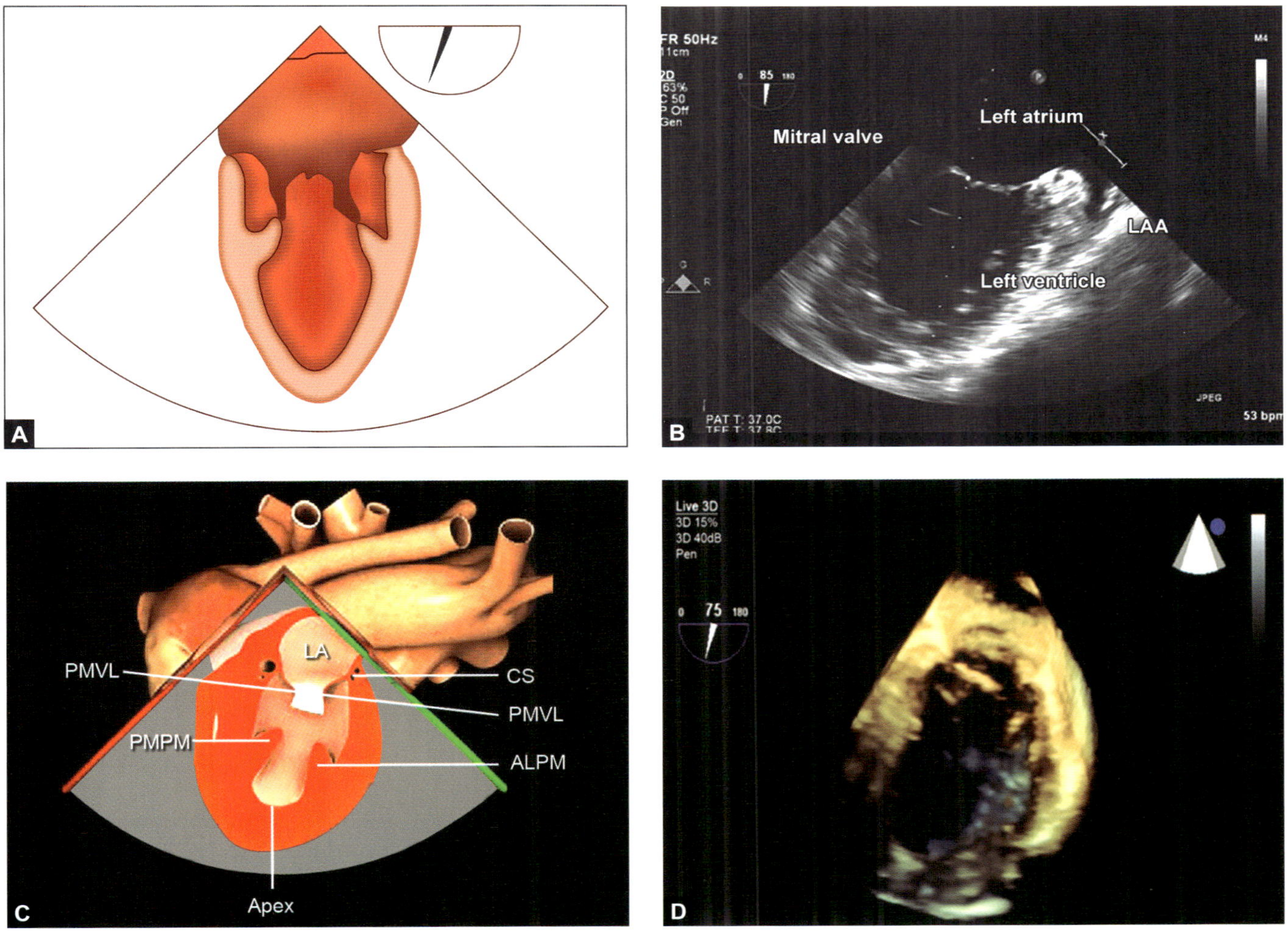

Figures 8A to D Midesophageal ME mitral commissural view

Abbreviations: ALPM, anterolateral papillary muscle; PMVL, posterior mitral valuve leaflet; PMPM, pulmonary papillary muscle; LA, left atrium; CS, coronary sinus

the intermittently seen "trap door." The probe is carefully manipulated to image both the posteromedial (PM) and anterolateral (AL) papillary muscles and LV apex.

- *Multiplane angle range:*
  - 60–70°
  - Sector depth: ~ 12 cm
- *Anatomy imaged:*
  - Left ventricle and atrium
  - Mitral valve
- *Clinical utility:*
  - *Left ventricle function:* Global and regional
  - *Left ventricle and atrial masses:* Thrombus, tumor, air; foreign bodies
  - Mitral valve evaluation: pathology, pathophysiology
  - Ventricular diastolic evaluation via transmitral Doppler flow profile analysis.

MIDESOPHAGEAL LONG-AXIS VIEW (FIGURES 9A TO D)

The ME long-axis (LAX) view is obtained by increasing the omniplane angle to 120° from the ME 4C (0°) or ME MC (45–60°) or ME 2C (90°) views. The more cephalad structures including the left ventricular outflow tract (LVOT), aortic valve (AV) and the proximal ascending aorta are lined up on the display right. The apex of the left ventricle (LV) and inferolateral (IL) and anteroseptal (AS) walls are seen.

- *Multiplane angle range:*
  - 120–160°
  - *Sector depth:* ~ 12–14 cm
- *Anatomy imaged:*
  - Left ventricle and atrium
  - Left ventricular outflow tract
  - Aortic valve

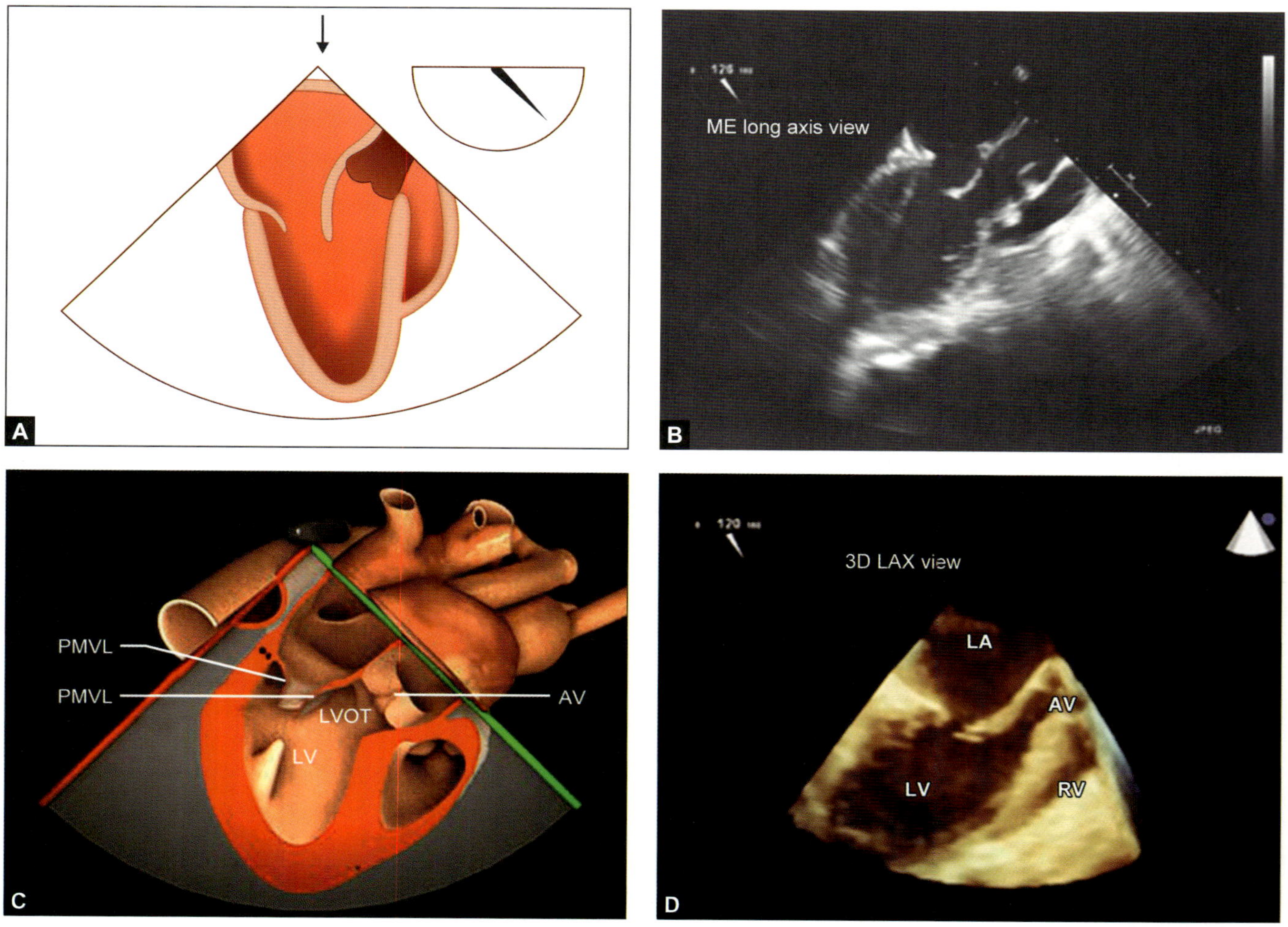

Figures 9A to D Midesophageal long axis view

Abbreviations: PMVL, posterior mitral valve leaflet; LVOT, left ventricular outflow tract; AV, aortic valve; LV, left ventricle; LA, left atrium

- Mitral valve
- Ascending aorta
- *Clinical utility:*
  - *Left ventricle function:* Global and regional
  - *Left ventricle and atrial masses:* Thrombus, tumor, air; foreign bodies
  - *Mitral valve evaluation:* Pathology, pathophysiology.
  - Ventricular diastolic evaluation via transmitral Doppler flow profile analysis
  - *Aortic valve evaluation:* Pathology, pathophysiology
  - *Ascending aorta pathology:* Atherosclerosis, aneurysms, dissections
  - Hypertrophic obstructive cardiomyopathy evaluation

MIDESOPHAGEAL AORTIC VALVE: LONG-AXIS VIEW (FIGURES 10A TO D)

The ME aortic valve (AV) LAX view is obtained by decreasing the display depth from the ME LAX view (120°). The left ventricular outflow tract (LVOT), AV and the proximal ascending aorta are lined up on the display right and the remainder of the mitral valve (MV) and left ventricle (LV) are eliminated from the image.

- *Multiplane angle range:*
  - 120–160°
  - Sector depth: ~ 8–10 cm
- *Anatomy imaged:*
  - Aortic valve
  - Proximal ascending aorta
  - Left ventricular outflow tract

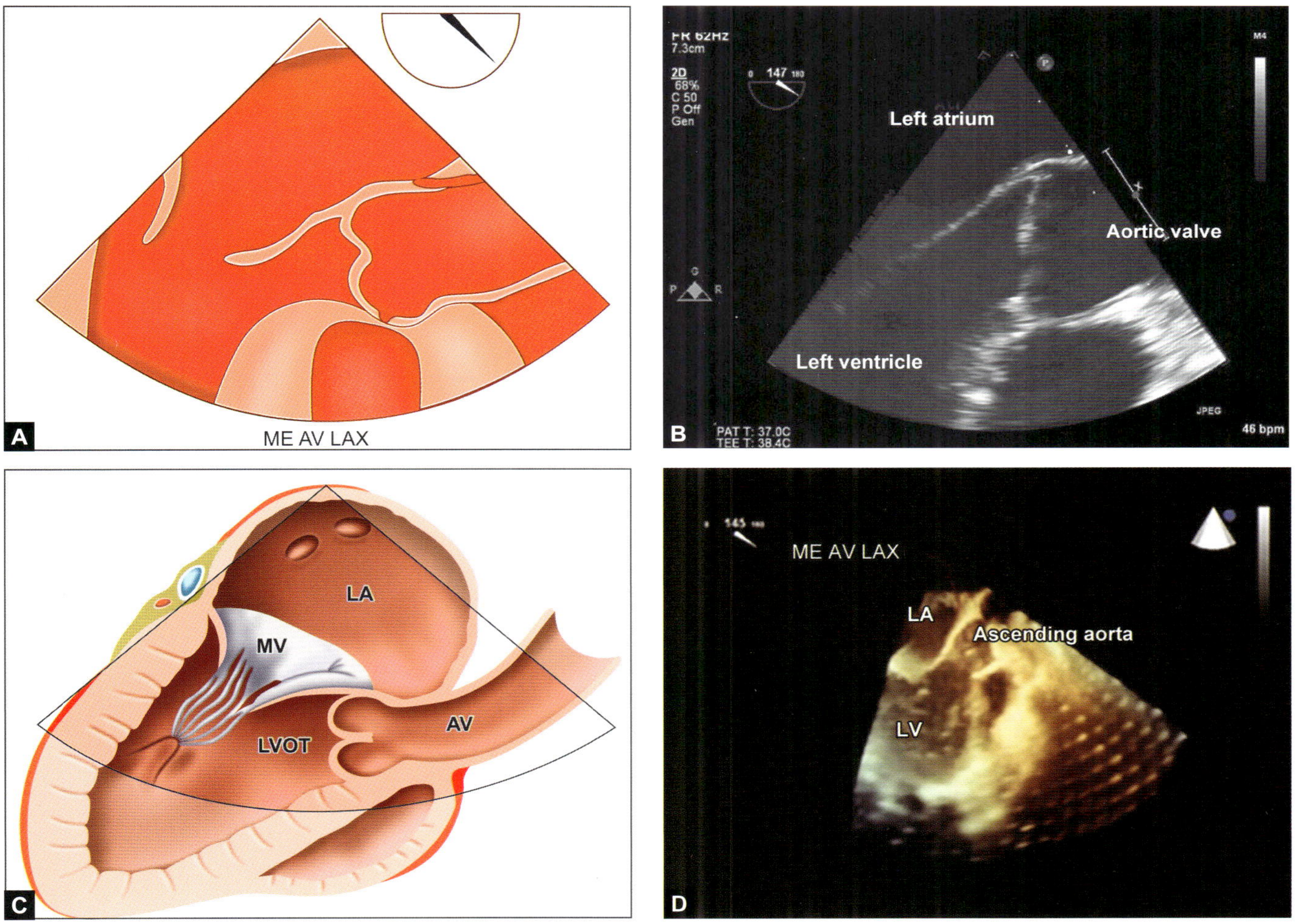

Figures 10A to D Midesophageal aortic long-axis valve

Abbreviations: ME, midesophageal; AV, aortic valve; LAX, long-axis; LA, left atrium; MV, mitral valve; LVOT, left ventricular outflow tract

- Mitral valve
- Right pulmonary artery
- *Clinical utility:*
  - *Aortic valve:* Pathology; pathophysiology
  - *Ascending aorta pathology:* Atherosclerosis, aneurysms and dissections
  - *Mitral valve evaluation:* Pathology, pathophysiology.

MIDESOPHAGEAL AORTIC VALVE: SHORT-AXIS VIEW (FIGURES 11A TO D)

From the ME 4C view, the probe is withdrawn until the aortic valve (AV) is positioned centrally. To obtain the ME AV SAX view, increase the omniplane angle to 30°–45° with slight anteflexion to align the imaging plane parallel to the AV annulus. All three aortic cusps appear symmetrical. Withdraw the probe to image the orifices of the left main and right coronary arteries.

- *Multiplane angle range:*
  - 30–60°
  - *Sector depth:* ~ 10–12 cm
- *Anatomy imaged aortic valve:*
  - Interatrial septum
  - Coronary ostia and arteries
  - Right ventricular outflow tract
  - Pulmonary valve
- *Clinical utility:*
  - *Aortic valve:* Pathology; pathophysiology
  - *Ascending aorta pathology:* Atherosclerosis, aneurysms and dissections

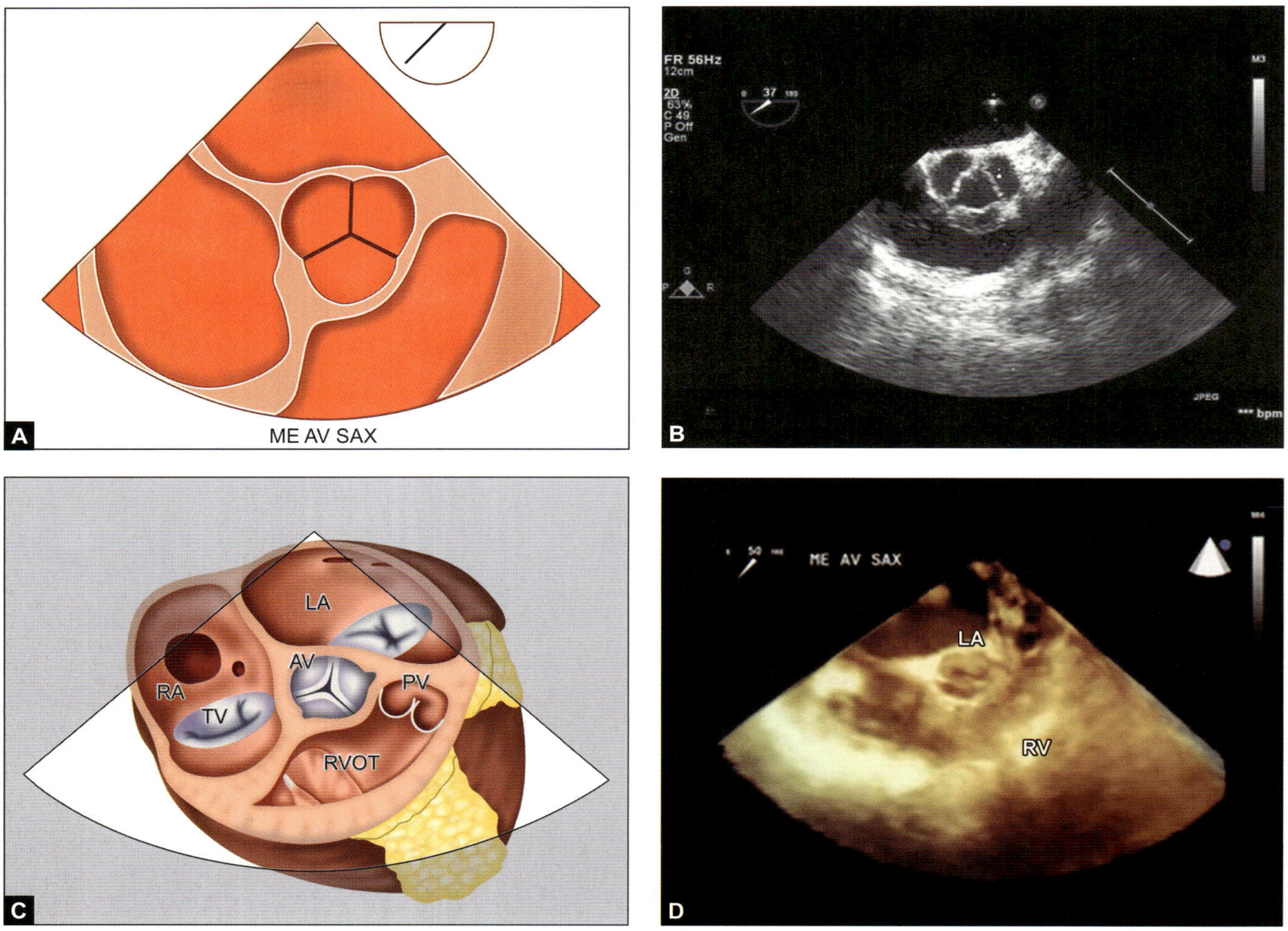

Figures 11A to D Midesophageal aortic valve: short-axis view
Abbreviations: ME, midesophageal; AV, aortic valve; LAX, long-axis; LV, left atrium; RV, right atrium; TV, tricuspid valve; PV, pulmonic valve; RVOT, right ventricular outflow tract

- *Left and right atrial masses:* Thrombus, embolus, air, tumor, foreign bodies
- Congenital or acquired interatrial septal defects evaluation.

MIDESOPHAGEAL BICAVAL VIEW (FIGURES 12A TO D)

The view is obtained from the ME 2C view (90°) by turning the entire probe to the patient's right towards the superior vena cava (SVC) and inferior vena cava (IVC). The transducer plane cuts through the left atrium (LA), right atrium (RA), and LAX of the IVC and SVC. The structures are displayed with the LA at the sector apex (closest to probe), RA in the far field and caudad IVC (left) and cephalad SVC (right).

- *Multiplane angle range*
  - 80–110°
  - *Sector depth:* ~ 8–10 cm
- *Anatomy imaged:*
  - Right and left atrium
  - Superior vena cava (long-axis)
  - *Inferior vena cava orifice:* Advance probe and turn to right to visualize inferior vena cava in the long-axis, liver, hepatic and portal veins
  - Interatrial septum
  - *Right pulmonary veins:* Turn probe to right
- *Clinical utility:*
  - *Right and left atrial masses:* Thrombus, embolus, air, tumor, foreign bodies
  - *Superior vena cava pathology:* Thrombus, sinus venosus atrial septal defect

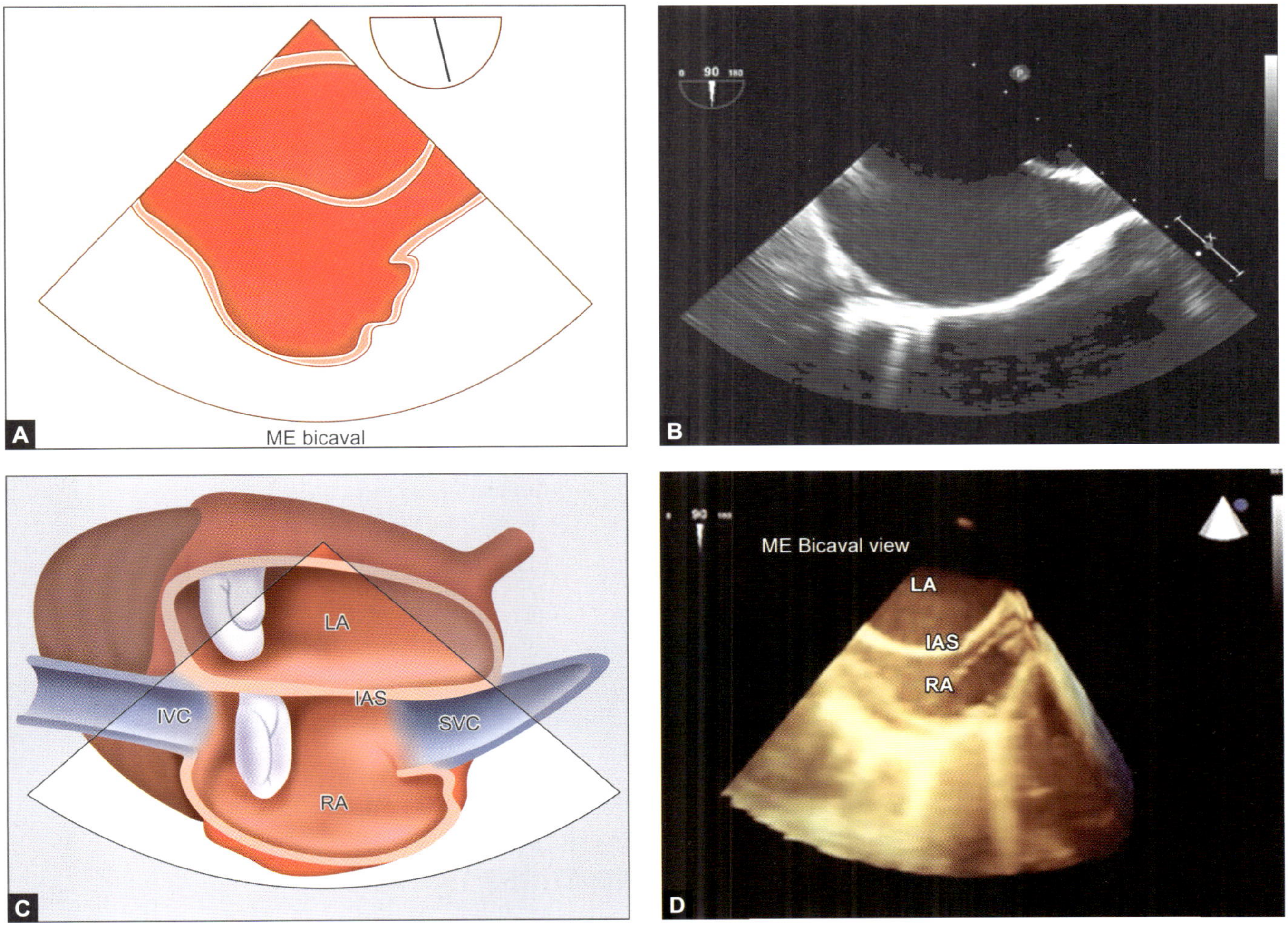

Figures 12A to D Midesophageal bicaval view

Abbreviations: ME, midesophageal; LA, left atrium; IVC, inferior vena cava; IAS, interatrial septum; SVC, superior vena cava; RA, right atrium

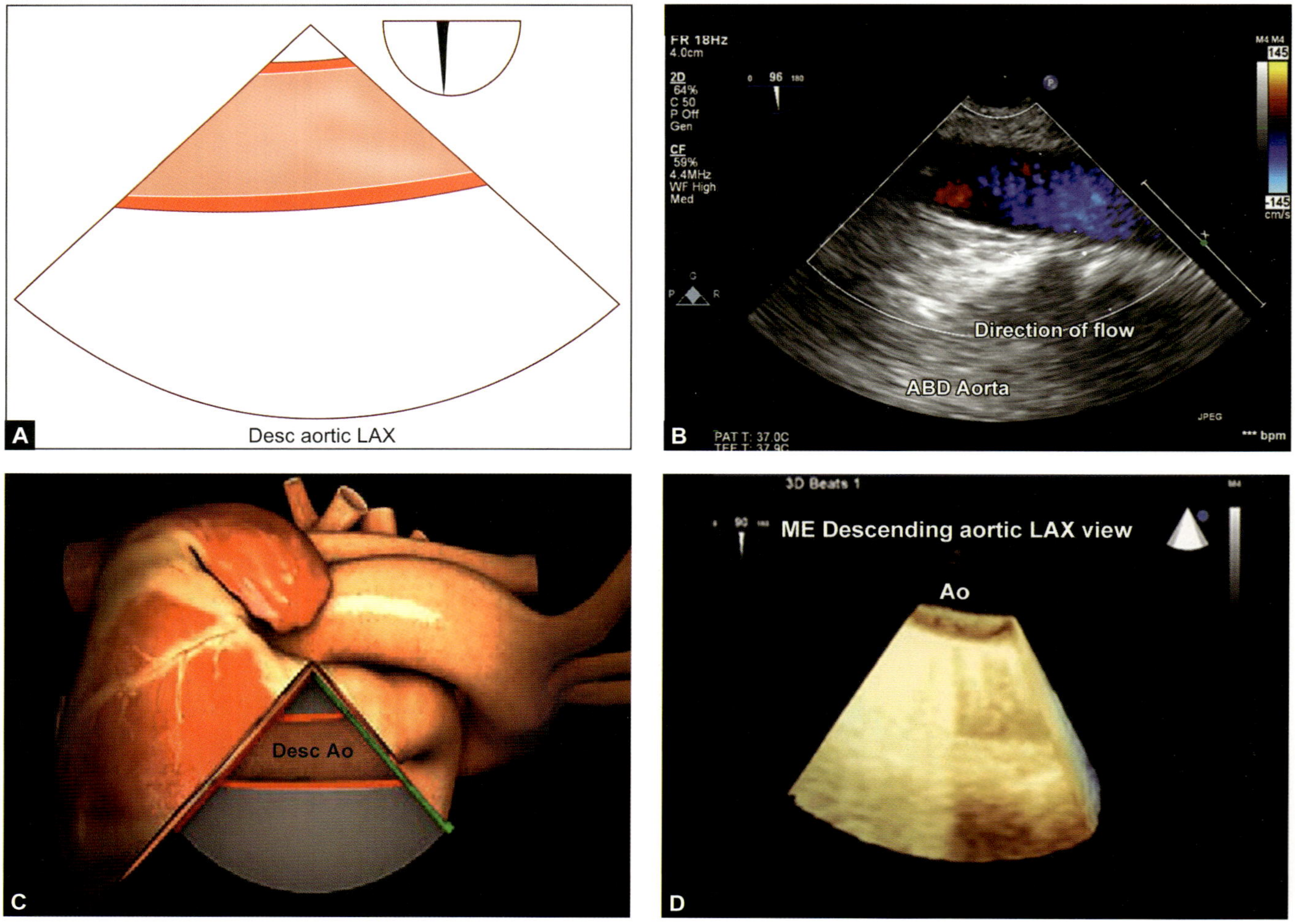

Figures 13A to D Midesophageal descending aorta: long-axis view
Abbreviations: Desc, descending; LAX, long-axis; Ao, aorta; ABD, abdominal

- Inferior vena cava pathology (thrombus, tumor)
- Femoral venous line placement
- Coronary sinus catheter line placement
- *Right pulmonary vein evaluation:* Anomalous return, Doppler evaluation for left ventricular diastolic function

MIDESOPHAGEAL DESCENDING AORTA: LONG-AXIS VIEW (FIGURES 13A TO D)

From the descending thoracic aorta SAX view (0°) the transducer angle is increased to 90° to obtain the descending aortic LAX view. The distal aorta is to the display left and the proximal aorta to the display right.

- *Multiplane angle range:*
  - 90–110°
  - Sector depth: ~ 6 cm
- *Anatomy imaged:*
  - Descending thoracic aorta
  - Left pleural space
- *Clinical utility:*
  - *Descending aorta pathology:* Atherosclerosis, aneurysms, and dissections
  - Intra-aortic balloon placement evaluation
  - Left pleural effusion

MIDESOPHAGEAL DESCENDING AORTA: SHORT-AXIS VIEW (FIGURES 14A TO D)

The descending thoracic aorta is visualized in SAX (0°) by turning the probe to the left from the ME 4C view (0°). The near field image of the circular aorta

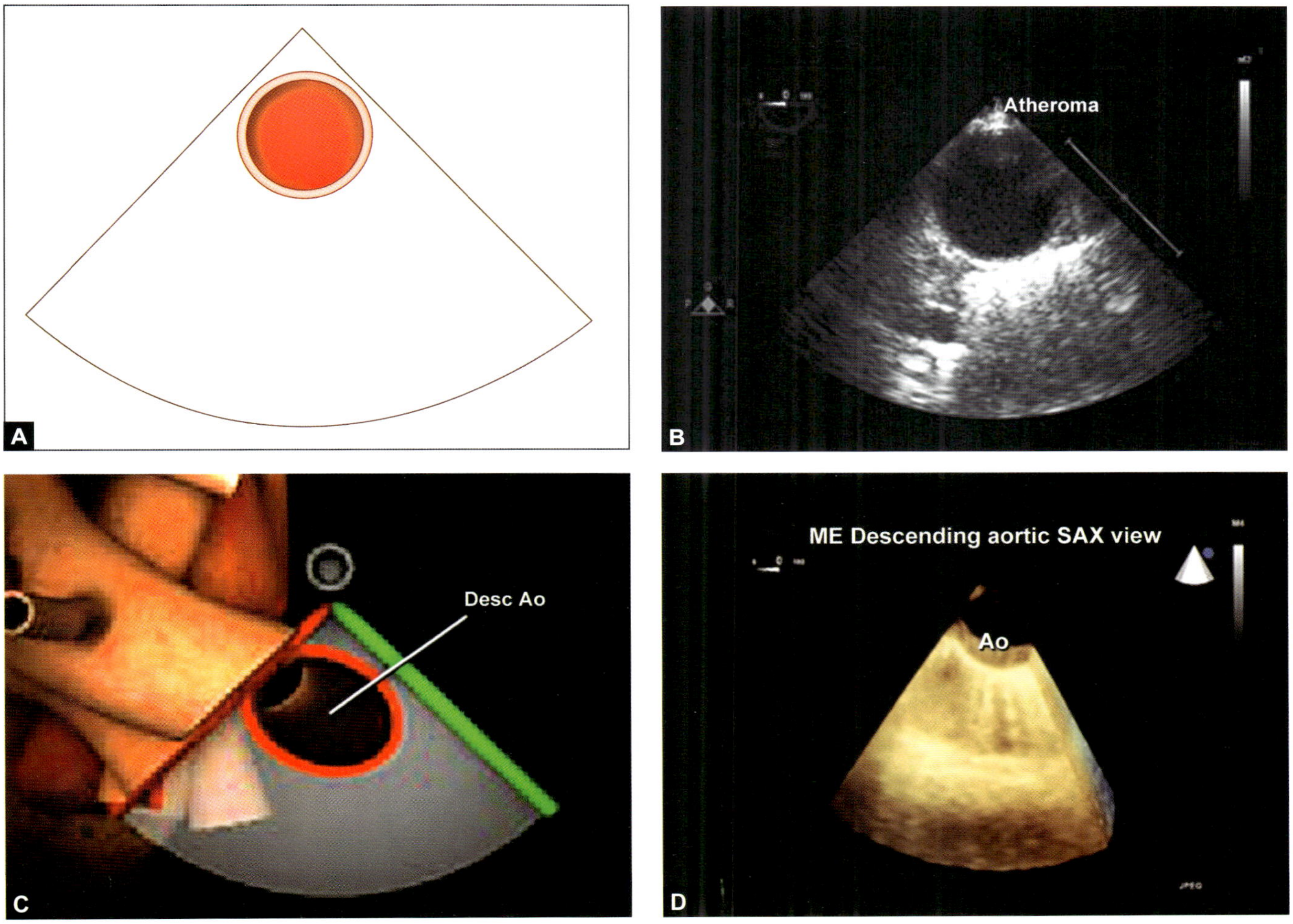

Figures 14A to D Midesophageal descending aorta: short-axis view
Abbreviations: Desc, descending; Ao, aorta

represents the right anterior wall of the aorta. Advance and withdraw the probe to image the entire descending aorta. Decrease the display depth.

- *Multiplane angle range:*
  - 0°
  - Sector depth: ~ 6 cm
- *Anatomy imaged:*
  - Descending thoracic aorta
  - Left pleural space
- *Clinical utility:*
  - *Descending aorta pathology:* Atherosclerosis, aneurysms, and dissections
  - Intra-aortic balloon placement evaluation
  - Left pleural effusion.

MIDESOPHAGEAL ASCENDING AORTA: LONG-AXIS VIEW (FIGURES 15A TO D)

The mid-ascending aorta (Ascending aorta) in LAX may be visualized from the ME AV LAX (120°), by withdrawing the probe to image the right pulmonary artery (RPA) in SAX.

- *Multiplane angle range:*
  - 100–150°
  - *Sector depth:* ~ 12 cm
- *Anatomy imaged:*
  - Ascending aorta
  - Right pulmonary artery

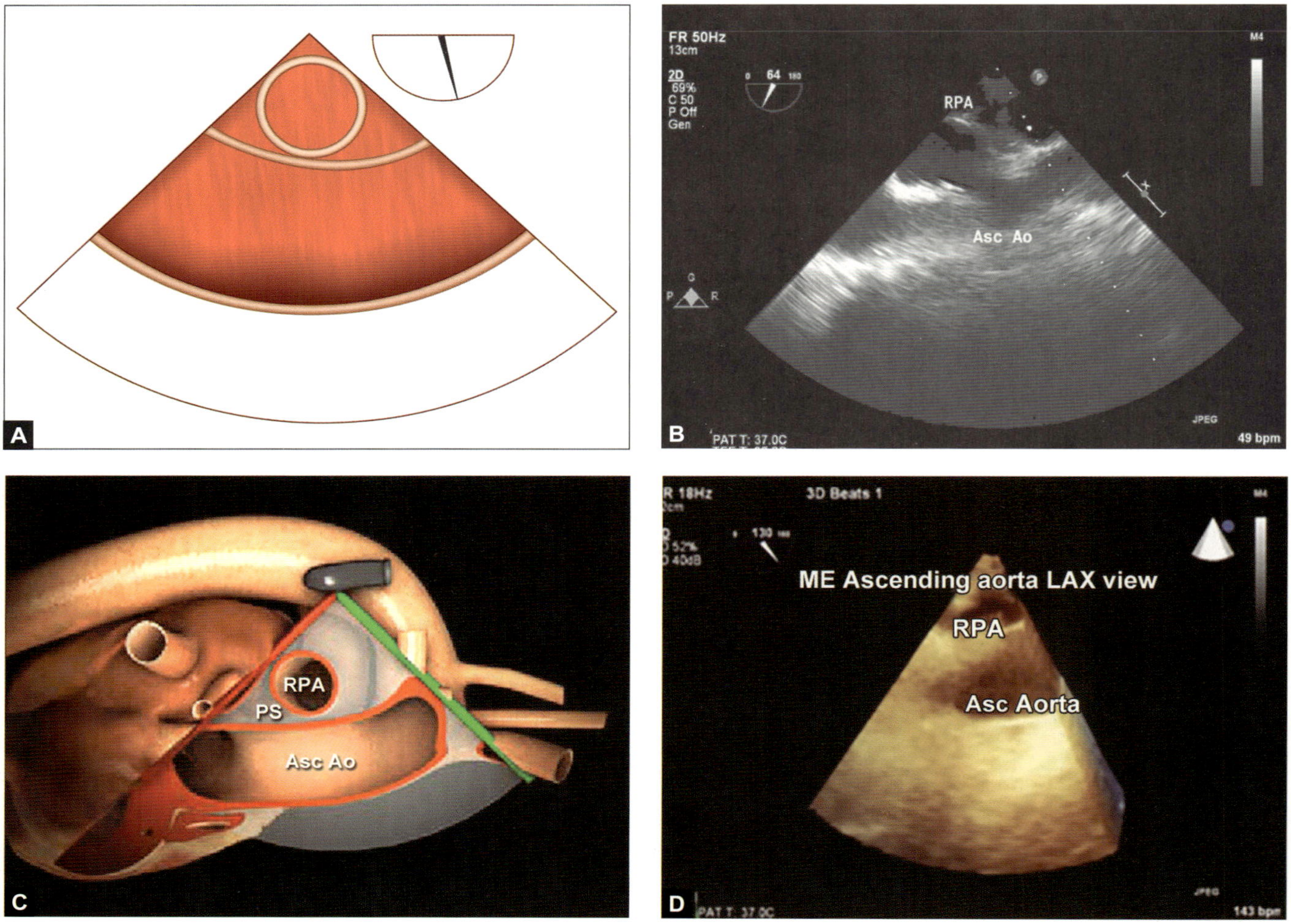

Figures 15A to D Midesophageal ascending aorta long-axis view
Abbreviations: RPA, right pulmonary artery; PS, pulmonary stenosis; Asc, ascending; Ao; aorta

- *Clinical utility:*
  - *Ascending aorta pathology:* Atherosclerosis, aneurysms, and dissections
  - Anterograde cardioplegia delivery evaluation
  - Pulmonary embolus/thrombus
- *Probe tip depth (from lips) upper esophageal (20–25 cm).*

MIDESOPHAGEAL ASCENDING AORTA: SHORT-AXIS VIEW (FIGURES 16A TO D)

The ME ascending aorta SAX view (0–10°) is obtained by withdrawing the probe from the ME aortic valve SAX view (30°) and rotating the omniplane angle back to 0°. This view is also obtained from the mid-ascending aorta LAX (120°) by decreasing the omniplane angle to 0–10° to image superior vena cava (SVC) in SAX, ascending aorta (Ascending aorta) in SAX and the right pulmonary artery (RPA) in LAX.

- *Multiplane angle range:*
  - 0–60°
  - *Sector depth:* ~ 12 cm
- *Anatomy imaged:*
  - Ascending aorta
  - Superior vena cava (short-axis)
  - Main pulmonary artery
  - Right pulmonary artery
  - Left pulmonary artery (turn probe tip to left)
  - Pulmonic valve

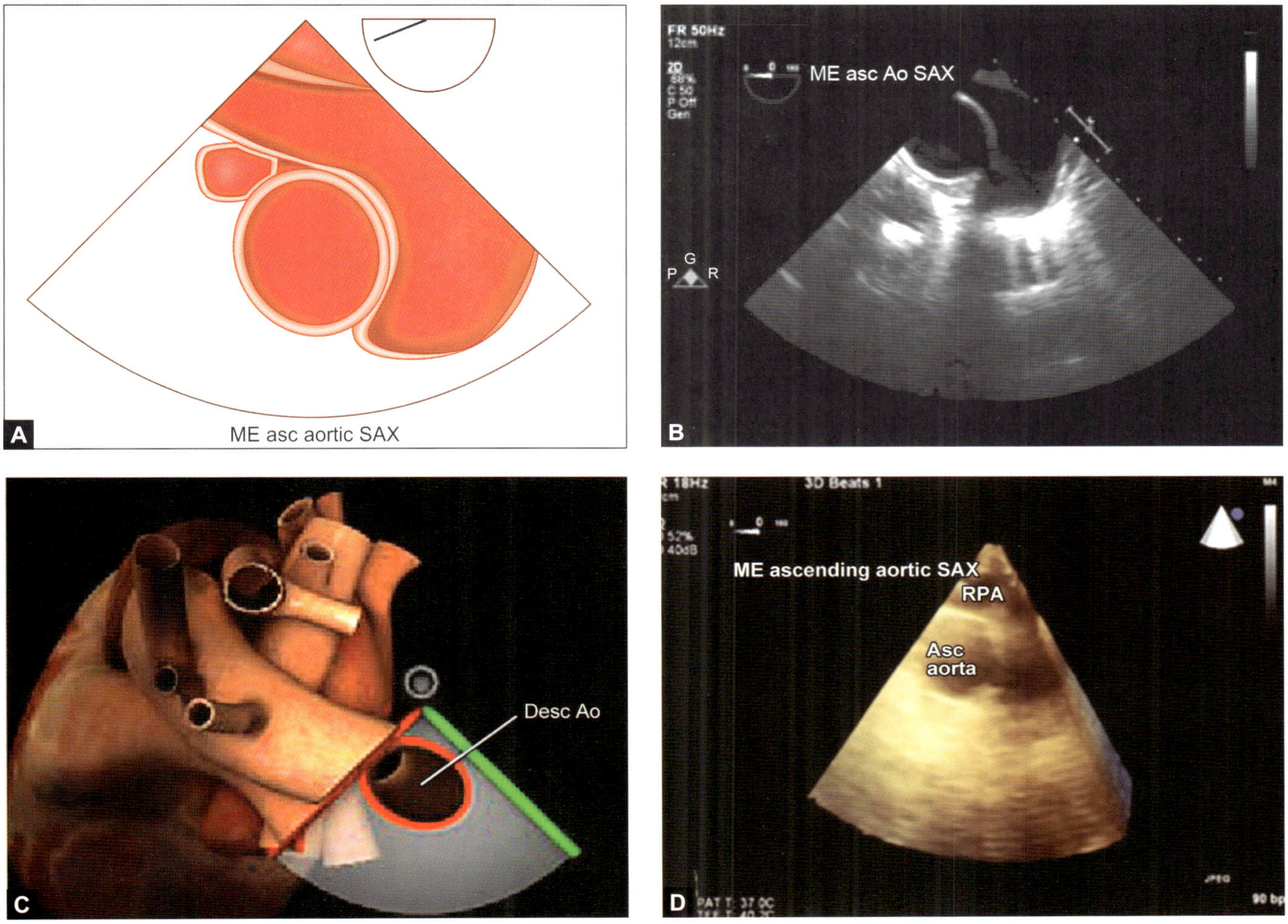

Figures 16A to D Midesophageal ascending aorta: short-axis view
Abbreviations: ME, midesdphageal; asc, ascending; desc, descending; SAX, shor-axis; Ao, aorta

- *Clinical utility:*
  - *Ascending aorta pathology:* Atherosclerosis, aneurysms, and dissections
  - *Pulmonic valve*: Pathology; pathophysiology
  - Pulmonary embolus/thrombus evaluation
  - *Superior vena cava pathology:* Thrombus, sinus venosus atrial septal defect
  - Pulmonary artery catheter placement.

MIDESOPHAGEAL LEFT ATRIAL APPENDAGE VIEW (FIGURES 17A TO D)

The left atrial appendage (LAA) view is obtained by reducing the image depth from the ME RVOT view and adjusting the omniplane angle between 60° and 80°. The LAA is seen above the mitral valve (MV) and aortic valve (AV). The left upper pulmonary vein (LUPV) is above, more posterior and closer to the probe.

- *Transducer angle:*
  - 90–110°
- *Level:*
  - Midesophageal
- *Maneuver (from prior image):*
  - Advanced
- *Clinical utility:*
  - Left atrial appendage
  - Left upper pulmonary vein.

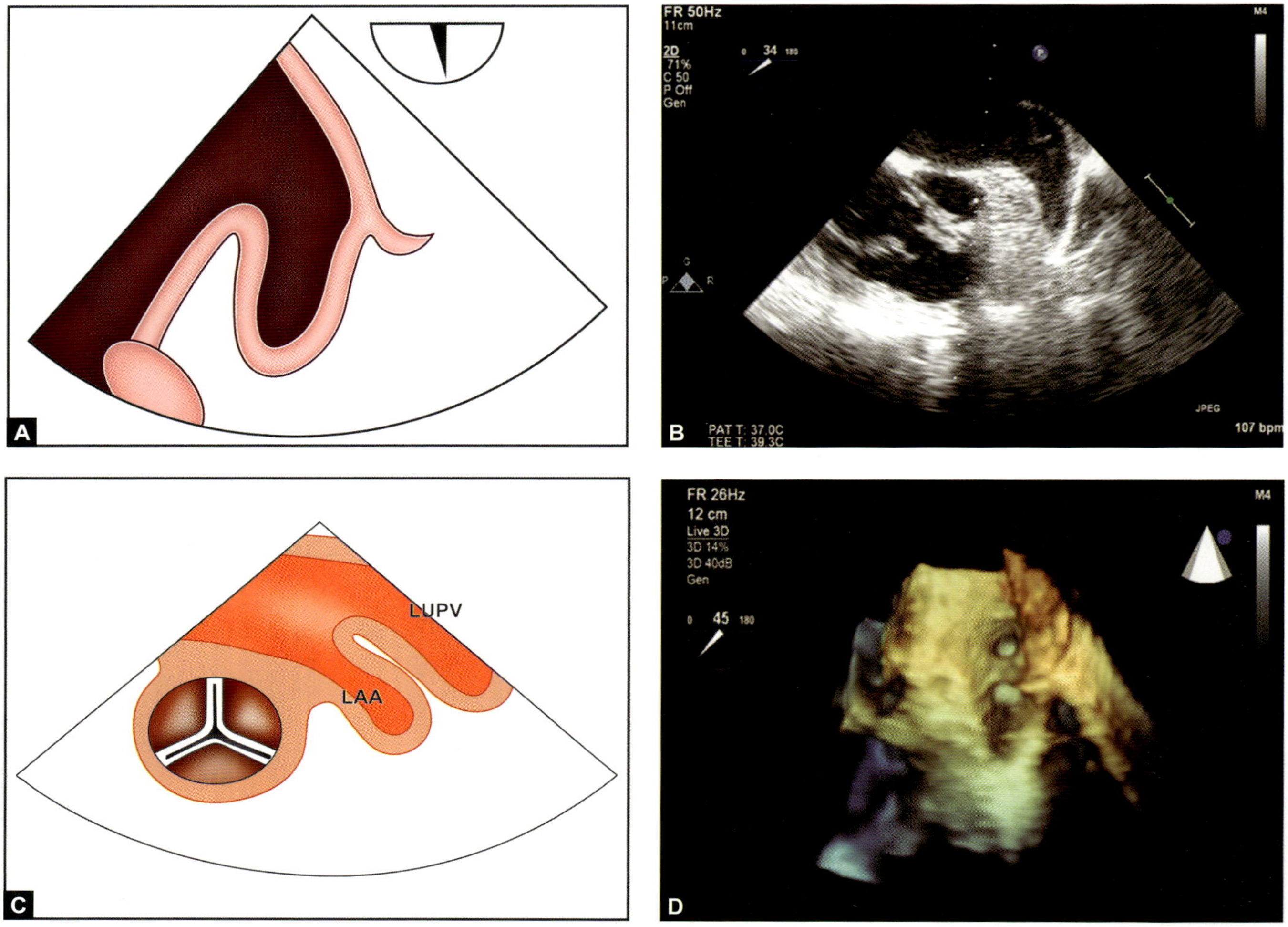

Figures 17A to D Midesophageal left atrial appendage view
Abbreviations: LUPV, left upper pulmonary vein; LAA, left atrial appendage

MIDESOPHAGEAL MODIFIED BICAVAL VIEW (FIGURES 18A TO D)

- *Structures imaged:*
  - Right atrium
  - LA
  - Interatrial septum
  - Inferior vena cava
  - TV
- *Probe adjustments:*
  - Probe rotated toward right as in bicaval view.
- *Clinical utility:*
  - For cannula placement in the SVC/IVC in all minimally invasive procedures, e.g. Robotic Group

MIDESOPHAGEAL RIGHT VENTRICULAR INFLOW-OUTFLOW VIEW (FIGURES 19A TO D)

Aptly named, this view images the right ventricular (RV) inflow from the tricuspid valve (TV) on the display left and RV outflow tract (RVOT) through the pulmonic valve (PV) on the display right in a single view. This view is obtained from the ME AV SAX view (30°) by increasing the omniplane angle to 60–75°. An off axis image of the aortic valve (AV) is displayed centrally.

- *Multiplane angle range:*
  - 60–90°
  - *Sector depth:* ~ 10–12 cm

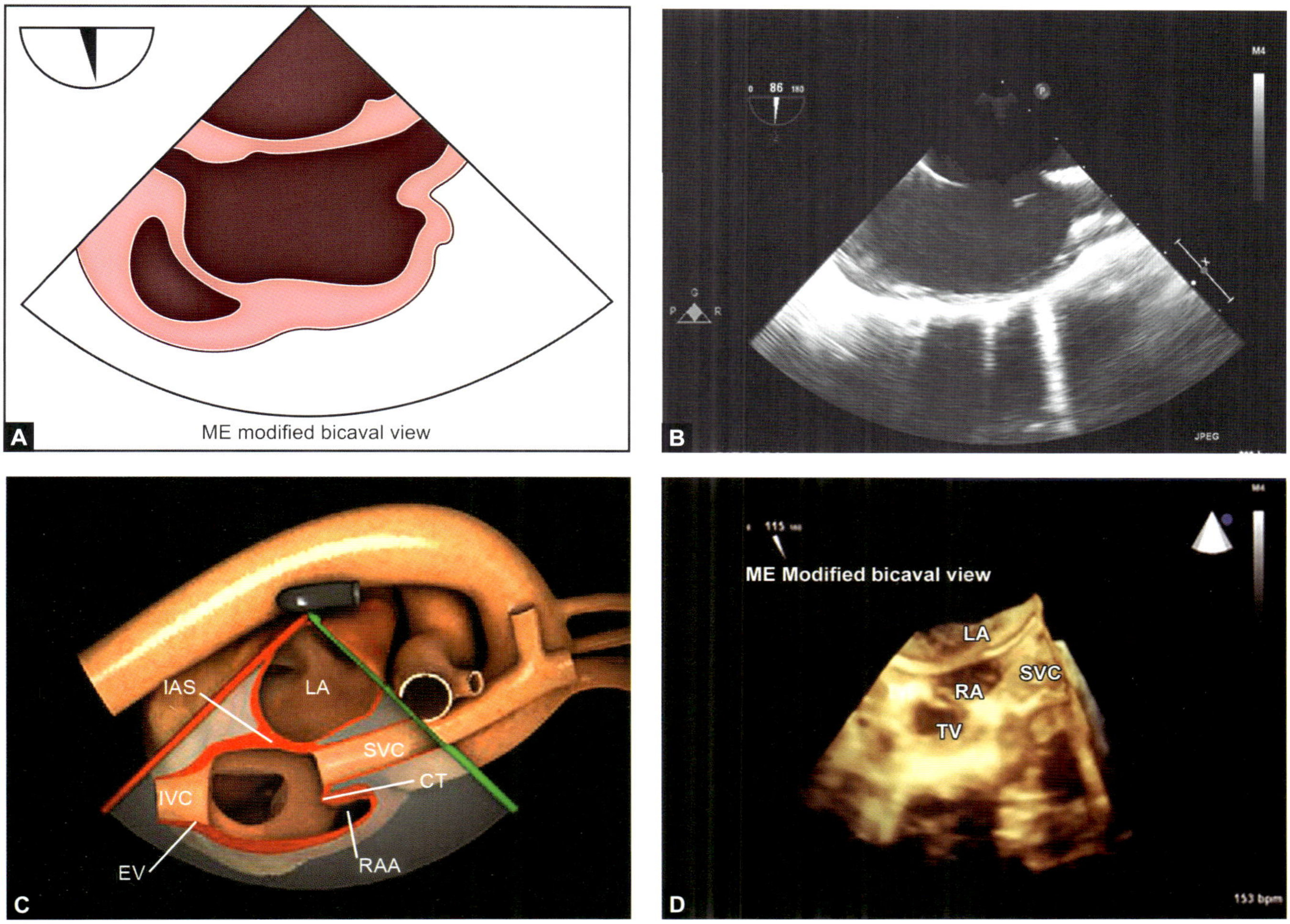

Figures 18A to D Midesophageal modified bicaval view

Abbreviations: ME, midesophageal; IAS, interatrial septum; LA, left atrium; IVC, inferior vena cava; SVC, superior vena cava; EV, eustachian valve; CT, crista terminalis; RAA, right atrial appendage

- *Anatomy imaged:*
  - Right ventricle and atrium
  - Left atrium
  - Tricuspid valve
  - Aortic valve
  - Right ventricular outflow tract
  - Pulmonic valve and main pulmonary artery
- *Clinical utility:*
  - *Right ventricle and atrial masses and left atrial:* Thrombus, embolus, tumor, foreign bodies
  - *Pulmonic valve and subpulmonic valve:* Pathology; pathophysiology
  - Pulmonary artery catheter placement
  - *Tricuspid valve*: Pathology; pathophysiology.

LOWER ESOPHAGEAL CORONARY SINUS VIEW

- *Image settings:*
  - Angle: ~ 0°–10°
  - *Sector depth:* ~12–14 cm
  - Retroflexed
- *Structures imaged:*
  - Coronary sinus in LAX
- *Clinical utility:*
  - Placement of retrograde cardioplegia cannula
  - Recognition of left superior vena cava (LSVC) in congenital heart disease
  - *Transgastric views:* Probe tip depth 40–45 cm.

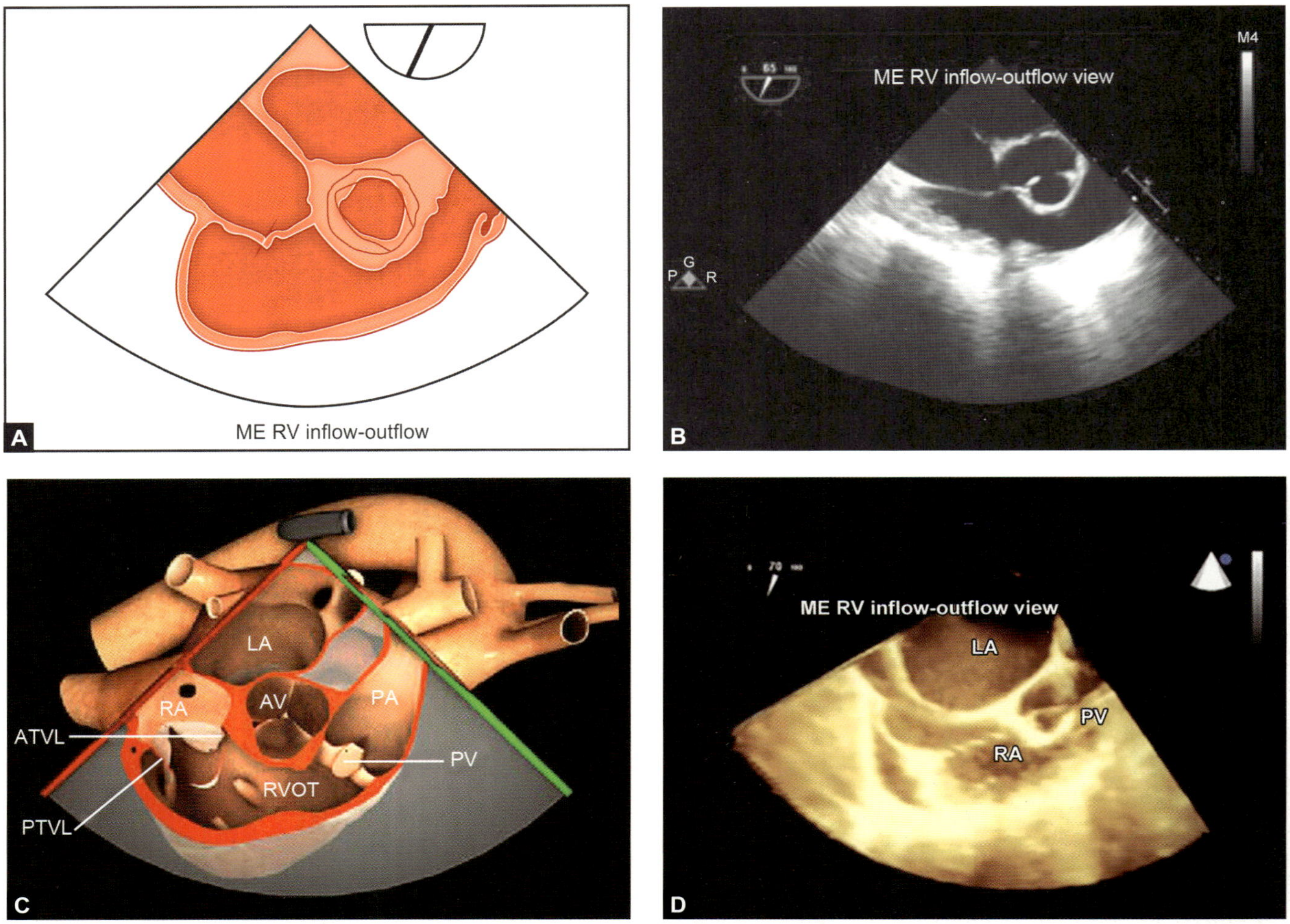

Figures 19A to D Midesophageal right ventricular inflow-outflow view

Abbreviations: ME, midesophageal, RV, right ventricle; ATVL, anterior tricuspid valve leaflet; PTVL, posterior tricuspid valve leaflet; LA, left atrium; RA, right atrium; AV, aortic valve; PA, pulmonary artery; PV, pulmonic valve; RVOT, right ventricular outflow tract

TRANSGASTRIC MODIFIED HEPATIC VEIN VIEW (FIGURES 20 AND 21)

- *Transducer angle:*
  - 0–20°
- *Level:*
  - Lower-esophageal
- *Maneuver (from prior image):*
  - Continuous wave (CW), advance
- *Clinical utility:*
  - Inferior vena cava (IVC)
  - Hepatic veins
  - Inferior vena cava (IVC) diameter for right atrium (RA) size.

TRANSGASTRIC TWO-CHAMBER VIEW (FIGURES 22A TO D)

The transgastric (TG) 2C view is obtained from the TG mid-papillary SAX view (0°) by increasing the transducer angle to 75°–90°. This images the left ventricle (LV) in LAX and the subvalvular structures of the mitral valve (MV). This view is similar to the ME 2C view now turned 90° with the probe closest to the inferior (Inf) wall of the LV (apex of sector).

- *Multiplane angle range:*
  - 80–100°
  - *Sector depth:* ~ 12 cm
- *Anatomy imaged:*
  - Left ventricle and atrium

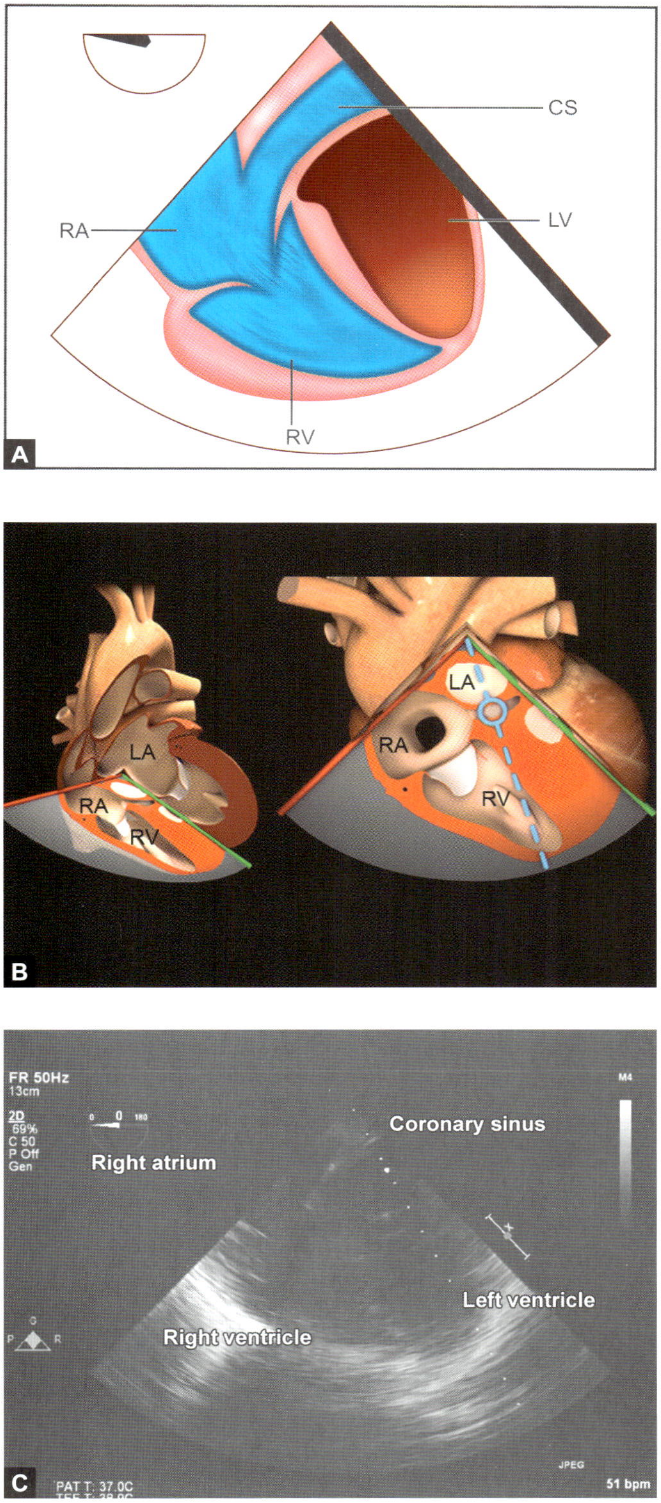

Figures 20A to C Transgastric modified hepatic vein view
Abbreviations: RA, right atrium; CS, coronary sinus; LV, left ventricle; RV, right ventricle

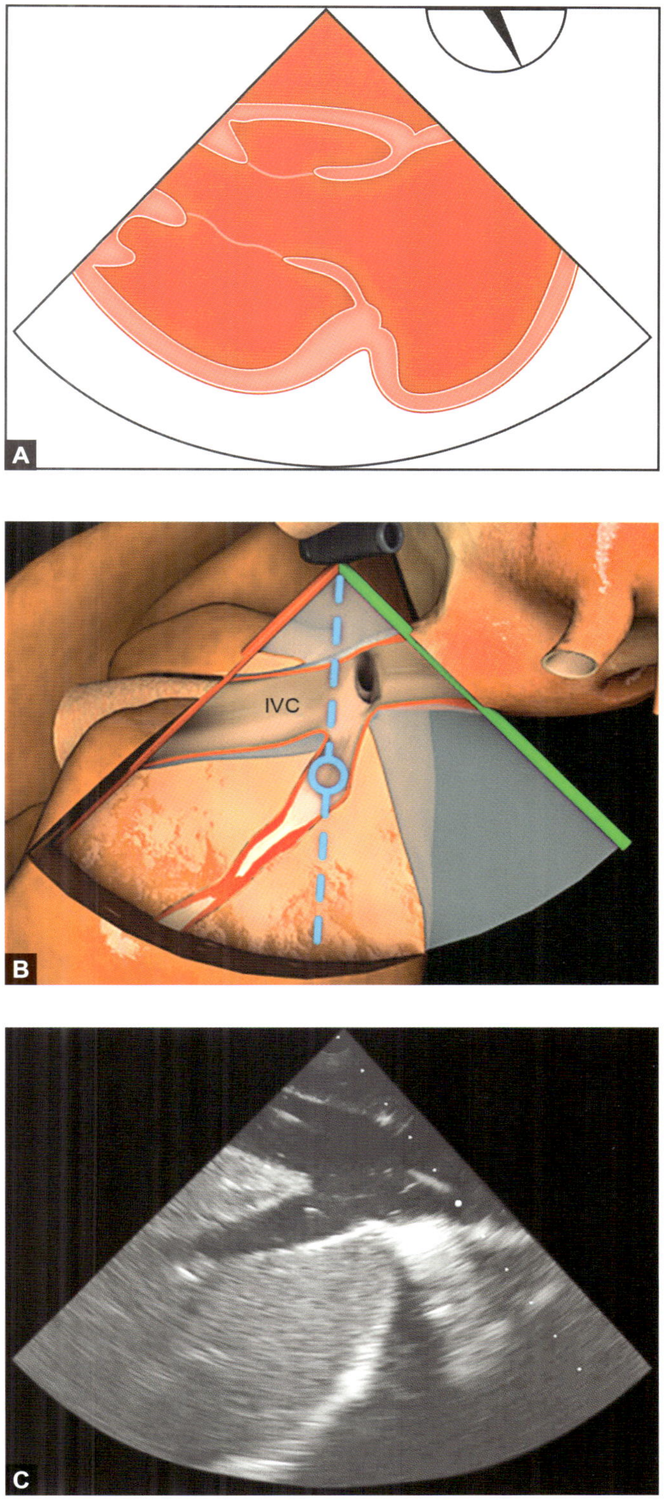

Figures 21A to C Transgastric modified hepatic vein view
Abbreviation: IVC, inferior vena cava

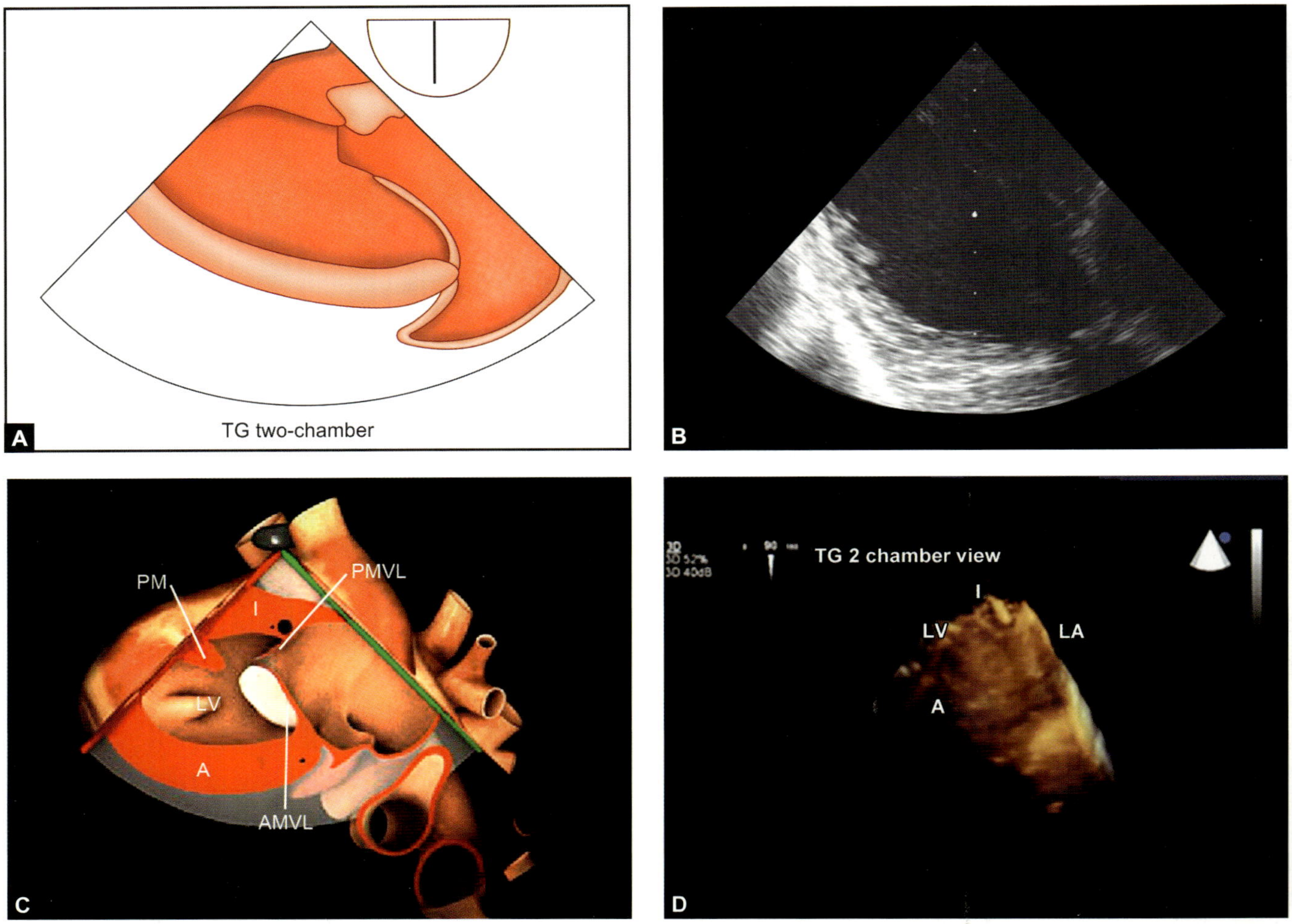

Figures 22A to D Transgastric two-chamber view
Abbreviations: TG, transgastric, PM, papillary muscles; PMVL, posterior mitral valve leaflet; AMVL, anterior mitral valve leaflet, LV, left ventricle; LA, left atrium; I, Inferior; A, Anterior

- *Mitral valve:* Chordae and papillary muscles
- Coronary sinus

- *Clinical utility:*
  - Left ventricular regional and global function (including apex)
  - *Left ventricular and atrial masses:* Thrombus, embolus, air, tumor, foreign bodies
  - *Mitral valve:* Pathology and pathophysiology

TRANSGASTRIC APICAL: SHORT-AXIS VIEW

- *Transducer angle:*
  - 0–20°
- *Transgastric*
  - Anatomy imaged
- *Left ventricle (apex)*
  - Right ventricle (apex)
- *Clinical utility:*
  - From the TG mid-papillary short-axis (SAX) view (0–20), the probe is advanced while maintaining contact with the gastric wall, to obtain the TG apical short-axis (SAX) view
  - The right ventricle (RV) apex is imaged from this view by turning to the right (clockwise). This view allows evaluation of the apical segments of the left and right ventricles.

TRANSGASTRIC BASAL: LONG-AXIS VIEW (FIGURES 23A AND B)

- *Multiplane angle range:*
  - 110–130°
- *Sector depth:* ~12 cm
  - Probe adjustments
  - Neutral leftward
- *Anatomy imaged:*
  - Mitral leaflets
  - Mitral subvalvular apparatus
  - Left ventricle (anteroseptal and inferolateral walls: basal and mid segments)
  - LV outflow tract
  - Aortic valve and proximal ascending aorta
- *Clinical utility:*
  - Left ventricular (LV) systolic dysfunction (anteroseptal and inferolateral walls)
  - Doppler interrogation of aortic valve.

TRANSGASTRIC BASAL: SHORT-AXIS VIEW (FIGURES 24A TO C)

The TG basal SAX view is obtained by withdrawing the probe from the TG mid-papillary SAX view or as the probe is advanced into the stomach at 0°. This permits a TG view of the mitral valve (MV) that is parallel to the MV annulus with the posterior mitral valve leaflet (PMVL) on the display right and the anterior mitral valve leaflet (AMVL) to the left. The posterior commissure (PC) is closest to the probe as are P3 and A3; the anterior commissure (AC) is in the far field.

- *Multiplane angle range:*
  - *0–20°*
  - *Sector depth:* ~ 12 cm
- *Anatomy imaged left and right ventricle:*
  - Mitral valve
  - Tricuspid valve
- *Clinical utility:*
  - *Mitral valve evaluation ("fish-mouth view"):* Pathology, pathophysiology
  - *Tricuspid valve evaluation:* Pathology, pathophysiology
  - Basal left ventricular regional function
  - Basal right ventricular regional function

TRANSGASTRIC MIDPAPILLARY: SHORT-AXIS VIEW (FIGURES 25 AND 26)

The TG views are obtained by advancing the probe in a neutral position into the stomach and applying varying degrees of anteflexion. In the TG mid-papillary SAX view (0°), the left ventricle (LV) is imaged in SAX with 6 LV segments (ASE/SCA 17 segment model) viewed at once. Manipulate the probe to center the LV cavity and slightly increase the transducer angle to obtain a symmetrical circular LV.

- *Multiplane angle range:*
  - 0–20°
  - *Sector depth:* ~ 12 cm
- *Anatomy imaged:*
  - Left and right ventricles
  - Papillary muscles

CHAPTER 9

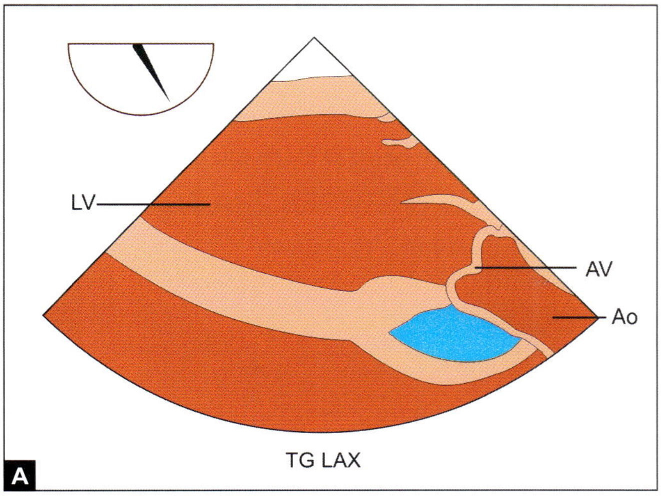

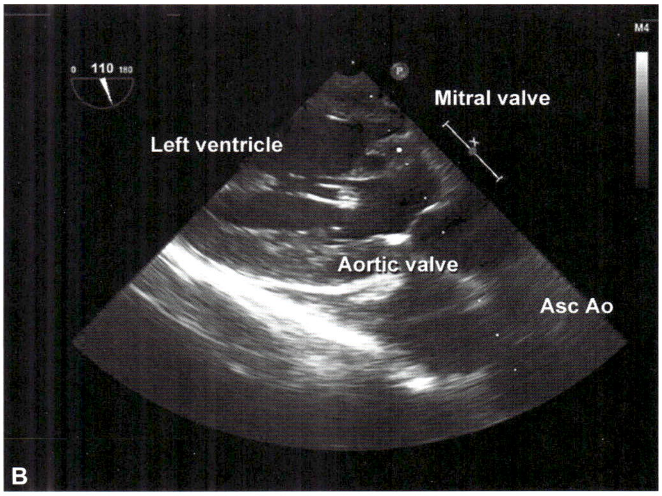

Figures 23A and B Transgastric basal long-axis view

Abbreviations: LV, left ventricle; AV, aortic valve; Ao, aorta; TG LAX, transgastric long-axis; Asc, ascending

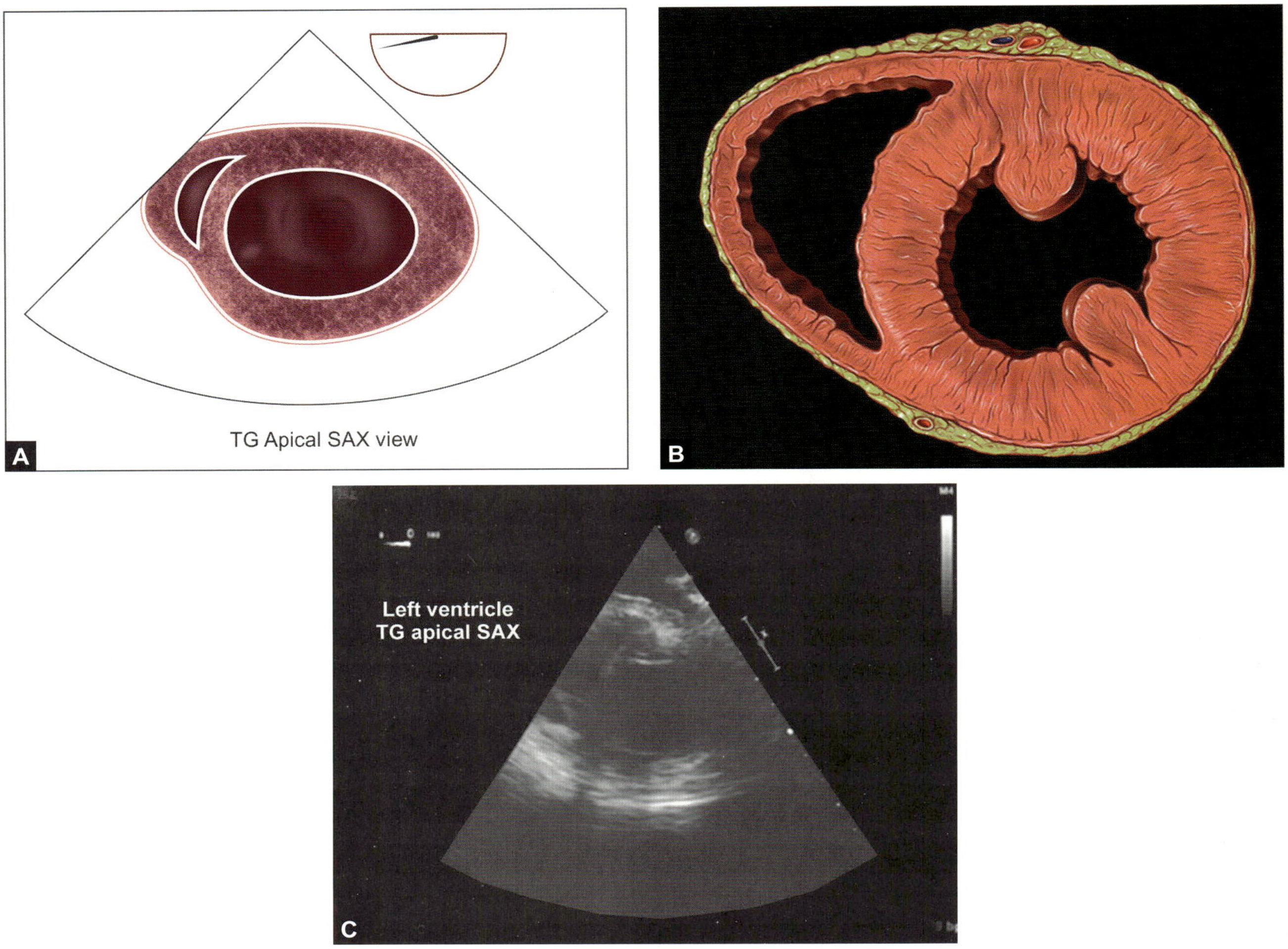

Figures 24A to C Transgastric basal: short-axis view
Abbreviations: TG, transgastric; SAX, short-axis

- *Clinical utility:*
  - Mid-left and right ventricular regional and global function
  - Intracardiac volume status.

TRANSGASTRIC RIGHT VENTRICULAR INFLOW-OUTFLOW VIEW (FIGURES 27A AND B)

- *Transducer angle:*
  - 0–20°
- *Level:*
  - Transgastric
- *Maneuver (from prior image):*
  - Right-flex
- *Clinical utility:*
  - Right atrium
  - Right ventricle
  - Right ventricular outflow tract
  - Pulmonary valve
  - Tricuspid valve.

TRANSGASTRIC RIGHT VENTRICULAR INFLOW VIEW (FIGURES 28A TO D)

The TG RV inflow view (120°) reveals a long-axis view of the right ventricle (RV), with the apex of the RV to the left and the anterior (Ant) free wall in the far field. It is obtained from the TG basal SAX view (0°), by turning the probe to the right to center the tricuspid valve (TV) and increasing the omniplane angle to 120°. The subvalvular structures of the TV are well seen.

- *Multiplane angle range:*
  - 100–120°
  - *Sector depth*: ~ 12 cm

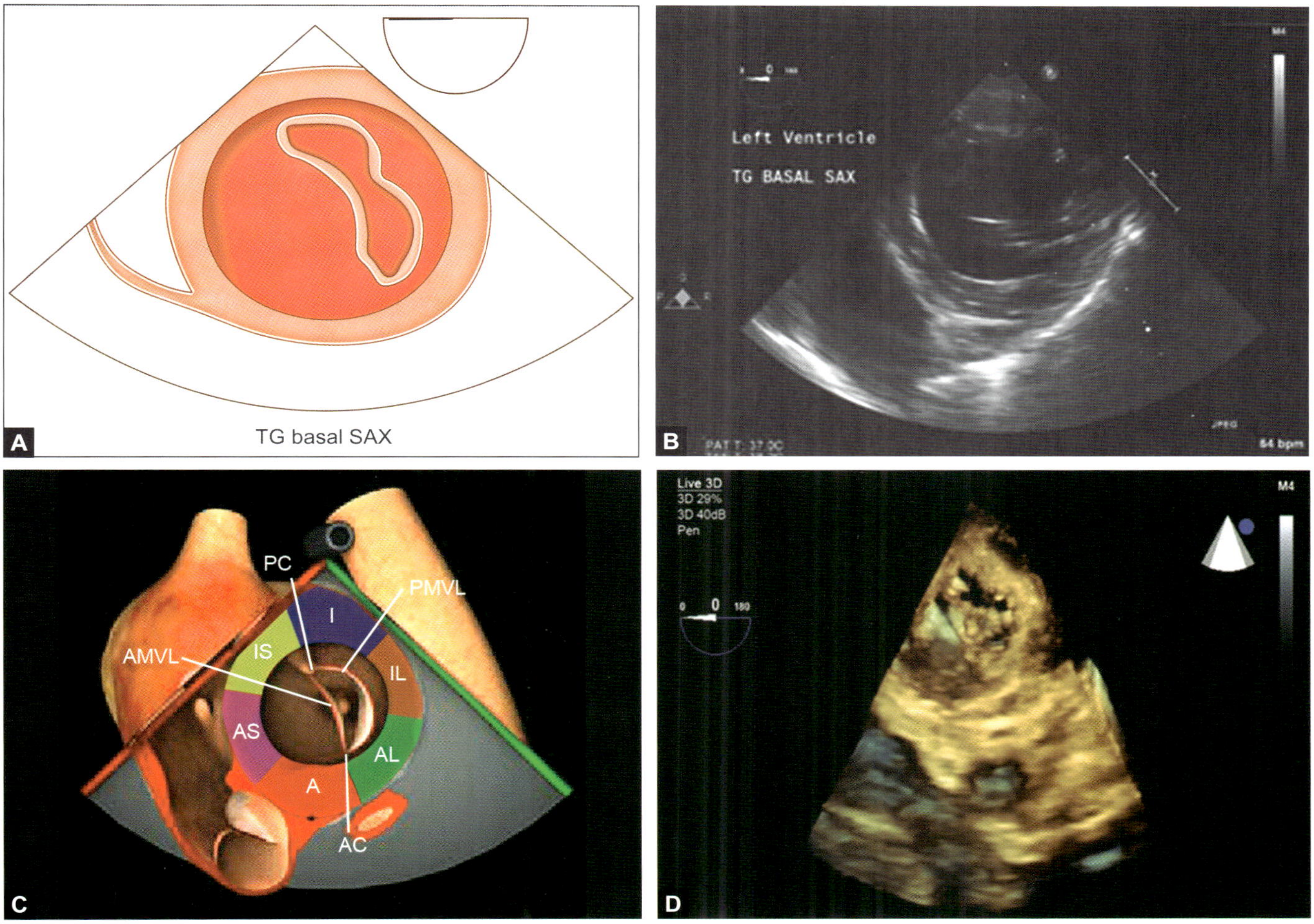

Figures 25A to D Transgastric midpapillary short-axis view

Abbreviations: TG, transgastric; SAX, short-axis; PC, posterior commissure; AMVL, anterior mitral valve leaflet; PMVL, posterior mitral valve leaflet; AC, anterior commissure; I, Inferior; IS, Interoseptal; AS, Anteroseptal; A, Anterior; AL, Anterolateral; IL, inferolateral

- *Anatomy imaged:*
  - Right ventricle and atrium
  - *Tricuspid valve:* Chordae and papillary muscles
- *Clinical utility:*
  - Right ventricular regional and global function
  - *Right ventricular and atrium masses*: Thrombus, embolus, tumor, foreign bodies
  - *Tricuspid valve:* Pathology and pathophysiology

Probe Tip Depth Deep Transgastric (45–50 cm)

TRANSGASTRIC BASAL RIGHT VENTRICULAR OUTFLOW VIEW (FIGURES 29A AND B)

- *Transducer angle:*
  - 0–20°
- *Level:*
  - Transgastric
- *Maneuver (from prior image):*
  - Anteflex
- *Clinical utility:*
  - Left ventricle (mid)
  - Right ventricle (mid)
  - Right ventricular outflow tract
  - Tricuspid valve (SAX)
  - Pulmonary valve.

DEEP TRANSGASTRIC: LONG-AXIS VIEW (FIGURES 30A TO D)

To obtain the deep TG LAX view (0°), the probe is advanced deep into the stomach and anteflexed.

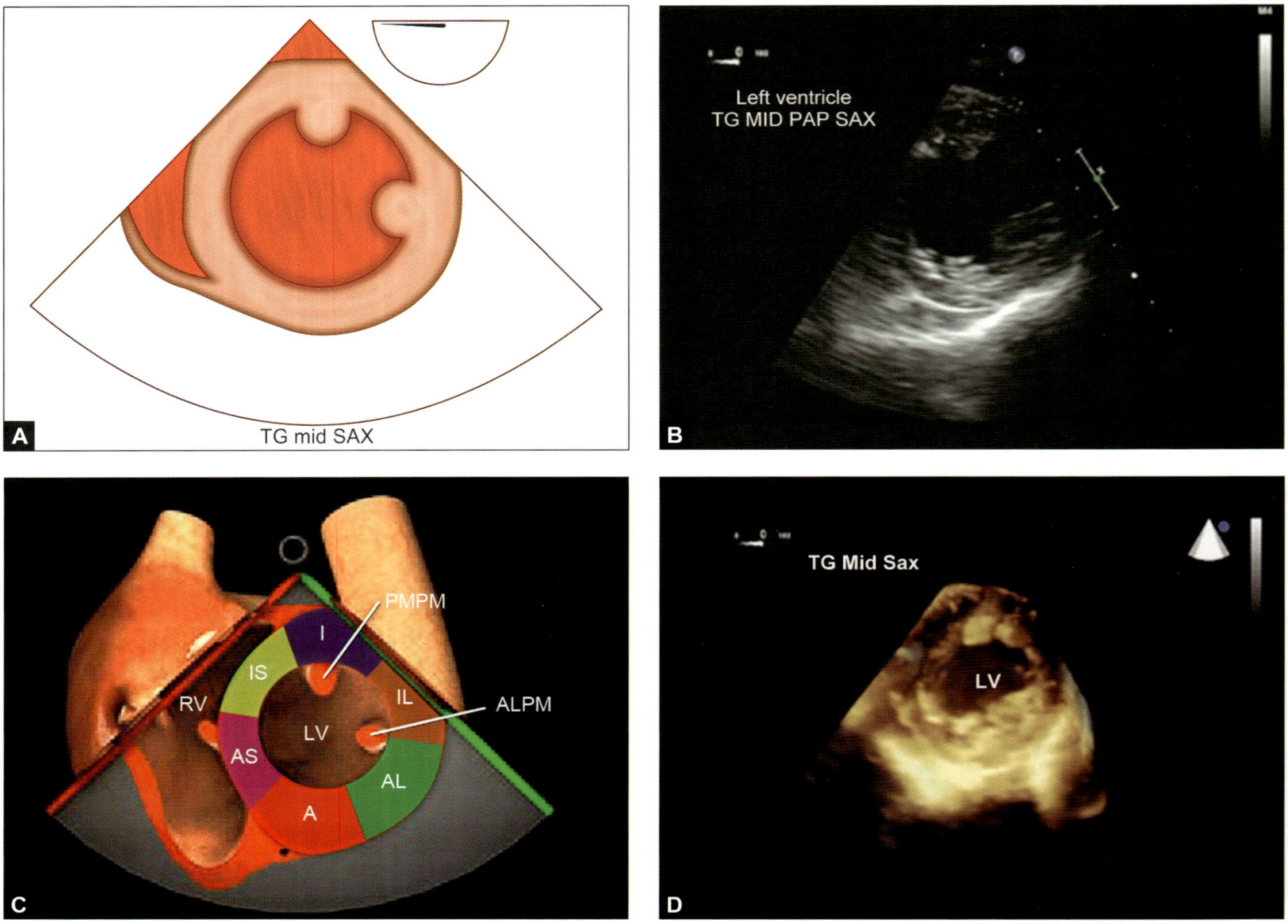

Figures 26A to D Transgastric midpapillary short-axis view

Abbreviations: RV, right ventricle; LV, left ventricle; PMPM, Pulmonary papillary muscle; ALPM, Anterolateral papillary muscle; I, Inferior; IL, Inferolateral; AL, Anterolateral; A, Anterior; AS, Anteroseptal; IS, Inferoseptal

Leftward flexion may be necessary to place the left ventricular outflow tract (LVOT) and aortic valve (AV) in the center of the screen. This image may be utilized in measuring the Doppler velocity of flow across the LVOT and the AV.

- *Multiplane angle range:*
  - 0–20° (anteflexion)
  - *Sector depth:* ~ 16 cm
- *Anatomy imaged:*
  - Left ventricle and outflow tract
  - Interventricular septum
  - Aortic valve and ascending aorta
  - Left atrium
  - Mitral valve
  - Right ventricle
  - Pulmonic valve
- *Clinical utility:*
  - Aortic valve and subaortic pathology and pathophysiology
  - Mitral valve pathology and pathophysiology
  - Left and right ventricle global function
  - *Left and right ventricle masses:* Thrombus, embolus, tumor
  - Foreign bodies
  - Congenital or acquired interventricular septal defect evaluation.

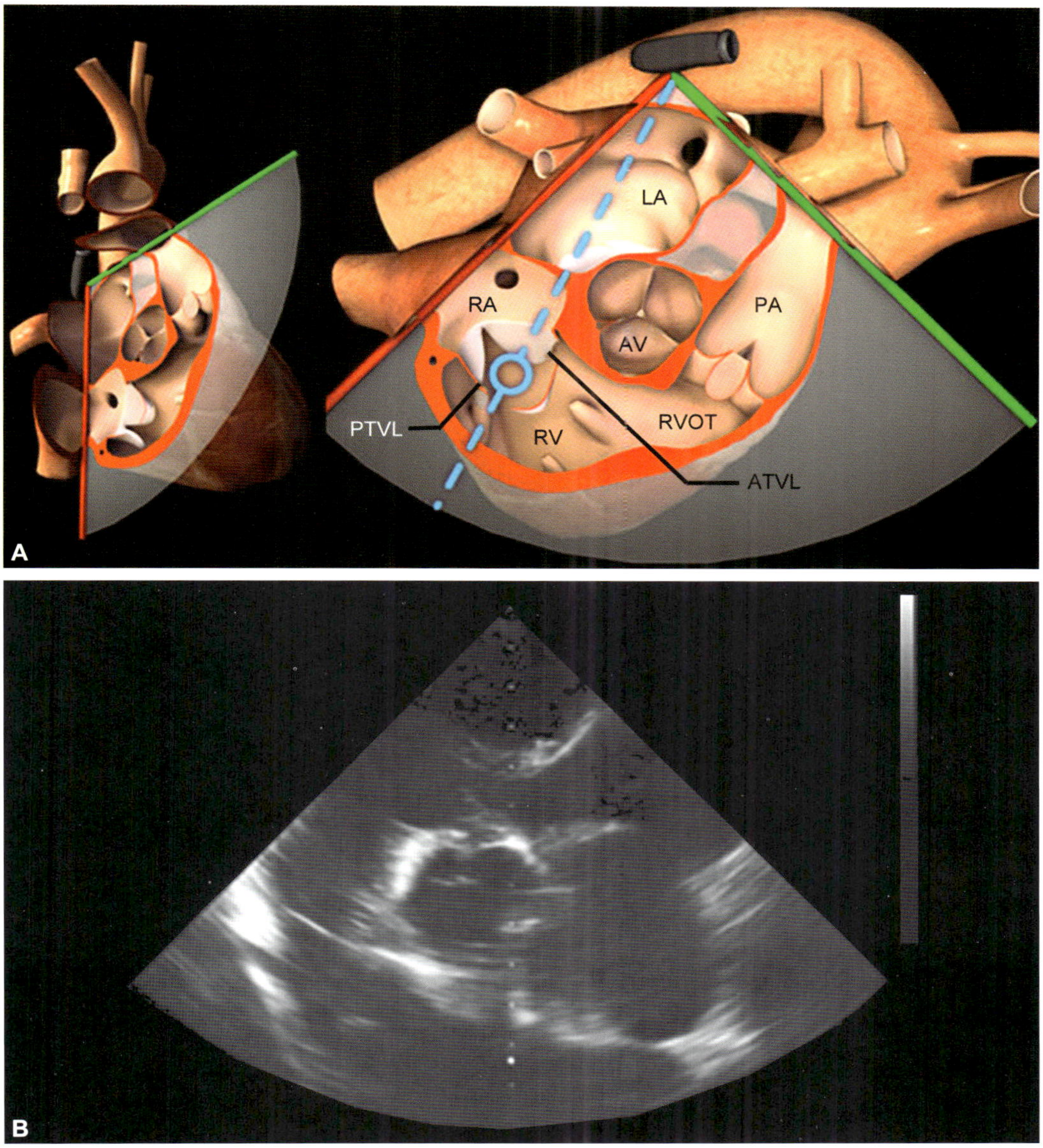

Figures 27A and B Transgastric right ventricular inflow-outflow view
Abbreviations: LA, left atrium; RA, right atrium, AV, aortic valve; PA, pulmonary artery; RV, right ventricle; PTVL, posterior tricuspid valve leaflet; RVOT, right ventricular outflow tract; ATVL, anterior tricuspid valve leaflet

UPPER ESOPHAGEAL AORTIC ARCH: LONG-AXIS VIEW (FIGURES 31A TO D)

From the descending thoracic aorta SAX view (0°), the probe is withdrawn cephalad to the upper esophagus (UE). The circular shape of the descending thoracic aorta changes to an oblong shape of the transverse aortic arch (0°). The proximal aortic arch is to the display left and the distal arch to the right. Further probe withdrawal may image the great vessels of the head and neck.

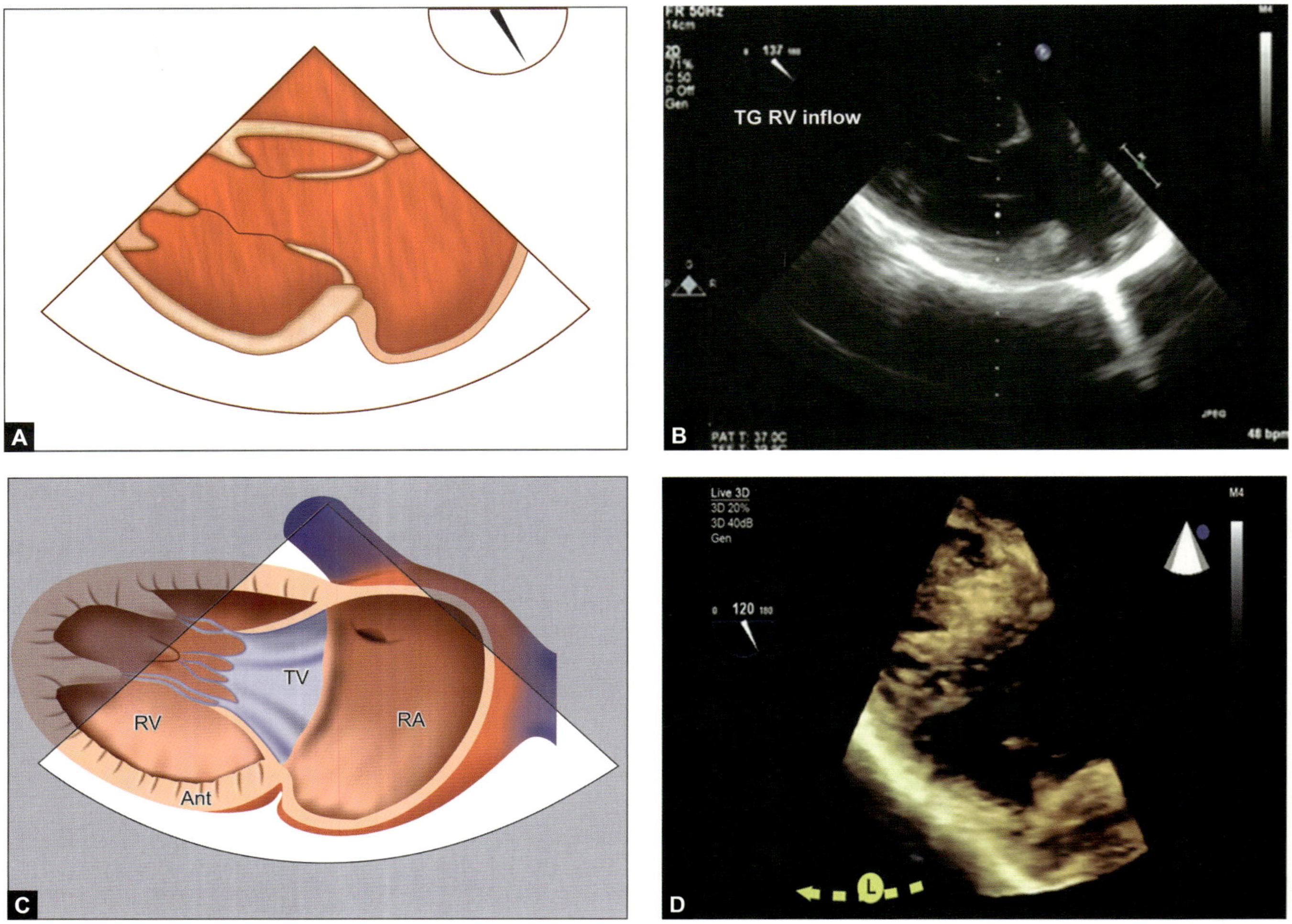

Figures 28A to D Transgastric right ventricular inflow view
Abbreviations: TG RV, transgastric right ventricle; TV, tricuspid valve; RA, right atrium; Ant, anterior

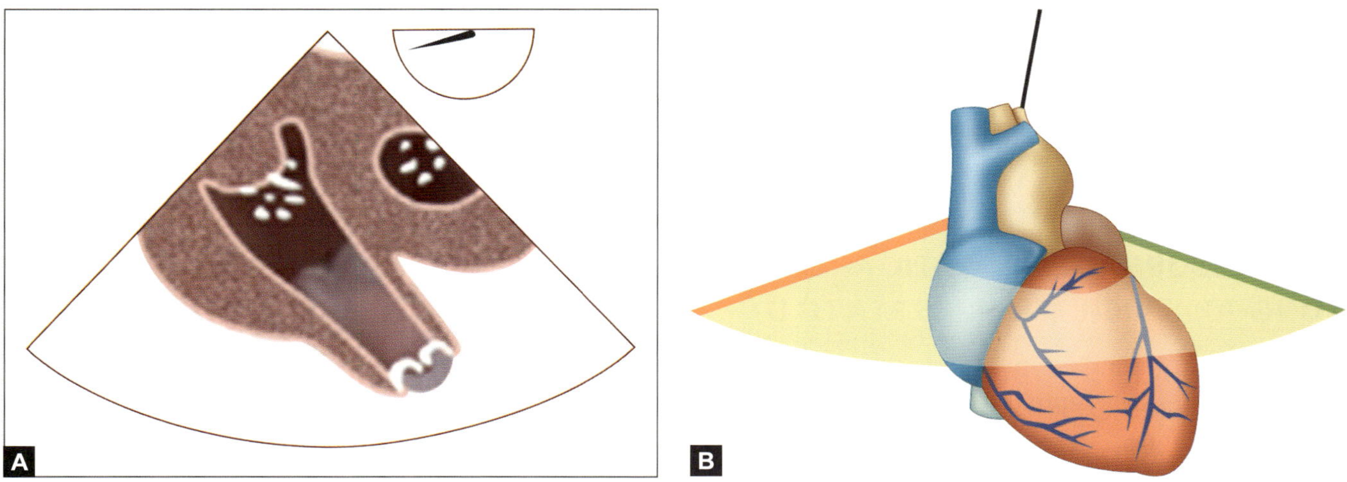

Figures 29A and B Transgastric basal right ventricular outflow view

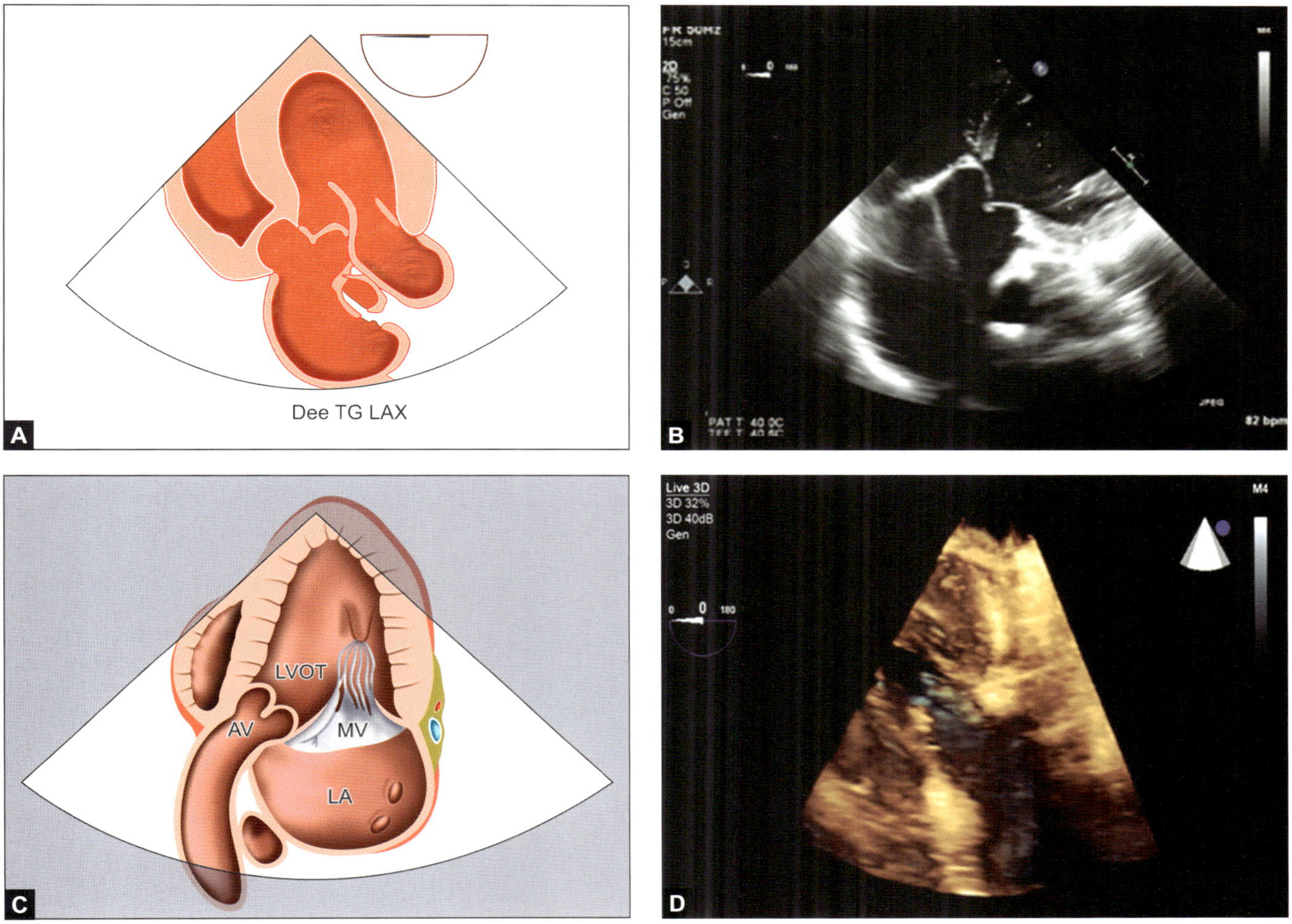

Figures 30A to D Deep transgastric long-axis view

Abbreviations: TG LAX, transgastric long-axis; LVOT, left ventricular outflow tract; AV, aortic valve; MV, mitral valve; LA, left atrium

- *Multiplane angle range:*
  - 0°
  - *Sector depth:* ~ 10 cm
- *Anatomy imaged:*
  - Aortic arch; left brachiocephalic vein; left subclavian and carotid arteries; right brachiocephalic artery
- *Clinical utility:*
  - *Ascending aorta and arch pathology*: Atherosclerosis, aneurysms and dissections; aortic cardiopulmonary bypass (CPB) cannulation site evaluation.

UPPER ESOPHAGEAL AORTIC ARCH: SHORT-AXIS VIEW (FIGURES 32A TO D)

From the upper esophageal (UE) aortic arch LAX view (0°), increasing the transducer angle to 60–90° obtains the UE aortic arch SAX view. With probe manipulation the proximal origin of the left subclavian artery and innominate vein is seen in the upper right display. The pulmonic valve (PV) and main pulmonary artery (PA) in LAX are seen in the lower left display.

- *Multiplane angle range:*
  - 90°
  - *Sector depth:* ~ 10 cm

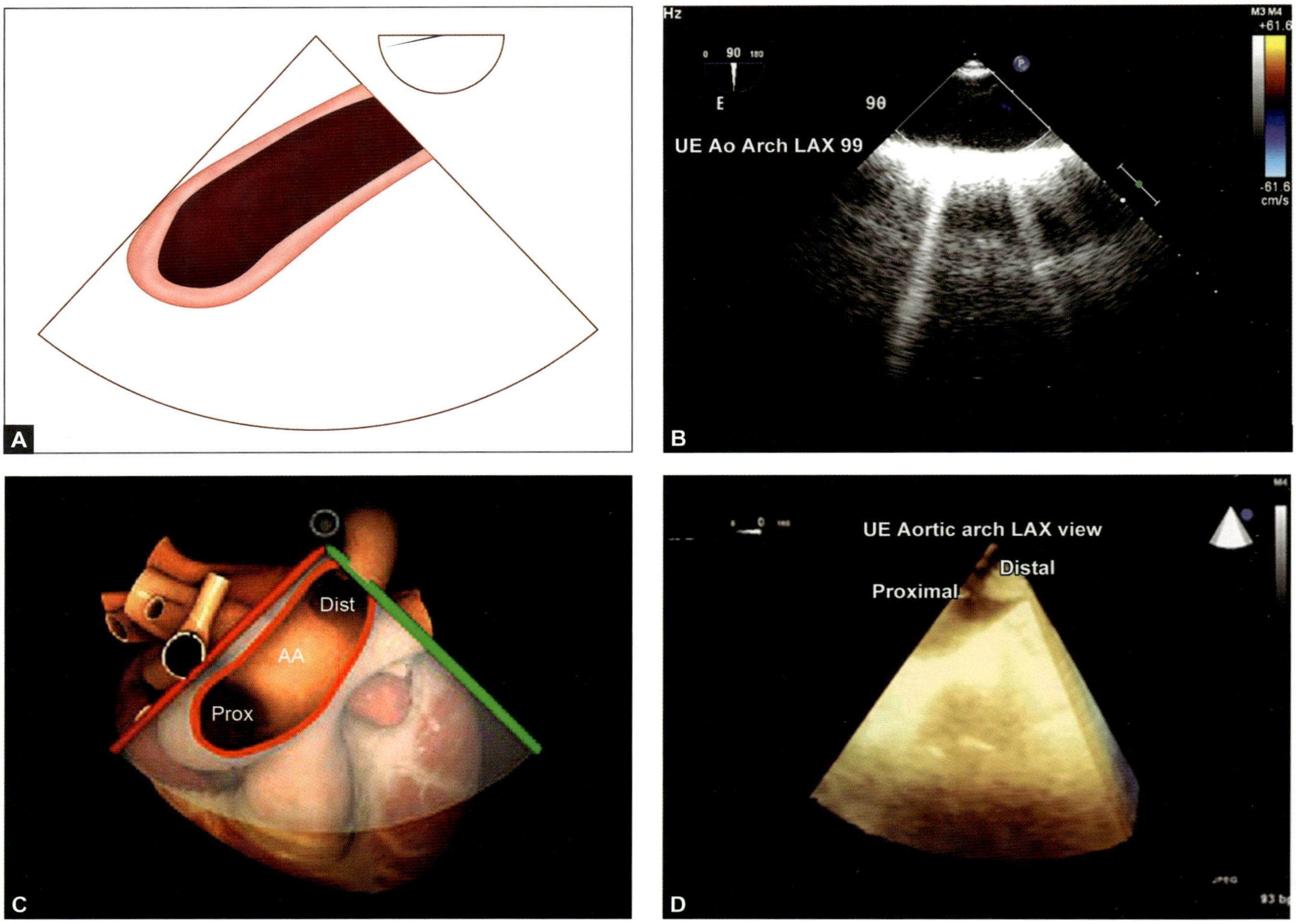

Figures 31A to D Upper esophageal aortic (UEAo) arch: long-axis (LAX) view
Abbreviations: Dist, distal; Prox, proximal

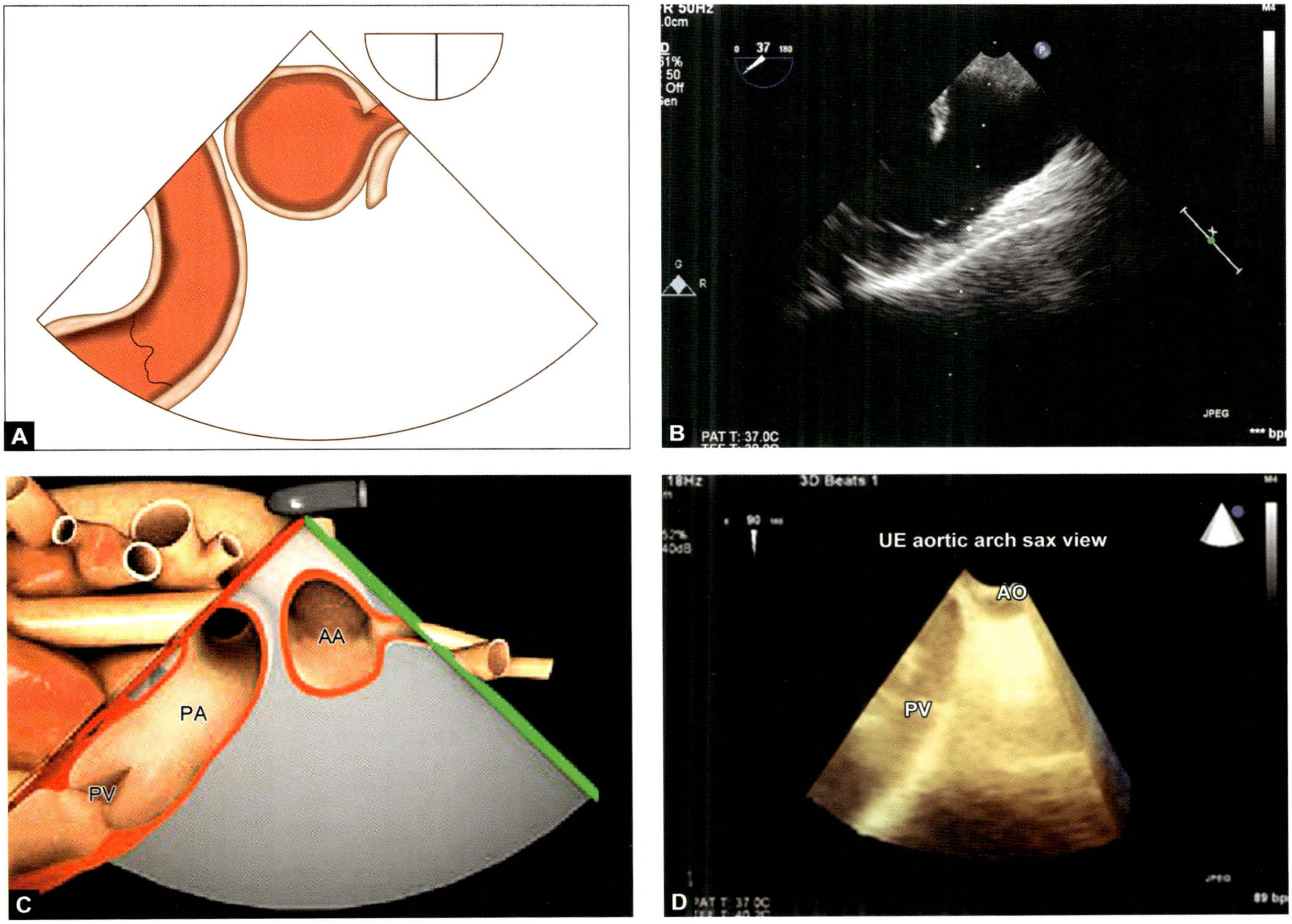

Figures 32A to D UE aortic arch: short-axis view
Abbreviations: AA, aortic arch, PA, pulmonary artery; PV, pulmonic valve

- *Structures imaged:*
  - Aortic arch; left brachiocephalic vein; left subclavian and carotid arteries; right brachiocephalic artery; main pulmonary artery and pulmonic valve
- *Clinical utility:*
  - *Ascending aorta and arch pathology*: Atherosclerosis, aneurysms and dissections; pulmonary embolus; pulmonary valve evaluation (insufficiency, stenosis, Ross procedure); pulmonary artery catheter placement.

Chapter 10

Simulation for Transesophageal Echocardiography of Mitral Valve

Naman Shastri

Chapter Outline

INTRODUCTION

Simulation-based medical education (SBME) was first introduced to the field of anesthesiology in the 1950s, when Dr. Bjorn Lind created the world's first medical mannequin, the "Resusci-Anne," for mouth-to-mouth ventilation training.The first "virtual" three-dimensional (3D) model of the heart was created in 1999 to facilitate teleconsultation in echocardiography. Soon afterwards a similar static, virtual heart model, that included a virtual transesophageal echocardiography (TEE) probe, was employed in what would become the first known echocardiography simulator to be used for training.

The mitral valve (MV) apparatus has a complex anatomical structure consisting of two asymmetric leaflets, a saddle-shaped annulus, chordae tendineae, and papillary muscles. It is important to assess the physiologic characteristics of the MV apparatus.

Three-dimensional (3D) echocardiography can provide detailed morphology of the MV leaflets and annulus contributing to our understanding of MV function and anatomy. It is more suitable to conduct 3D assessment for the evaluation of MV function because of the complex MV structure.

Surgeons are now using 3D transesophageal echocardiography (TEE) prior to MV repair to evaluate MV geometry and focus the surgical procedure, particularly for MV prolapse. Current clinical 3D echocardiography can demonstrate excellent volumetric morphology of the MV apparatus and provide information on the regurgitated flow jet across the MV leaflets using Doppler ultrasound in realtime allowing evaluation of mitral regurgitation.

But prior to that excellent Hands on training is very important for the operator to have complete idea about the complex structure of the mitral valve in real time so simulation has played the important role.

HOW SIMULATION WORKS FOR TEE?

The beating heart is freely controlled by the computer keyboard and mouse; it can be viewed from any angle both internally and externally and through a range of zoom. It can be rotated around any axis and sliced in any plane to allow maximal flexibility in the display of cardiac structures.

Incorporated into the system is a comprehensive anatomy text with over 150 separate intracardiac structures labelled and described. Any selected structure can be simultaneously highlighted in the text and displayed within the 3D model. A number of predefined areas of the heart can be displayed separately or in combination to demonstrate anatomical relationships. The arrangement of the display windows on the screen can be adjusted by the operator according to personal preference.[1]

Selected screen displays, still or animated, may be stored as slides, with impressive automatic transition between images within a slideshow. All image output can be displayed on the system monitor or relayed to an external projector to add a dramatic enhancement to lecture presentations.

In the **Ultrasound Simulator Package** the on-screen introduction of a virtual TEE probe generates simulated ultrasound images that are derived directly and continuously from the 3D model. Ultrasound plane positioning is controlled using the computer keyboard and mouse via screen icons representing the standard flexion, rotation and angulation capabilities of a multiplane TEE probe.

In the **Manikin Simulator Package** a realistic TEE probe with authentic controls inserts into the mouth of a life-size upper-body manikin. With easy USB connection to the computer system, the hand held probe controls the position of the on-screen simulated TEE probe and ultrasound plane.

The 3D model can be set to display the 'cut surface' at the level of the TEE ultrasound plane to further clarify the plane orientation. This mode allows students of TEE to visualize clearly the relationship between the 2D TEE image represented on the screen and the underlying 3D anatomy of the heart. Any structure selected in the 3D model is highlighted in the simulated TEE image, and vice versa, so that the user can easily identify any intracardiac region.

As with the core anatomy package, the arrangement of windows displaying the heart, the TEE image and descriptive text may be adjusted by the user. In this package the slideshow feature incorporates the ability to capture the simulated ultrasound images.

A key to the success of this technology is the use of tiny electromagnetic sensors by Ascension Technology, Milton, VT, that are embedded in the model ultrasound probe. The sensors track the position of the TEE probe head in real time, in much the same way that a GPS system can track the location of a moving object. Ascension makes 3D tracking devices for medical guidance, real-time visualization, and minimally invasive surgery and target acquisition.

SIMULATION AND MITRAL VALVE

Simulation in mitral valve is useful tool to get educated and have better understanding. It can be useful in many ways **(Figures 1A and B)**. Like, to see the complex structure in computed generated images, which is nearly the same in real life without limitation of timing and duration of procedure. It can also simulate the various pathology such as mitral valve prolapse, cardiac tamponade and intracardiac tumors, and disease states such as congestive heart failure and chronic obstructive pulmonary disease that the trainee can expect to encounter in actual clinical settings and some software can allow us to get Doppler analysis done.

All the different views of the mitral valve by TEE can be clearly seen with simulation like real time seen in patients **(Figures 2A and B)**.

Most of the TTE simulator is available in both transthoracic and transesophageal echocardiography capacity **(Figures 3A and B)**. So we can compare both images and have both idea at the same time.The simulator's interface comprises of an anatomically correct beating 3D virtual heart model and scan plane on one side and a two-dimensional (2D) ultrasound image corresponding to the position of the scan plane on the other. The imagery on the screen changes with the trainee's probe-manipulations on the mannequin. The virtual heart model can be rotated and viewed from many different perspectives to better understand the anatomic basis of image acquisition.

The simulator has introduced another feature to help assess trainee progress: metrics. Metrics are based on target cut planes (TCP)of Mitral valve that are actually expert-acquired "ideal" images of standard echocardiographic views of Mitral valve stored in the system. During metrics training, a TCP is displayed on the screen and the trainee is asked to attain the same

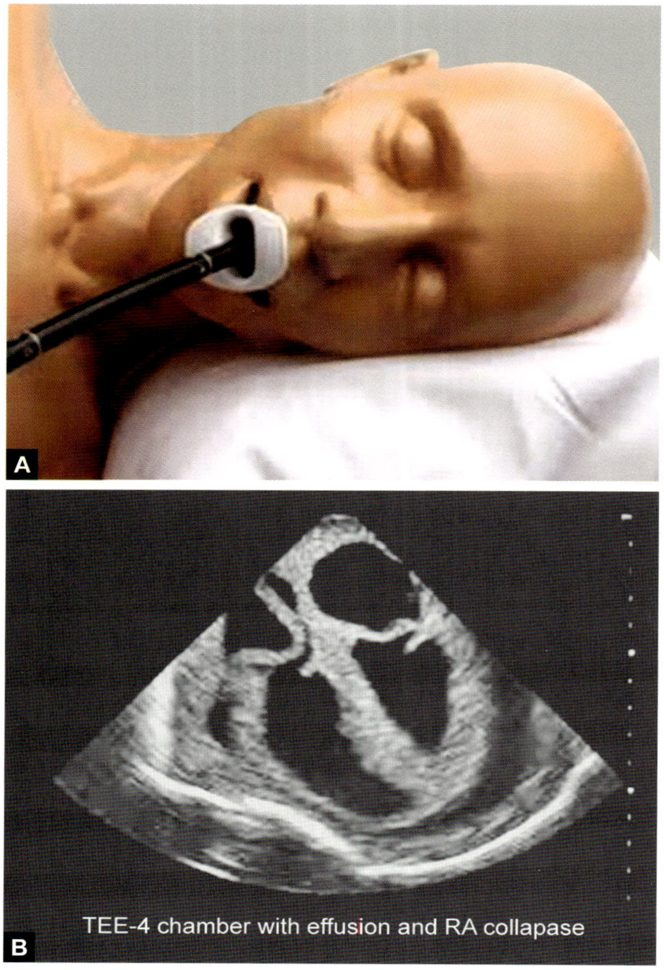

Figures 1A and B The TEE probe insertion and the classical TEE view

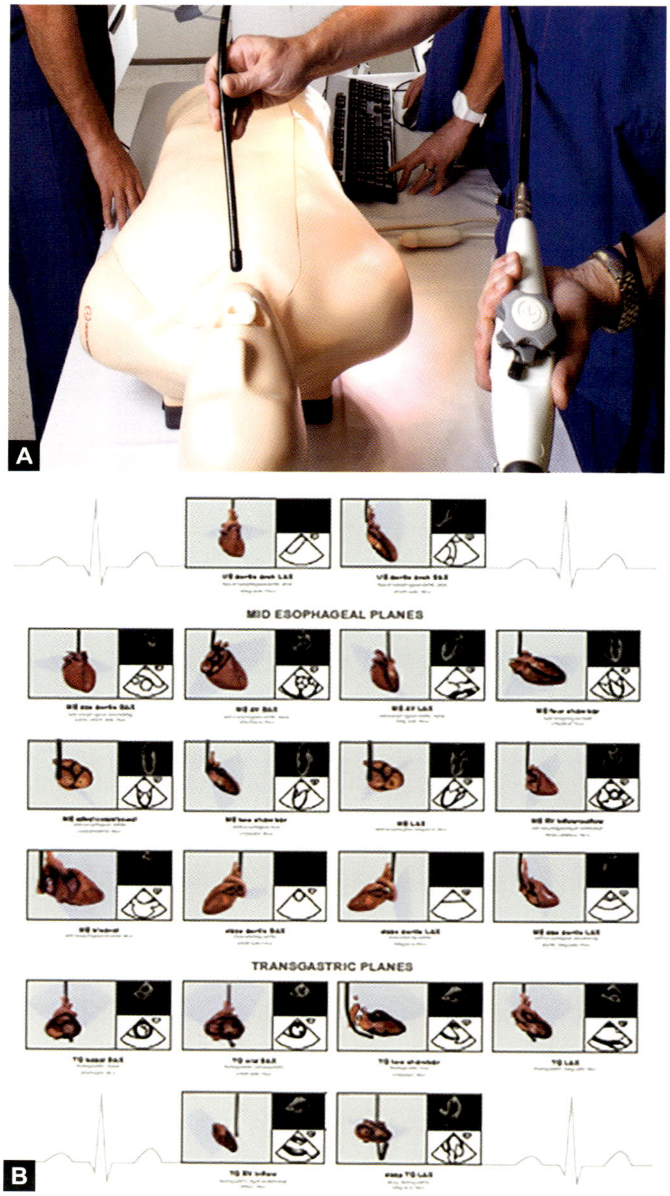

Figures 2A and B Different TEE views on simulators

using his cognitive understanding of cardiac anatomy and manual dexterity.

OTHER ADVANCED USE OF SIMULATION FOR MITRAL VALVE BY COMPUTATIONAL SIMULATION

As per recent advances in echocardiography regarding 3D echocardiography nowadays it is very easy to understand the normal and different pathology of complex mitral valve geometry. So recently many simulated software developed from the acquiring the 3D images form real time 3D echocardiography and date acquired form real time images and those images are placed in the simulated software to simulate the real time complex mitral valve in to reality.[2]

Precise 3D geometry of the MV apparatus acquired from 3D echocardiography can be utilized for computational evaluation of MV functional characteristics. Computational simulation combined with 3D echocardiography can help us better understand the features of dynamic morphologic and structural alterations of the MV apparatus capturing the consequences of valve function in microseconds.

Moreover, the use of patient-specific MV apparatus geometry may be a crucial factor to determine the

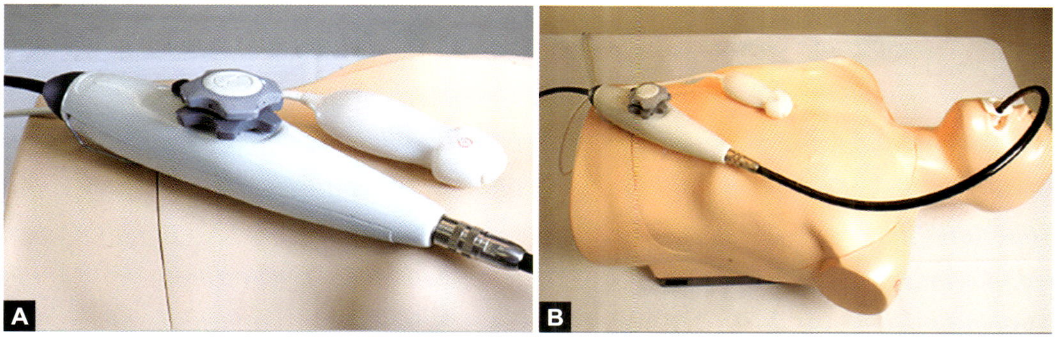

Figures 3A and B The TEE heartworks simulator for TEE and TTE

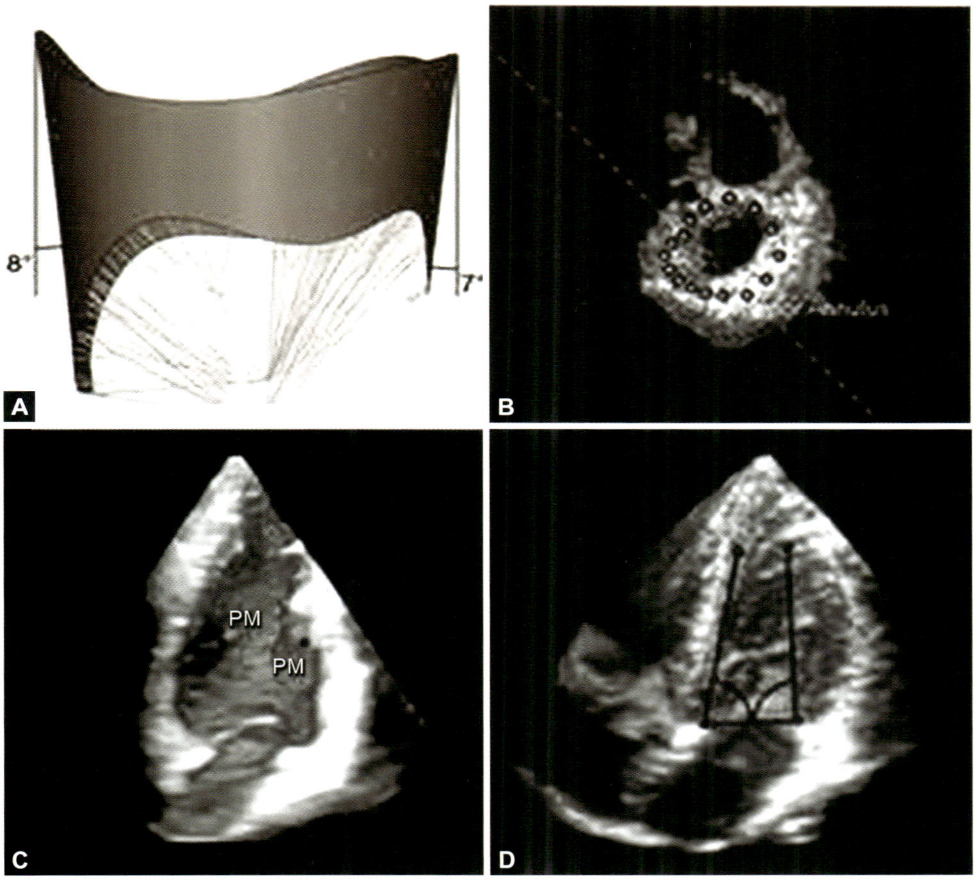

Figures 4A to D Precise 3D geometry of the mitral valve detected on the ultrasound frame
Abbreviation: PM, papillary muscles.

extent and severity of abnormality of each structural component, such as extreme local stress concentration in the leaflets, annulus, or chordae tendineae during valve function. The integrated modeling platform developed in this study allows us to create a geometrical MV apparatus model from patient 3D TEE data for computationally accurate and physiologic evaluation of the MV function.

In Figure 4: (A) Valve geometrical model, (B) Annular profile, (C) papillary muscles and (D) leaflets inclination are detected on the end diastolic ultrasound frame **(Figures 4A to D)**. These few images are acquired and functioning mitral valve simulator model is formed and various functional profile are created like annular movement, papillary muscle movement. Even the sear stress faced by commissures are calculated by the simulated mitral valve module.

Simulation of Blood Flow through the Mitral Valve (Figure 5)

There have been attempts to test the effectiveness of surgical repairs in vitro based on pressure drop required to cause mitral valve prolapse which have been carried out in many experiments. As many surgeon are not comfortable with certain technique and always doubt the hemodynamic date obtain from the repair technique they use, so various simulator have been use in the experimental model to evaluate the different repair technique and flow dynamics through that mitral valve orifice. So according to patient pathology and same pathology created in the porcine valve simulated model and flow dynamic is studied.

The heart valves are extracted from porcine hearts which are then stored in the refrigerator before use. The mitral valve is removed by extracting a section with the mitral valve annulus and the anterior and posterior leaflets papillary muscles.The papillary muscles of the mitral valve specimen are attached to a wire set-up which is connected to the ring structure.

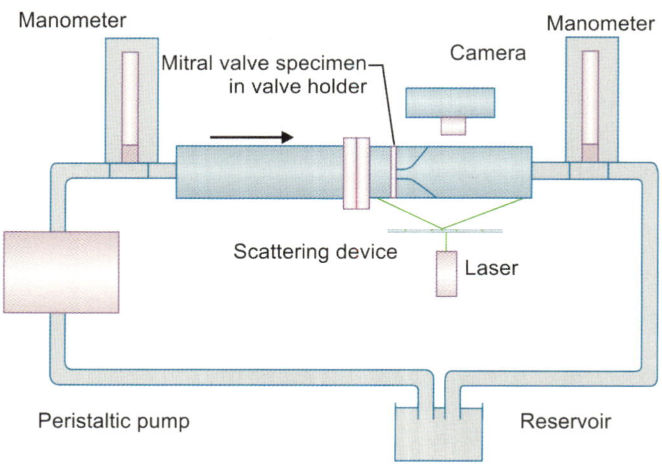

Figure 5 Simulation of blood flow through the mitral valve

Flow through a Healthy Mitral Valve (Figures 6A and B)

Velocity increases as water passes through the mitral valve annulus. The flow decelerates as the cross sectional area increases when the flow emerges from the annulus. The boundary layer separates when water passes through the leaflets causing flow in opposite directions, thus generating vortices. The formation of vortices is important in the flow of blood in the heart. The energy generated by the swirl helps propel the flow out of the ventricle. The set-up can be further developed to test various mitral valve patient's mitral valve failure can be evaluated through various medical imaging methods and the data obtained may be used to simulate a physical model which can be used as an analogue to

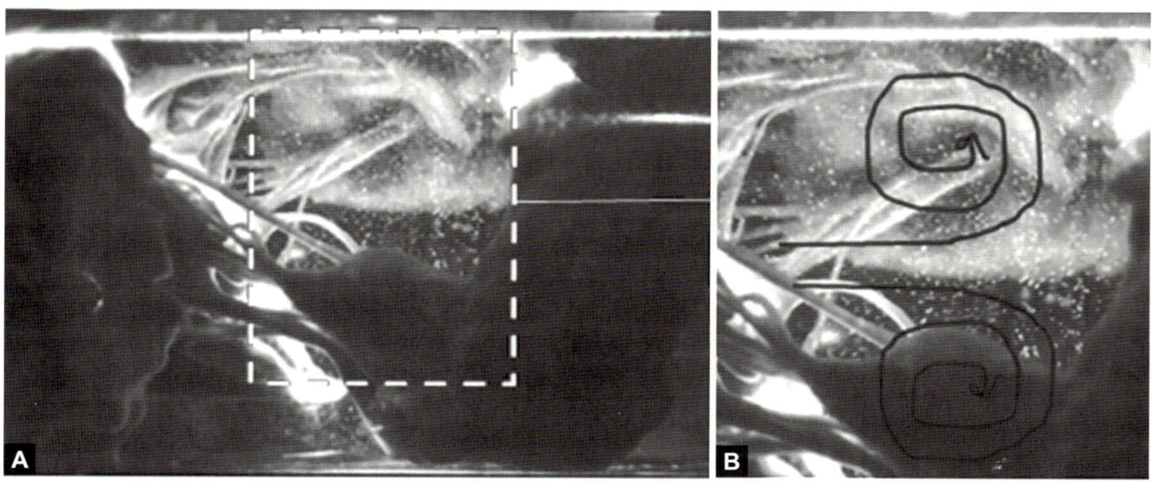

Figures 6A and B Flow through a healthy mitral valve

be placed inside the chamber. Various repair methods may be tested on the damaged mitral valve analogue. The method which yields the flow structure closest to a healthy mitral valve will be chosen for the patient.

EVALUATION OF MITRAL VALVE DYNAMICS

Current clinical 3-dimensional (3D) transesophageal echocardiography (TEE) can demonstrate volumetric morphology of the MV apparatus. However, biomechanical information is not available from 3D echocardiography. If imaging techniques can be combined with appropriate computational MV evaluation methods, then improved diagnosis and therapeutic approaches to MV repair can be developed **(Figures 7A and B)**.

Virtual MV models is created by utilizing 3D TEE data of patients with normal and pathological MVs followed by computational simulations of MV function.

Computational simulations clearly demonstrated deformation and stress distribution of the MV structure across the cardiac cycle at a microsecond scale and corresponded well to 3D TEE data **(Figures 8 and 9)**. Here we present 4 case studies (1 normal and 3 different types of pathological MVs) **(Figures 10 to 13)**.[3-5]

CONCLUSION

The availability of reality-enhanced TEE simulation is a significant departure from traditional training models that rely on a combination of didactics and real time clinical teaching particularly in assessing mitral valve as it is complex structure amongst all structure of heart. While more 'real world' in application, the challenges of simultaneous clinical management may place additional burden on educators in the operating room. Simulation in TEE provides a more controlled environment in which to assess the efficacy of this training methodology over conventional approaches while also providing objective data of different pathology to justify its routine use.

This technology can also be used by trainees in several disciplines such as anesthesiology, cardiology, cardiac surgery and critical care to improve proficiency

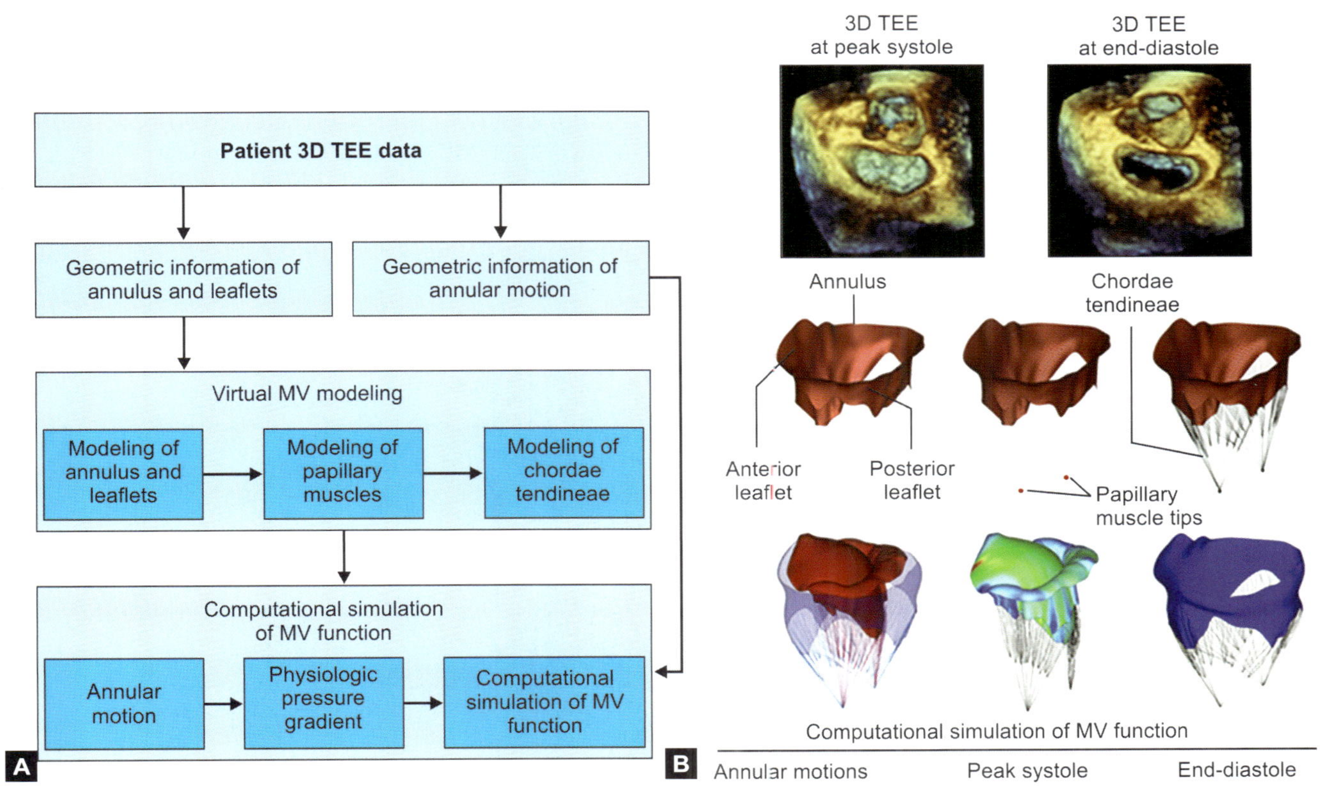

Figures 7A and B Flow chart for virtual MV modeling and computational simulation of MV function (A) Flow chart for the mitral valve (MV) evaluation protocol using 3-dimensional (3D) transesophageal echocardiography (TEE) data and computational simulation; (B) Representative image of the MV evaluation protocol described in (A)

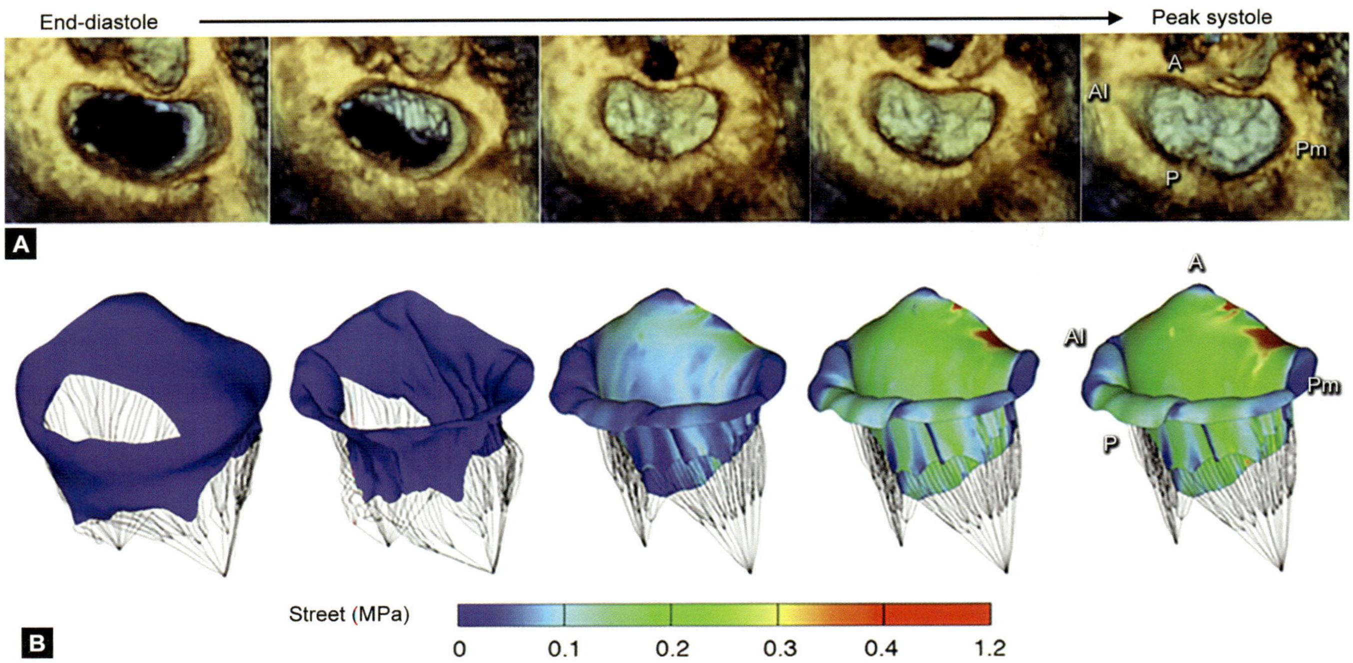

Figures 8A and B Images of a normal MV (A) Volumetric MV images from 3D TEE data demonstrating normal leaflet coaptation (atrial view); (B) Virtual MV model demonstrating dynamic motion of the annular morphology and stress distribution over the leaflets

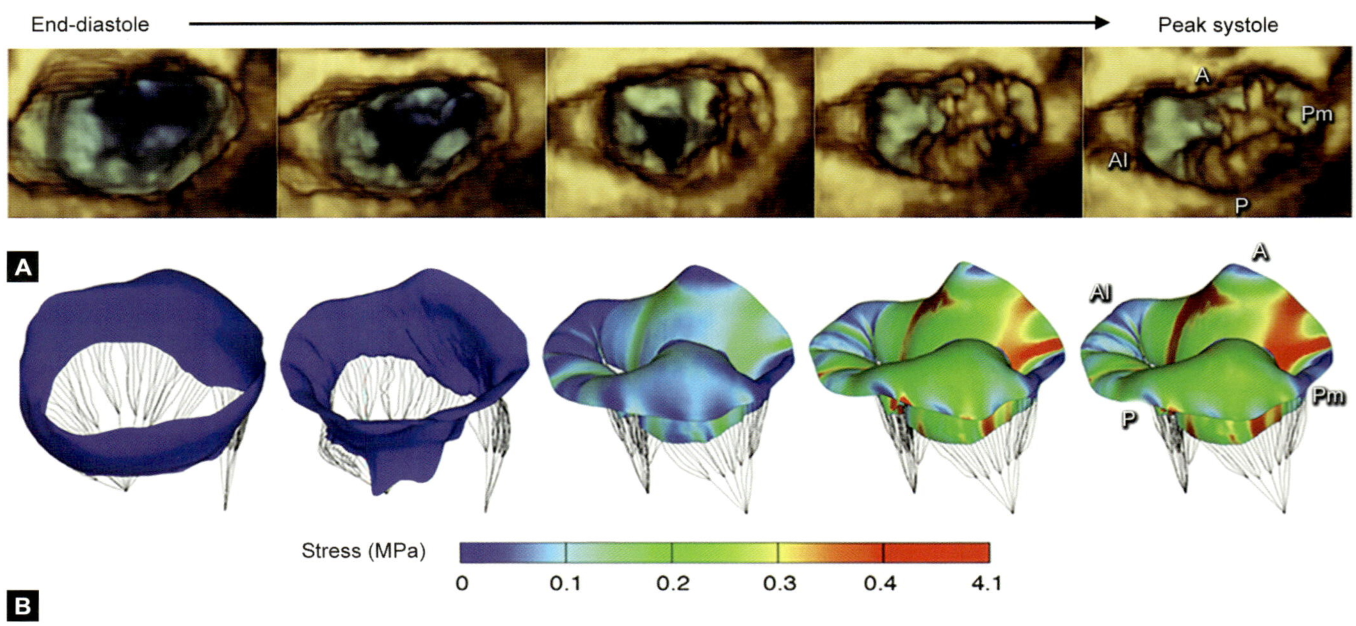

Figures 9A and B Images of a pathological MV with posterior chordal rupture (A) Volumetric MV images from 3D TEE data demonstrating posterior leaflet prolapse (atrial view). The scallops in the flail leaflet were involved with chordal rupture; (B) Virtual MV model with ruptured chordae demonstrating flail posterior leaflet prolapse and excessive leaflet stress concentration

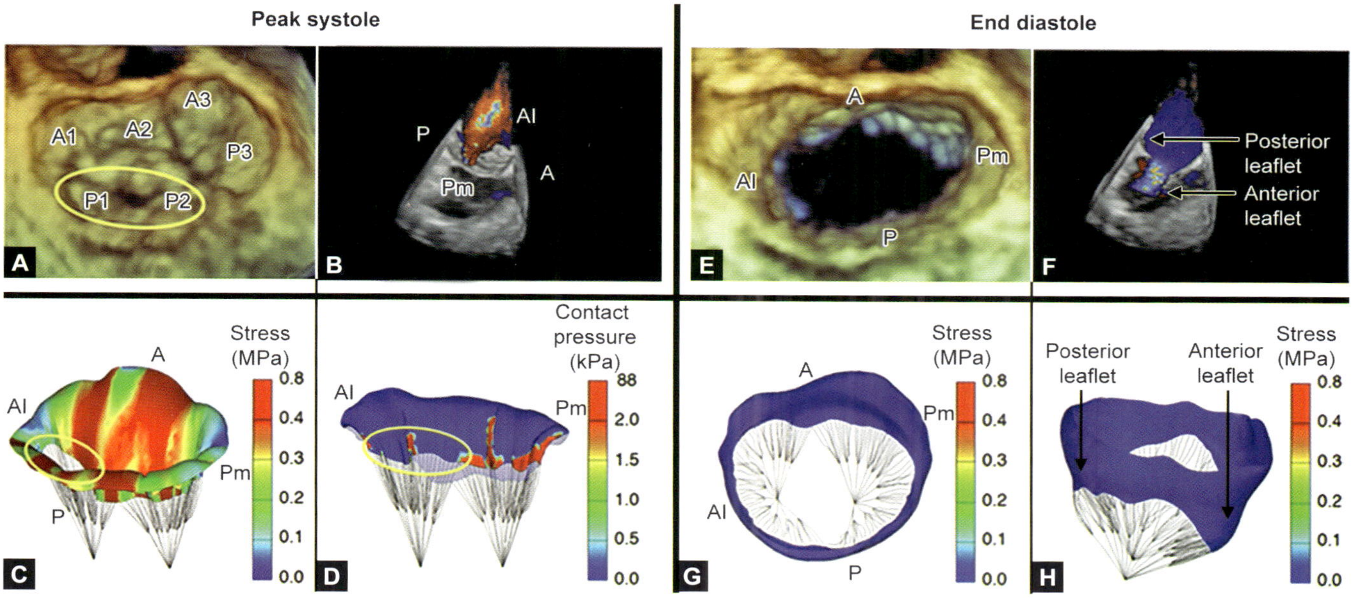

Figures 10A to H Case 1: A normal MV with complete coaptation; A to D (peak systole), E to H (end-diastole) (A) Volumetric MV image from 3D TEE data demonstrating normal leaflet coaptation at peak systole (ventricular view); (B) Two-dimensional (2D) Doppler TEE image at 60° demonstrating a cross-sectional commissural (Al-Pm) view; (C) Leaflet stress distribution demonstrating relatively symmetric stress distribution (atrial view); (D) Contact pressure distribution between the leaflets demonstrating complete coaptation (posterior view); (E) Volumetric MV image from 3D TEE data demonstrating 2 fully open leaflets at end-diastole (ventricular view); (F) 2D TEE image at 0°; (G) Leaflet stress distribution (atrial view); (H) Leaflet morphology corresponding to (F)

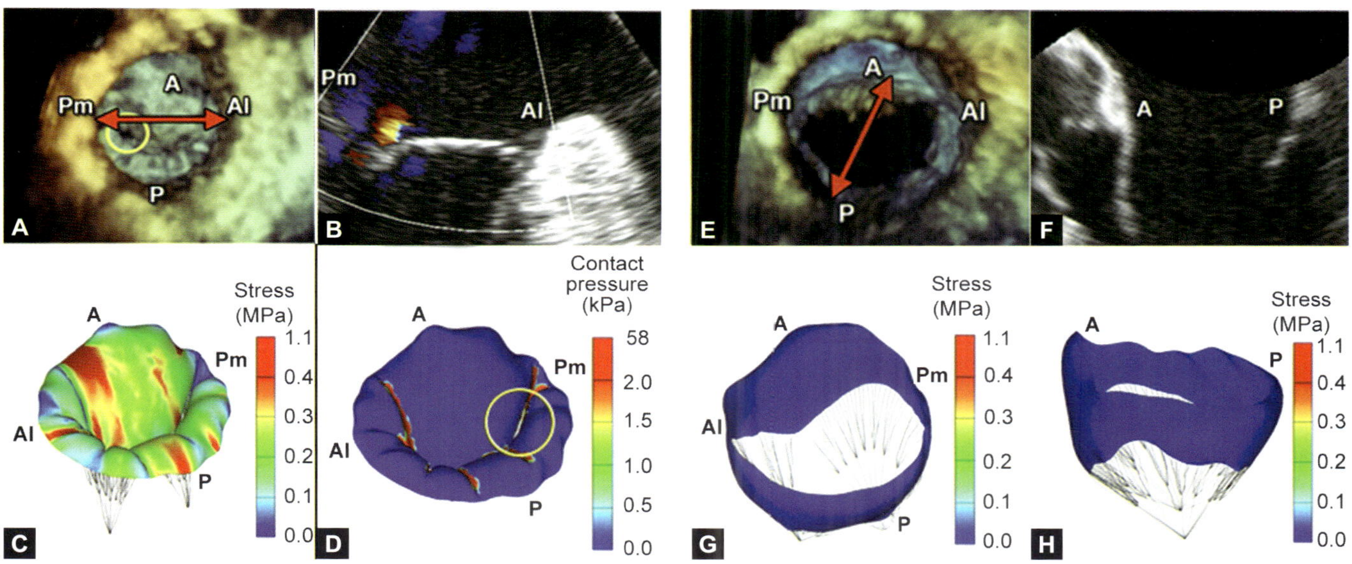

Figures 11A to H Case 2: A Degenerative MV with mild regurgitation and small annular dilation; A to D (peak systole), E to H (end-diastole) (A) Volumetric MV image from 3D TEE data demonstrating defective coaptation at peak systole (ventricular view); (B) 2D Doppler TEE image at 60° demonstrating the mild regurgitant jet (red arrow in [A]); (C) Leaflet stress distribution demonstrating asymmetrically distributed large stress values (atrial view); (D) Contact pressure distribution demonstrating faulty leaflet contact; (E) 3D TEE MV image data at end-diastole (ventricular view); (F) 2D TEE image at 0° (red arrow in [E]); (G) Leaflet stress distribution (atrial view); (H) Leaflet morphology corresponding to (F)

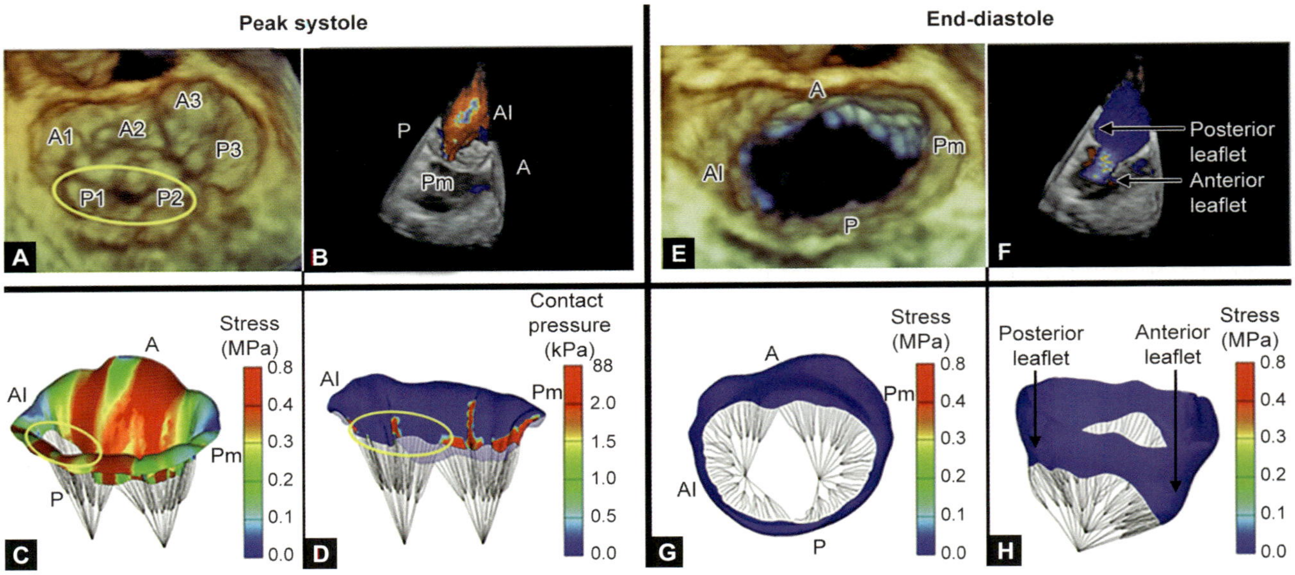

Figures 12A to H Case 3: A degenerative MV with severe regurgitation and large annular dilation; A to D (peak systole), E to H (end-diastole) (A) Volumetric MV image from 3D TEE data demonstrating defective coaptation (P1 and P2 scallops) at peak systole (atrial view); (B) 3D Doppler TEE image demonstrating severe regurgitation which corresponds to (A); (C) Leaflet stress distribution demonstrating defective coaptation and widely spread large stress distribution (atrial view); (D) No contact pressure between 2 leaflets in the scallops (posterior view); (E) 3D TEE MV image data at end-diastole (atrial view); (F) 3D Doppler TEE image; (G) Leaflet stress distribution (atrial view); (H) Leaflet morphology corresponding to (F)

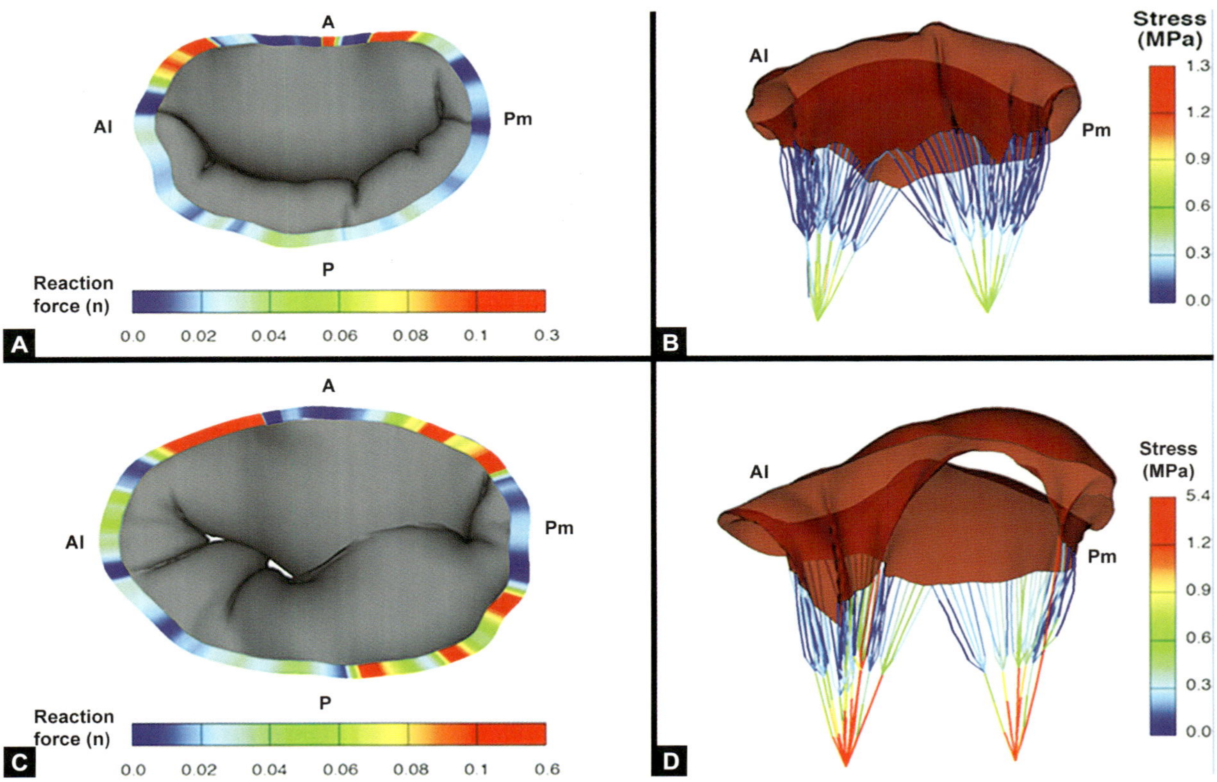

Figures 13A to D The mitral valve dynamics on computational simulator when reaction force "Stress" is applied to the valve

in basic TEE image acquisition and interpretation. At the present time, exposure to intraoperative TEE is challenging for trainees outside the operating room environment. The development of cardiac pathology will greatly help trainees develop the recommendations.

REFERENCES

1. Simulators for transesophageal echocardiography training. SCA Bulletin; 2013;12(2):124-5.
2. The transesophageal echocardiography simulator based on computed tomography images. IEEE transactions on biomedical engineering. 2013;60(2):292-9.
3. Simulator training for transesophageal echocardiography: Anesthesiology. 2014;121(2):430.
4. From real-time 3D echocardiography to mitral valve finite element analysis: A novel modeling approach. Computers in Cardiology. 2008;35:1-4.
5. Three-dimensional asymmetrical modeling of the mitral valve: A finite element study with dynamic boundaries. J Heart Valve Dis. 2005;14:386-92.

Chapter 11

Transesophageal Echocardiography in Intensive Care Unit

Kanchi Muralidhar

Chapter Outline

USEFULNESS ECHOCARDIOGRAPHY FOR CRITICAL CARE

Echocardiography is an important diagnostic and monitoring bed-side imaging modality which has transformed the care of critical ill patients. Many investigators have reiterated that echocardiography is of immense value in the critical ill patients; this modality of patient management is immediately available, portable, and importantly, relatively noninvasive and provides diagnosis fairly quickly without having to move the patient out of the intensive care unit. The list utility of echocardiography in intensive care unit is listed in the **Table 1**.

FOCUS ASSESSED TRANSTHORACIC ECHOCARDIOGRAPHY PROTOCOL FOR RAPID DIAGNOSIS IN INTENSIVE CARE UNIT

Using the FATE protocol, the cardiac structures are visualized through the chest wall. The FATE protocol is performed using the following four positions of the probe as shown in the diagram below **(Figures 1A and B)**:

1. *Subcostal view:* The transducer is placed in the epigastrium, a little to the right of the midline. The cardiac chambers are visualized as shown in (a); this imaging is easier to obtain in patients with chronic obstructive lung disease and those on positive pressure ventilation.
2. *Apical view:* This imaging is obtained by placing the transducer at the point of maximal cardiac impulse; please see (b) in the figure below.
3. *Parasternal view:* The transducer is placed in the left parasternal region either in the third of fourth intercostal space with the marker directed to the right shoulder. The long-axis of the left ventricle is visualized as shown in the figure (c); turning the probe by 90° at the same position clockwise will produce short axis of the LV as shown in the figure (d) below.
4. *Pleural view*: This view is obtained by placing the transducer probe on the lateral side of the chest to look for pleural effusion **(Figures 2A and B)**.

TABLE 1 Usefulness of echocardiography in the intensive care unit

• Hemodynamic management of hemodynamically unstable patient with hypotension
– Assess volume status
– Left ventricular function
– Regional wall motion abnormality
– Global myocardial dysfunction
– Right ventricular function
– Outflow tract obstruction
– Valvular stenosis/insufficiency
– Pericardial effusion/tamponade
– Pulmonary embolism
– Diastolic dysfunction
• Determination of cause of persistent hypoxia
– Right ventricular function
– Right ventricular pressure
– Intracardiac shunt
– Pulmonary embolus
• Diagnosis of aortic dissection
• Lung scan e.g. for pneumothorax
• Hemodynamic calculations
• Diagnosis and management of intracardiac infections
– Bacterial endocarditis
• Monitoring and surveillance
– Confirm/exclude pre-existing/current cardiac disease

The FATE protocol is followed the identity **(Figures 1A and B)**:[1]

- Obvious pathology.
- Assess wall thickness and chamber dimensions.
- Assess contractility.
- Image pleura on both sides.
- Relate findings to the clinical context.

However, the transthoracic echocardiography has significant limitations in the ICU settings especially in situations listed in the **Table 2**.

TABLE 2 Limitations of transthoracic imaging in intensive care unit

• Mechanical ventilation and intermittent positive pressure ventilation (IPPV)
– Especially PEEP > 15 cm H_2O
• Inaccessible/unobtainable windows
– Surgical dressing and drains
– Chest tubes
– Sternotomy/Thoracotomy/or upper abdominal incisions
• Surgery–induced fluid collections or edema of chest wall
• Inability to position patient optimally
• Obesity
• Severe chronic obstructive pulmonary diseases
• Pneumothorax, pneumopericardium
• Surgical/subcutaneous emphysema
• Lack of patient cooperation for respiratory maneuvers

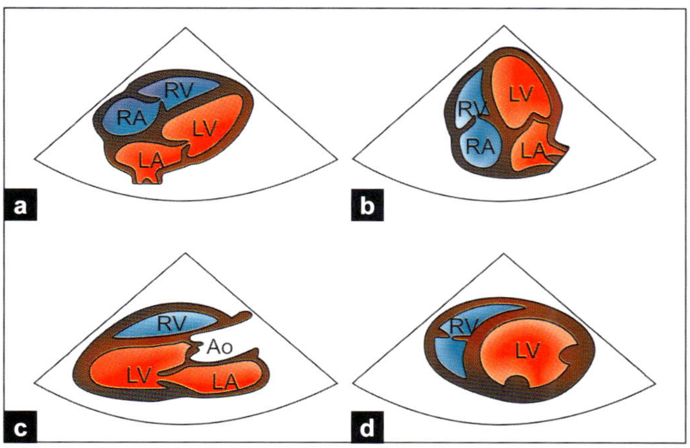

Figure 1A A schematic representation of FATE protocol (a) subcostal view (b) apical view (c) parasternal long axis view (d) parasternal short axis view

Abbreviations: RA, right atrium; RV, right ventricle; LA, left atrium; LV, left ventricular; Ao, aorta

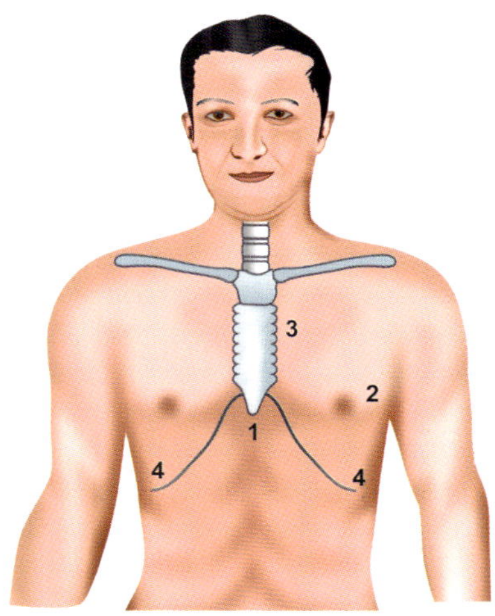

Figure 1B Transducer positions for FATE protocol (1) subcostal (2) apical (3) parasternal (4) pleural

Transesophageal Views Useful for Critical Care Units

In patients with poor acoustic windows using the transthoracic approach, the only alternative is to use the transesophageal approach. The following views are particularly useful in the ICU setting with the TEE approach.

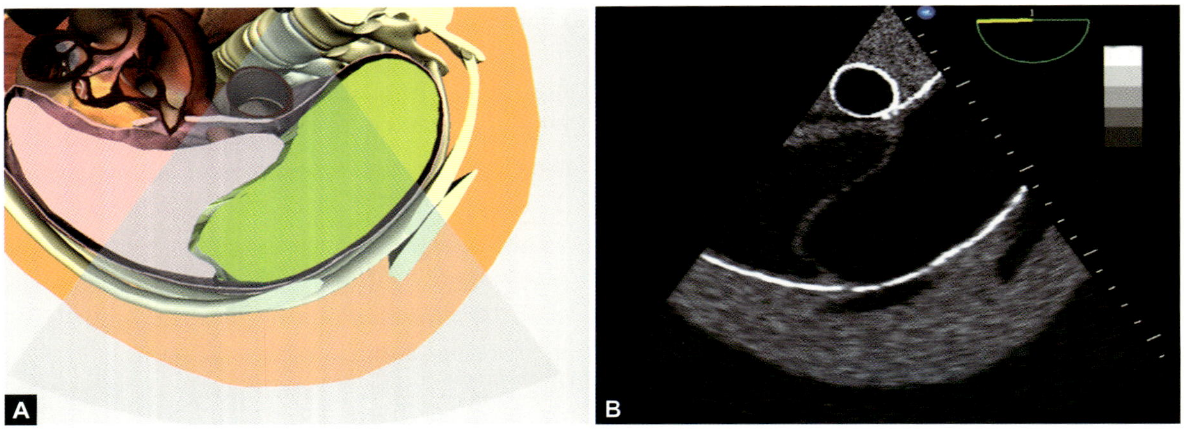

Figures 2A and B Left sided pleural effusion with collapsed left lung

Transgastric (TG) Midpapillary Short Axis (SAX) View

Required structures:
- Left ventricular (LV) cavity
- LV walls (at least 50% of the circumference with visible endocardium)
- Papillary muscles (approximately equal in size and distinct from ventricular wall)
- *Image settings:*
- *Angle:* ~0°
- *Sector depth:* ~12 cm
- *Probe adjustments:* Anteflexed

- *Primary diagnostic uses:*
- Hemodynamic instability
- LV enlargement
- LV hypertrophy
- LV preload, volume status of the patient
- LV systolic dysfunction
- LV regional wall motion (mid-segments)

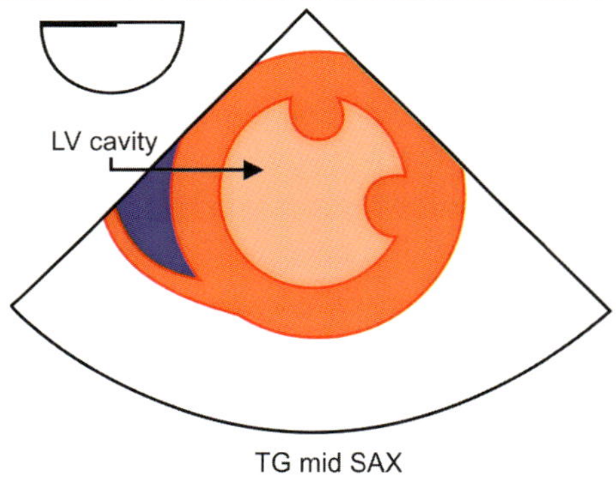

Midesophageal (ME) Four Chamber View

Required structures:
- Left atrium (LA)
- Left ventricular (LV)
- Right atrium
- Right ventricle (RV)
- Mitral valve
- TV

Image settings:
- *Angle:* ~ 0–10°
- *Sector depth:* ~12–14 cm

Probe adjustments:
- Neutral—retroflexed

- *Primary diagnostic uses:*
- Chamber enlargement/ dysfunction
- Left ventricular (LV) regional wall motion (inferoseptal and anterolateral walls)
- Mitral valve disease
- Tricuspid valve (TV) disease
- Detection of intracardiac air/ mass including thrombus and atrial septal defect

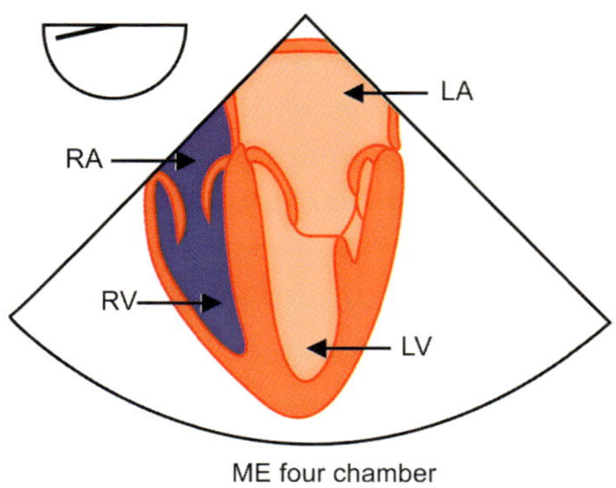

Abbreviations: LA, left atrium; LV, left ventricular; RV, right ventricle; RA, right atrium

Midesophageal (ME) Left Ventricular Long Axis (LAX) View

Required structures:	*Primary diagnostic uses:*	
• LA • Mitral valve • LV • LV outflow tract • Aortic valve (AV) and proximal ascending (ASC) aorta *Image settings:* • *Angle:* ~110–130° • *Sector depth:* ~12–14 cm *Probe adjustments:* • Neutral	• Mitral valve pathology • LV outflow tract pathology • LV ventricular wall motion (anteroseptal and inferolateral walls) • Systolic anterior motion of anterior mitral leaflet	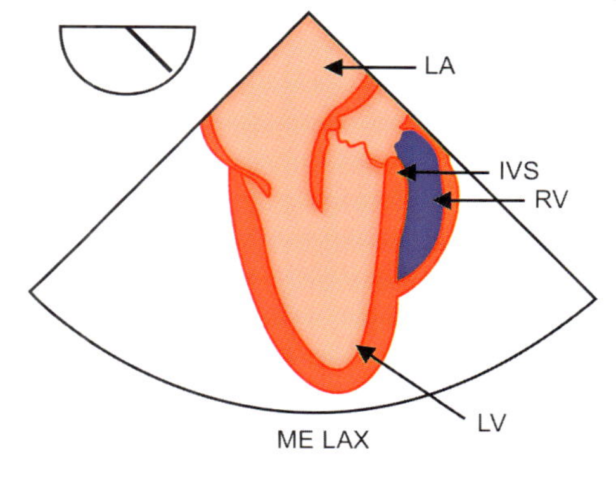

Abbreviations: LA, left atrium; LV, left ventricle; RV, right ventricle; IVS, interventricular septum

Midesophageal (ME) Ascending Aortic Short Axis (SAX) View

Required structures:	*Primary diagnostic uses:*	
• Aorta in cross-section in the transverse plane • Pulmonary artery (PA) (main and proximal right) *Image settings:* • *Angle:* ~10–30° • *Sector depth:* ~12 cm *Probe adjustments:* • Withdraw probe slowly by 1–2 cm from the AV SAX view	• Aortic atherosclerosis • Aortic dissection/aneurysm • PA pathology (emboli, dilatation, etc.)	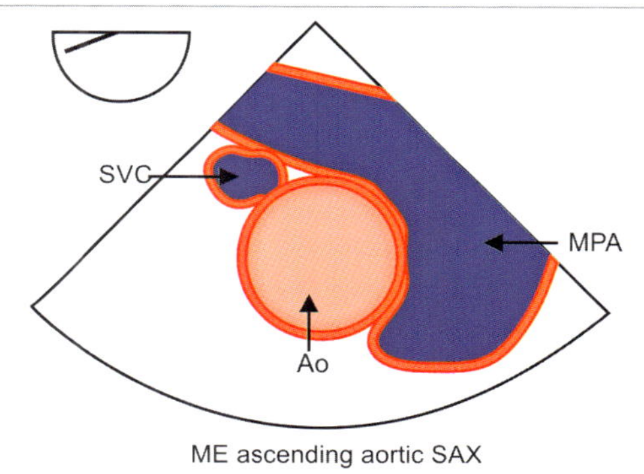

Abbreviations: Ao, aorta; MPA, main pulmonary artery; SVC, superior vena cava

Differential Diagnosis of Hypotension in Critical Care Unit

Use of TEE is a category I indication in the evaluation of life-threatening hemodynamic disturbances; **Table 3** shows the differential diagnosis of hypotension in the ICU setting.

Diagnosis of Cause of Persistent Hypoxia (Figures 3 and 4)

In patients with persistent or refractory hypoxemia, the presence of intracardiac shunt must be excluded by injecting agitated saline through the right side of the heart e.g. upper limb vein: intracardiac shunt results in saline contrast appearing in the left side of the heart instantaneously where as in case of an intrapulmonary shunt, e.g. pulmonary arteriovenous malformation, the contrast appears on the left side after about 3–5 cardiac cycles. Calculation of right atrial pressure is most required **(Table 4)** in all cases in the ICU.

EVALUATION OF LEFT VENTRICULAR SYSTOLIC FUNCTION (FIGURES 5A AND B)

Left ventricular (LV) global systolic performance is commonly expressed in terms of one or more of the following, all of which can be determined by echocardiography by TTE or TEE. The parameters are (i) fractional shortening (FS), (ii) fractional area change (FAC) (iii), ejection fraction (EF), (iv) cardiac output.

Fractional Shortening

Fractional shortening (FS) is determined by the formula:

LVIDd−LVIDs/LVIDd × 100

TABLE 3 Differential diagnosis of hypotension in critical care unit

Condition	*TEE findings*	*Useful views*
Hypovolemia	Decreased EDA Increased FAC "Kissing" papillary muscles	TG SAX of LV TG LAX of LV
Vasodilatation	Normal EDA Increased FAC	TG SAX of LV ME 4 ch, 2 ch, LAX
Impaired LV systolic function	Increased EDA, decreased FAC Increased ESA, decreased FAC	TG SAX of LV TG LAX of LV
Pericardial tamponade	Effusion Diastolic collapse of right-sided chambers	ME 4 ch; TG SAX and LAX of LV
Aortic dissection	Intimal flap Two lumens in aorta (one true and other false), aortic regurgitation, Pericardial effusion	ME 5 ch; and LAX; ascending/ descending Ao
Pulmonary embolism	Dilated RA and RV TR/PR jets, flow through PFO, echogenic density in PA	ME 4 ch; RV in/outflow; PA views (upper E)

Abbreviations: EDA, end-diastolic area; ESA, end systolic area; TG SAX, transgastric short axis; TG LAX, transgastric long axis; FAC, fractional area change; ME, midesophageal; 2ch, two chamber; 4ch, four chamber; RA, right atrium; LV, left ventricle; RV, right ventricle; Ao, aorta; LA, left atrium; PA, pulmonary artery; E, esophageal; TR, tricuspid regurgitation; PR, pulmonic regurgitation; PFO, patent foramen ovale

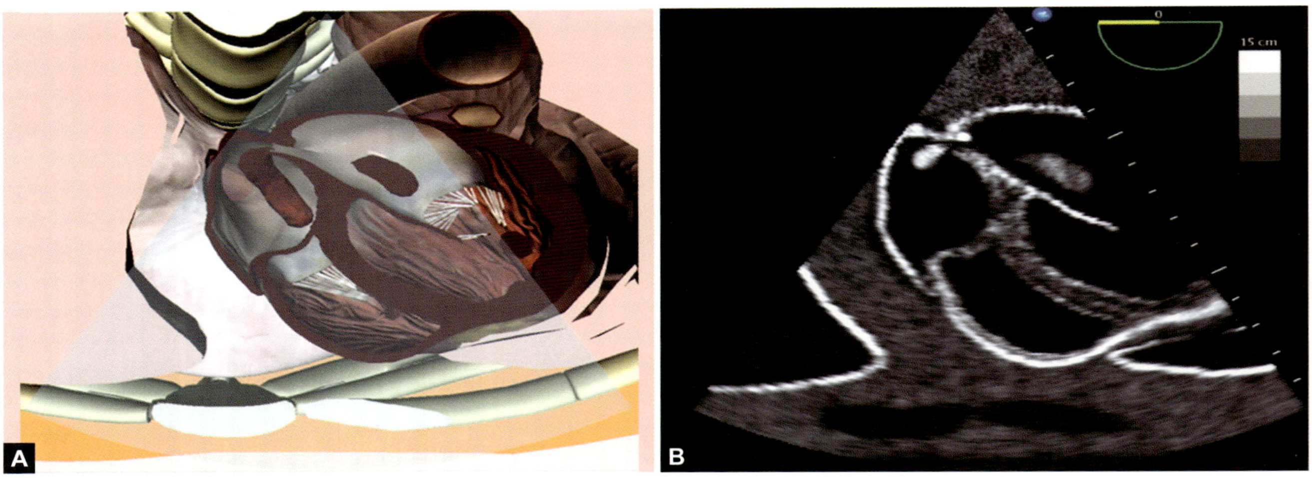

Figures 3A and B Simulation picture of movement of a thrombus across a patent foramen ovale (PFO) from left atrium (LA) to right atrium (RA)

Where IDs refers to internal diameter in systole and IDd refers to internal diameter in diastole. Using TEE the LV systolic function is best estimated by using the transgastric-mid papillary short axis. FS is heavily afterload dependent and slightly preload dependent.

Fractional Area Change

Fractional area change (FAC) is a relatively simple parameter to determine that is obtained from the transgastric mid papillary view. FAC is the relation between LV diastolic area to the systolic area obtained from the following equation: FAC%= end diastolic area– end *systolic area*/end diastolic area × 100.

Ejection Fraction

Ejection fraction is calculated by using the equation EDV–ESV/EDV × 100, where EDV refers to end-diastolic volume and ESV refers to end-systolic volume. However, please note that all geometric methods make assumptions on shape of ventricle and presence of wall

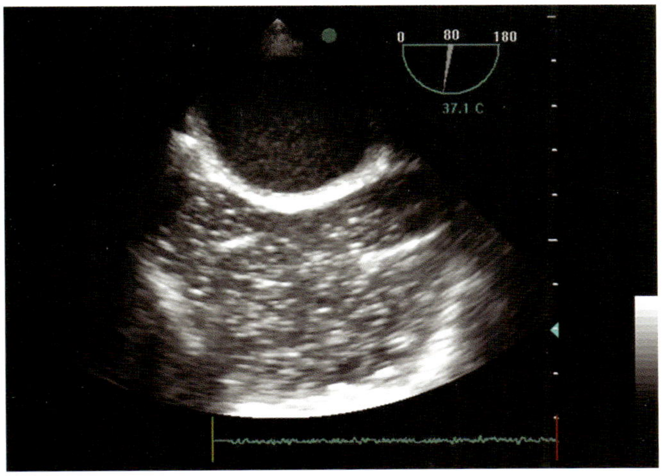

Figure 4 ME bi-caval view showing saline contrast in RA with intact interatrial septum

TABLE 4 Measurement of right atrial pressure (RAP)

Inferior vena cava diameter	*Change with negative inspiration (i.e. sniff)*	*Estimated RAP (mm Hg)*
Small (< 1.5 cm)	Collapse	0–5
Normal (1.5–2.5 cm)	Decrease by > 50%	5–10
Normal (1.5–2.5 cm)	Decrease by < 50%	10–15
Dilated (> 2.5 cm)	Decrease by < 50%	15–20
Dilated (with dilated hepatic veins)	No change	> 20

motion abnormality makes the determination of EF untenable.

Estimation of Cardiac Output (Figure 6)

Flow across a fixed orifice is the product of the cross sectional area (CSA) and the velocity of flow through the orifice. The cardiovascular system is pulsatile and hence the velocity of instantaneous blood flow varies. The integration of the instantaneous flow rate over the entire flow period through a given orifice is called the velocity-time integral (VTI). Stroke volume (SV) is derived as a product of CSA and VTI as shown below. Cardiac output in turn is the product of the SV and the heart rate. The preferred site of measurement of SV and cardiac output is the LV outflow tract (LVOT).

Diagnosis of Infective Endocarditis (Figure 7)

Echocardiography is necessary for the diagnosis and management of patients suffering from infective endocarditis (IE). The two essential components of echocardiographic features of IE are (i) oscillating intracardiac mass or vegetation (ii) annular abscess, dehiscence of prosthetic valve or acute valvular regurgitation.

Detection of Myocardial Ischemia (Figure 8)

Recognition and identification of regional wall motion abnormality can be readily achieved by

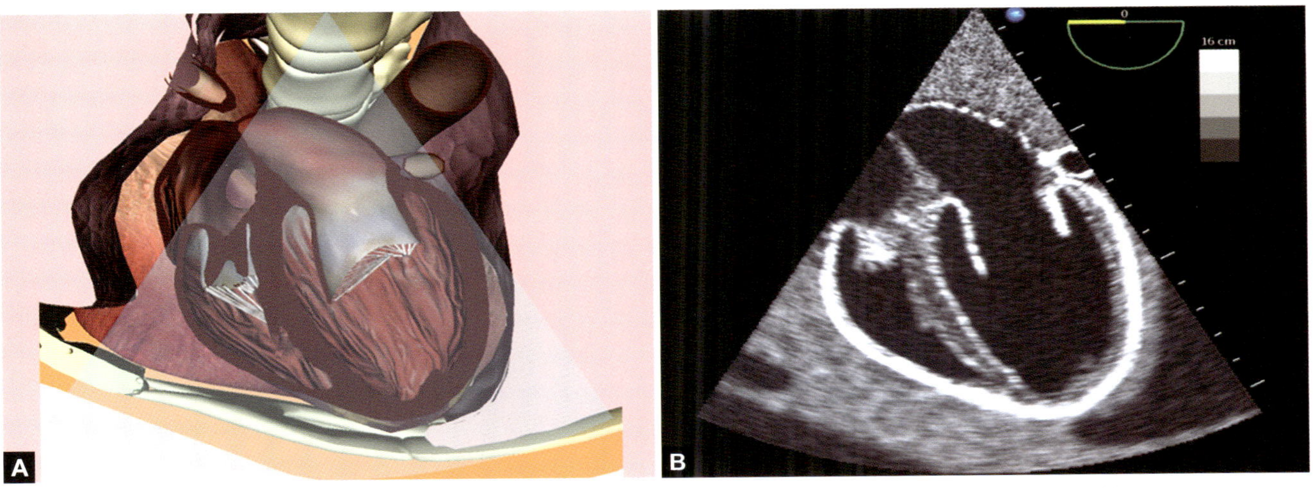

Figures 5A and B Simulation picture of midesophageal 4-chamber view showing left ventricular dilation

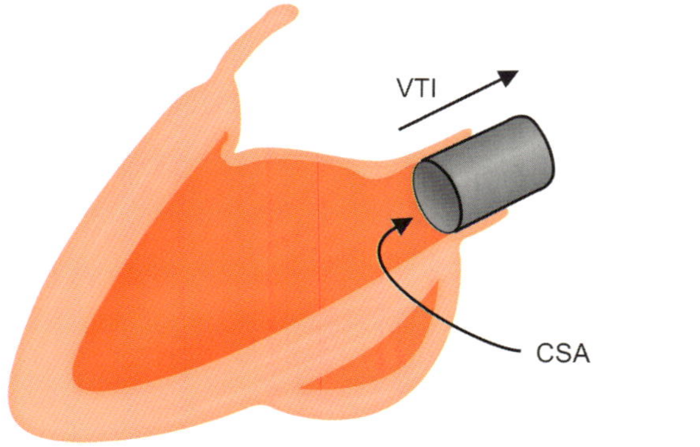

Figure 6 Use of Doppler echocardiography in calculation of stroke volume (SV). The VTI of the Doppler velocity curve can be conceptualized as the length of a cylinder of blood (stroke distance) ejected through a CSA on one heart-beat. SV is calculated as the product of CSA and VTI; SV (cm^3) = CSA (cm^2) × VTI (cm)
Abbreviations: CSA, cross-sectional area; VTI, velocity time integral

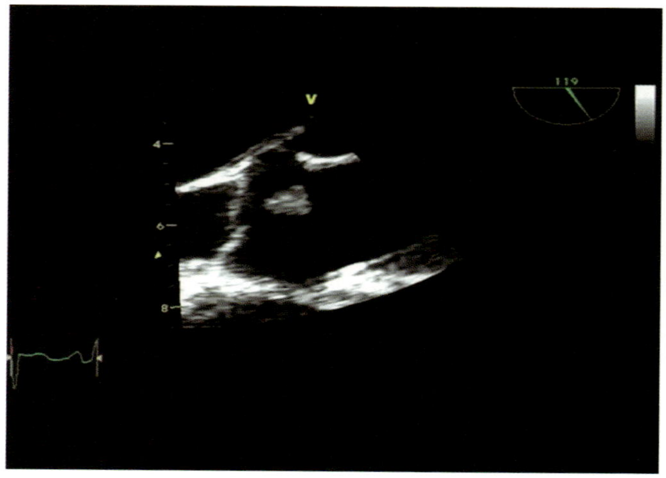

Figure 7 ME long axis of aortic valve showing vegetation attached the downstream of aortic value

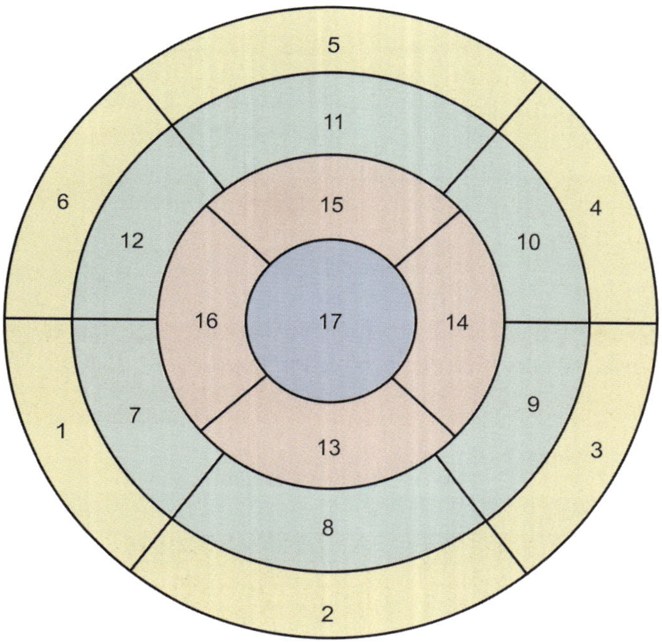

1 = Basal anteroseptal
2 = Basal anterior
3 = Basal anterolateral
4 = Basal inferolateral
5 = Basal inferior
6 = Basal inferoseptal
7 = Mid anteroseptal
8 = Mid anterior
9 = Mid anterolateral
10 = Mid inferolateral
11 = Mid inferior
12 = Mid inferoseptal
13 = Apical anterior
14 = Apical lateral
15 = Apical inferior
16 = Apical septal
17 = Apex

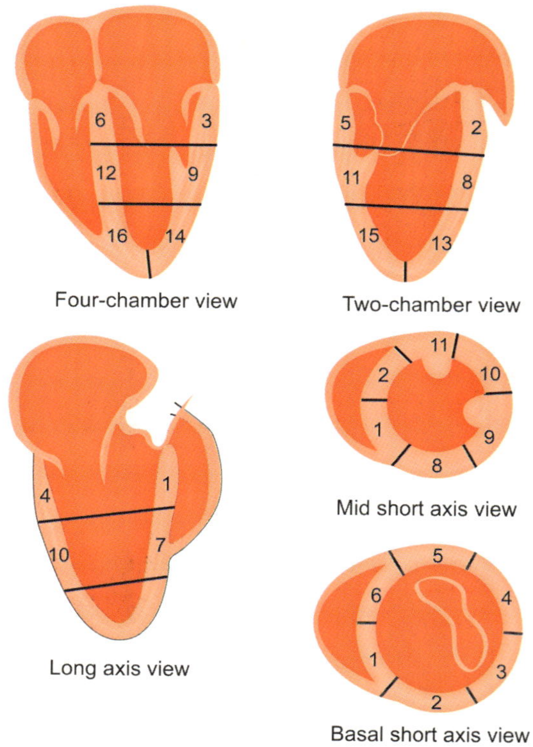

Basal segment
1 = Basal anteroseptal
2 = Basal anterior
3 = Basal anterolateral
4 = Basal inferolateral
5 = Basal inferior
6 = Basal inferoseptal

Mid segments
7 = Mid anteroseptal
8 = Mid anterior
9 = Mid anterolateral
10 = Mid inferolateral
11 = Mid inferior
12 = Mid inferoseptal

Apical segments
13 = Apical anterior
14 = Apical lateral
15 = Apical inferior
16 = Apical septal

Figure 8 17-segments model of regional LV assessment; the basal and midlevel and divided into six segments and apex into four segments

two-dimensional echocardiography in the ICU setting. Serial echocardiography is useful in monitoring the success of reperfusion therapy and extent of myocardial viability.

Diagnosis of Aortic Pathology (Figures 9 and 10)

Transesophageal echocardiography is an extremely useful modality for the diagnosis and classification of thoracic aortic pathology namely aneurysm, dissection and atheromatous lesion.[2,3] A thoracic aortic aneurysm is a permanent localized dilatation of thoracic aorta that has at least a 50% diameter increase involving all the three layers of the vessel wall. Less than 150% of normal localized dilatation of the thoracic aorta is termed 'ectasis'. Annuloaortic ectasia is defined as isolated dilatation of the ascending aorta, aortic root, and aortic valve annulus. A false aneurysm or a pseudoaneurysm is a localized dilation of the aorta that does not contain all three layers of the vessel wall; instead a false aneurysm consists of connective tissue and clot.

TEE is particularly useful in diagnosis of an aortic dissection with a complete picture of origin/location of dissection flap, involvement of coronary ostia with an associated risk of myocardial ischemia, degree of aortic insufficiency and pericardial effusion.

Diagnosis of Pericardial Tamponade (Figures 11A and B)

Quick and rapid accumulation of pericardial fluid in the closed pericardial cavity can precipitate hemodynamic instability and cardiovascular collapse.

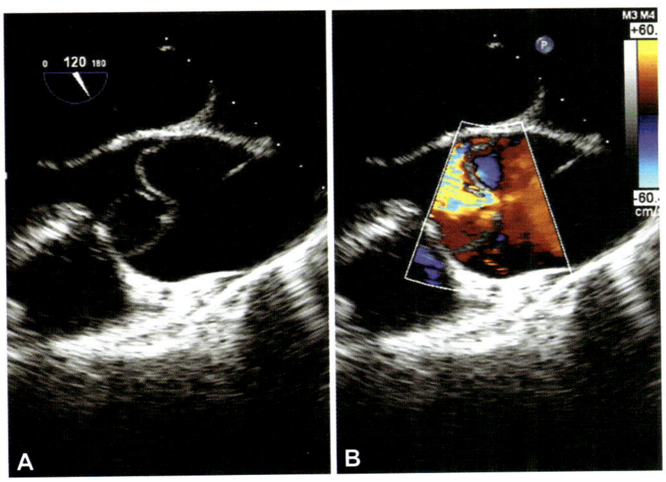

Figures 9A and B ME long axis of aortic valve showing intimal flap in the aortic lumen

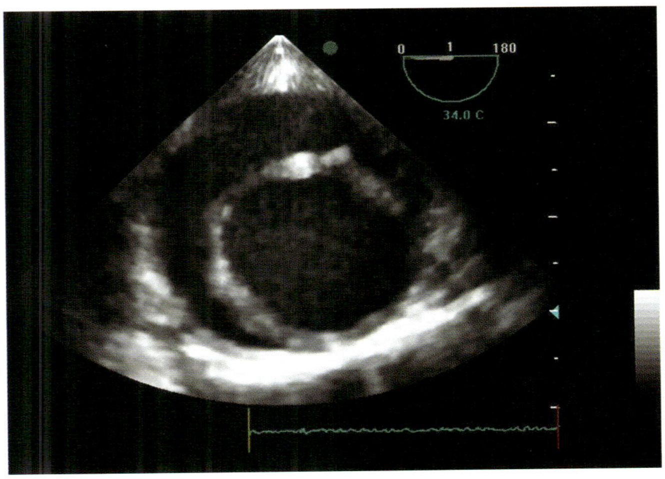

Figure 10 Short axis of descending thoracic aorta showing aortic dissection

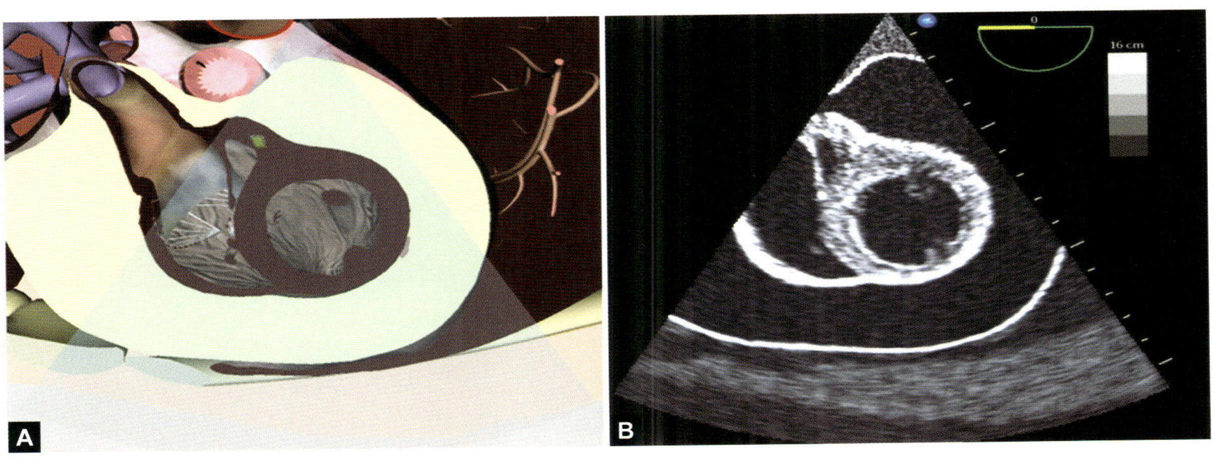

Figures 11A and B Simulation picture of transgastic short axis showing global pericardial effusion

Echocardiographic findings consistent with pericardial effusion and tamponade are listed in the **Table 5**.

TABLE 5 Diagnostic criteria for pericardial effusion/tamponade

Clinical	
Elevated jugular venous pressures	
Pulsus paradoxus	
Hypotension	
Low cardiac output	
2D Echo	
Swinging heart (electrical alternans)	
RA collapse late diastole	
RV collapse early diastole	
Dilated IVC without inspiratory collapse	
LA collapse in late diastole and early systole	
Doppler (Spontaneous ventilation)	
Respiratory variation in mitral and tricuspid inflow	
Inspiration	Increased tricuspid E-wave velocity
	Decreased mitral E-wave velocity
Expiration	Decreased tricuspid E-wave velocity
	Increased mitral E-wave velocity
Hepatic flow	Expiration severely decreased diastolic forward flow or flow reversal
	Atrial component flow reversal

Diagnosis of Pulmonary Embolism (Figures 12A and B)

The 2D echocardiography either using TTE or TEE is useful to provide supportive evidence of acute pulmonary embolism. McConnel and colleagues demonstrated that patients with acute pulmonary thromboembolism have a distinct regional pattern of RV dysfunction with akinesis of mid-free wall but preserved contractility of the RV apex.[4] The echocardiographic indicators of acute pulmonary embolism are shown in the **Table 6**.

TABLE 6 Echocardiographic indicators of acute pulmonary embolism

Direct	Evidence of clot
Indirect	Right heart strain
	RV dilation
	McConnell's sign
	Abnormal septal motion
	Tricuspid regurgitation
	Pulmonary hypertension
	Inferior vena cava dilation
	Pulmonary artery dilation

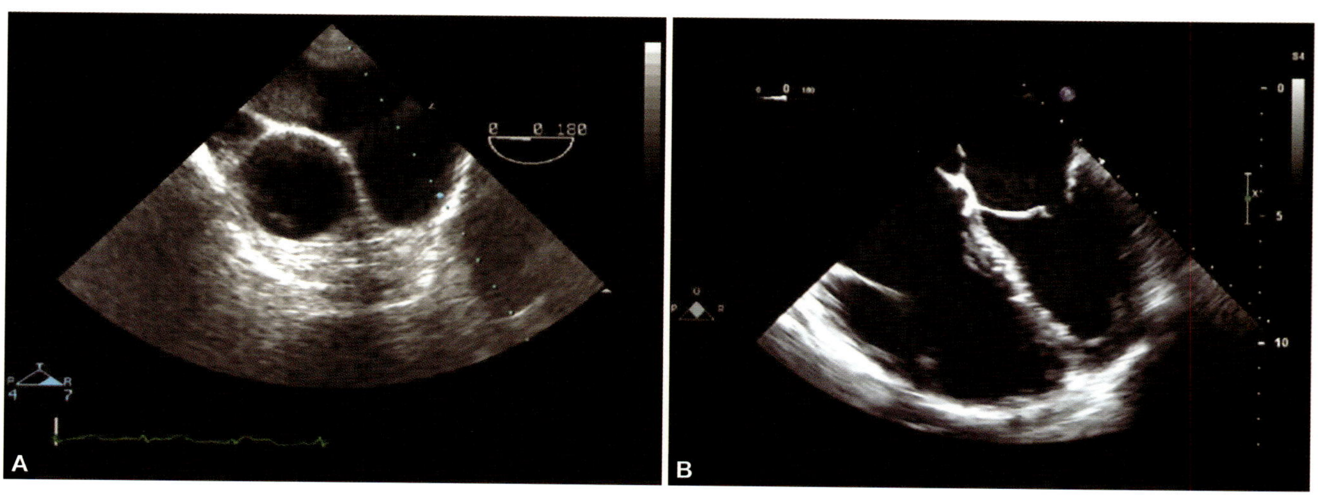

Figures 12A and B (A) ME ascending aortic short axis showing embolism in right pulmonary artery; (B) ME 4-chamber view showing right ventricle dilation in pulmonary embolism

CONCLUSION

Hemodynamic instability associated with hypotension in the ICU is a class I indication for performing TEE. The advantage of TEE is that it provides better acoustic windows than that with TTE in almost all mechanically ventilated patients. It has been demonstrated that TEE leads to a change in management in more than 50% of ICU patients when performed for hemodynamic instability. TEE is especially of proven value assessment of suspected infective endocarditis and diagnosis of aortic dissection.

REFERENCES

1. Focus Assessed Transthoracic Echo—Fate-Protocol. *www.fate-protocol.com/130067GE_Fate_Card.pdf*
2. Keren A, Kim CB, Hu BS, et al. Accuracy of biplane and multiplane transesophageal echocardiography in diagnosis of typical acute aortic dissection and intramural hematoma. J Am Coll Cardiol. 1996;28:627.
3. Willens HJ, Kessler KM. Transesophageal echocardiography in the diagnosis of diseases of the thoracic aorta: part 1. Aortic dissection, aortic intramural hematoma, and penetrating atherosclerotic ulcer of the aorta. Chest. 1999;116:1772.
4. Rosenberger P1, Shernan SK, Body SC, Eltzschig HK. Utility of intraoperative transesophageal echocardiography for diagnosis of pulmonary embolism. Anesth Analg. 2004;99(1):12-6.

Chapter 12

Simulation for Transesophageal Echocardiography of Tricuspid and Pulmonary Valves

Dharmesh Agarwal, Poonam Malhotra Kapoor

Chapter Outline

- Pulmonary Valve
- Pulmonary Stenosis
- Pulmonary Regurgitation
- Tricuspid Valve
- Etiology of Tricuspid Disease
- Tricuspid Regurgitation
- Tricuspid Stenosis

PULMONARY VALVE

Anatomy

It is a trileaflet valve with three semilunar cusps (one anterior and two posterior (right and left)). It is similar to the aortic valve in basic structure and function with thinner leaflets and larger area in comparison to aortic valve. In relation to the aortic valve it is located anterosuperior and to the left. The leaflets are directly connected to the musculature of the RV. The pulmonary valve (PV) is roughly perpendicular to the aortic valve.

Transesophageal Echocardiography Views

The PV is sometimes difficult to visualize by transesophageal echo because of its anterior location.[1]

1. *Midesophageal right ventricular (ME RV) inflow-outflow view (multiplane angle ≈50°–70°)* **(Figure 1)**: This view is obtained by increasing the multiplane angle (≈50°–70°) from midesophageal (ME) aortic valve short axis view without changing the probe position and keeping the aortic valve in the center of the image. PV valve will be seen in long axis in this view since it is oriented perpendicular to the aortic valve. PV will be seen in the far field adjacent to the right coronary cusp-left coronary cusp (RCC-LCC) commissure.[2-4] This view cannot be utilized for Doppler assessment due to non-alignment of ultrasound beam to the blood flow **(Figure 2)**.
2. *Upper esophageal (UE) aortic short axis view (multiplane angle ≈0°–30°)*: This view is obtained by keeping the probe in upper esophagus with multiplane angle ≈0°–30°. Main pulmonary artery branching into the right pulmonary artery (RPA) and left pulmonary artery (LPA) will be seen in the long axis, while aorta and superior vena cava in the

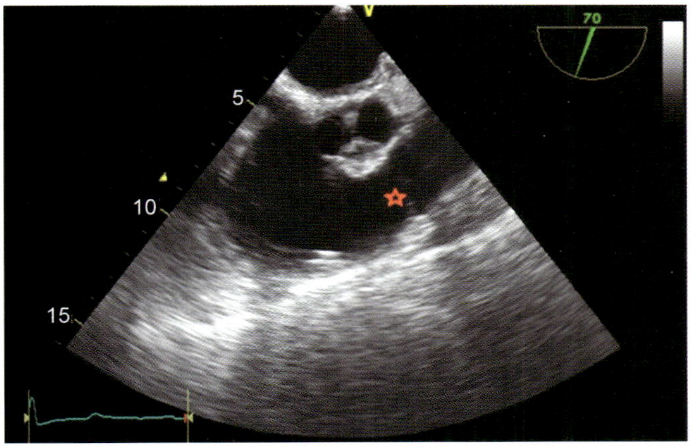

Figure 1 Midesophageal right ventricular (ME RV) inflow-outflow view, pulmonary valve is seen next to star

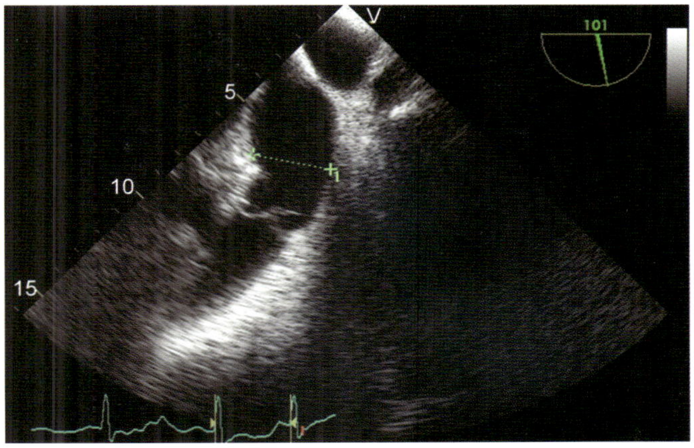

Figure 3 Upper esophageal (UE) aortic arch short axis (SAX) view

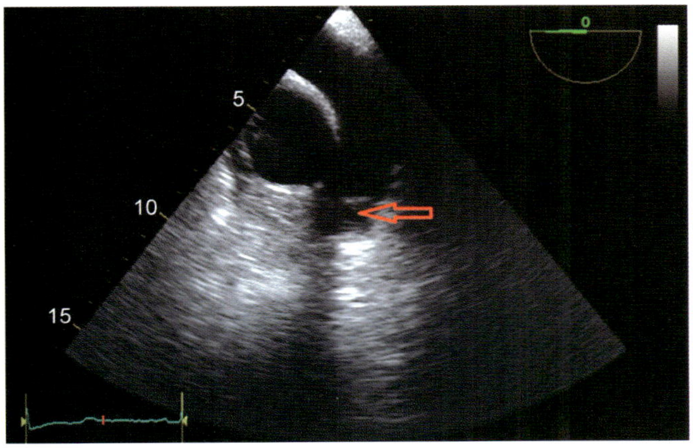

Figure 2 Upper esophageal (UE) ascending aorta SAX view, next to arrow PV is seen

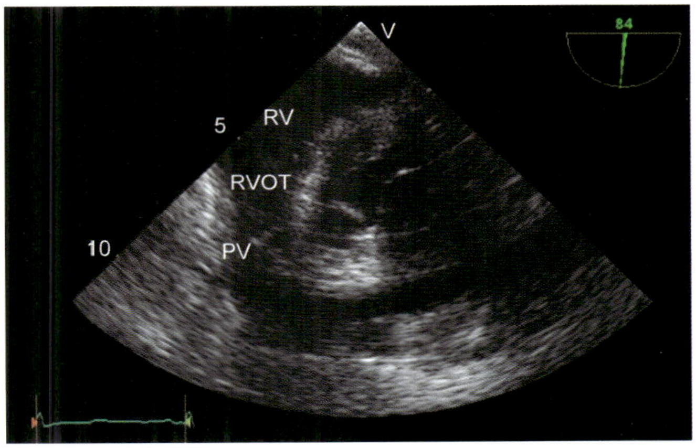

Figure 4 Transgastric pulmonary valve (TG PV) view
Abbreviations: RV, right ventricle; RVOT, right ventricular outflow tract; PV, pulmonary valve

short axis. PV can be seen in some patients in the farfield to the left of image. This is important view for Doppler assessment of main pulmonary artery (MPA) and PV (if visible) **(Figure 3)**.

3. *Upper esophageal aortic arch short axis (SAX) view (multiplane angle ≈70°–90°):* This view is obtained by changing multiplane angle ≈70°–90° from UE aortic arch long axis view. One can easily locate the level of stenosis and as well grade the severity of it. This view is excellent for examination of proximal part of pulmonary artery **(Figure 4)**.
4. *Transgastric PV view (multiplane angle ≈60°–90°)*: To obtain this view one need to increase multiplane angle ≈60°–90° with right flexion from deep transgastric aortic valve (TG AV) view until right ventricular ouflow tract (RVOT) and PV is seen in the far field on the right of image. This view is very important for Doppler assessment of the RVOT and PV. One can easily identify the level of obstruction (mid RV, infundibular or valvular) and grade the severity of it.

PULMONARY STENOSIS

The most common cause is congenital which can be subvalvular, valvular or supravalvular. It can be due to rheumatic heart disease, carcinoid, or infective endocarditis. The severity of stenosis is evaluated through Doppler examination **(Table 1)**.

CHAPTER 12

TABLE 1 Grading severity of pulmonary stenosis

Severity of pulmonary stenosis	*Peak systolic gradient across PV (MM of Hg)*
Mild	≤ 29
Moderate	30–60
Severe	>60

Two-dimensional Echocardiography (Figures 5 and 6)

There will be abnormal systolic leaflet motion and doming of leaflets into the pulmonary artery. Long standing stenosis will lead to poststenotic dilatation of pulmonary artery.[5] Two-dimensional echocardiography has some clear advantages over M-mode, because it can gather and display anatomic data in a form that all physicians are familiar with. Its spatial characteristics are such that target recognition is greatly enhanced, resulting in rapid, accurate identification of valves and chambers.

Its ability to localize and identify such cardiac structures as the recesses or commissures of valves or portions of the right and left ventricles is superior to that of M-mode. This is of particular value when sound transmission qualities are impaired. The spatial morphology of structures is readily appreciated by the two-dimensional approach, so that vegetative lesions may not only be detected, but also sized and characterized morphologically.

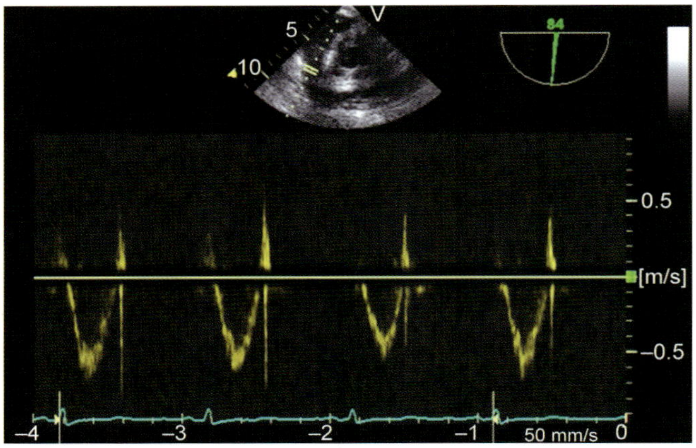

Figure 5 Pulsed wave (PW) Doppler across pulmonary valve

Doppler Echocardiography (Figures 7 and 8)

There will be increased flow velocities through the valve and turbulence beyond the orifice on color Doppler. It is the severe pulmonary stenosis which will require treatment. Use color Doppler to look for any coexistent tricuspid regurgitation. The color jet can also help in obtaining correct alignment of the probe for continuous wave (CW) and pulsed-wave (PW) Doppler recordings. Use Doppler to record forward flow through the tricuspid valve from a modified ME 4 chamber view. Ignore traces obtained from ectopic beats (and the beat following an ectopic), and if the patient is in AF, average

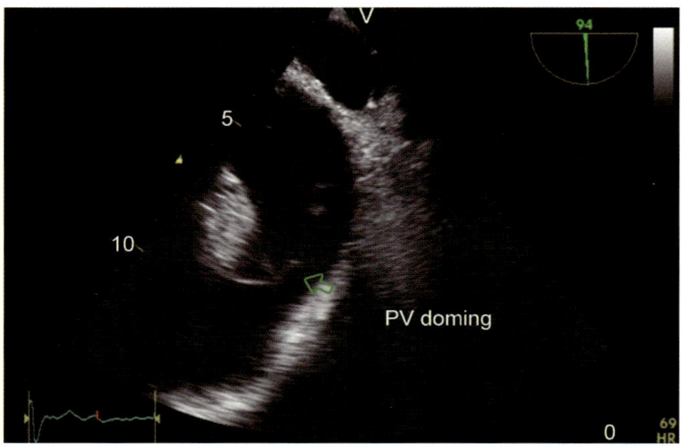

Figure 6 Thickened pulmonary valve (PV) in upper esophageal (UE) aortic arch SAX view

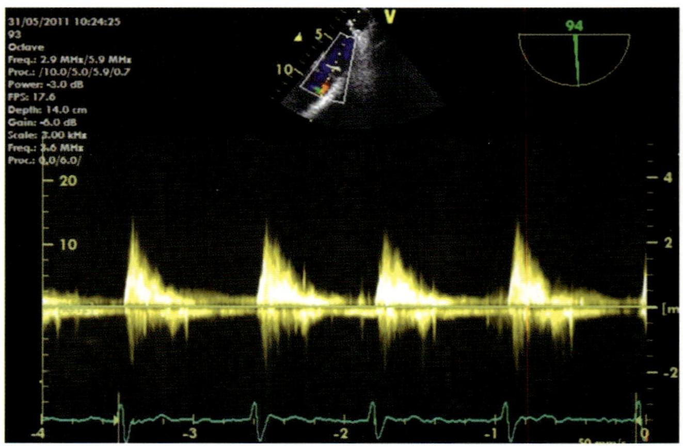

Figure 7 Continuous wave (CW) Doppler across pulmonary valve; mild pulmonary stenosis

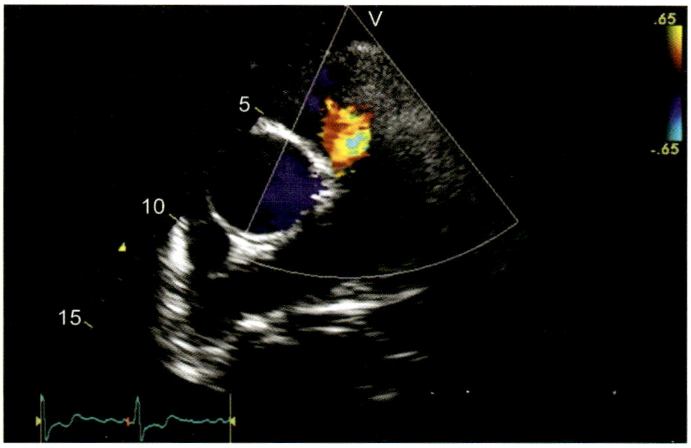

Figure 8 PR color Doppler jet, transthoracic echocardiography (TTE)

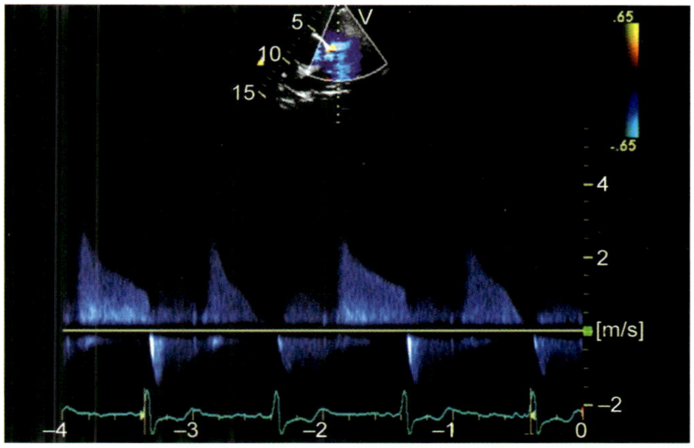

Figure 9 PW across PV in case of PR, TTE

the measurements taken from several beats. From the trace, measure the mean tricuspid valve gradient (trace the velocity time integral (VTI) of the tricuspid inflow).

PULMONARY REGURGITATION

Most common reason of pulmonary regurgitation is acquired either from surgical correction of tetralogy of Fallot (especially with transannular patch) or pulmonary hypertension (leading to dilated pulmonary artery and pulmonary annulus). Other cause includes rheumatic, carcinoid, infective and congenital.

Quantification and Grading

Pulmonary regurgitation is assessed by semiquantitative methods like regurgitant jet size, continuous wave (CW) Doppler jet density and velocity time integral (VTI) across pulomary valve.[6] PR is the most neglected among all regurgitation and grading of which is not so well defined so far, however roughly it can be assessed **(Figure 9 and Table 2)**.

Conclusion

Although in clinical practice disease involving right sided valves is less common in comparison to the left sided valves, one should not neglect these valves during transesophageal echocardiography (TEE). However imaging right sided valves can be difficult by TEE due to their anterior location, but can be examined by little modification of standard views if needed.

TABLE 2 Grading severity of pulmonary regurgitation

	Mild	*Moderate*	*Severe*
PV	Normal	Normal/ abnormal	Abnormal
RV Size	Normal	Variable	Dilated
Color Doppler jet size	Thin (<10 mm in length)	Intermediate	Large and wide origin
CWD jet density	Faint	Dense, variable deceleration	Dense with steep deceleration
PV VTI:AV VTI	Little more than AV VTI	Intermediate	Significantly higher PV VTI

Abbreviations: PV, pulmonary valve; RV, right ventricle; CWD, continuous wave Doppler; VTI, velocity time integral

TRICUSPID VALVE

Anatomy

The tricuspid valve has a largest orifice area of >7 cm^2. It is a trileaflet valve with larger anterior, septal and posterior leaflet (unequal size). Either septal or posterior leaflet can be smallest. Rarely can it be bicuspid or quadricuspid. Tricuspid valve apparatus is similar to mitral valve and comprises of leaflet, annulus, chordae tendinae, papillary muscle and right ventricular myocardium. Tricuspid annulus is a three dimensional irregular and saddle shape structure with

CHAPTER **12**

annular highs and lows.[7] One can miss the major axis of annulus on two-dimensional echocardiography and for the same reason largest possible annular diameter should be obtained in more than one view.[8] It is more apically located in comparison to mitral valve. Apical displacement is exaggerated in Ebstein anomaly and absent in endocardial cushion defect or septum primum atrial septal defect. Anterior papillary muscle is the largest of all and originates from moderator band. Moderator band is very important for maintenance of right ventricular function and geometry.

Transesophageal Echocardiography Views

1. *Midesophageal 4 chamber view* **(Figure 10)***:* This is obtained by keeping the probe in mid-esophagus with multiplane angle 0°–15°. To the left of image is septal leaflet and to the right is anterior leaflet. With further advancement of the probe in esophagus posterior leaflet will appear on the right of the image when coronary sinus is visible in the long axis. The whole tricuspid valve can be quickly screen with probe moving up and down while keeping color Doppler on.
2. *The ME RV inflow-outflow view* **(Figure 11)** *(multiplane angle ≈50°-70°):* This view is obtained by increasing the multiplane angle (≈50°–70°) from ME aortic valve short axis view without changing the probe position and keeping the aortic valve in the center of the image. The tricuspid valve will be seen on right of the image adjacent to noncoronary and right coronary cusp of the aortic valve.
3. *Midesophageal modified bicaval view* **(Figure 12)***:* Clockwise rotation of the probe from ME left ventricle long axis view will lead to ME modified bicaval view with tricuspid valve seen in the far field **(Figure 13)**. This is an excellent view for Doppler assessment due to parallel alignment of blood flow with ultrasound beam. This view will be useful for placement of coronary sinus catheter.
4. *Transgastric tricuspid valve short axis view* **(Figure 14)***:* Clockwise rotation of the probe from TG midpapillary short axis view with anteflexion will produce TG tricuspid valve short axis view ("en face view"). This is the only view where all three leaflets of valve are visible at the same time, which will be helpful in locating regurgitant orifice and leaflet identification. This enface view is very important for leaflet identification since all schemes for identification of

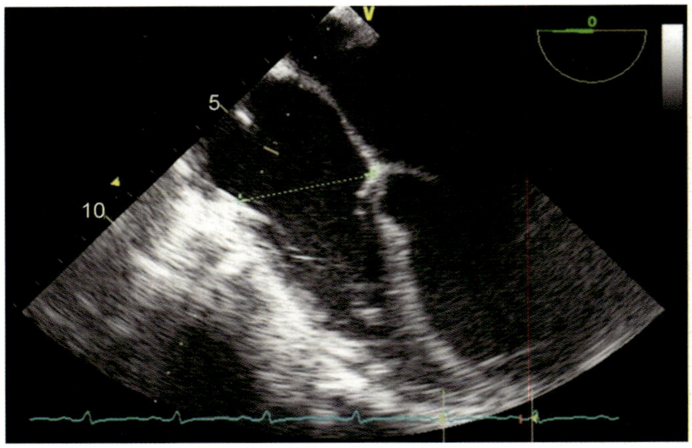

Figure 10 Midesophageal 4 chamber view showing tricuspid annulus measurement

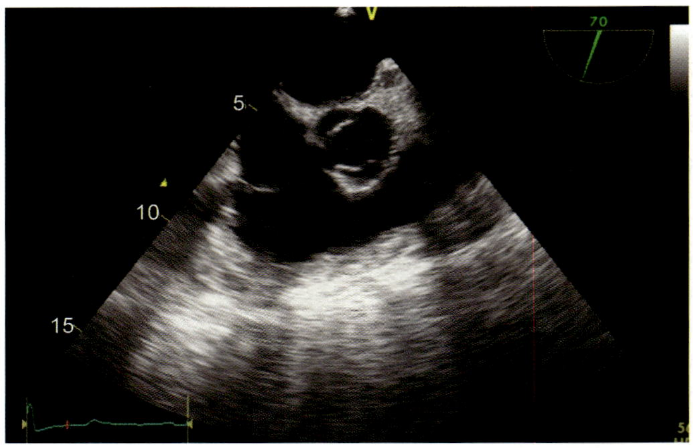

Figure 11 Midesophageal right ventricular (ME RV) inflow-outflow view

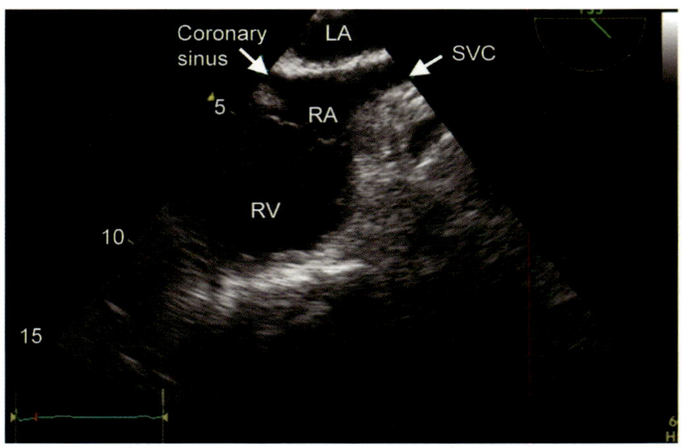

Figure 12 Midesophageal modified bicaval view
Abbreviations: RV, right ventricle; RA, right atrium; LA, left atrium; SVC, superior vena cava

the tricuspid valve leaflets are partially correct and conflicting due to the complex structure and wide variation in anatomy. Only septal leaflet can be idenitified with good accuracy rate in ME 4ch view **(Figure 15)**.

5. *Transgastric right ventricle inflow* **(Figures 16 and 17)***:* Clockwise rotation of the probe from TG two chamber view will result in TG RV inflow view. This is very important for assessment of subvalvular apparatus and measurement of tricuspid annular plane systolic excursion (TAPSE) and S[1] (peak systolic velocity at lateral annulus of tricuspid valve). Anterior and posterior leaflet are visible in this.
6. *Transgastric hepatic vein view* **(Figures 18A and B)***:* Hepatic vein will be visible in the far feild in liver

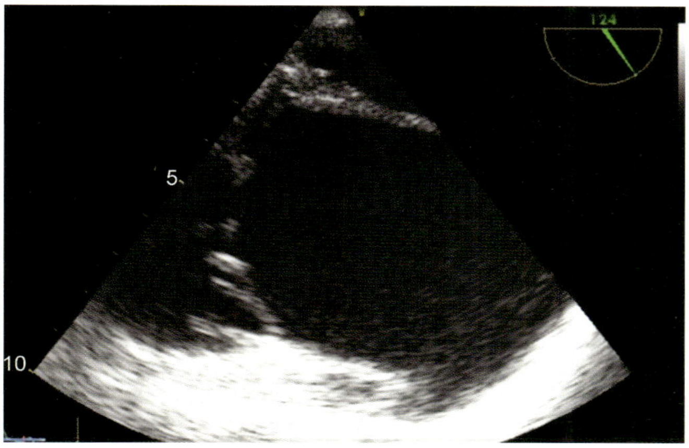

Figure 13 Thickened tricuspid leaflet in midesophageal modified bicaval view

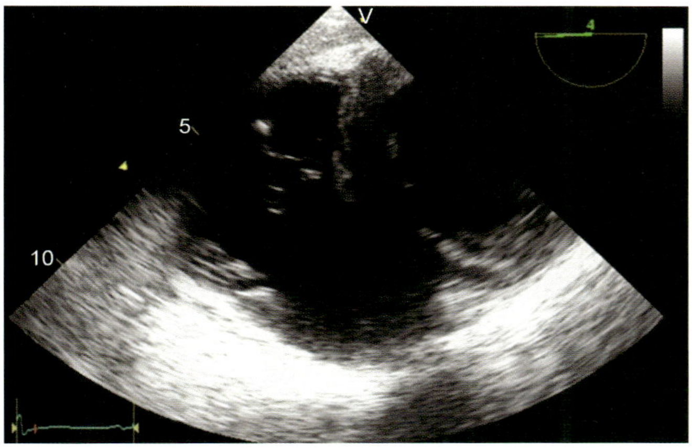

Figure 14 Transgastric tricuspid valve (TG TV) short axis view

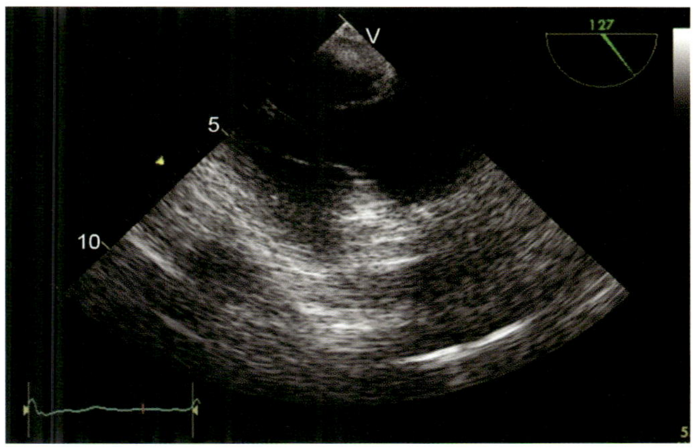

Figure 16 Transgastric right ventricle (TG RV) inflow view

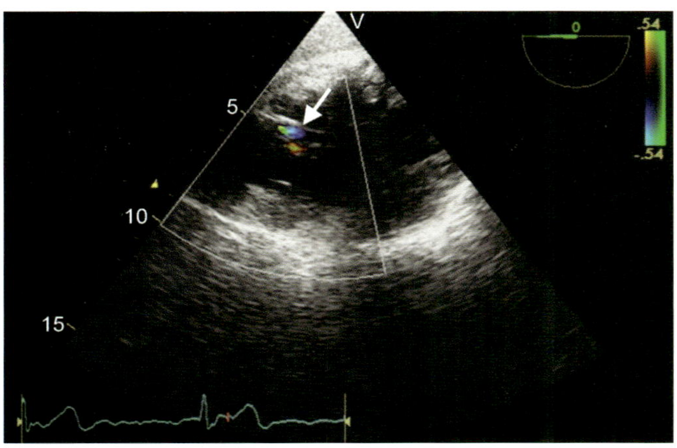

Figure 15 Transgastric tricuspid valve (TG TV) short axis view with color Doppler showing regurgitant jet location

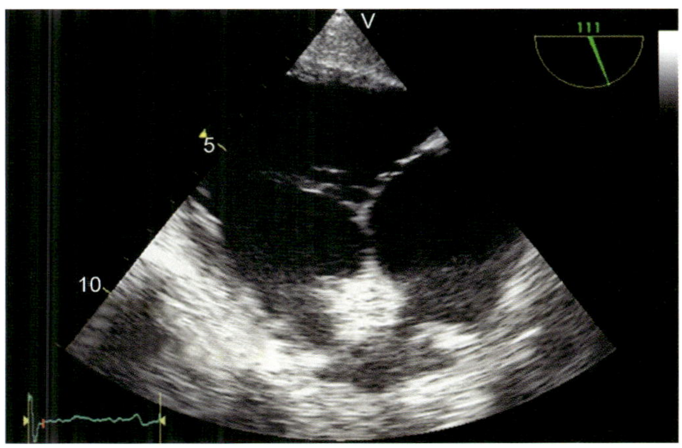

Figure 17 Transgastric right ventricle (TG RV) inflow view showing normal subvalvular apparatus

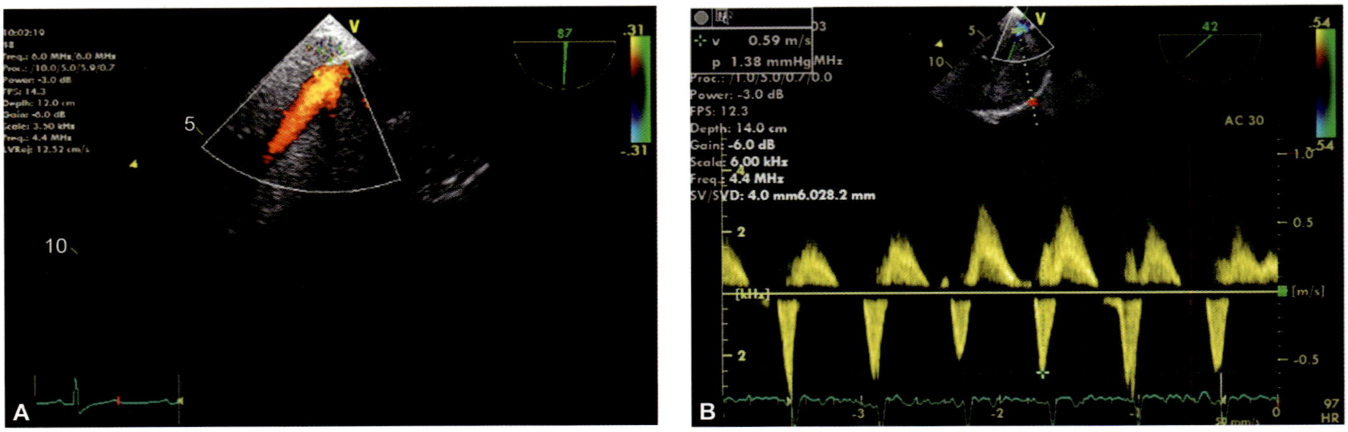

Figures 18A and B (A) Transgastric hepatic venous color Doppler; (B) Normal pulsed wave Doppler

texture with change in multiplane angle (≈50°–60°) and clockwise rotation of the probe from TG IVC long axis view. Hepatic venous flow will be assessed, while keeping sample volume in hepatic vein. Systolic reversal of hepatic venous flow is sign of severe tricuspid regurgitation.

Annular measurement done on a single 2D echo view will not be correct due to irregular shape annulus. One should measure annulus in both septolateral and anteroposterior axis.

ETIOLOGY OF TRICUSPID DISEASE

Annular Dilation

Tricuspid regurgitation (TR) in the absence of leaflet pathology is called functional TR and is the most commonly seen TR in clinical practice. Functional TR is secondary to pulmonary arterial hypertension which can be primary or secondary to left sided heart disease. Moderate to severe functional TR needs to be addressed during the surgical procedure for providing better symptomatic outcomes and probably better survival rates.

Rheumatic Disease

Usually there is secondary tricuspid regurgitation due to rheumatic mitral valve disease, however sometime it can directly affect the tricuspid valve in addition to mitral valve. Rheumatic tricuspid valvulitis will lead to incompetent valve due to fibrosis and scarring leading to restricted leaflet movement. Rarely commissural fusion in closed position can lead to stenosis.

Endocarditis

It is the most common cause of direct involvement of the tricuspid valve. Typically vegetations are seen as oscillating, echo-dense masses attached to the atrial side of the tricuspid valve. Sometimes endocarditis can lead to destruction of the valve leaflet or chordae that result in flail leaflet.

Carcinoid Syndrome

It is due to release of vasoactive substances (serotonin, bradykinins, histamine, prostaglandins) from carcinoid tumors located in gut. These vasoactive substances can damage the right sided heart valves (PV, TV) and spares left sided due to inactivation of tumor secretions in the lung by monoamine oxidase. There will be thickening and fibrosis of the right sided valve leading to variable degree of regurgitation and stenosis.

Ebstein Anomaly

It is a rare congenital anomaly with malformed tricuspid valve. Typically septal leaflet is displaced more apically and the portion of morphological right ventricle is atrialized. Septal leaflet of tricuspid valve will be displaced apically by ≥ 8mm/m^2 body surface area from the level of anterior mitral leaflet. Feasibility of repair depends on the severity of tricuspid valve malformation.

TRICUSPID REGURGITATION

It is the most common right sided valvular lesion. It is most commonly secondary to left sided heart disease or pulmonary hypertension. Less commonly, it can be primarily involved by endocarditis, rheumatic heart disease, Ebstein anomaly. Very rarely, it can be due to blunt trauma or carcinoid syndrome.

Two-dimensional Echocardiography

There will be varying degree of dilatation of right atrium and ventricle depending on severity of TR. Depending on etiology, one can find dilated annulus, incomplete coaptation of the leaflets, prolapsed or restricted thickened or normal leaflet, vegetations on atrial side of the TV. Pulmonary artery is usually dilated in secondary TR **(Figures 19 to 24 and Table 3)**.

Color Flow Doppler

Regurgitant jet area is a sensitive and semiquantitative technique for grading the severity of valvular regurgitation. TR is usually severe when regurgitant jet area fills more than half of RA. It is widely used method with important limitations such as dependence of hemodynamic conditions and machine settings. One needs to assess the severity of TR in awake patient with optimized gain settings.

Vena contracta is the narrowest part of jet area just distal to flow convergence and has good correlation with effective regurgitant orifice area. A vena contracta width >0.65 cm is indicative of severe regurgitation.

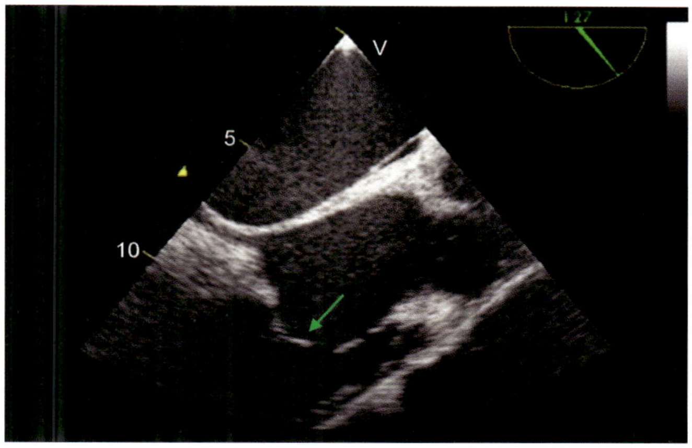

Figure 20 Midesophageal modified bicaval view showing noncoapting leaflet

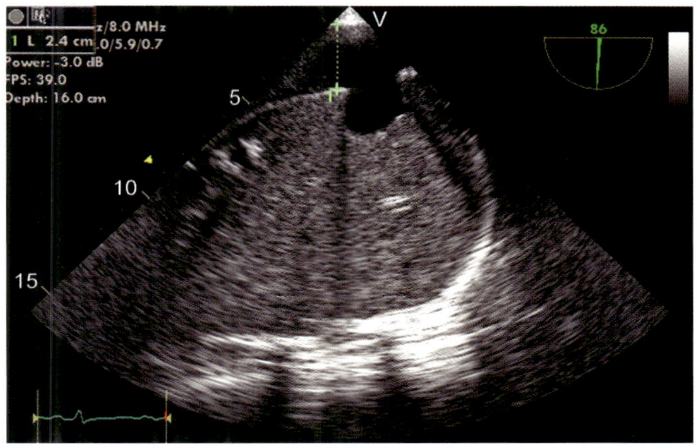

Figure 21 Transgastric long axis inferior vena cava (IVC) view showing dilated IVC

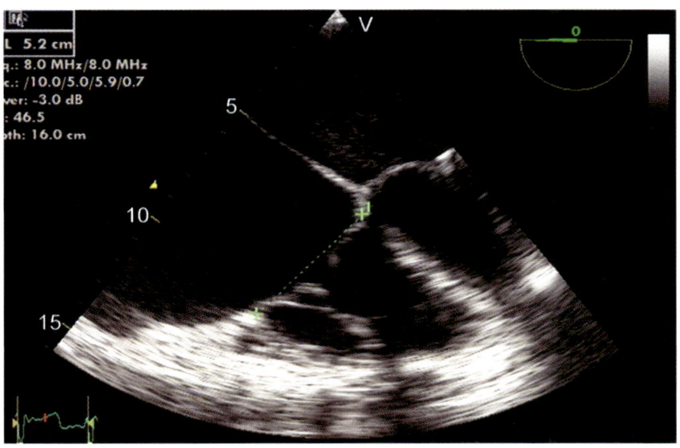

Figure 19 Dilated tricuspid annulus with dilated right atrium

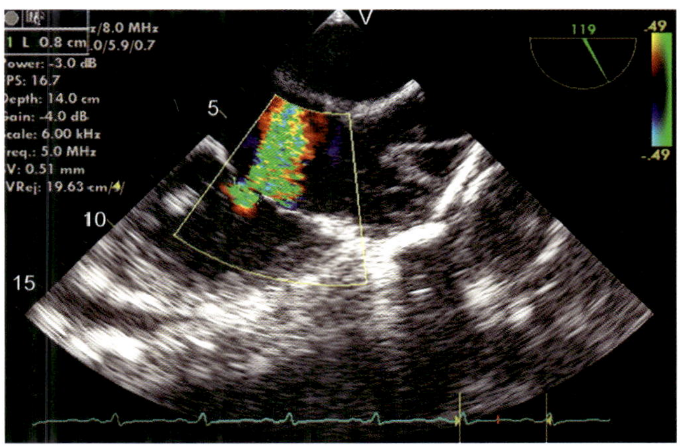

Figure 22 Midesophageal modified bicaval view with color Doppler showing vena contracta width of 8 mm

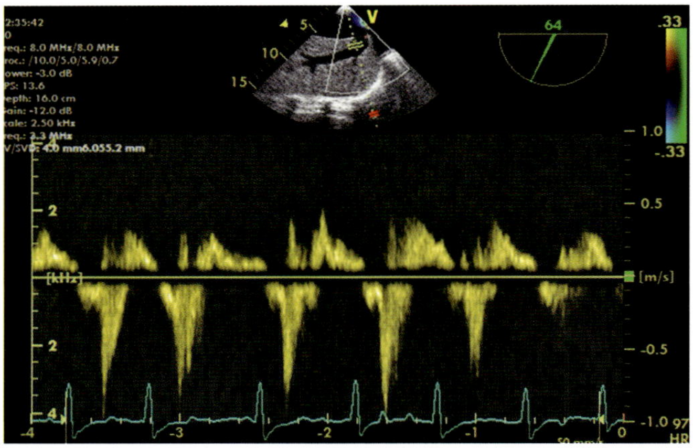

Figure 23 Systolic reversal on hepatic venous flow suggestive of severe TR

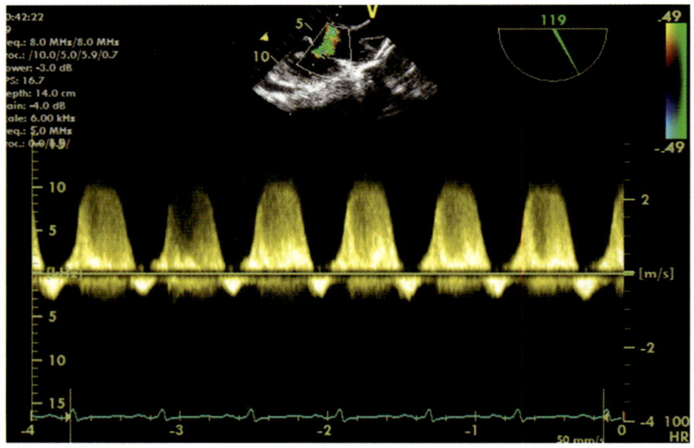

Figure 24 Continuous wave (CW) Doppler of TR jet

TABLE 3 Tricuspid leaflet identification with 3D transthoracic echocardiogram

	4 chamber view	*Parasternal SAX view*	*RV inflow view (without left ventricle in scan)*
Anterior leaflet	Towards RV free wall (81%)	Adjacent to aortic valve (68%)	Anteriorly placed (100%)
Posterior leaflet	Towards RV free wall (19%)	Towards RV free wall (100%)	Other (77%)
Septal leaflet	Towards septum (100%)	Adjacent to aortic valve (32%)	Other (23%)

Abbreviations: SAX, short axis; RV, right ventricle

Pulsed Wave Doppler (Figures 18A and B)

A systolic reversal of hepatic venous flow is a sign of severe TR. Hepatic venous flow velocities are very low and possible with proper alignment of ultrasound beam with blood flow while keeping aliasing velocities around 30 cm/second.

Continuous Wave Doppler

It is used to measure the TR jet velocity. Peak TR jet velocity will give systolic pressure gradient between right ventricle and right atrium by modified Bernoulli equation. Addition of estimated right atrial pressure to this will give right ventricular systolic pressure (RVSP). RVSP is same as systolic pulmonary arterial pressure in absence of right ventricular outflow tract obstruction. Any of the TEE view can be used to measure RVSP provided Doppler beam is well aligned with TR jet.

TRICUSPID STENOSIS

It is most commonly due to rheumatic heart disease and relatively uncommon. On two dimensional echocardiography there will be diastolic doming with thickening of leaflets and reduction in TV orifice. Dilated right atrium and inferior vena cava are supportive findings. Normal flow velocities across the TV are typically less than 0.7 meter/second, which in stenosis is increased to > 1 meter/second. Continuous wave Doppler allows the measurement of transvalvular pressure gradient. A mean pressure gradient of >5 mm Hg and/or pressure half time >190 milli seconds is suggestive of hemodynamically significant tricuspid stenosis **(Figure 25 and Table 4)**.

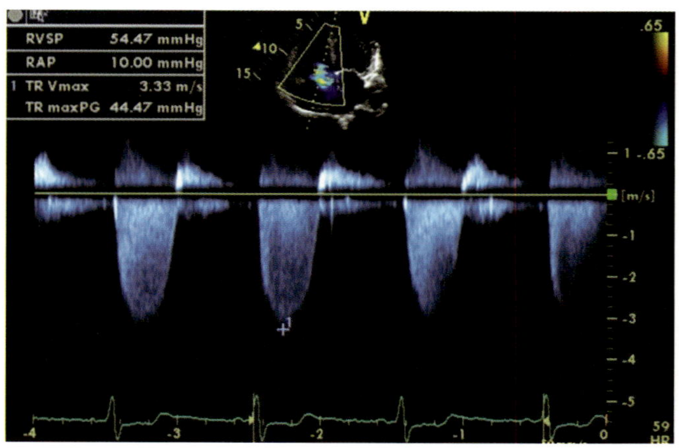

Figure 25 Right ventricular systolic pressure (RVSP) measurement from TR jet, TTE

TABLE 4 Grading severity of tricuspid regurgitation

	Mild	*Moderate*	*Severe*
Leaflet morphology	Usually normal	Normal/abnormal	Abnormal
RA/RV/IVC	Normal	Normal/dilated	Dilated
Regurgitant jet area (cm^2)	<5	5–10	>10
Regurgitant jet area/RA area	≤19 %	20–40%	>41 %
VC width (mm)	Not defined	Not defined but <7	>7
PISA radius in cm (V_A $28_{cm/sec}$)	<0.6	0.6–0.9	>0.9
CW Doppler Jet density	Soft	Dense	Dense
Hepatic vein Doppler	Systolic dominance	Systolic blunting	Systolic reversal

Abbreviations: RA, right atrium; RV, right ventricle; IVC, inferior vena cava; VC, vena contracta; CW, continuous wave; PISA, proximal isovelocity surface area

CONCLUSION

Like pulmonary valve, anterior location of the tricuspid valve makes it more difficult for transesophageal echocardiography. All schemes for identification of the tricuspid valve leaflets are partially correct due to complex structure and variable anatomy in addition to transducer position. For the same reason tricuspid valve short axis view is valuable for identifying the diseased leaflet. One should grade the severity of tricuspid valve disease on awake patient.

REFERENCES

1. Anwar AM, Geleijnse ML, Soliman OI, McGhie JS, Frowijn R, Nemes A, et al. Assessment of normal tricuspid valve anatomy in adults by real-time three-dimensional echocardiography. Int J Cardiovasc Imaging. 2007;23(6):717-24.
2. Perrino, Albert C, Reeves, Scott T. Practical Approach to Transesophageal Echocardiography, 2nd Edition. Lippincott Williams & Wilkins; 2008.pp.281-95.
3. Robert F, John K, Marco R. Core topics in Transesophageal Echocardiography, Cambridge University; 2010. pp.135-44.
4. Fukuda S, Saracino G, Matsumura Y, Daimon M, Tran H, Greenberg NL, et al. Three dimensional geometry of the tricuspid annulus in healthy subjects and in patients with functional tricuspid regurgitation: a real-time, 3-dimensional echocardiographic study. Circulation. 2006;114(1 Suppl):I492-98.
5. Baumgartner H, Hung J, Bermejo J, Chambers JB, Evangelista A, Griffin BP, et al. Echocardiographic assessment of valve stenosis: EAE/ASE recommendations for clinical practice. J Am Soc Echocardiogr. 2009; 22(1):1-23
6. Lancellotti P, Tribouilloy C, Hagendorff A, Popescu BA, Edvardsen T, Pierard LA, et al. Recommendations for the echocardiographic assessment of native valvular regurgitation: an executive summary from the European Association of Cardiovascular Imaging. European Heart Journal–Cardiovascular Imaging. 2013;14:611-44.
7. Mahmood F, Kim H, Chaudary B, Bergman R, Matyal R, Gerstle J, et al. Tricuspid annular geometry: a three-dimensional transesophageal echocardiographic study. J Cardiothorac Vasc Anesth. 2013;27(4):639-46.
8. Stankovic I, Daraban AM, Jasaityte R, Neskovic AN, Claus P, Voigt JU. Incremental value of the en face view of the tricuspid valve by two-dimenional echocardiography for accurate identification of tricuspid valve leaflets. J Am Soc Echocardiogra. 2014;27(4):376-84.

Chapter 13

Transesophageal Echocardiography Simulation for Left Ventricular Systolic Function

Sanjay Goel

Chapter Outline

- Use of Simulator for Transesophageal Echocardiography Training
- Assessment of Left Ventricular Systolic Function
- Regional Left Ventricular Function
- Transesophageal Echocardiography Views Used for Left Ventricular Assessment
- Normal Regional Function of Left Ventricle
- Assessment of Global Left Ventricular Function
- Preload
- Left Ventricle Dimensions
- Quantitative Methods
- Ejection Fraction
- Cardiac Output
- Qualitative Methods
- Myocardial Performance Index or Tei Index

USE OF SIMULATOR FOR TRANSESOPHAGEAL ECHOCARDIOGRAPHY TRAINING

The traditional training of transesophageal echocardiography (TEE) encompasses studies performed on cardiac surgery patients in the operating room under supervision of the anesthesiologist. The high-stress environment of the operating room may not always conducive for teaching and unpredictable clinical presentation prevents standardization of clinical experience for all trainees. Possible risk of injury to the patient is another important ethical consideration. Echocardiography training has benefitted tremendously from the introduction of simulators by dealing with several of these shortcomings. Simulation-based echocardiography training is trainee-focused as compared to the patient-focused nature of the conventional model where any emergency during the procedure take precedence over resident training. The conventional model is limited to a one patient-one procedure and patients are at risk of potential injury at the hands of an inexperienced trainee. Use of simulator minimizes risk of harm to the patient and allows the trainee to refine his/her skills in a stress-free environment. Furthermore, addition of different pathologies to simulators helps the trainees to understand the commonly encountered echocardiographic abnormalities. Most commercially available simulators consist of a life-sized mannequin, dummy TEE and dedicated workstations. The simulator's interface comprises of an anatomically correct beating 3D virtual heart model and scan plane on one side and a two-dimensional (2D) ultrasound image corresponding to the position of the scan plane on the other. The imaging plane on the screen changes with the trainee's probe-manipulations on the mannequin. The virtual heart model can be rotated and viewed from many different perspectives to better understand the anatomic basis of image acquisition. The trainee's performance can be compared with his/her past performance or with other trainees for an objective evaluation of his/her proficiency in achieving the target image of acceptable quality.

ASSESSMENT OF LEFT VENTRICULAR SYSTOLIC FUNCTION

After completion of comprehensive examination of the heart, left ventricle (LV) systolic function assessment is usually the first priority of the cardiac anesthesiologist. It is beyond doubt that TEE is an invaluable tool for cardiac monitoring during intraoperative period as it can be performed without interfering the surgery and also produces superior images as compared to transthoracic echocardiography. Systolic function of the LV is a powerful predictor of clinical outcome after cardiac surgery. This chapter will help the beginner to learn how to assess the systolic function of LV using different imaging views and Doppler techniques. However, it is important to remember that systolic function of the LV includes both regional and global function of the LV.

REGIONAL LEFT VENTRICULAR FUNCTION

As per guidelines by the American Society of Echocardiocarphy, LV is divided into 17 segments, six segments both in the basal and mid portions (anteroseptal, inferoseptal, anterior, anterolateral, inferolateral, and inferior walls) and five at the apex (septal, anterior, lateral, inferior, and apical). As these segments can be assessed in both midesophageal **(Figures 1A to C)** and transgastric views **(Figures 2A to C)**, one should evaluate the segments in more than one view before documenting upon the regional wall motion abnormality (RWMA).

TRANSESOPHAGEAL ECHOCARDIOGRAPHY VIEWS USED FOR LEFT VENTRICULAR ASSESSMENT

Global and regional functions of LV can be assessed in following TEE views:

- Midesophageal (ME) 4-chamber view (0°) **(Fig. 1A)**.
- ME 2-chamber view (60°–90°) **(Figure 1B)**.
- ME long axis view (90°–120°) **(Figure 1C)**.
- Transgastric (TG) basal short axis view (0°) **(Figure 2A)**.
- TG midpapillary short axis view (0°) **(Figure 2B)**.
- TG apical short axis view (0°) **(Figure 2C)**.

In addition, TG long axis view and deep TG view are used for Doppler techniques. ME 4-chamber, 2-chamber, and long axis views are used to assess the LV regional wall contractility. On the other hand, TG midpapillary short axis view provides information regarding volume status, contractility and thickening of each segment. Measurement of LV cavity area and dimensions during systole and diastole calculate both fractional area change (FAC) and fractional shortening (FS), the surrogates of ejection fraction (EF), respectively. In addition, distributions of the three coronary arteries can be seen in this view, making it particularly useful for monitoring of RWMA. Three coronary arteries which supply blood to the heart are left anterior descending (LAD) artery, left circumflex (LCx) artery, and right coronary artery (RCA). LAD artery supplies segments (1, 2, 7, 8, 13, 14, 17), RCA supplies segments (3, 4, 9,19, 15) and LCx artery supplies segments (5, 6, 11, 12, 16). These segments are shown in **Figures 1 and 2**.

During the assessment of LV using TEE examination, one must avoid foreshortening of the LV. Whenever imaging plane passes through the myocardial wall **(Figures 3A and B)**, true LV apex is lost and myocardium appears falsely thickened in the image. This is called LV foreshortening. This can be corrected by retroflexing the tip of the probe or changing the angle from 0 to 30 degree **(Figure 3B)**.

NORMAL REGIONAL FUNCTION OF LEFT VENTRICLE

During systole, endocardial border of the LV segment moves towards the center of the ventricle (endocardial excursion) resulting in reduced cavity area and increased

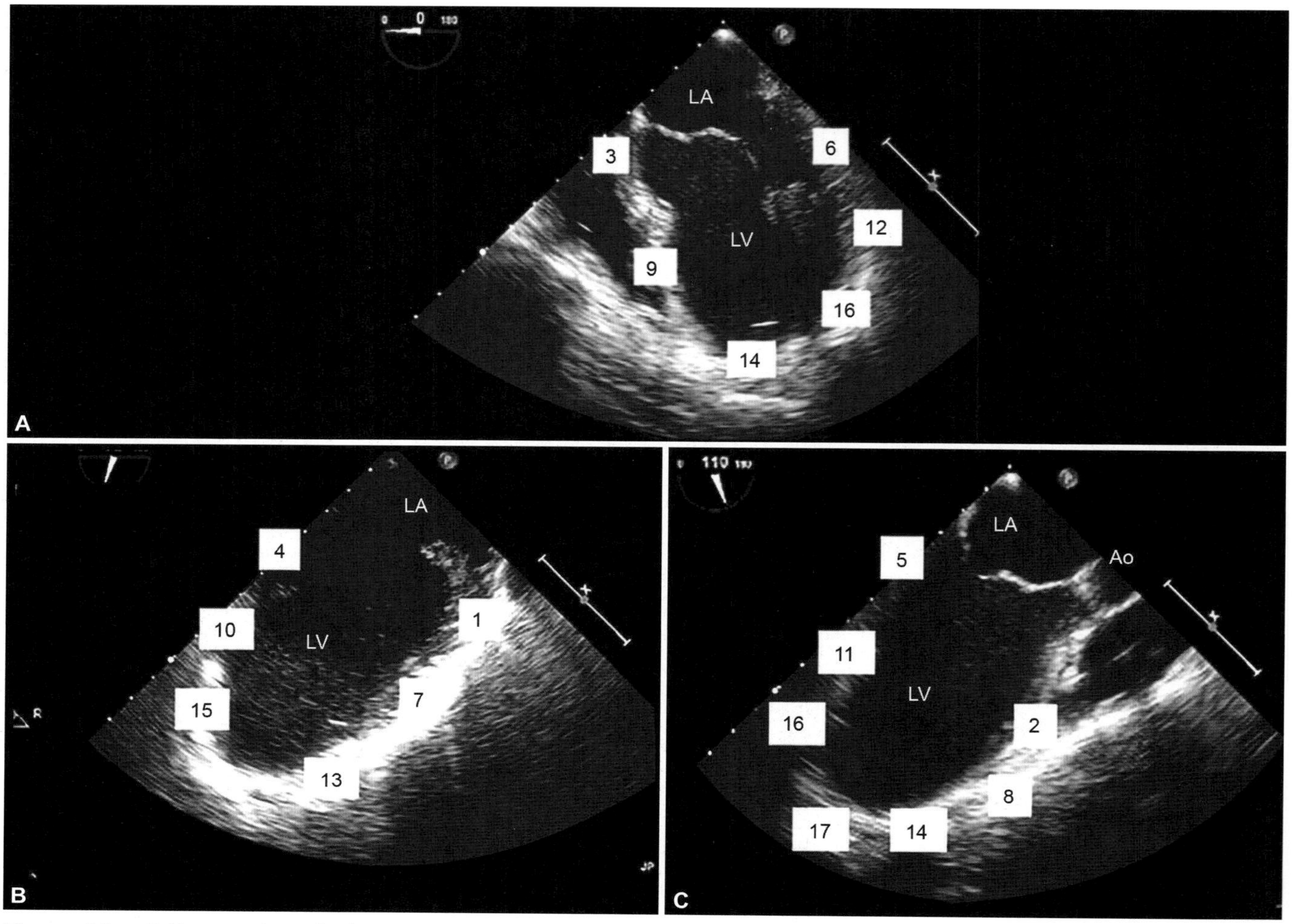

Figures 1A to C Transesophageal echocardiographic midesophageal views to evaluate the 17 segments of the left ventricle (LV). (A) Midesophageal four chamber view; (B) Midesophageal two chamber view; (C) Midesophageal long axis view. 1. Basal anterior; 2. Basal anteroseptal; 3. Basal inferoseptal; 4. Basal inferior; 5. Basal inferolateral; 6. Basal anterolateral; 7. Midanterior; 8. Midanteroseptal; 9. Midinferoseptal; 10. Midinferior; 11. Midinferolateral; 12. Midanterolateral; 13. Apical anterior; 14. Apical septal; 15. Apical inferior; 16. Apical lateral; 17. Apex

distance between the endocardial and epicardium (wall thickening). A normally contracting myocardium is characterized by a contractility of 30% and myocardial wall thickening of 30–50% during systole. Segments of the LV wall are labeled as mild hypokinetic (contractility 10–30%, and thickening 30–50%), severe hypokinetic contractility <10%, and thickening <30%), akinetic (contractility 0%, and thickening <10%), and dyskinetic (contractility 0% or none, and thickening none or thinning), based on their contractility and thickening during systole.

During assessment of the myocardial wall contractility, one must remember that thickening of basal inferior wall and basal interventricular septum is asynchronous and often reduced as compared to the other ventricular segments. Moreover, it may be difficult to assess the ventricular septal motion in the presence of a left bundle branch block, right volume overload, constrictive pericarditis, or the postoperative state after cardiac surgery. Decrease in the endocardial excursion, i.e. contractility of a particular segment should not be used as the sole criterion for the presence of ischemia as the contractility of the segment may be affected by the rotation and the translation of the heart, and as well as tethering. Decreased myocardial thickening is more specific for ischemia.

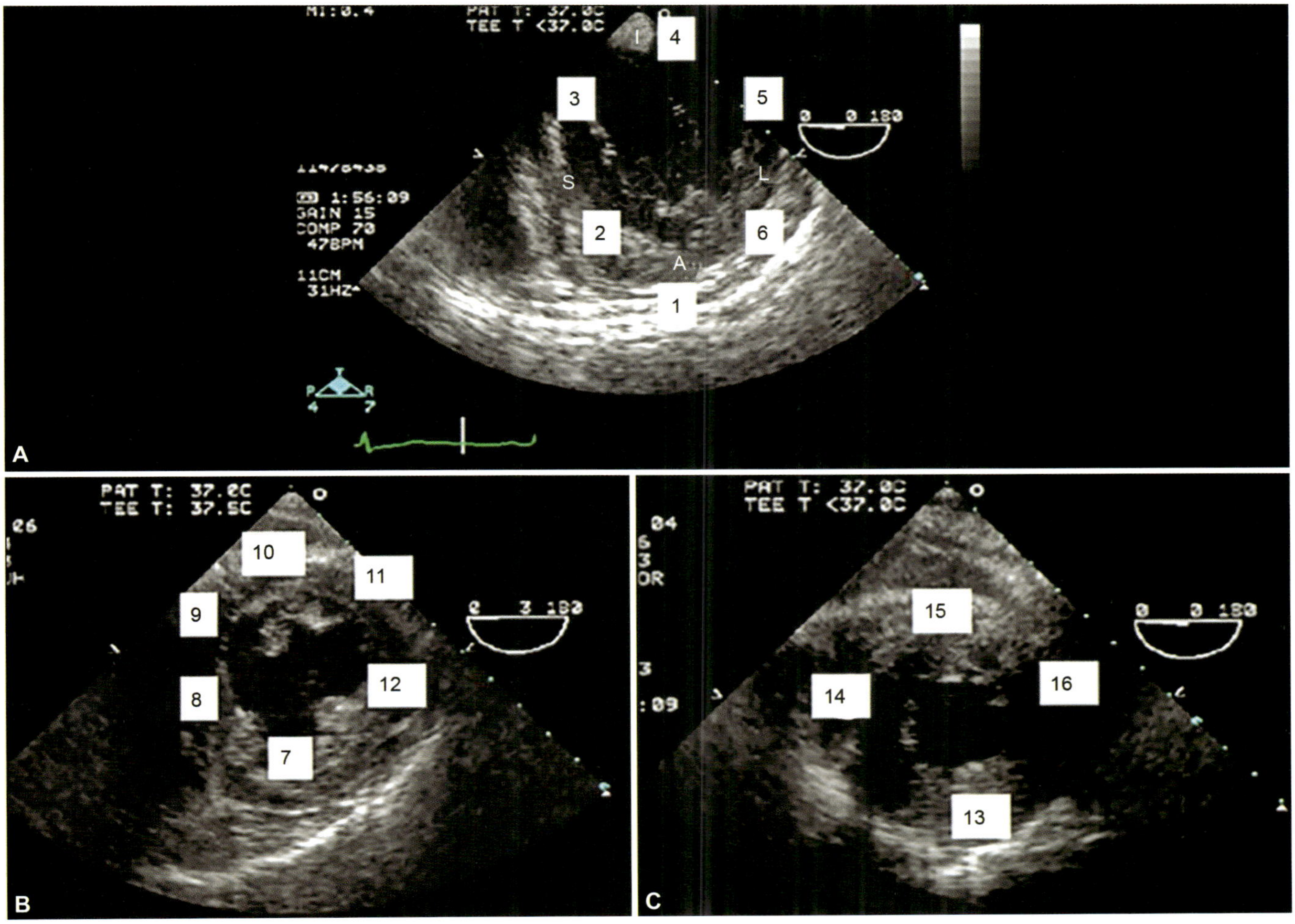

Figures 2A to C Transesophageal echocardiographic transgastric views to evaluate the 17 segments of the left ventricle. (A) Transgastric basal short axis view; (B) Transgastric mid papillary short axis view; (C) Transgastric apical view 1. Basal anterior; 2. Basal anteroseptal; 3. Basal inferoseptal; 4. Basal inferior; 5. Basal inferolateral; 6. Basal anterolateral; 7. Mid anterior; 8. Mid anteroseptal; 9. Mid inferoseptal; 10. Mid inferior; 11. Mid inferolateral; 12. Mid anterolateral; 13. Apical anterior; 14. Apical septal; 15. Apical inferior; 16. Apical lateral. 17. Segment, the apex of the left ventricle is not shown here

If the intraoperative TEE examination reveals new RWMA, the anesthesiologist must use all the previously mentioned views to confirm the diagnosis. Intraoperative team must determine the cause and then plan the treatment accordingly. One must rule out nonischemic causes of RWMAs such as conduction abnormalities (left bundle branch block or ventricular pacing). Occlusion of coronary graft should be revised where as coronary embolism due to air, calcium or atheromatous material requires increase in coronary perfusion pressure and administration of coronary dilators such as nitroglycerin and diltiazem. Coronary spasm need to be dealt with vasodilators.

ASSESSMENT OF GLOBAL LEFT VENTRICULAR FUNCTION

Global LV function can be assessed by either quantitative or qualitative methods. Quantitative methods are based on volume measurements and thus, depend upon the loading conditions like preload and afterload. Therefore, this technique is limited by variation in both preload and afterload during intraoperative period. On the other hand, qualitative assessment of the LV function is less dependent on the preload and afterload, and proved to be useful during the intraoperative period.

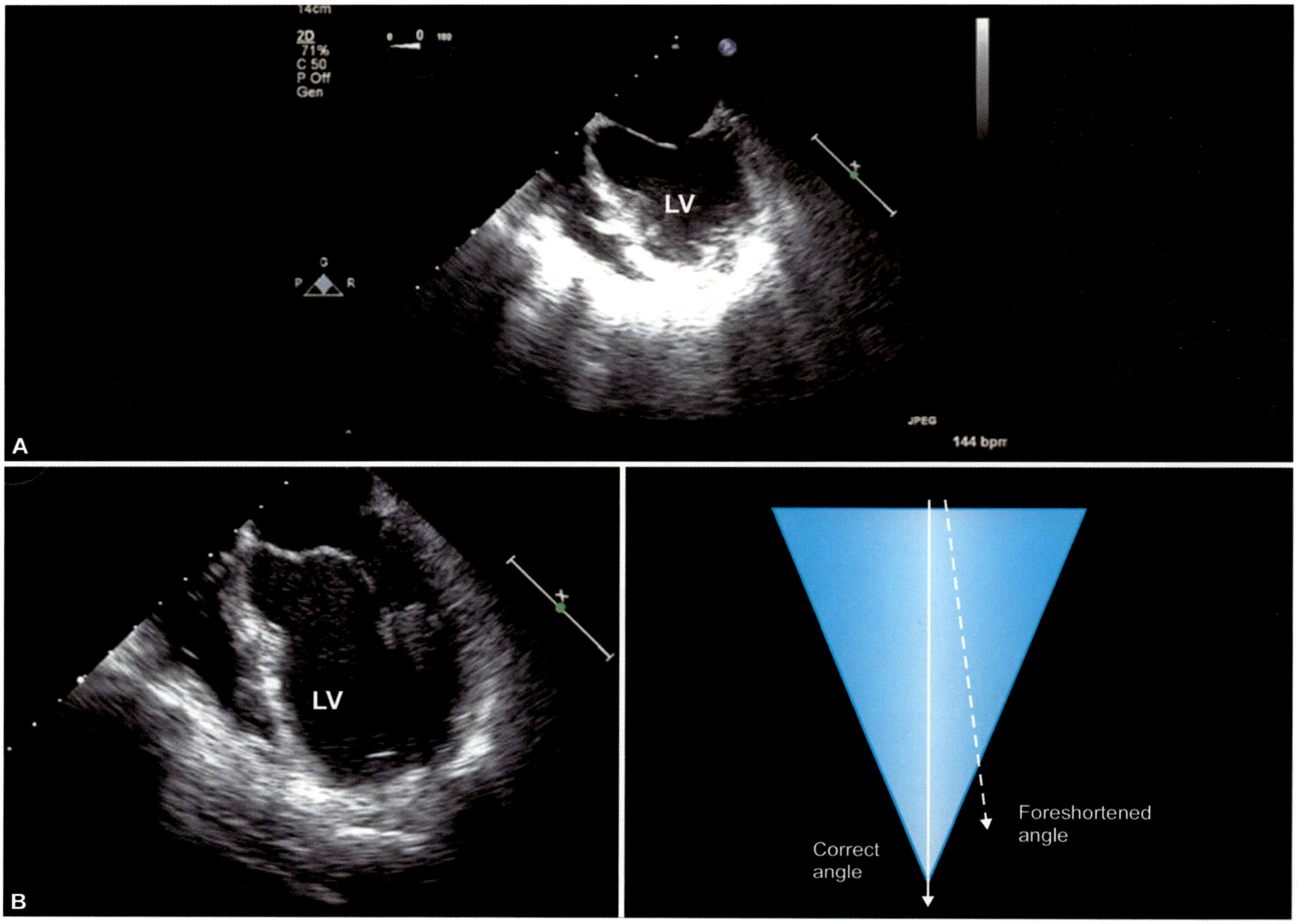

Figures 3A and B Transesophageal midesophageal 4 chamber view showing left ventricle (LV) foreshortening (A) and correction of foreshortening (B)

PRELOAD (FIGURES 4A AND B)

TG midpapillary short axis view is used to assess the volume status of the LV. LV end diastolic area (LVEDA) is used as surrogate for preload. During severe hypovolumic state, cavity area reduces so much that both posteromedial and anterolateral papillaries nearly touch each other (Kissing papillaries). There is poor correlation between LVEDA and pulmonary capillary wedge pressure or pulmonary artery diastolic pressure due to variations in chamber compliance. In situations like patients with hypertrophic ventricle and chronic obstructive airway disease, where assessment of volume status using pulmonary artery pressure can be difficult during intraoperative period as well as immediate postoperative period especially in presence of inotropes, TEE can be helpful in guiding the volume status in such conditions.

LEFT VENTRICLE DIMENSIONS (FIGURE 5)

Left ventricle dimension should be measured in the ME 4 chamber view at the end of diastole. An imaginary line should be drawn along the long axis of the ventricle passing through the apex. Then another line should be drawn perpendicular to the long axis of LV at the level of maximum dimension **(Table 1)**.

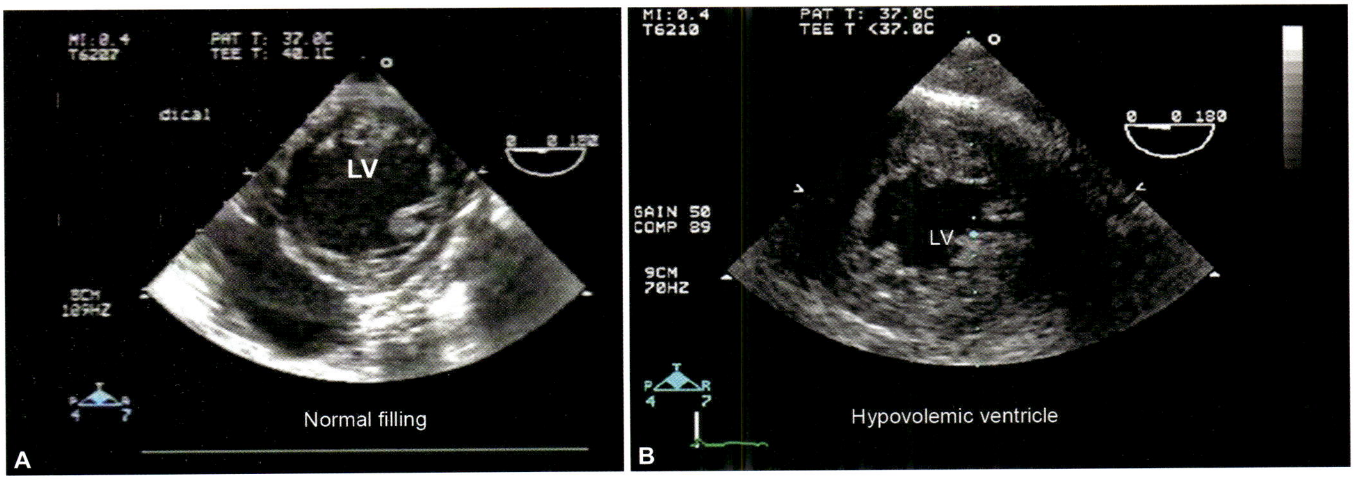

Figures 4A and B Preload: (A) Transgastric midpapillary short axis view showing normal left ventricle (LV); (B) Transgastric midpapillary short axis view showing obliteration of left ventricle cavity (Kissing papillaries) due to hypovolemia

TABLE 1 Mentions the measurements of the mild, moderate and severe dilated LV

LVEDD (mm)	*Normal*	*Mild*	*Moderate*	*Severe*
Male	42–59	60–63	64–68	>69
Female	39–53	54–57	58–61	>62

QUANTITATIVE METHODS

Quantitative methods are based on volume of the cardiac chamber during systole and diastole. It include measurement of EF and cardiac output (CO).

EJECTION FRACTION

It is the ejection phase of LV contractility. It is calculated as follows.

EF = {LVEDV-LVESV}/LVEDV

LVEDV: Left ventricular end-diastolic volume (in mL)

LVESV: Left ventricular end-systolic volume (in mL).

The normal LVEF is 55–75%.

EF represents the contractility of the LV. It also represents the efficiency of the global cardiac pump to eject part of its end-diastolic volume which may be affected by preload, afterload, and myocardial contractility. Different techniques are used to measure EF such as eye balling, FS, FAC, and modified Simpson's method. Amongst them, use of eye balling is more commonly used by intraoperative echocardiographer.

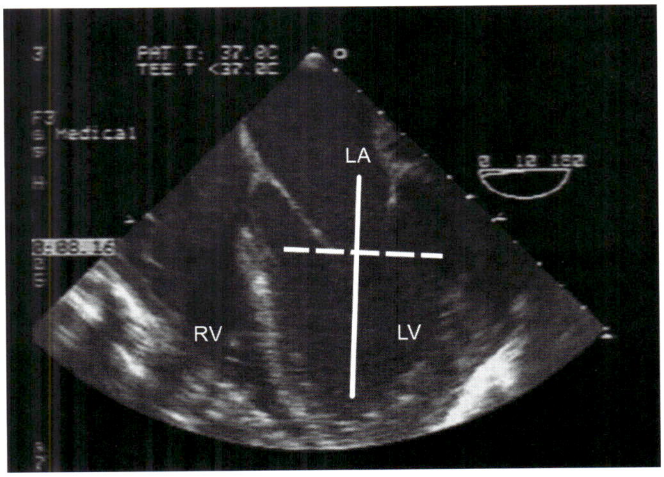

Figure 5 Midesophageal view showing how to measure the end-diastolic dimension of left ventricle (LV). First a longitudinal line is drawn a ong the long axis of LV and then transverse line is drawn perpendicular to long axis at the level of maximum dimension

Eye Balling

In the clinical setting, visual estimation of the left ventricular EF as well LV contractility is the common practice. This method is good but requires experience and has a learning curve. In the beginning, performer can calculate EF using both quantitative and qualitative methods and correlate them with the visual estimation. The correlation between the visual echocardiographic estimation (eye balling) and other methods have been found good, especially in patients with impaired EF.

Fractional Shortening (Figure 6)

Fractional shortening (FS), a linear measurement is the surrogate measure of EF. The interobserver variation is less with linear measurement (FS) as compared to the planimetric (FAC) and volumetric method (modified Simpson's method) but it ignores the regional variation of LV function and is not reliable in presence of RWMA. The M mode tracing of TG short axis view just above the papillary muscle is usually done and the internal diameters are measured during systole and diastole.

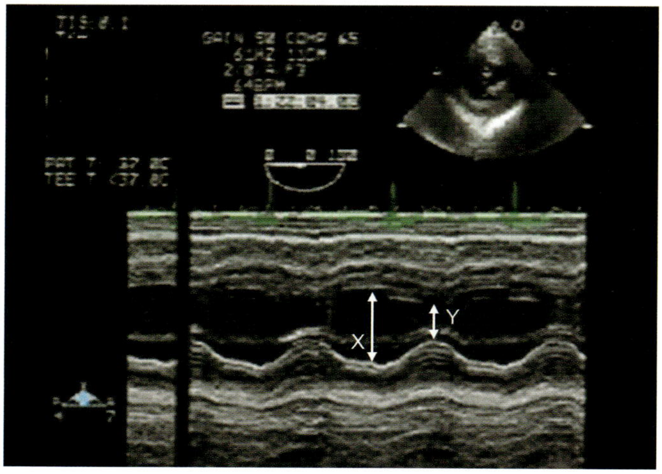

Figure 6 M-mode across the short axis of left ventricle to calculate the fractional shortening (FS) using the left ventricular end-diastolic diameter "X" and left ventricular end-systolic diameter (Y) FS= X-Y/X

FS = LVIDd–LVIDs/LVIDd, where LVIDd is the LV internal diameter during diastole and LVIDs is the LV internal diameter during systole.

Normal values: For men 25–43%, for women 27–45%.

Fractional Area Change (Figures 7A and B)

It is the planimetric method where LV end diastolic area and end systolic area is measured by tracing the edges of the endocardial border of the LV at the end diastole and end systole respectively in TG midpapillary short axis view. In case of ME 4 chamber view, tracing of the endocardial border starts from the medial annulus of the mitral valve, along the free wall to the apex, and then back to lateral annulus of the mitral valve. This modality of systolic function determination is both preload and afterload dependant.

FAC is equal to LVEDA–LV end-systolic area (LVESA) divided by LVEDA.

The normal values varies from 36% to 64%, depending on the level where it is measured (40% for the base, 50% at the midpapillary muscle, and 60% at the apical levels).

Method of Discs (Modified Simpson's Biplane Method) (Figures 8A and B)

Both FS and FAC do not represent the true EF but are good surrogate representative of EF. Modified Simpson's method is volumetric method where both end-diastolic

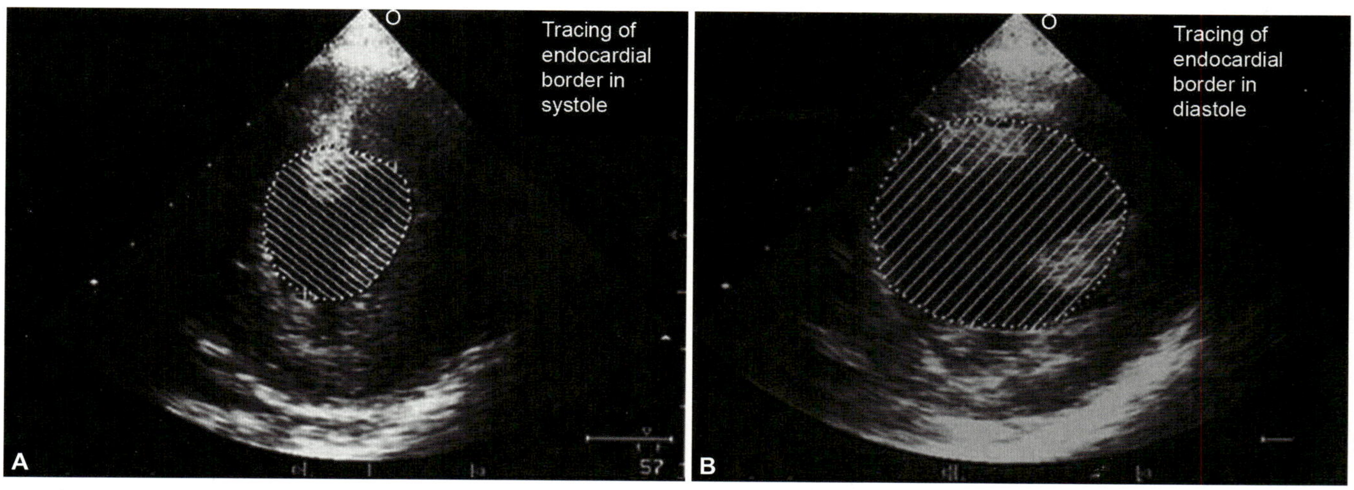

Figures 7A and B Fractional area change (FAC) is measured using transgastric mid-papillary view of the left ventricle in diastole (A) and systole (B). FAC = EDA – ESA/EDA. Note that papillary muscle are included in the tracing

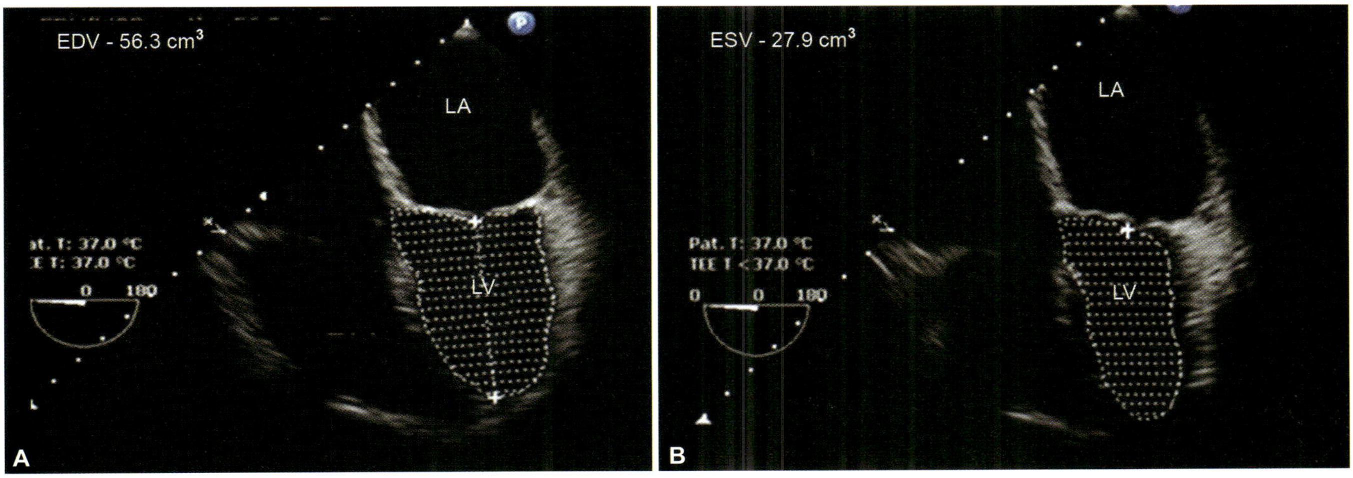

Figures 8A and B Modified Simpson's biplane method: Mid-esophageal four chamber view showing how to calculate the left ventricle (LV) volume during diastole (A) and systole (B). Ejection fraction = (EDV – ESV/EDV = 56.3 – 27.9/56.3% = 50%) where EDV is end-diastolic volume and ESV is end-systolic volume

and the end-systolic volumes are measured to calculate the EF.

The Simpson's rule states that the volume of a cavity is equal to the sum of the volumes of a series of smaller slices (disc summation method). The volume of each slice (disc) is obtained by its surface area and thickness. The modified Simpson's biplane method applies this algorithm to estimate LV volume using both ME 4 and 2-chamber views. In this technique, LV endocardial border is manually traced in the four and two-chamber views during systole and diastole and machine would calculate the EF. Tracing should start at the medial annulus of mitral valve and continue up to lateral annulus of the mitral valve. Papillary muscles are included in the tracing.

The advantage of this method is that it can be used in patients with RWMA as well as patients with dilated heart, i.e. low EF.

However, certain problems are encountered during the measurement of the EF.

- Lateral border of the LV many a times is not well defined making it difficult to trace. It is because of echocardiographic beam parallel to the lateral wall.
- Presence of calcium on the mitral annulus creates image drop out making it difficult to visualize ventricular wall.
- As this method assumes that the length of the LV is similar in the two orthogonal views, its accuracy decreases if the measurements of the major axis of the LV in the four and the two chamber views differ by 20%.

CARDIAC OUTPUT (FIGURES 9A AND B)

The cardiac output (CO) is the amount of blood pumped by the heart per minute. It is measured in liters per minute.

CO (L/min) = SV × HR, where SV is the stroke volume (in mL); and HR is the heart rate (in beats per minute).

The cardiac index (CI) is obtained by the following equation:

CI = CO/BSA, where CI in L/min per m^2 and BSA is the body surface area (m^2).

SV is the blood volume ejected from the LV during each systole so it is LVEDV-LVESV.

SV can also be measured using Doppler volumetric method where cross sectional area (CSA) of the cylindrical vessel and the stroke distance reached by the column of blood during the flow period, i.e. velocity time integral (VTI) are calculated. Product of CSA and VTI calculate the SV.

However, there are certain assumptions to be remembered for accurate measurement of SV using Doppler technique.

- Blood flow should be laminar. Smooth spectral signal obtained with pulse wave Doppler is evidence of laminar flow in the great vessels and across normal cardiac valve.

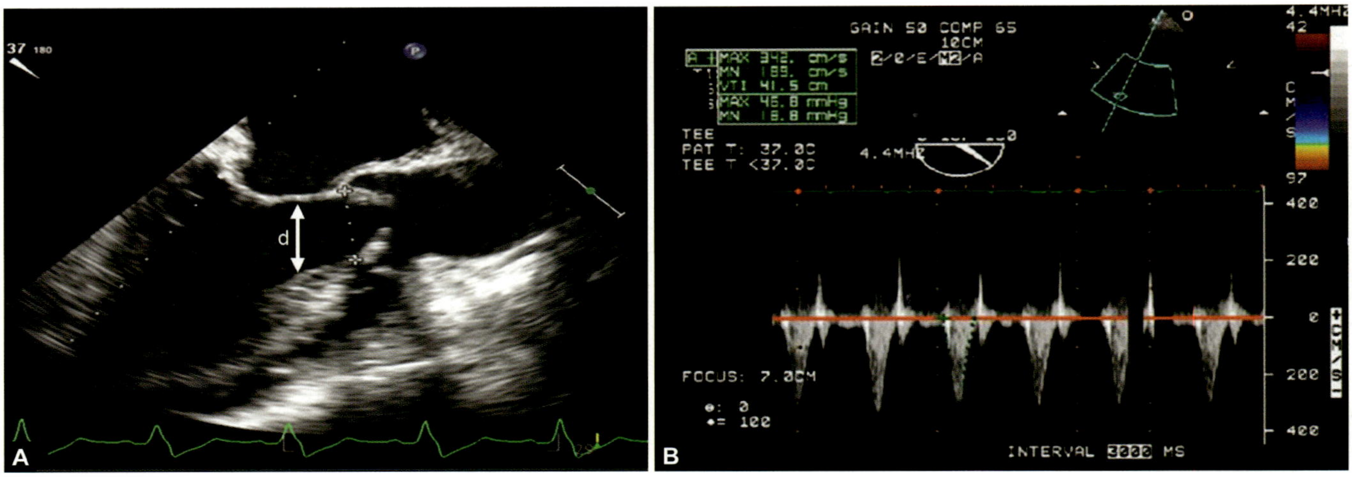

Figures 9A and B Cardiac output: (A) Firstly measure the left ventricular outflow tract (LVOT) diameter (d) using midesophageal aortic valve long axis view. (B) Transgastric long axis view showing aortic outflow tract velocities measured using continuous wave Doppler across the aortic valve. Tracing the envelope calculates the velocity time integral (VTI). Heart rate (HR) is calculated by putting calliper at the two consecutive QRS waves. Machine automatically calculates the HR. CO = 0.785 d^2 x VTI x HR

- Diameter is measured most accurately when the ultrasound beam is perpendicular to the blood tissue interface, i.e. ME long axis view of aortic valve, whereas VTI is accurately measured when ultrasound beam is parallel to blood flow, i.e. TG long axis view of LV or deep TG view.
- Average VTI (3–4 measurements in normal sinus rhythm, and 8–10 in atrial fibrillation) should be obtained.
- The VTI is measured with Doppler beam parallel to blood flow, i.e. angle is zero or less than 20% in the Doppler equation in order to avoid underestimation.

How to do the Measurements?

- The diameter, i.e. "d" of the left ventricular outflow tract is obtained from the ME long axis view of the aortic valve at level of 1 cm proximal to aortic valve. Any error in measurement at this point magnifies the error by second power.
- In TG long axis view or Deep TG view, Doppler beam is aligned to the blood flow across the aortic valve, pulse wave Doppler icon is pressured just above (approximately 1 cm) the aortic valve, i.e. left ventricular outflow tract so as to obtain the spectral envelope. VTI is obtained by tracing the best defined margins of the envelope and machine will calculate the VTI.

CSA can be calculated with using the formula for the area of a circle (of radius 'r') after measuring the orifice diameter (d) in cm.

CSA (cm^2) = $\Pi \times r^2 = \Pi \times (d/2)^2 = 0.785 \times d^2$, where CSA in "$cm^2$", r in "cm", and d in "cm".

SV = CSA × VTI = 0.785 d^2 × VTI

Aortic valve and ascending aorta are the most common sites for calculating CSA and VTI due to it accuracy. Calculations can also be performed at mitral valve and pulmonary valve but they are not as accurate as aortic valve and ascending aorta.

Doppler technique does not make any geometric assumptions about the LV cavity, therefore this technique is better than 2D technique of measuring SV especially in the asymmetrical LV.

QUALITATIVE METHODS

Mitral Annular Plane Systolic Excursion (MAPSE) or Mitral Annular Motion (MAM) (Figure 10)

It is an indirect measure of LV systolic function. It is usually measured in the ME four-chamber view where distance from mitral annulus to apex is measured during systole and diastole. The difference in the distance during systole and diastole, i.e. MAM is usually 12±2 mm. If it is less than 8 mm, it has sensitivity of 98% and specificity of 82% in indentifying EF less than 50%. EF can also be calculated using formula.

EF = 16.08 + 3.42 × MAM, where, MAM is Mitral annular motion in mm.

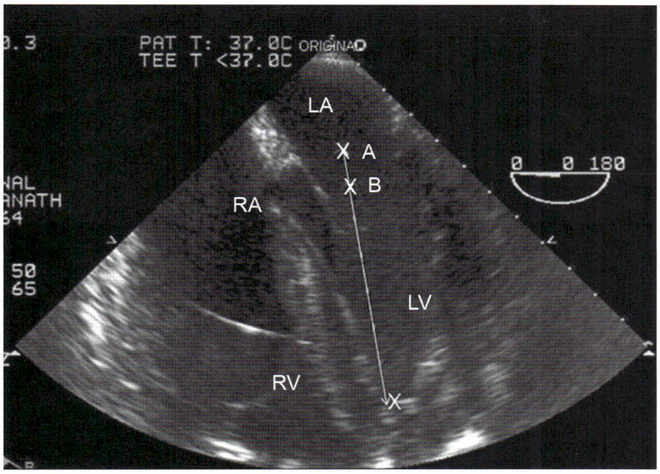

Figure 10 Mitral annulus plane systolic excursion (MAPSE) can be calculated in the midesophageal four chamber view. Distance from the mitral valve (MV) to the apex is calculated during the diastole and systole. Difference between the two, i.e. mitral annular motion (MAM) calculates the MAPSE

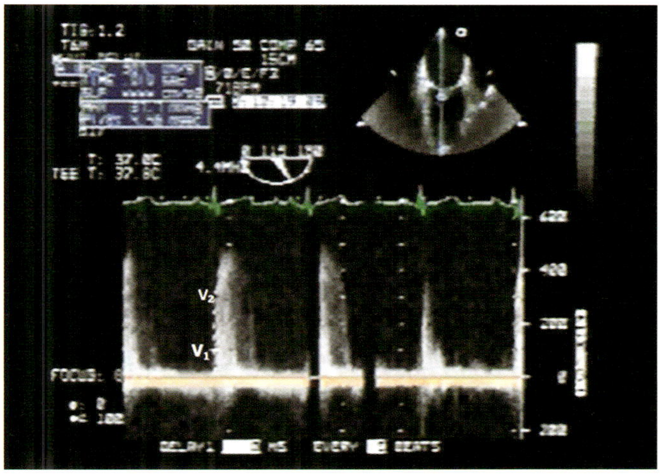

Figure 11 LV dP/dt is measured using continuous wave across the mitral valve. Presence of mitral regurgitation leads to formation of spectral envelope above the baseline. Calliper is placed at velocity 1m/s and second Calliper at 3 m/s at the ascending limb of the spectral envelope (see V_1 and V_2). Machine would calculate the time required to rise in ventricular velocity from 1 m/s to 3 m/s

LV dP/dt (Figure 11)

LV dP/dt is the rate of rise in LV pressure during early systole. It is obtained from MR jet velocity profile. LV dP/dt is a simple technique but is load dependent. dP is change in MR jet velocity from 1 m/s (V_1) to 3 m/s (V_2) and calculated by simplified Bernoulli equation $[4 \times (V_2^2 - V_1^2)]$.

$dP = 4V_2^2 - 4V_1^2 = 4(3)^2 - 4(1)^2 = 36-4 = 32$ mm Hg

Thus, dP/dt = 32/dt.

dt is obtained by calculating the time taken by the MR jet velocity to rise from 1.0 m/s to 3.0 m/s. (dP/dT) value > 1200 mm Hg depicts normal LV function, whereas LV dP/dt less than 1000 mm Hg depicts LV dysfunction.

MYOCARDIAL PERFORMANCE INDEX OR TEI INDEX

The myocardial performance index (MPI) can be calculated using 2D echo with Doppler technique, i. e. pulse wave Doppler of the transmitral flow velocities (conventional method) as well as tissue Doppler imaging (TDI). 2D Doppler imaging uses high velocity moving objects like red blood cells, whereas, myocardial tissue velocity is usually less than 20 cm/sec and approximately 10 times slower than blood. Thus, myocardium has high amplitude and low frequency. TDI measures myocardial tissue velocities, allowing a quantitative assessment of myocardial function during the entire cardiac cycle. The technique is less dependent on chamber geometry and no endocardial border delineation is needed, making it useful even in presence of suboptimal echocardiographic image quality. However, appropriate alignment of the ultrasound beam is very important in TDI technique. Angle more than 20º yields erroneous results, though, alignment can be difficult in dilated LV. Parameter derived from TDI to estimate the global LV function are mitral transannular velocity and Tei index.

Mitral Transannular Velocity (Figure 12)

Systolic mitral annular velocity (S') is quick and easy way of estimating LVEF. S' more than 8 cm/s represents EF at least 50%. S' has been found to be closely related to LVEF. EF can be calculated by S' using following formula.

EF (%) = $8.0 + 5.5 \times S'^{1}$ (cm/sec), S' is systolic mitral annular velocity.

MPI or Tei Index (Figures 13 and 14)

It is the sum of isovolumic contraction time (IVCT) and isovolumic relaxation time (IVRT) divided by ejection time (ET). Prolongation of IVCT and shortening of ET occurs during systolic dysfunction while IVRT is

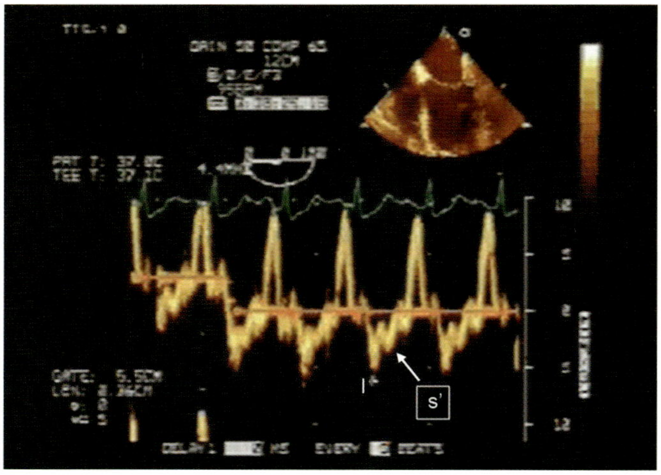

Figure 12 Mitral annular velocity (S') is calculated using tissue Doppler at lateral annulus of the mitral valve. S' more than 8 cm/s represents ejection fraction (EF) at least 50%. Please note that first negative waveform "I" is the isovolumic contraction (IC) and second negative waveform is systolic mitral annular velocity (S')

prolonged during early stage of diastolic dysfunction. Thus both systolic and diastolic dysfunction leads to increase in MPI. Both systolic and diastolic phases are thus involved in the assessment of global LV function. MPI is obtained by using transmitral flow (a = End of A wave to the beginning of E wave signifying IVRT + IVCT + ET) **(Figure 13A)** and ET = Aortic ejection time calculated in the TG long axis view or deep TG view **(Figure 13B)**.

MPI = a – ET/ET. Normal value of MPI for LV is 0.39 ± 0.05.

Value more than 0.5 signifies LV dysfunction **(Table 2)**.

Normally this is obtained in two views, "a" is obtained in ME 4 chamber view whereas "ET" is obtained in TG long axis view. Thus cardiac cycle is different in this case leading to error in measurement because hemodynamics may be different in two cardiac cycle. However, if good image of deep TG view is obtained then both 'a" and "ET" can be obtained in same view, i.e. in same cardiac cycle. Pulse wave in normal valve patient and continuous wave in patients with valvular heart disease can be used to calculate the MPI.

The advantage of using TDI is that measurements are done during single beat at the lateral mitral annulus **(Figure 14)**.

SUMMARY

TEE has proved to be an important cardiac monitoring tool during perioperative period. It has altered the surgical plan due to presence of unexpected finding prior to surgery. During perioperative setting, it is the rapid diagnostic tool to detect RWMA and thus, prompt identification and swift intervention for intraoperative

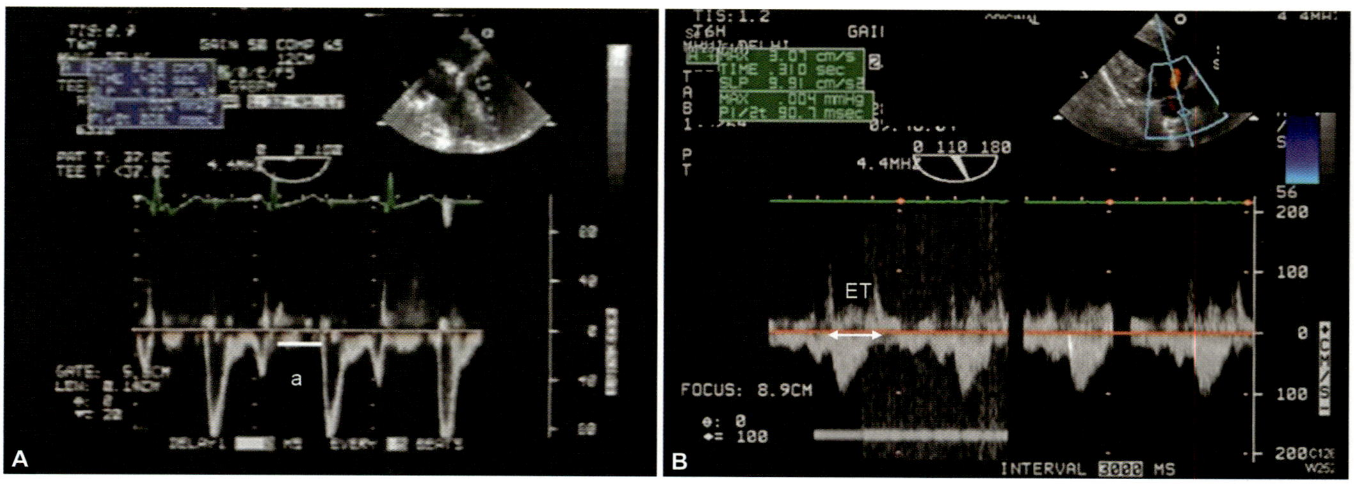

Figures 13A and B Myocardial performance index (Tei index) using pulse wave Doppler (conventional method). (A) Pulse wave across the mitral valve produces two negative wave (E and A). Time from end of wave A to beginning of E wave is calculated (a). (B) Ejection time (ET) is calculated in the transgastric long axis view using continuous wave across the aortic valve. Distance from the onset of spectral envelope to end of the envelope measures the ET (ET). Tei index = a-ET/ET. Normal Tei index is 0.39 ± 0.05. Left ventricle systolic function is abnormal if Tei index is more than 0.42

TABLE 2 Different TEE views for detecting left ventricular (LV) function

Views	*Purpose of the view*
Midesophageal 4 chamber view	Assessment of the segments of LV, MAPSE FAC, modified Simpson's method, tissue Doppler imaging at the lateral annulus of the mitral valve
Midesophageal 2 chamber view	Assessment of the segments of LV, FAC Modified Simpson's method
Midesophageal long axis view	Assessment of the segments of LV Measurement of diameter of left ventricular outflow tract
Transgastric midpapillary short axis view	Contractility of segments of LV, volume status, FAC, FS
Transgastric basal short axis view	Segments of LV
Transgastric apical view	Segements of LV
Transgastric long axis view and deep transgastric view	For measurement of VTI of blood flow across the aortic valve

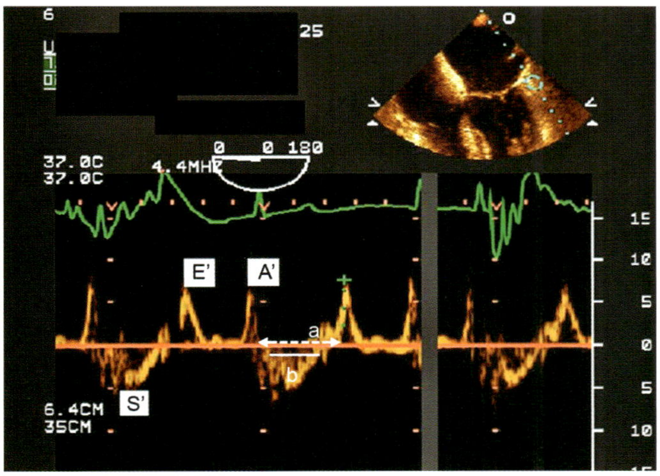

Figure 14 Myocardial performance index or Tei index using tissue Doppler method: "a" is measured from end of wave A' to beginning of the wave E'. "b" is calculated from the onset of the wave S' to end of this wave. Tei index = a-b/b. In this method, both "a" and "b" are calculated in single beat

myocardial ischemia with TEE has played key role in improving early CABG outcome. Apart from that, echocardiographer can not only do the eye ball examination of the LV but also perform the both quantitative and qualitative methods to validate his findings. In addition, use of TEE in hemodynamically unstable patient in surgical intensive care can lead to early detection of problem and its management. **Table 2** summaries vary views to evaluate the LV regional and global systolic function.

RECOMMENDED READING

1. Cerqueira MD, Weissman NJ, Dilsizian V, et al. Standardized myocardial imaging of the heart: a statement for healthcare professional from the cardiac imaging committee of the council on clinical cardiology of the American Heart Association. Circulation. 2002;20:213-33.
2. Goel S. Evaluation of the left ventricular function. In: Tempe DK, Subramaniam B, Subramaniam K, Ramakrishna H (Eds). Problem based transesophageal echocardiography, First. CBS Publisher, New Delhi. 2014.pp.28-36.
3. Hahn TR, Abraham T, Adams MS, et al. Guidelines for performing a comprehensive transesophageal echocardiographic examination: recommendations from the American Society of Echocardiography and the Society of Cardiovascular Anesthesiologists. J Am Soc Echocardiogr. 2013;26:921-64.
4. Lang RM, Bierig M, Devereux RB, et al. Recommendations for chamber quantification. Eur J Echocardiogr. 2006;7:79-108.
5. Skubas N. Intraoperative Doppler tissue imaging is a valuable addition to cardiac anaesthesiologist's armamentarium: a core review. Anesth Analg. 2009;108:48-66.

Chapter 14

Evaluation of Aorta by Simulated Transesophageal Echocardiography

TA Patil, Dattatreya Prabhakumar, Praveen Kalligudd

Chapter Outline

- Simulation in Transesophageal Echocardiography
- Evaluation of Aorta
- Anatomical Considerations
- Echocardiographic Evaluation of the Thoracic Aorta
- Thoracic Aortic Diseases

Medical simulation is well-established in anesthesia and is considered an important educational tool. Patient simulation is now a part of regular and recurrent training curriculum in anesthesiology in the United States, United Kingdom and some European nations.

Simulators are commonly used for teaching and training and their popularity could be attributed to various reasons:

1. Simulate a high degree of reality
2. No risk for a real patient
3. Predictable, programmable and reproducible scenarios
4. Repetition possible; can be stopped or restarted
5. Practice for life-threatening and rare clinical scenarios.

SIMULATION IN TRANSESOPHAGEAL ECHOCARDIOGRAPHY (FIGURE 1)

During and after training, anesthesia residents are allowed to perform procedures on patients under supervision. Simulation would be a far more effective training tool to teach skills necessary to perform invasive procedures and TEE.

Traditionally, TEE training is achieved by practicing on cardiac surgical patients in the operating room (OR) under supervision. The environment of the OR is not always conducive for teaching and unpredictable clinical situations prevent standardization of clinical teaching. Risk of injury to the patient is another reality which must be borne in mind. TEE simulators provide solutions for several of these shortcomings.

EVALUATION OF AORTA

Atherosclerosis of the ascending aorta and aortic arch is recognized as one of the important predictors of postoperative stroke after cardiac surgery. Aortic dissection and rupture are emergent situations requiring rapid, accurate diagnosis in order to reduce the morbidity and mortality.

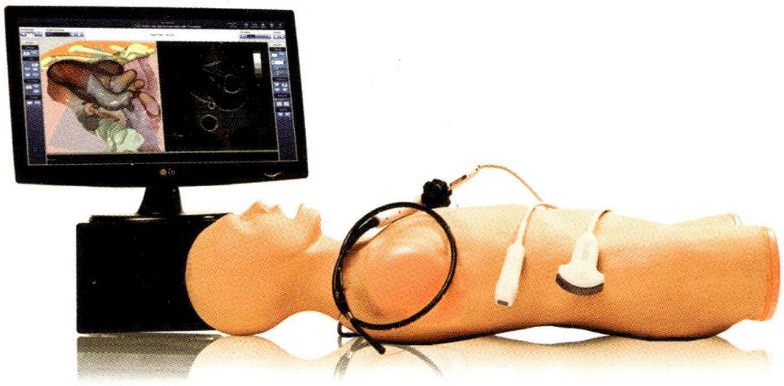

Figure 1 Realistic TEE environment for simulated training

ANATOMICAL CONSIDERATIONS

The thoracic aorta is divided into four segments surgically: aortic root, ascending aorta, aortic arch and the descending thoracic aorta **(Figure 2)**. Aortic root consists of the aortic annulus, aortic cusps, sinuses of valsalva and the sinotubular junction (STJ). The aortic diameter varies between 33 mm and 35 mm with a wall thickness of 2 mm. The ascending aorta with a length of about 7–11 cm originates from the aortic annulus at the level of STJ crossing beneath the main pulmonary artery, and then courses in an anterior and rightward direction over the origin of the right pulmonic artery which terminates and continues as the aortic arch at the origin of the innominate artery.

The aortic arch courses in a posterior and leftward direction giving rise to the innominate (brachiocephalic artery), left common carotid, and left subclavian artery. It is difficult to visualize the distal ascending aorta and the proximal aortic arch with TEE because of the underlying trachea.

The descending thoracic aorta begins distal to the left subclavian artery at the level of the ligamentum-arteriosum and courses anteriorly and caudally towards the diaphragmatic hiatus. The aorta courses in a smooth curved fashion from the anterolateral side of the 4th thoracic vertebra to the anterior surface of the 11th vertebral body. At the distal level the descending thoracic aorta lies directly posterior to the esophagus.

ECHOCARDIOGRAPHIC EVALUATION OF THE THORACIC AORTA

The following imaging planes are recommended for imaging the thoracic aorta:

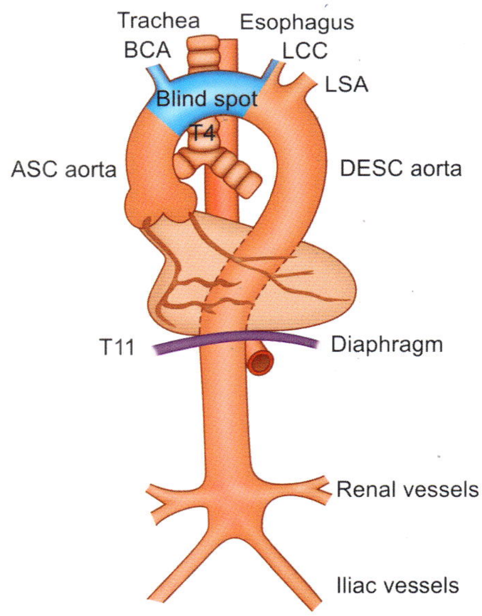

Figure 2 Anatomy of the aorta (Illustrations by Dr Srinivasa Holla)

1. Midesophageal aortic valve long axis
2. Midesophageal ascending aorta short axis and long axis view
3. Descending aortic short and long-axis views
4. Upper esophageal aortic arch long and short axis views

Midesophageal Aortic Valve Long Axis View (Figures 3A and B)

The midesophageal aortic valve long axis view (ME-AV LAX) is important in evaluating the aortic valve and the proximal ascending aorta. Measurements can be made of the left ventricular outflow tract, the annulus, sinuses of valsalva, STJ and ascending aorta if valve replacement and/or root reconstruction is being planned.

Midesophageal Ascending Aorta Short Axis and Long Axis Views (Figures 4A and B)

These views are crucial to exclude dissections of the aorta. Artifacts are commonly encountered within the ascending aorta, hence the priority to distinguish artifacts from true dissections to prevent needless, expensive interventions.

From the ME 4C view withdraw the probe to obtain the ME 5C view, continue to withdraw to a point where

CHAPTER 14

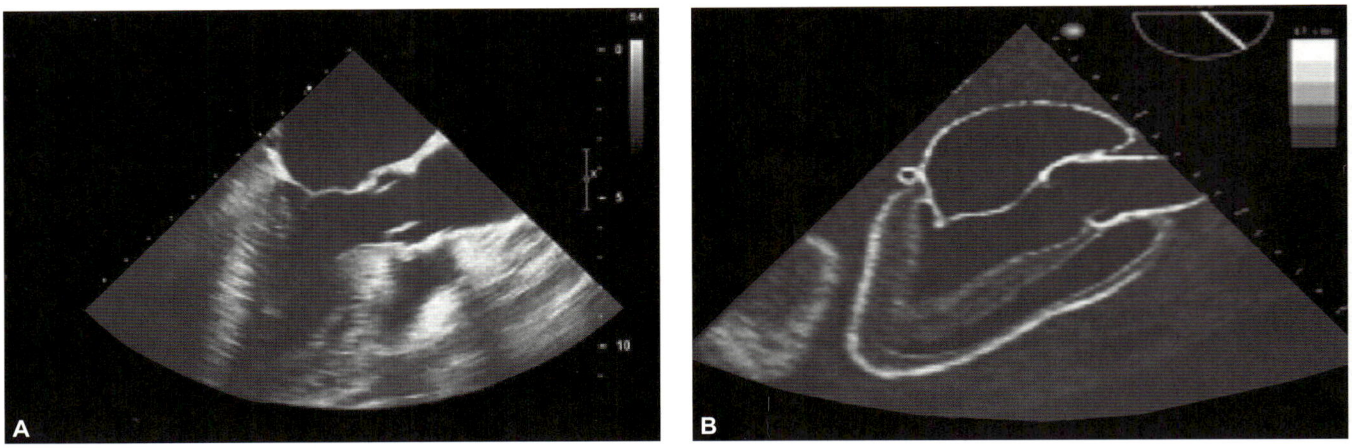

Figures 3A and B (A) 2D view of ME-AV LAX; (B) Simulated view of ME-AV LAX

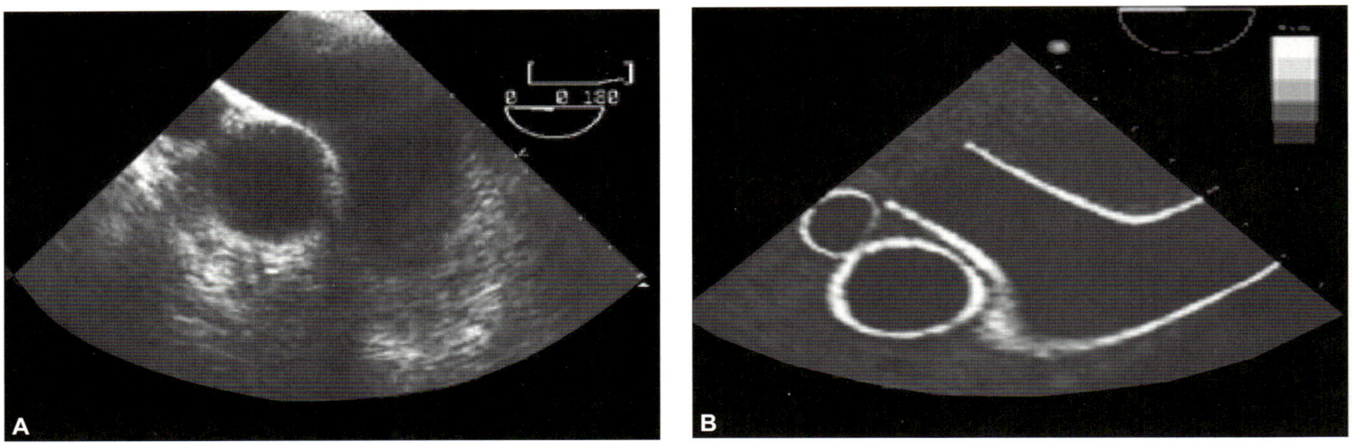

Figures 4A and B (A) 2D view of ME-ASC aortic SAX; (B) Simulated view of ME-ASC aortic SAX

the ascending aorta disappears, anteflex the probe to obtain the ME-ASC aorta SAX view. Increasing the multiplane angle to 90 degrees the ME-ASC aortic LAX view is obtained.

Midesophageal Descending Aorta Short and Long Axis Views (Figures 5 and 6)

At the midesophageal level from the four chamber view rotating the probe in an anticlockwise direction or to the left and optimizing the depth to 4–6 cm results in descending aortic short axis view. This is an important view to evaluate many diagnostic issues like the presence of an atheromatous plaque,dissection,aneurysm, left pleural effusion, confirming the severity of aortic insufficiency and the position of intra-aortic balloon **(Figures 7A and B)**. Increasing the multiplane angle to 90 degrees the long axis view is visualized.

Upper Esophageal Aortic Arch Long Axis and Short Axis Views (Figures 8 and 9)

Withdrawing the TEE probe from the descending aortic short axis view with simultaneous clockwise rotation of the probe, the main aim being is to retain the descending aortic view in the center of the image, the upper esophageal aortic arch long axis view is obtained. Increasing the multiplane to 90 degree the short axis

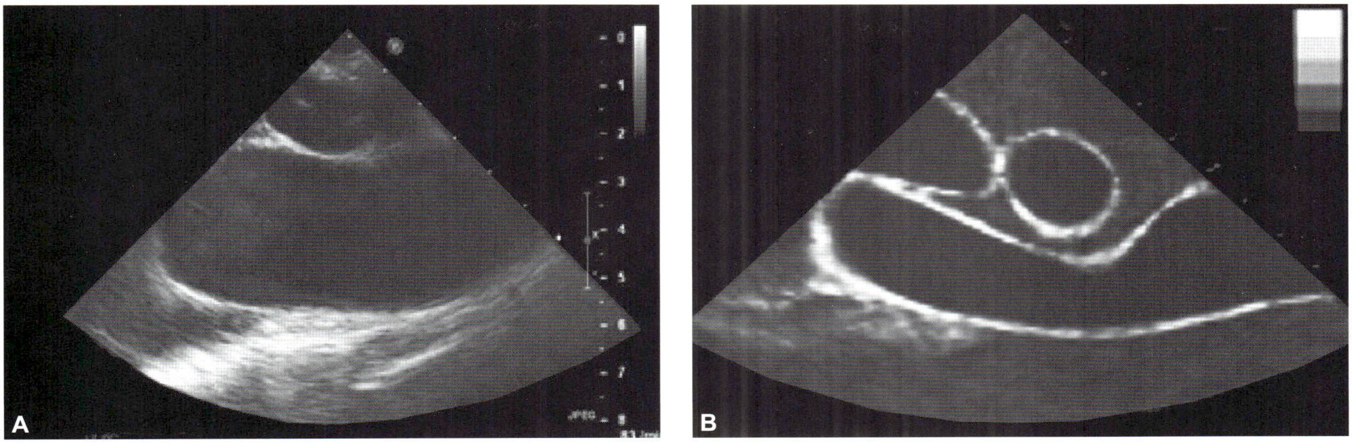

Figures 5A and B (A) 2D view of ME-ASC aortic LAX; (B) Simulated view of ME-ASC aortic LAX

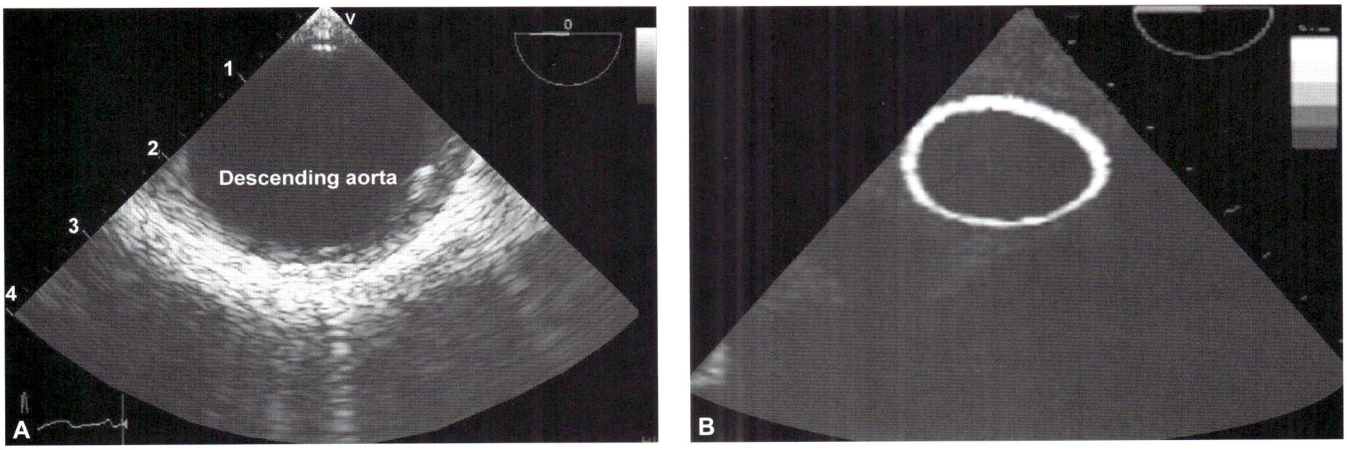

Figures 6A and B (A) 2D view of ME-DESC aortic SAX; (B) Simulated view of ME-DESC aortic SAX

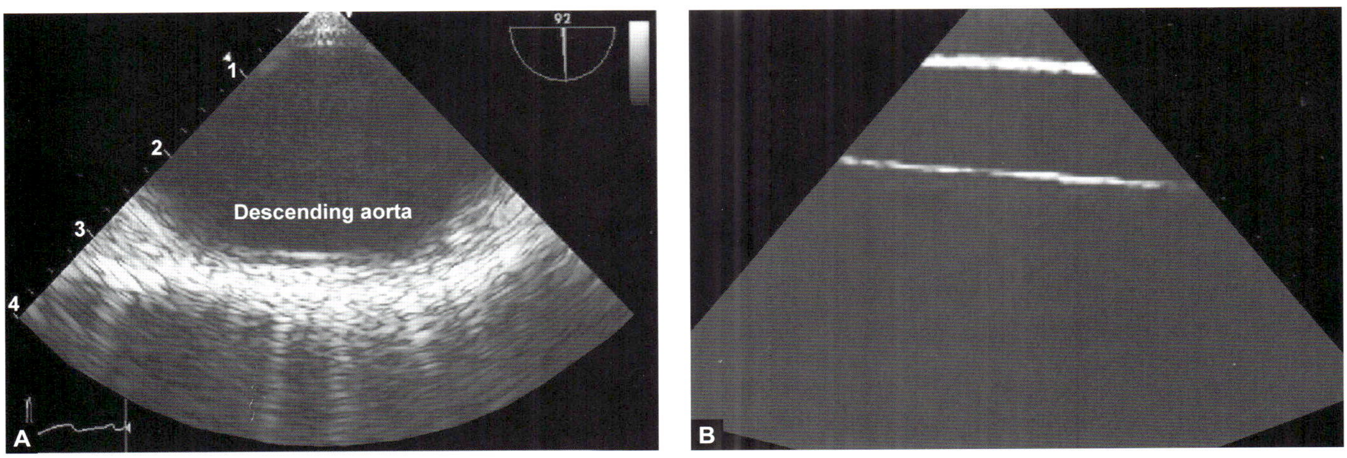

Figures 7A and B (A) 2D view of ME-DESC aortic LAX; (B) Simulated view of ME-DESC aortic LAX

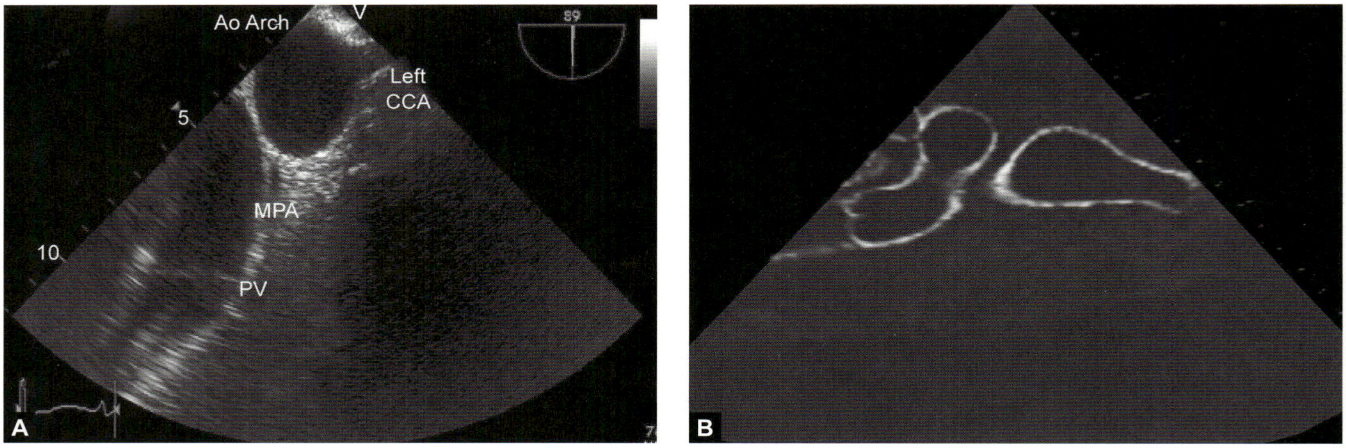

Figures 8A and B (A) 2D view of UE-aortic arch SAX; (B) Simulated view of UE-aortic arch SAX

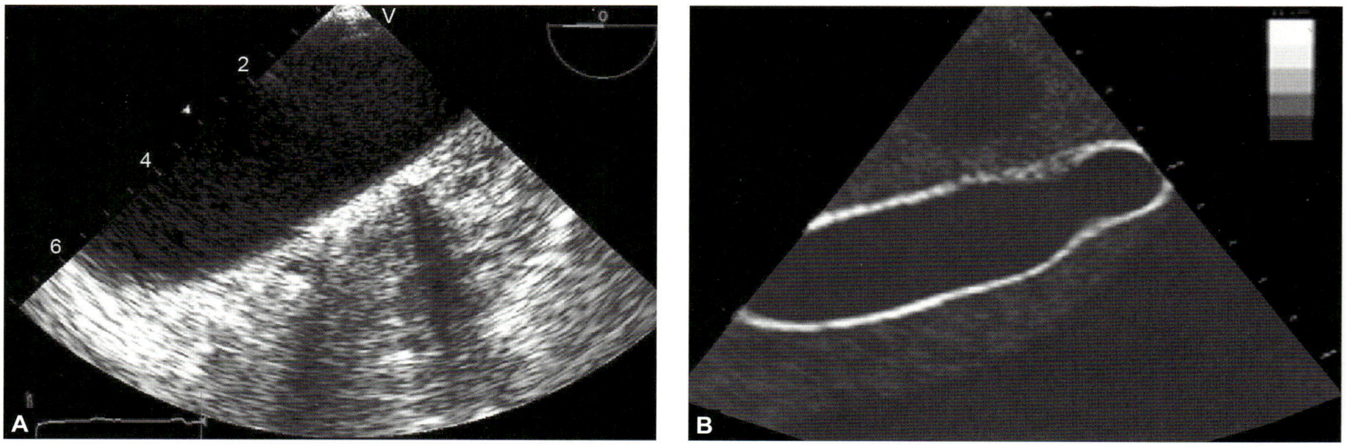

Figures 9A and B (A) 2D view of UE-aortic arch LAX; (B) Simulated view of UE-aortic arch LAX

view of the upper esophageal aortic arch is obtained. The aorta changes its appearance from circular to longitudinal in the long axis view.

The diagnostic issues related to this view include recognition of patent ductus arteriosus, spectral Doppler of the pulmonary artery and presence of atheromatous plaques in the aortic arch. The origins of the left subclavian, left common carotid and the bracheocephalic arteries can be visualized frequently by minimal rotation of the TEE probe.

THORACIC AORTIC DISEASES

The main diseases of the aorta are—Aortic aneurysm, atherosclerosis and aortic dissection.

Atherosclerosis

Atherosclerosis of the ascending aorta and aortic arch is one of the important predictor of postoperative stroke after cardiac surgery occurring in 1–6% of the patients. Echocardiography should be used to identify aortic atherosclerosis prior to anticipated surgical manipulations. Identification of significant disease by TEE permits alterations in the surgical procedure **(Figures 10A and B)**.

Lesions of the ascending aorta and arch have been identified as risk factors for stroke, peripheral embolization, perioperative stroke, as well as neuropsychological dysfunction after open heart surgery. Atheroemboli, thromboemboli, and plaque thickness >4 mm correlate with significant embolic risk. Although

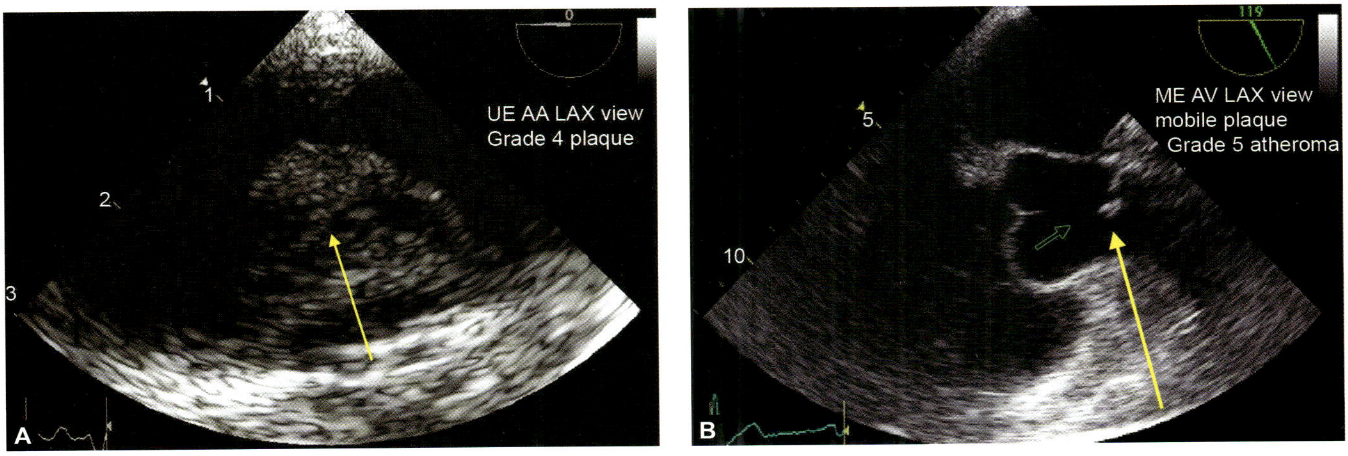

Figures 10A and B (A) UE-aortic arch LAX view, arrow (yellow) indicating grade 4 atheroma; (B) ME-AV LAX view, arrow (yellow) indicating grade 5 atheroma in the proximal ascending aorta

TEE evaluation of the lesions is sensitive and specific, one of the important limitations is inadequate visualization of distal ascending aorta and proximal aortic arch because of the interposed airfilled trachea.

Aortic Aneurysms

An aneurysm is defined as dilatation of aorta more than 50% of normal aortic diameter involving all the three layers of the vessel wall. The aorta is considered to be dilated if its diameter varies between 3.7 cm–5.0 cm, aneurysmal if the diameter is more than 5.0 cm and dissected if it presents with a intimal flap. Aortic aneurysm is either saccular or fusiform. A fusiform aneurysm has a uniform shape with a symmetrical dilatation that involves the entire circumference of the aortic wall while saccular aneurysm is a localized out pouching of the aortic wall.

Thoracoabdominal aneurysms are grouped into four types based on the **Crawford classification (Figure 11)**.

Type 1—involves the descending aorta just distal to the origin of left subclavian artery to the abdominal aorta above the renal arteries.

Type 2—involves the descending aorta terminating distal to the renal arteries.

Type 3—involves the distal half of the descending aorta and the abdominal aorta to its bifurcation.

Type 4—involves the abdominal aorta to its bifurcation.

TEE can be used to define the size, location, and extent of the aortic aneurysm as well as the presence of a hematoma or thrombus. It can also be useful to identify associated aortic valve disease, which helps the surgeon in formulating the surgical plan. TEE may also be used to evaluate the patency aortic arch branches to confirm the presence of organ malperfusion. It is an important monitoring tool of cardiac function during aortic aneurysm surgeries.

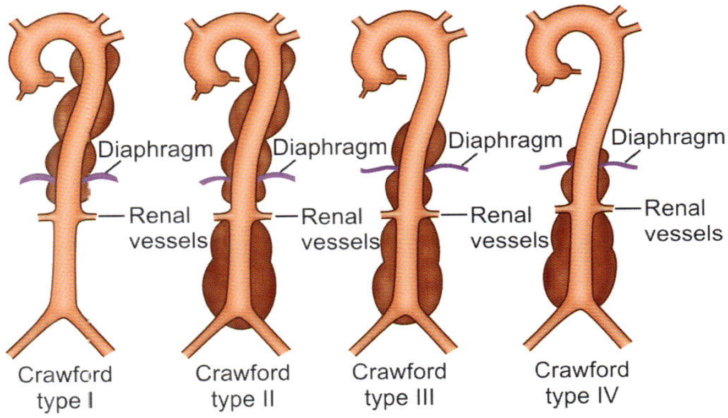

Figure 11 Crawford classification of thoracoabdominal aneurysms (Illustration by Dr Srinivasa Holla)

Aortic Dissections (Figures 12A and B)

Aortic dissection is formed by an intimal tear which is contained by the media leading to the development of a true and false lumen. The false lumen may extend into branches of the aorta in the chest or abdomen, causing malperfusion, ischemia, or occlusion with resultant

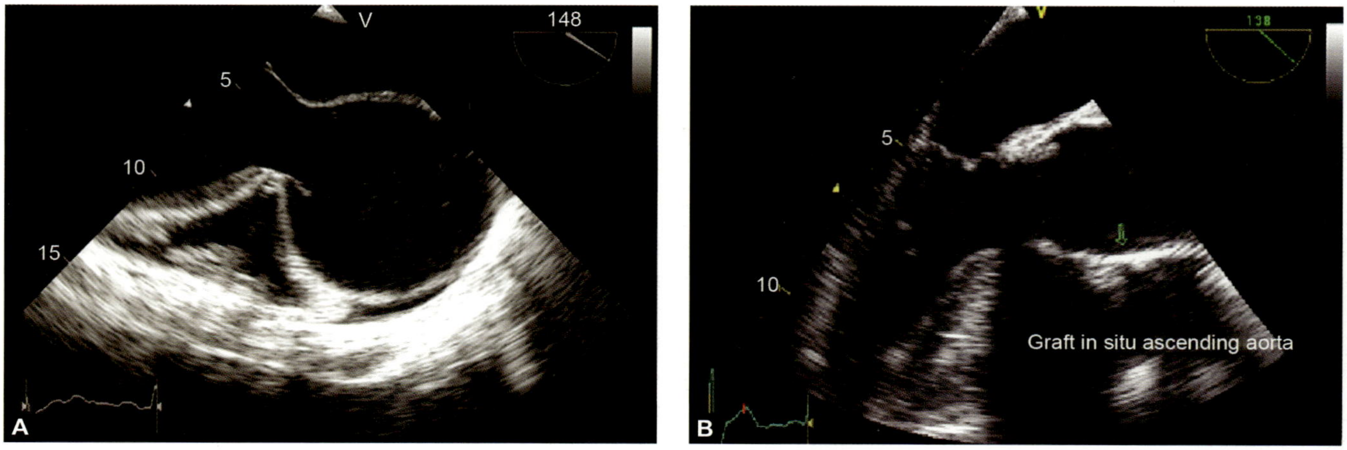

Figures 12A and B (A) ME-AV-LAX view showing dilated annulus and ascending aorta; (B) ME-AV-LAX view showing a Dacron graft in-situ in the ascending aortic position

complications. The dissection can also progress proximally involving the aortic sinus, aortic valve leading to aortic insufficiency and may also involve the coronary arteries resulting in ischemic events.[1,2]

TEE also has 98% sensitivity and 100% specificity for diagnosing dissections, hence is an ideal imaging modality especially in unstable patients. **The Debakey classification and the Stanford classification systems are used to describe aortic dissections.**

Type 1—originates in the ascending aorta extending distally up to the aortic bifurcation.

Type 2—originates in the ascending aorta up to the brachiocephalic trunk.

Type 3a—originates distal to the left subclavian artery terminating just above the diaphragm.

Type 4a—originates distal to the left subclavian artery up to the aortic bifurcation.

Stanford classification is divided into two types, Type A involving the ascending aorta (Debakey type 1, 2), Type B the ascending aorta is spared (Debakey Type 3a, 3b). This classification is simple and clinically important **(Figure 13)**.

Aortic dissections can be evaluated by TEE using the standard views. The presence of an intimal flap is the most important evidence of an aortic dissection. Presence of an intimal flap, true and a false lumen and forward systolic flow in the true lumen are sensitive features of dissection. Other findings are complete thrombosis of the false lumen, central displacement of intimal calcification and separation of intimal layers from the thrombus.[3-5]

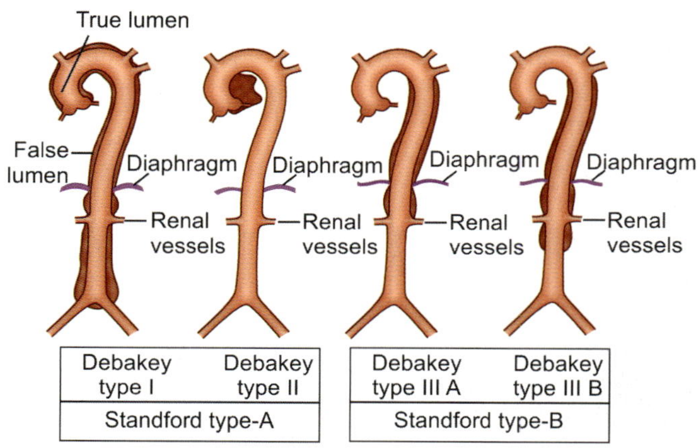

Figure 13 Thoracoabdominal dissections (Illustrations by Dr Srinivasa Holla)

Entry and Exit Sites of Aortic Dissections

Transesophageal echocardiography is a valuable imaging modality to locate the intimal tear site which is of extreme importance for the success of surgical repair and also to determine the type of dissection. Resection of the primary site decreases the incidence of complications and redoes surgeries. Intimal tear occurs in the ascending aorta 1 to 3 cm above the right or left sinus of valsalva in about 70% of the cases and at the site of ligamentum arteriosum in about 30% of the cases. In the ascending and aortic arch the dissection plane is along the greater curvature but in the descending aorta it is located lateral to the true lumen.

TEE plays an important role in the identification of the true and false lumen. True lumen expands during systole and compressed during diastole. M-mode placed through the dissection helps in identifying the systolic expansion of the true lumen **(Figures 14 to 18)**.

True lumen is smaller than the false lumen, has a less echogenic thin layer compared to the false lumen which has a bright echogenic layer. In the false lumen variable amounts of thrombus and spontaneous echo contrast are frequently present. True lumen exhibits a forward systolic color flow pattern, sometimes flow can be seen from the true to the false lumen. Thickening of the aortic wall more than 15 mm is considered to be a sign of dissection indicating massive thrombosis of the false lumen making it difficult to identify the intimal flap.

Descending Aortic SAX View Showing the Dissection Flap (Figures 17A and B)

It is of great importance to examine the midesophageal aortic valve long axis view carefully to detect proximal ascending aortic dissections. It is in this view a Swan-Ganz catheter appears as an artifact. Hence, it is very important to differentiate an artifact from a true dissection lest the patient may be subjected to a needless expensive surgical procedure thereby increasing the

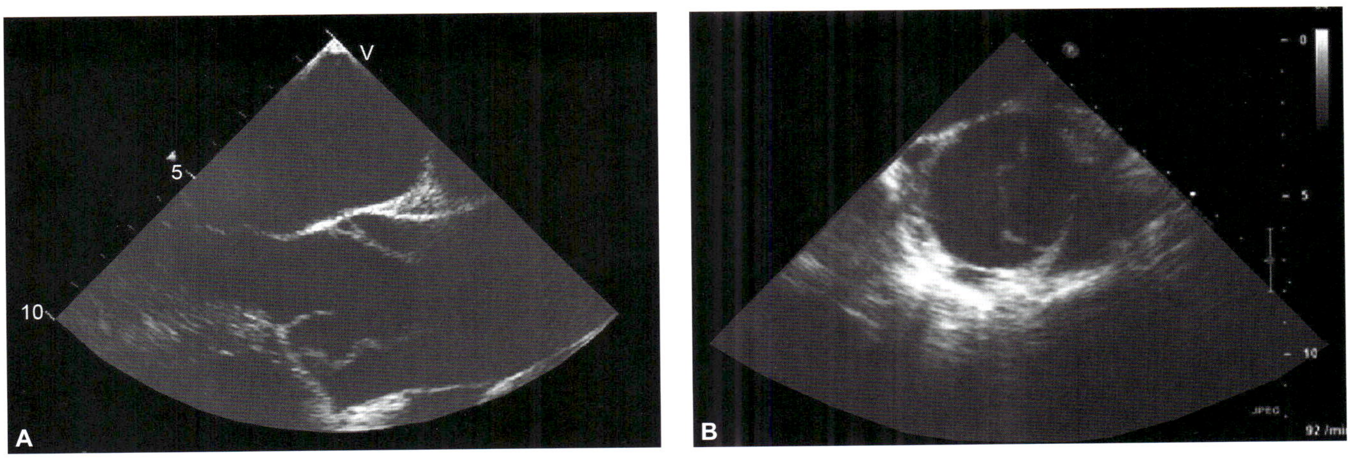

Figures 14A and B (A) ME-AV-LAX showing the intimal flap arising from the STJ; (B) ME-AV-SAX showing the intimal flap

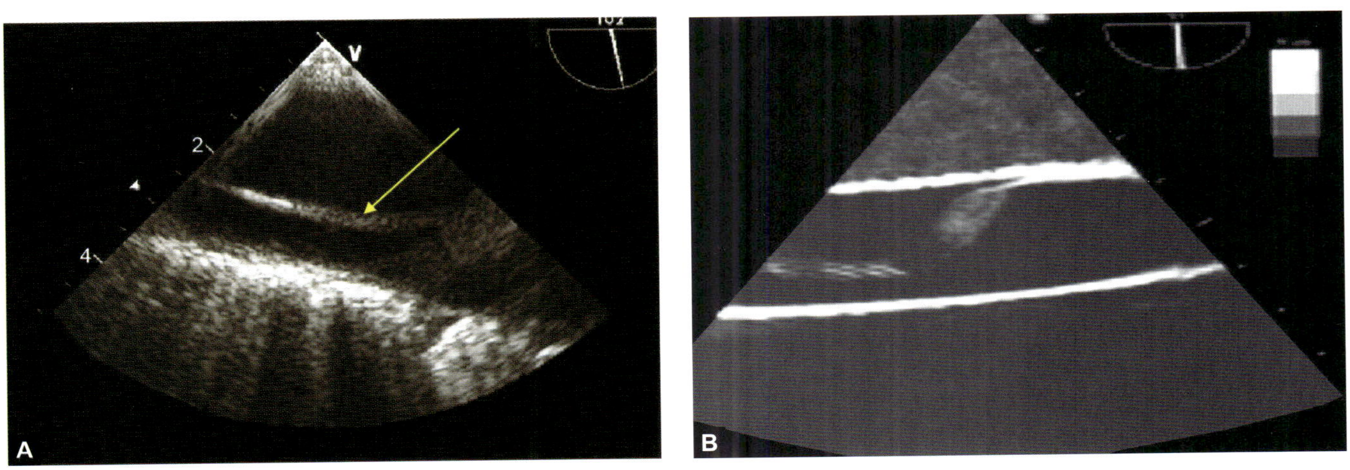

Figures 15A and B (A) DESC-aortic LAX showing the dissection flap; yellow arrow indicates true lumen; (B) Simulated view of DESC-aortic LAX showing the dissection flap

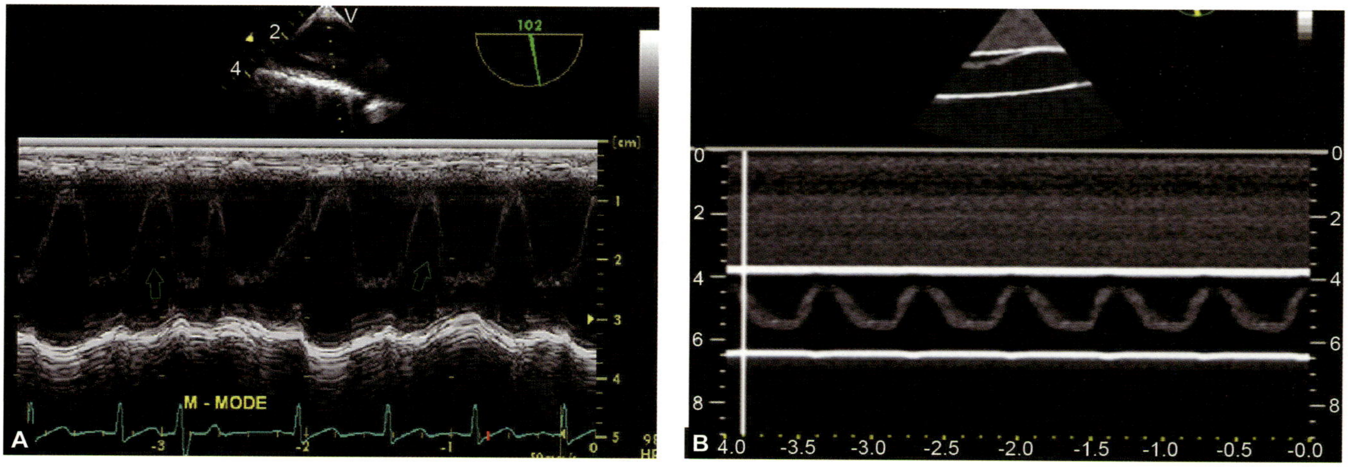

Figures 16A and B (A) M-mode showing systolic movement of the intimal flap towards the false lumen; (B) Simulated M-mode showing systolic movement of the intimal flap towards the false lumen

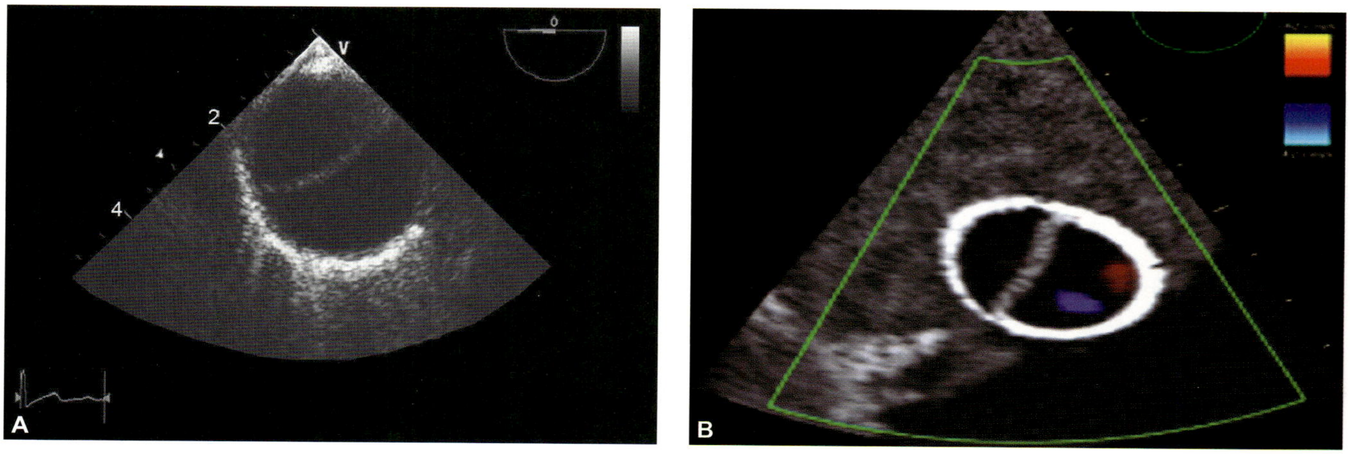

Figures 17A and B (A) Descending aortic SAX view showing the dissection flap; (B) Color flow Doppler, simulated descending aortic SAX view showing the dissection flap

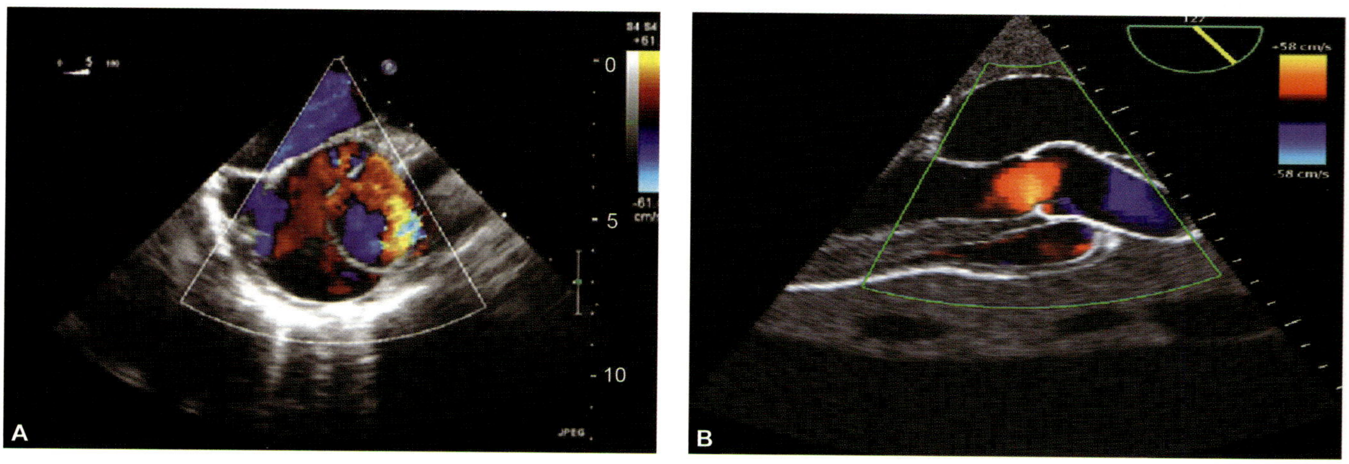

Figures 18A and B (A) 2D ME-AV-SAX view, color flow Doppler illustrating the intimal flap and severe aortic insufficiency; (B) Simulated ME-AV-LAX view, illustrating severe aortic insufficiency

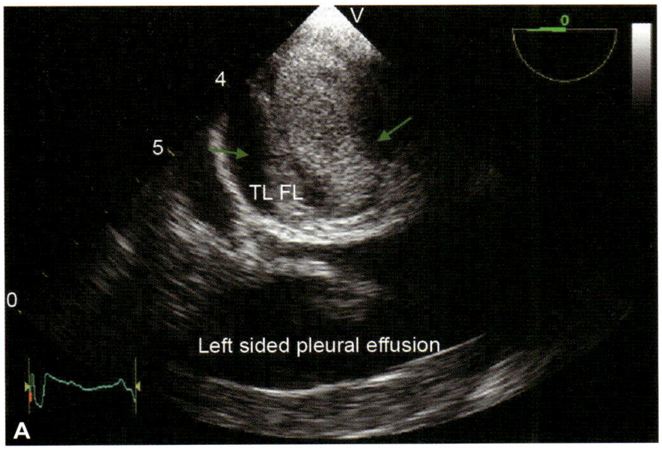

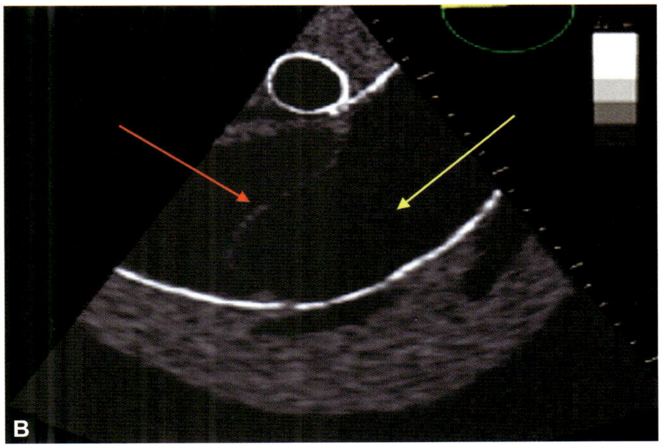

Figures 19A and B (A) 2D descending aortic SAX view with the dissection flap, complete thrombosis of the false lumen with left sided pleural effusion (TL—True lumen, FL—False lumen); (B) Simulated view of descending aortic SAX view. Arrow (yellow) indicating left sided pleural effusion and collapsed lung (red arrow)

morbidity. A linear artifact of the ascending aorta can be distinguished from an intimal flap by (1) indistinct borders, (2) lack of rapid oscillatory movements, (3) extension of the artifact through the aortic wall as a straight line, (4) presence of color flow on both sides of the artifact. Artifacts can also occur in the descending aorta. These are mirror image artifacts caused by a highly reflective aorta which occur at twice the distance from the transducer appearing as a double-lumen aorta.

Complications of Aortic Dissections

Complications associated with dissections are aortic insufficiency occurring in about 50–70% of the cases, coronary dissections in 10–20% of the cases, pleural and pericardial effusion and global left ventricular dysfunction. TEE can be used to determine the cause of aortic insufficiency which helps to formulate the surgical plan. TEE is a reliable tool to evaluate the coronary anatomy in the presence of dissection in the midesophageal aortic valve short axis view. LV dysfunction may be secondary to ischemia following coronary dissection or due to severe aortic insufficiency presenting in about 10–15% of the cases. Pericardial effusion is due to transudation of fluid from the wall of the false lumen into the pericardial cavity. Another routine finding is the presence of left pleural effusion causing a hemothorax **(Figures 19A and B)**.

Intramural Hematoma (Figure 20)

Intramural hematomas are characterized by thickened aortic walls without an intimal flap involving the ascending or the descending aorta probably due to rupture of the vasa vasorum leading to a hemorrhagic vessel wall. Hematomas involving the ascending aorta need emergent surgical therapy, while those involving the descending aorta are managed medically. Intramural hematomas as described by Mohr-Kahaly are characterized by thickening of the aortic wall of more than 7 mm with a longitudinal length of 1–20 cm and absence of intimal tear.

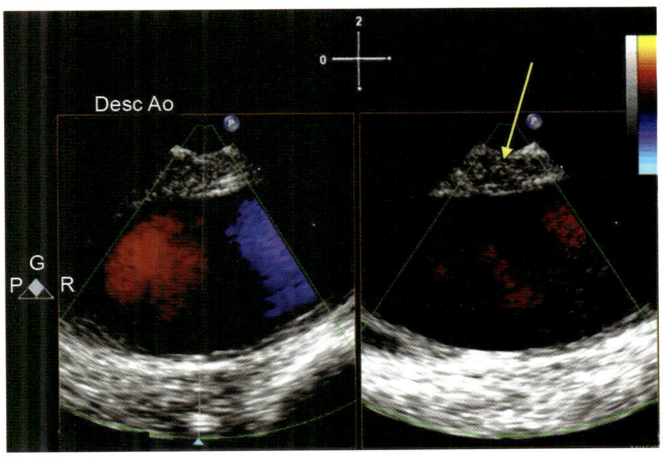

Figures 20 2D biplane view of the descending aortic SAX, arrow (yellow) indicating intramural hematoma of the anterior wall

CHAPTER 14

CONCLUSION

A simulation-based TEE curriculum can improve the knowledge and technical skills of echo learners, both beginners and advanced. The simulator-based teaching model for TEE is a probably better method of teaching concepts of TEE like anatomic correlation, structure identification, and image acquisition.

Simulators allow understanding of a wide range of normal or pathological cases scenarios with multiple hemodynamic and level variables on-demand. The greatest advantage being the risks and inconvenience associated with learning on real patients are avoided.

Simulators provide users with a real-time 3D graphic representation of the cardiac structures, cross-sectional anatomy, and transducer location. This augmented reality feature provides users with a better understanding of their current scanning location, cross-sectional anatomy, preferred imaging planes, structural anatomy and their position relative to the ultrasound transducer's location. The process of learning image optimization with the simulator is also possible.

The authors acknowledge the help of Mr. Pradeep K, CAE Healthcare, India for providing the simulated material, and Dr Srinivas Holla for his illustrations.

REFERENCES

1. Kouchoukos NT, Dougenis D. Surgery of the thoracic aorta. N Engl J med. 1997;336:1876-88.
2. Kamp TJ, Goldschmidt-Clermont PJ, Brinker JA, Resar JR. Myocardial infarction, aortic dissection, and thrombolytic therapy. Am Heart J. 1994;128:1234-7.
3. Hartnell GG. Imaging of aortic aneurysms and dissection: CT MRI. J Thorac Imaging. 2001;16:35-46
4. Mehta RH, Suzuki T, Hagan PG, et al. Predicting death in patients with acute type A aortic dissection. Circulation. 2002;105:200.
5. Erbel R, Alfonso F, Boileau C, et al. Task force on aortic dissection diagnosis and management of aortic dissection. Eur Heart J. 2001;22:1642-81.

Chapter 15

Evaluation of Aortic Valve by Simulated Transesophageal Echocardiography

Raghu B

Chapter Outline

- Aortic Valve Anatomy
- Aortic Stenosis
- Aortic Regurgitation

INTRODUCTION

Every complete transesophageal echocardiographic examination should include a careful assessment of aortic valve. Aortic valve disease is very common in western populations. About 25% of people over 65 years of age have aortic sclerosis and 3% over 75 years have severe calcific aortic stenosis. Aortic valve replacement has been until recently the standard surgical procedure for the treatment of AV disease. However this trend is progressively changing towards surgical repair in selected cases.

AORTIC VALVE ANATOMY

Aortic valve (AV) apparatus is composed of valve cusps, sinuses of Valsalva, proximal ascending aorta. Abnormalities involving any of these structures can lead to aortic valve dysfunction. Proximal to the aortic valve, the left ventricular outflow tract consists of the inferior surface of the anterior mitral leaflet, ventricular septum and posterior left ventricular free wall.

The aortic valve is a complex, intricate structure with remarkable durability. It is composed of three cusps of equal size, each of which is surrounded by a sinus. The cusps are separated by three commissures and supported by a fibrous annulus. Each cusp is crescent shaped and capable of opening fully to allow unimpeded forward flow, then closing tightly to prevent regurgitation. The free edge of each cusp curves upward from the commissure and forms a slight thickening at the tip or midpoint, called the nodule of Arantius. When viewed from a conventional echocardiographic short axis projection, these three lines of closure are recorded as an inverted Y shape. Behind each cusp is its associated Valsalva sinus. The sinuses represent out pouchings in the aortic root directly behind each cusp. They function to support the cusps during systole and provide a reservoir of blood to augment coronary artery flow during diastole. The sinus and its corresponding cusp share the same name. The left and right coronary arteries arise from the left and right sinuses, respectively, and are associated with the left and right aortic cusps. The non coronary sinus is associated with the non coronary aortic cusp. At the superior margin of the sinuses, the aortic root narrows at the sinotubular junction.[1]

Normal Values

- *Aortic valve area (AVA):* 2–4 cm^2
- *Aortic antegrade velocity, Vmax:* 0.9–1.7 m/sec
- *Left ventricular outflow tract (LVOT) velocity:* 0.9–1.1 m/sec.

Echocardiographic Examination

Five standard views are recommended for systematic examination of aortic valve apparatus:

1. Midesophageal AV long axis view **(Figure 1)**
2. Midesophageal AV short axis view **(Figures 2A and B)**
3. Deep transgastric (TG) long axis view **(Figures 4A and B)**
4. Transgastric long axis view **(Figures 5A and B)**
5. Midesophageal five chamber view **(Figures 6A and B).**

Midesophageal AV Short Axis View (ME-AV-SAX)

- Ideal view to assess morphology **(Figures 7A and B)**
- Leaflet closure line
- Presence of specific leaflet pathology (bicuspid value, calcific degeneration) **(Figures 8A and B)**

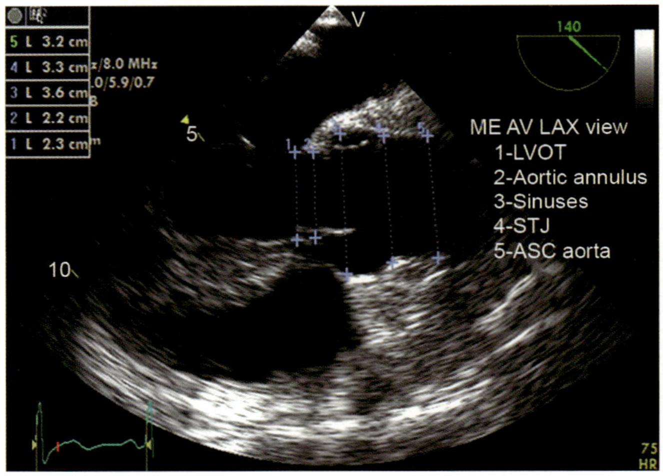

Figure 1 Measurements of AV apparatus

- Diastolic coaptation defect with color flow Doppler can locate and assess the severity of aortic regurgitation (AR)
- Calculation of the valve area by planimetry
- Can measure the vena contracta.

Midesophageal AV Long Axis View (ME-AV-LAX) (Figures 3A and B)

- Sinus of Valsalva anatomy
- Measurement of annuals diameter, sinuses, sino-tublar junction
- AR (with Doppler)
- Proximal aortic root (withdraw probe 1–2 cm)
- Leaflet motion (diastolic leaflet prolapse or impaired systolic).

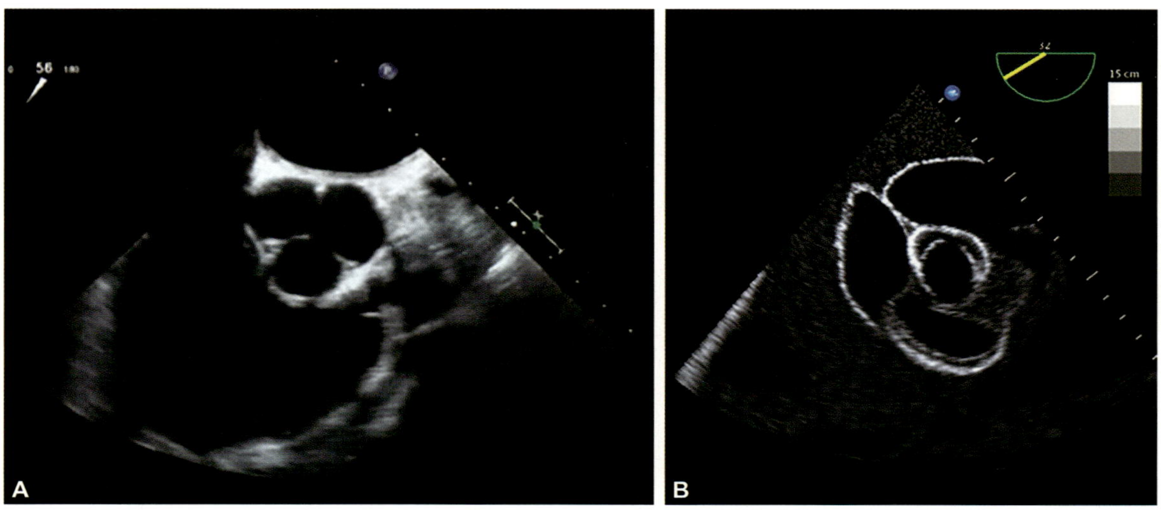

Figures 2A and B (A) 2D ME AV SAX view; (B) Simulated view of ME AV SAX view

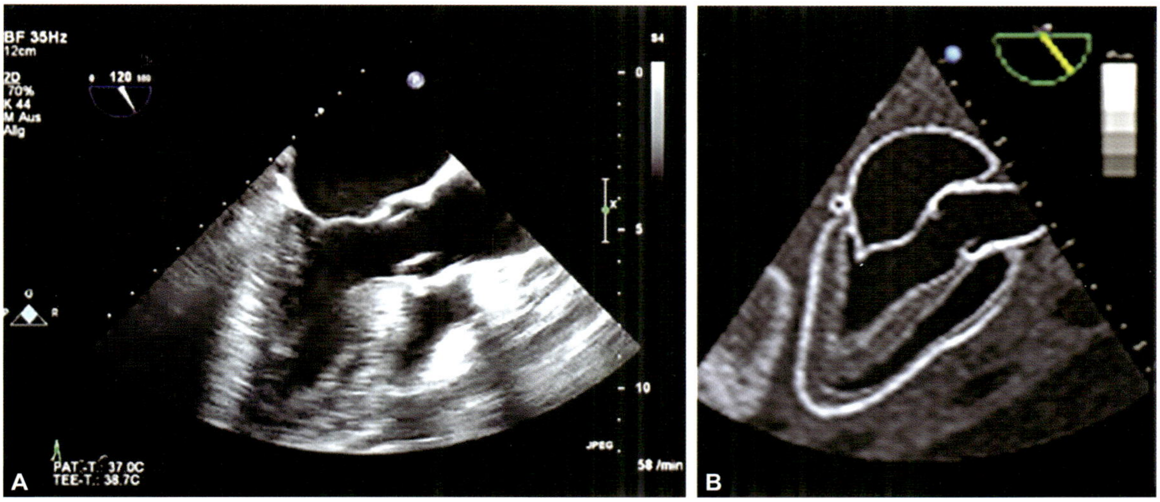

Figures 3A and B (A) 2D view of ME AV LAX; (B) Simulated view of ME AV LAX

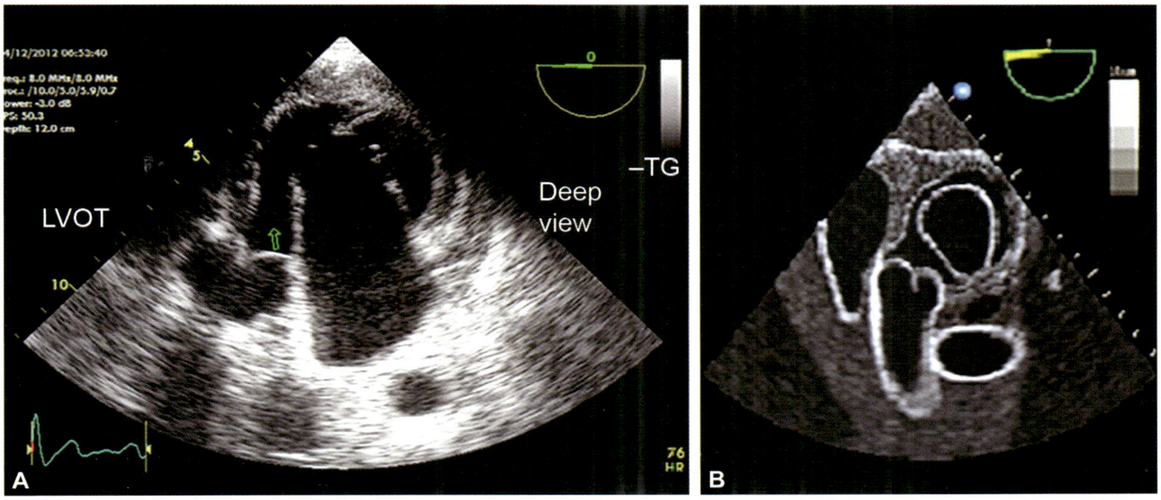

Figures 4A and B (A) 2D deep transgastric view; (B) Simulated deep transgastric view

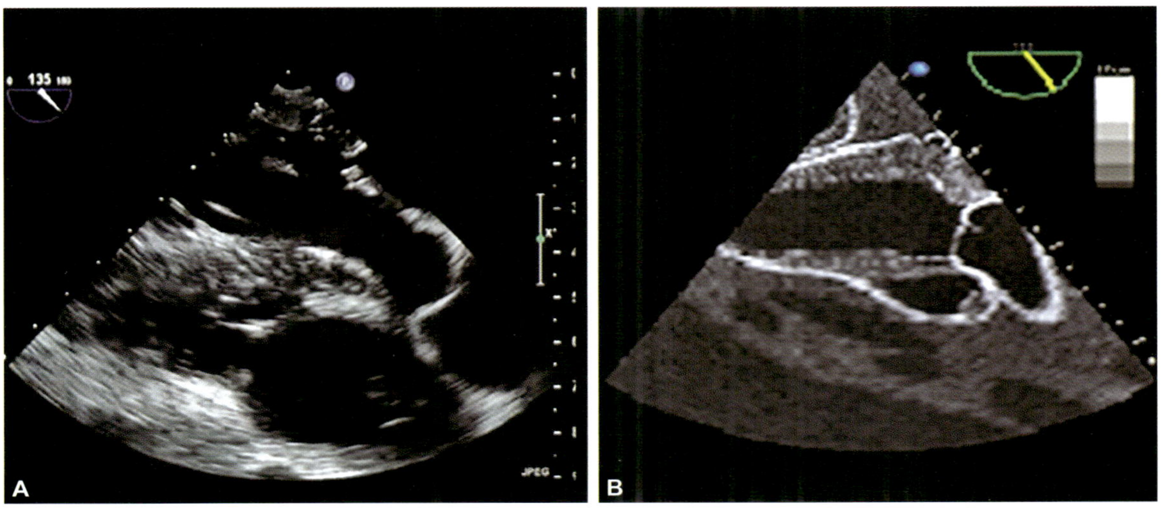

Figures 5A and B (A) 2D view of transgastric LAX; (B) Simulated view of transgastric LAX

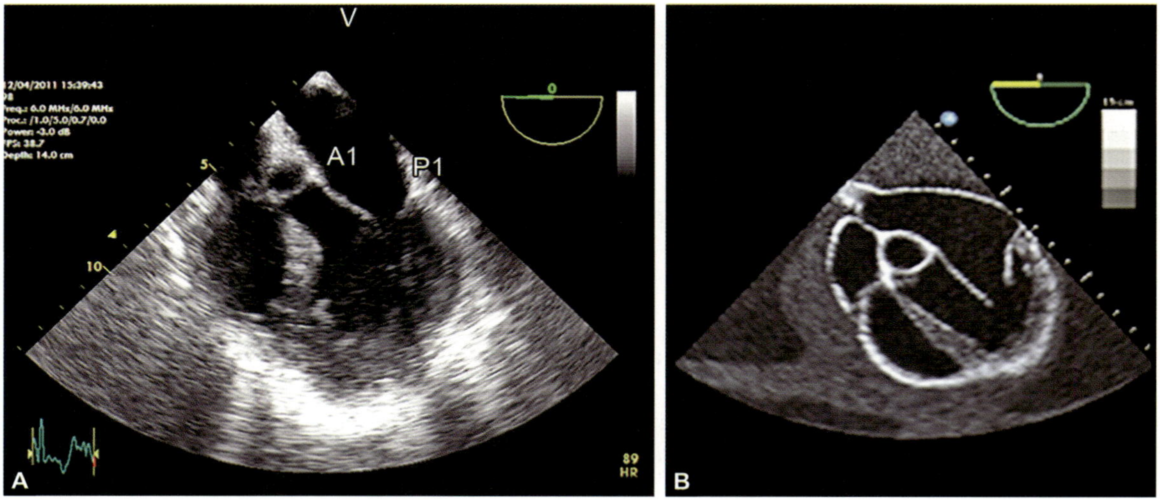

Figures 6A and B (A) 2D ME-5C view; (B) Simulated ME-5C view

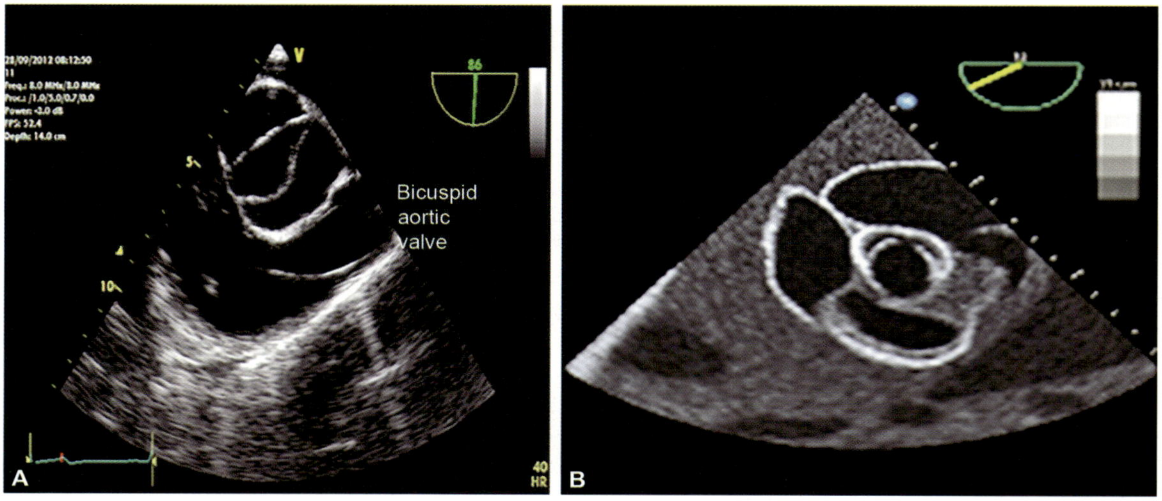

Figures 7A and B (A) 2D ME AV SAX view; (B) Simulated ME AV SAX view

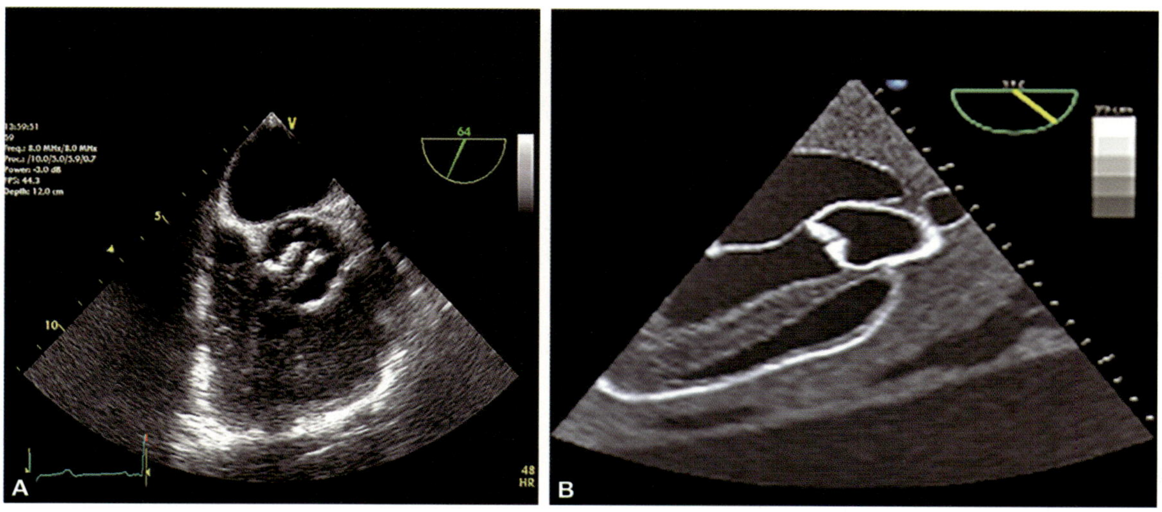

Figures 8A and B (A) 2D ME AV SAX view depicting calcific leaflets; (B) Simulated ME AV LAX view depicting aortic stenosis

Deep Transgastric View

- Flow directed measurement gradient
- AR color flow Doppler (quantitative)
- AR continuous wave Doppler (CWD)

Transgastric Long Axis View (Figures 5A and B)

Flow directed measurement gradient

- AR color flow Doppler (quantitative)
- AR continuous wave Doppler

In patient with prosthetic valves in the aortic or mitral position imaging the LVOT from mid-esophageal windows may be impossible owing to acoustic shadowing in the far field. In such situations transgastric long axis views are recommended to assess the prosthetic valves.

Midesophageal Five Chamber (5C) Views

Leaflet motion or perforation of leaflets and AR can be assessed.

AORTIC STENOSIS

Aortic stenosis may consequence of calcific degeneration of normal trileaflet valve, rheumatic aortic disease or congenital valve abnormality.

Calcific Aortic Stenosis

More common form of aortic stenosis and tends to occur in patients over age of 70 years. It is characterized by fibro-calcific changes in the body and along the free edges of the leaflet resulting in marked increase in echogenicity and restriction of leaflet motion. The leaflet may be effected asymmetrically and there may be a fusion of one or more of the commissure. Calcification may extend down in to LVOT (tear drop calcification) and to the base of the anterior mitral leaflet.

Typical progression of aortic stenosis is by increase in the mean pressure gradient by 7 mm of Hg/year and decrease in the aortic valve area by 0.1cm^2/year.[2]

Bicuspid Aortic Valve

Occurs in approximately 2% of the normal population and may be familial. Secondary calcification occurs in a significant number of cases and usually leads to onset of symptoms in the fourth to sixth decade.

The characteristic echocardiographic sign is that the two leaflet opening in systole resulting in an elliptical rather that starshaped orifice. A raphe or fibrous ridge is usually present on one of the leaflet perpendicular to the orifice and is typically more sclerotic than the leaflet themselves.

If a bicuspid AV is detected it is important to rule out other associated abnormalities, including coartation of aorta, subaortic obstruction and dilatation of the aortic root.

Very rarely occasionally an AV may be congenitally unicuspid or quadricuspid.

Rheumatic Aortic Stenosis

Rheumatic valvulitis tends to produce thickening of the free edges of the AV leaflets and fusion of the commissures, causing a circular rather than a star-shaped orifice, which may be eccentric **(Figure 9)**.

Assessing Aortic Valve Severity (Table 1)

Visual appearance using 2D (ME AV SAX; ME AV LAX)

- Thickened leaflets, restricted mobility
- Commissural fusion (2D). Mean and peak gradients **(Figures 10A and B)**
- Secondary changes include LVH,LV dialation, poststenotic dilatation.

Other Imaging Modalities [M-mode and Color Flow Doppler (CFD)]

- Systolic leaflet doming inward;<15 mm leaflet separation (M-mode)

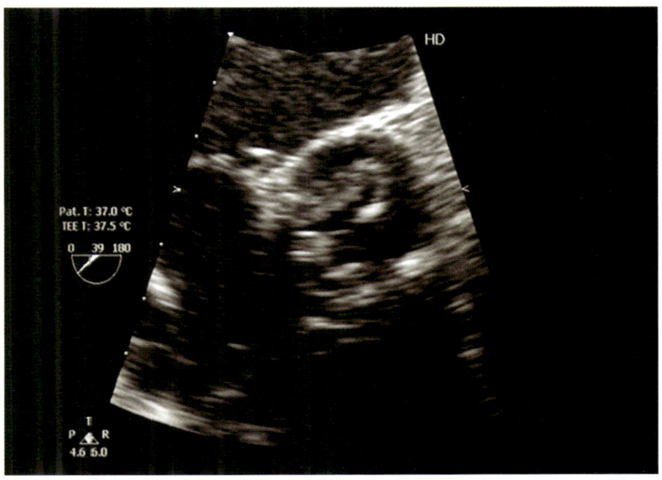

Figure 9 ME AV SAX view depicting stenotic aortic valve with commissural fusion

CHAPTER 15

TABLE 1 Comparison of mild, moderate and severe aortic stenosis

Severity	*Mild*	*Moderate*	*Severe*
Mean AVG (mm Hg)*	< 25	25–40	> 40
Mean AVG (mm Hg)**	< 30	30–50	> 50
Vmax (m/sec)	2.6–3.0	3.0–4.0	> 4.0
AVA (cm^2)	> 1.5	1.0–1.5	< 1.0
Indexed AVA (cm^2/m^2)	> 0.85	0.60–0.85	< 0.6
Velocity ratio	> 0.5	0.25–0.5	< 0.25

*AHA/ACC Guidelines **ESC Guidelines

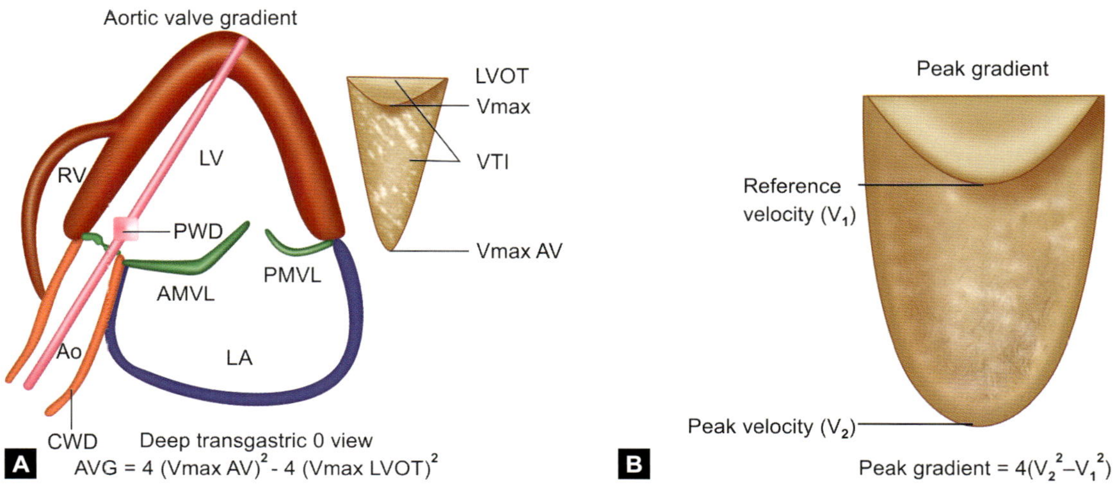

Figures 10A and B Calculation of peak gradient from velocity

Abbreviations: AMVL, anterior mitral valve leaflet; PMVL, posterior mitral valve leaflet; VTI, velocity-time integral; LVOT, left ventricular outflow tract; LV, left ventricle; RV, right ventricle; LA, left atrium; AV, atrioventricular; CWD, continuous wave Doppler; PWD, pulsed wave Doppler; Ao, aorta

- High velocity turbulent flow post-stenosis (mosaic appearance with CFD)

Transvalvular Gradient Using CWD (Deep TG LAX; TG LAX between 90–120 Degrees) (Figure 14)

- **Step 1:** Obtain a continuous wave Doppler of the aortic valve.[3]
- **Step 2:** Obtain a pulse wave Doppler of the LVOT.

Note: Typically, the PWD of the LVOT will yield a maximum velocity less than 1 m/sec. Therefore, its peak gradient is insignificant compared to the aortic valve peak velocity.

- Simplified Bernoulli equation = $4v^2$
- Peak velocity (m/sec) = instantaneous gradient
- Mean velocity (VTI) = mean gradient

Obtaining Aortic Valve Area

1. Planimetry using 2D (ME AV SAX) **(Figures 11 to 13)**
   - Visualize all cusps simultaneously
   - Trace orifice in systole
   - Measure the length of side and calculate AVA = cusp length^2 × 0.433.

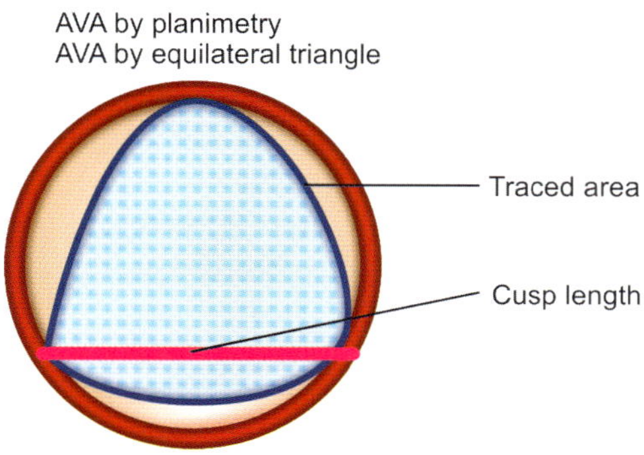

Figure 11 SAX of aortic valve

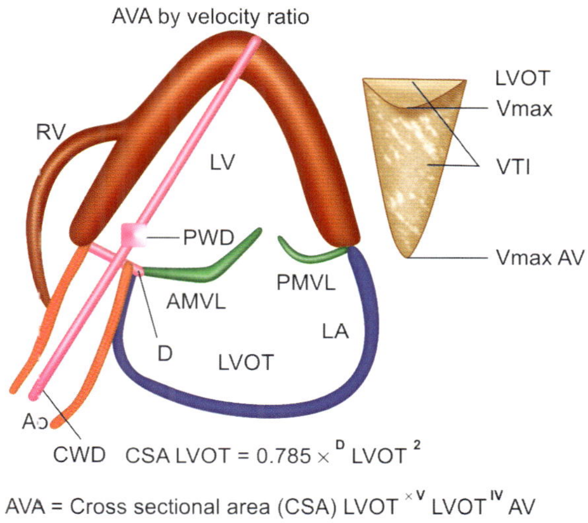

Figure 13 Section through LVOT and aortic valve

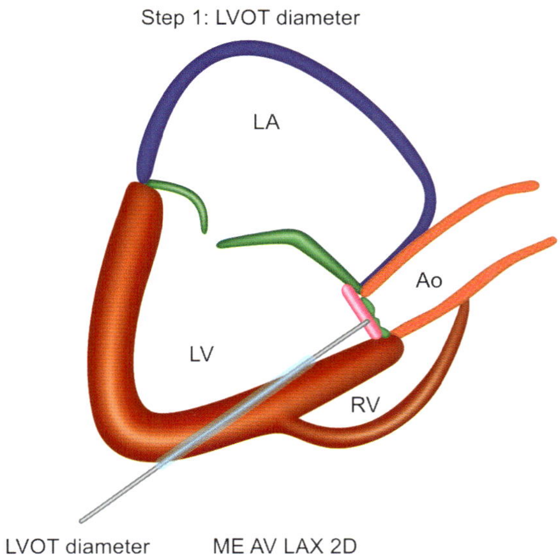

Figure 12 Section through ME AV LAX view on 2D

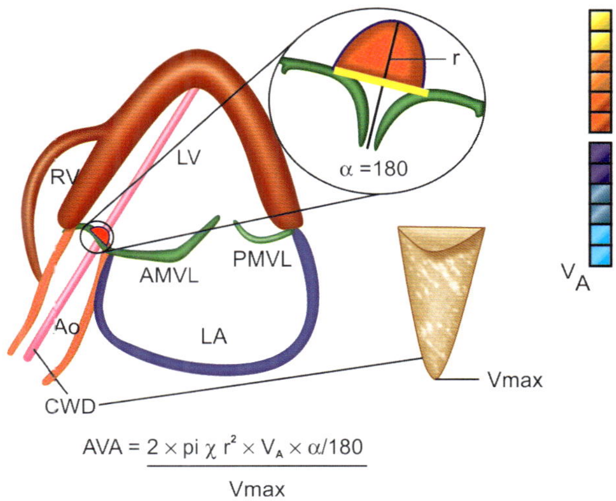

Figure 14 Deep transgastric section of aortic valve

Continuity Equation Using Peak Velocities or VTI (Deep TG LAX or TG LAX and LVOT Diameter) (ME AV LAX)

Measurement LVOT diameter in midsystole.
Area of LVOT = $0.785 \times (D/2)^2$

Flow across LVOT = Flow across AV
Flow = Velocity × Area
Velocity LVOT × Area LVOT = Velocity AV × Area AV
AVA = Velocity LVOT × Area LVOT/Velocity AV

2. **AVA by Gorlin formula**
   AVA = CO/square root of mean AVG
   CO = $0.785 \times (\text{LVOT diameter}/2)^2 \times$ VTI AV

3. **AVA by PISA**
   PISA radius (r)(cm):
   Aliasing velocity (V_A)(cm/sec)
   Vmax (m/sec)
   Angle (α)°

Aortic Valve

Normal area	2.5–4.5 cm^2
Mild stenosis	1.0–2.5 cm^2
Moderate stenosis	0.75–1.0 cm^2
Severe stenosis	< 0.75 cm^2

AORTIC REGURGITATION

Aortic regurgitation may result from abnormalities of the AV leaflet and the aortic root.

Etiology

- Leaflet pathology
  - Congenital
  - Rheumatic
  - Infective
  - Myxomatous.
- Aortic root pathology
  - Aortic aneurysm
  - Aortic dissection
  - Marfan's syndrome.

Assessing Severity (Table 2)

2D Imaging

- Structural abnormalities of the leaflet:
  - Congenital abnormalities (bicuspid AV)
  - Acquired defects (vegetations, abscess formation, myxomatous valves)
  - Leaflet thickening, distortion of cusps and abnormalities in coaptation
  - Evidence of prolapse, sinotubular junction for dilatation (ME AV LAX)
- Associated dilation
- Early diastolic closure of MV, flutter of anterior MV leaflet.

Color Flow Doppler

- **Jet length** (ME LAX) **(Figures 15A and B)**
  - *Mild:* < 2 cm length (not past anterior mitral leaflet)
  - *Moderate:* To tip of anterior mitral leaflet
  - *Severe:* Beyond tip of anterior mitral leaflet
- **Jet width (height) to LVOT diameter**
  - ME AV LAX view
  - Regurgitant jet height/LVOT height % (color M-mode)

    Mild: 25–45%

    Moderate: 46–64%

    *Severe:*w> 65
- **ME AV SAX view**
  - Regurgitant jet area/AV area

    Mild: <30%

    Moderate: 30–50%

    Severe: > 50%
- **Diastole flow reversal**
  - *Mild:* Flow reversal in ascending aorta
  - *Moderate:* Flow reversal in arch of aorta
  - *Severe:* Flow reversal in abdominal aorta

Measure slope or pressure half-time of regurgitation jet. This is the time it takes for the systolic pressure gradient between the aorta and the LV to increase by 50% of its initial value.[4] The more severe the AR, the faster the pressure equilibrates with the LV pressure and shorter the pressure half time and steeper the slope **(Figures 16A and B)**.

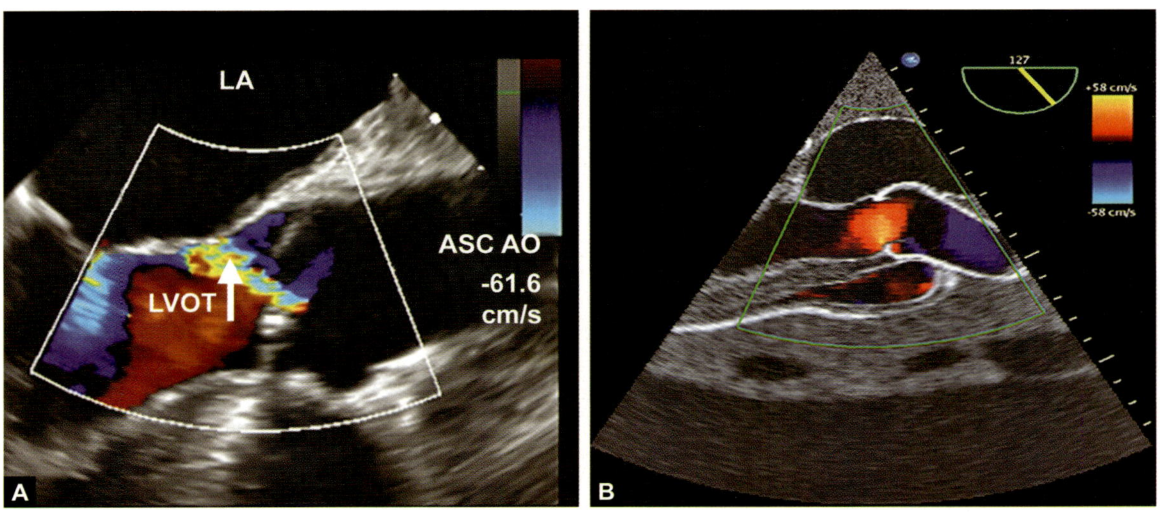

Figures 15A and B ME LAX view for AR jet length simulated image

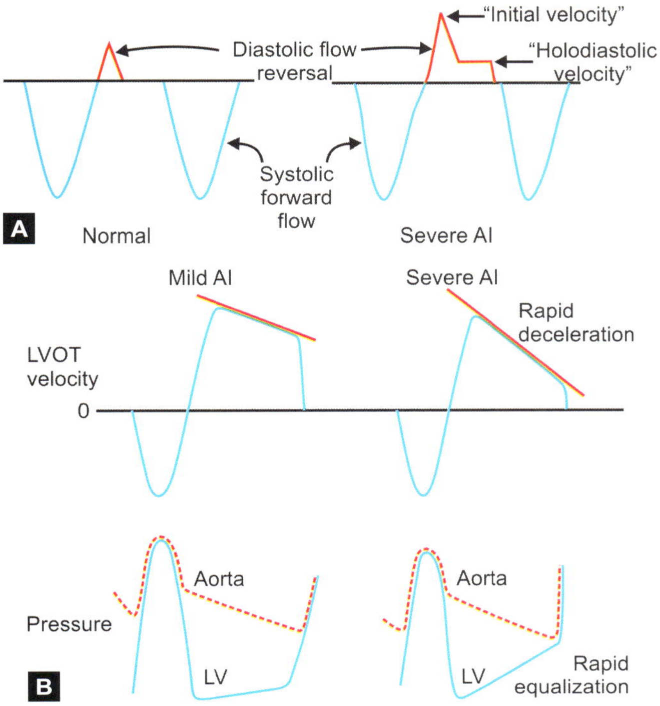

Figures 16A and B Illustration of deceleration slope is steeper and approaches zero velocity more rapidly with severe regurgitation

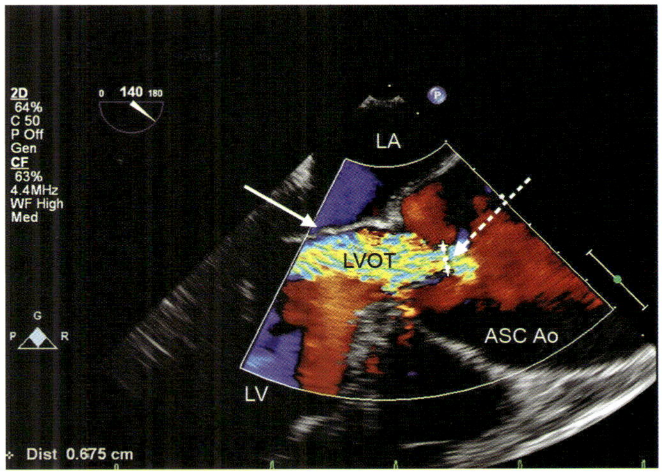

Figure 17 Illustration of vena contracta

AR Severity

Vena contract width (cm) **(Figure 17)**

- *Mild:* <0.3
- *Moderate:* 0.3-0.6
- *Severe:* > 0.6

The clinical scenario and pretest probability of disease should guide the use of transesophageal versus transthoracic imaging. Those at high risk for endocarditis or its complications in particular should undergo early TEE. Serial studies may be required to guide management. In the setting of an initially negative echocardiographic study, a repeat examination is indicated if the clinical suspicion of endocarditis persists or if the clinical picture changes **(Figures 18A and B)**.[5] Combined transthoracic echocardiography and TEE may supply complementary information useful in management and follow-up **(Figures 19A and B)**.

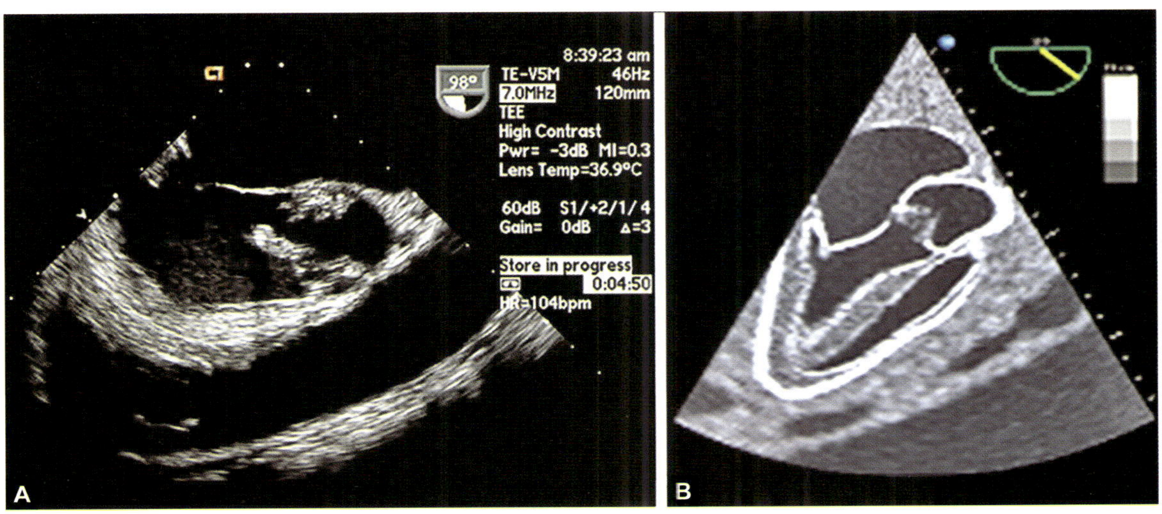

Figures 18A and B Aortic valve endocarditis: (A) 2D Modified AV-LAX view depicting endocarditis of the AV; (B) Simulated view of modified AV-LAX view depicting endocarditis of the AV

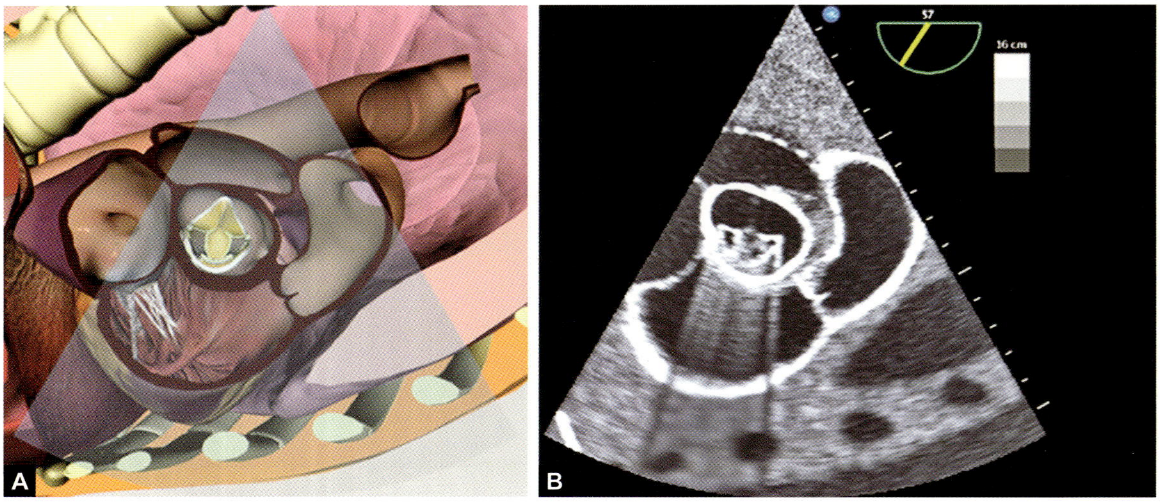

Figures 19A and B Simulated image of bioprosthetic valve in aortic position

TABLE 2 Quantification of aortic valve regurgitation based on DT and pressure-half time

	DT (Slope)	*Half-time*
Mild	< 2 m/sec	>500 msec
Moderate	2–3.5 m/sec	200–500 msec
Severe	>3.5 m/sec	<200 msec

Calculation of Regurgitation Volume (RV), Regurgitation Fraction (RF) and Effective Orifice Area (EOA)

SV = CSA × VTI
Volume = SV [LVOT]-SV [mv]
RF = Volume/SV [LVOT]
ERO = Volume/VTI [ARjet]
R.V>60 mL, RF>50%, ERO>0.3 cm^2 indicate severe AR

CONCLUSION

Assessment of the AV remains a challenge. In clinical practice, the integration of patient data is essential, and a good correlation of the clinical and echo findings remains essential. Accordingly, we must be thoroughly familiar with the application of all these techniques for an optimal assessment of AV in the operating room. Simulation of the AV helps in training and understanding the TEE views and associated pathological lesions of the AV.

REFERENCES

1. Reeves ST, Glas KE, Eltzschig H, et al. Guidelines for performing a comprehensive epicardial echocardiography examination: recommendations of the American Society of Echocardiography and the Society of Cardiovascular Anesthesiologist. Anesth Analg. 2007;105(1):22-28.
2. Maslow AD, Mashikian J, Haering JM, et al. Tranesophageal echocardiographic evaluation of native aortic valve area: Utility of the double-envelope technique. J Cardiothorac Vasc Anesth. 2001;15:293-9.
3. Oh JK, Taliercio CP, Holmes DR, et al. Prediction of the severity of aortic stenosis by Doppler aortic valve area determination: prospective Doppler-catheterization correlation in 100 patients. J Am Coll Cardiol. 1988;11(6):1227-34.
4. Maslow AD, Regan MM, Haering JM, et al. Echocardiographic predictors of left ventricular outflow tract obstruction and systolic anterior motion of the mitral valve after mitral valve reconstruction for myxomatous valve disease. J Am Coll Cardiol. 1999;34(7):2096-104.
5. Tadros TM, Klein KD, Shapira OM. Ascending aortic dilatation associated bicuspid aortic valve: pathophysiology, molecular biology, and clinical implications. Circulation. 2009;119:880-90.

Chapter 16

Simulation for Transesophageal Echocardiography for Aortic Valve Stenosis

Poonam Malhotra Kapoor, Kalpana Irpachi, Arindam Choudhury, Ujjwal Chowdhury, Jitin Narula

Chapter Outline

- Introduction to Normal Aortic Valve
- Transesophageal Echocardiography Views of Aortic Valve
- Causes and Anatomic Presentation
- How to Assess Aortic Stenosis?
- Dobutamine Stress Echo

INTRODUCTION TO NORMAL AORTIC VALVE

It is important to diagnose and treat diseases of the aortic valve. Simulation helps to make it easier and better **(Figures 1A to E)** untreated aortic valve disease can eventually result in heart failure, severe infection, and even sudden death. Some patients present with severe symptoms, whereas others have few, if any symptoms. The diagnosis may be made on a routine physical examination. Regular medical follow-up, treatment to prevent infection of the valve (infective endocarditis), and optimal timing of surgery are necessary to avoid the severe consequences of improper function of the aortic valve.

The aortic valve consists of three half-moon-shaped pocket-like flaps of delicate tissue, referred to as cusps **(Figures 2A to D)**. When the aortic valve is closed, the cusps are perfectly aligned and separate the large pumping chamber of the heart (the left ventricle) from the large artery (aorta) that supplies blood to the body. During the period when the left ventricle contracts and pumps the blood (systole), the aortic valve opens widely and blood flows freely from the left ventricle to the aorta. When the left ventricle then relaxes (diastole), the aortic valve closes completely so that the blood remains in the aorta. During diastole, blood flows into the left ventricle from the lungs through the left atrium across the mitral valve, thus refilling the ventricle for the next contraction.

TRANSESOPHAGEAL ECHOCARDIOGRAPHY VIEWS OF AORTIC VALVE (FLOW CHART 1)

Midesophageal AV: Short Axis View

Multiplane angle range aortic value—30°-60° **(Figures 3A to D)**.

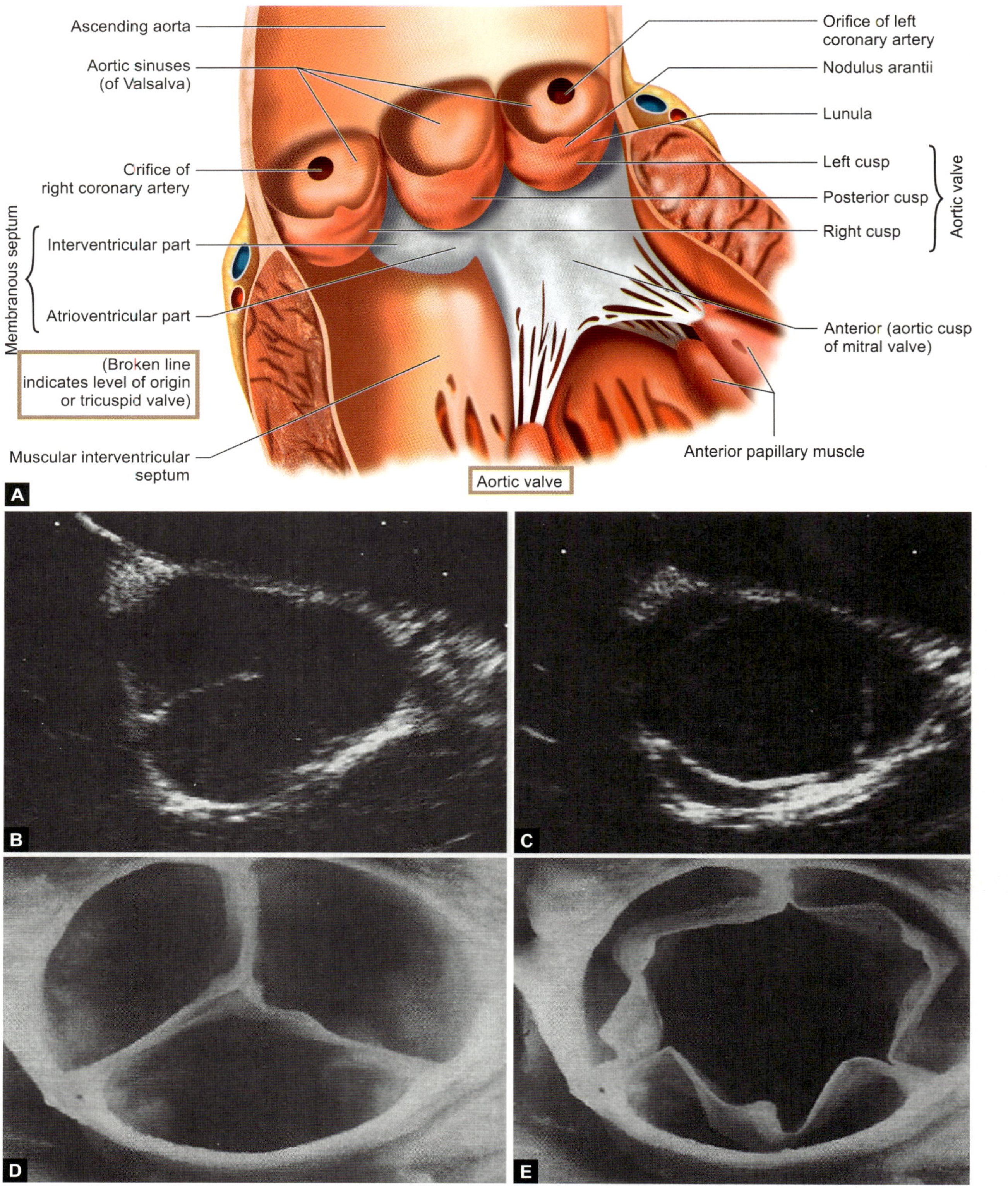

Figures 1A to E (A) The aortic valve apparatus with three cusps and origin of different coronary arteries; (B to E) The typical Mercedes Benz sign showing the three cusps, three sinuses and three commissures supported by fibrous annulus of the normal aortic valve

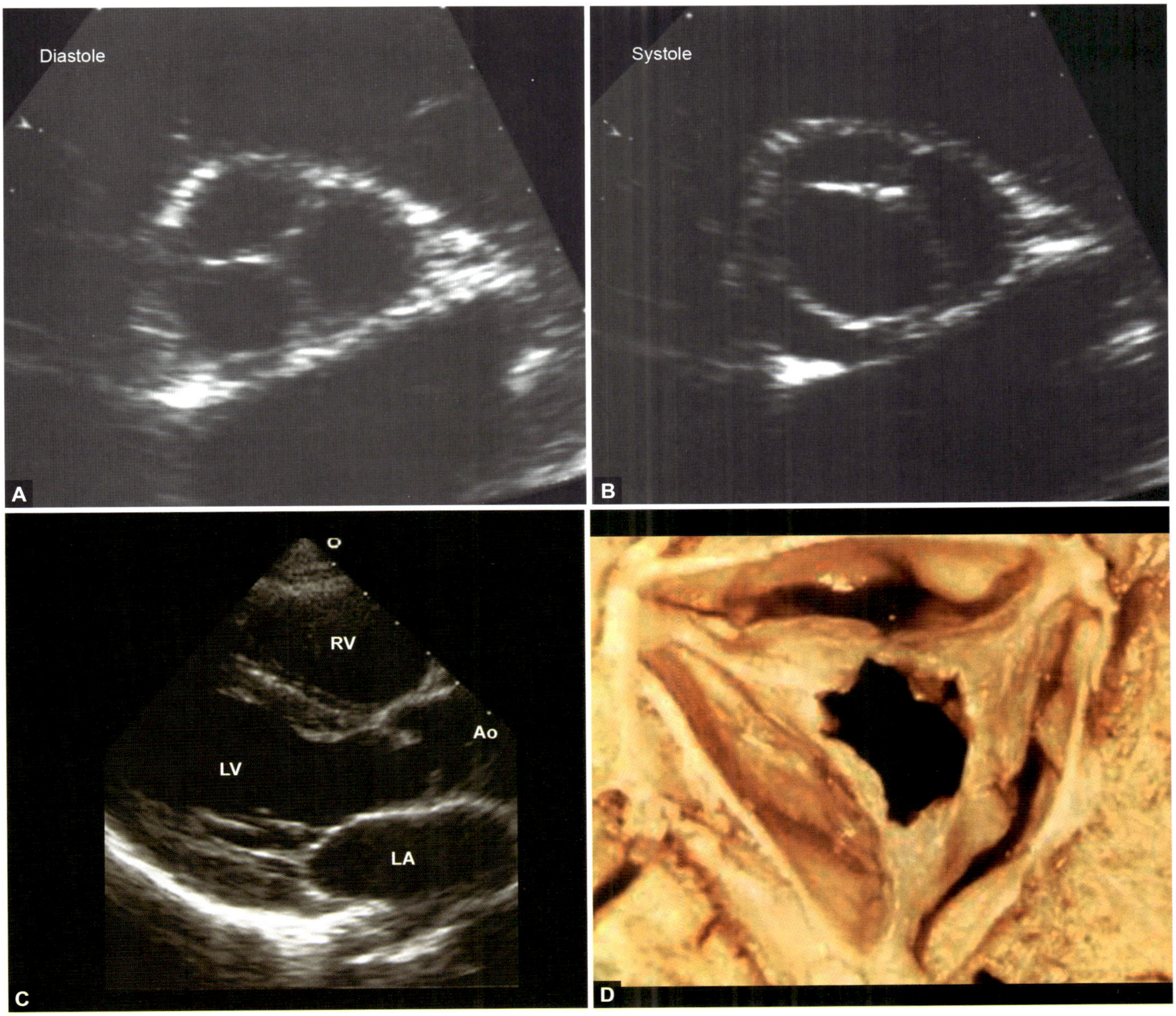

Figures 2A to D (A and B) Three cusps are seen in diastole and systole of aortic valve; (C) Commissural fusion, thickening and calcification of aortic valve; (D) Narrowed, calcific aortic valve lumen
Abbreviations: LV, left ventricle; LA, left atrium; RV, right ventricle; Ao, aorta

Clinical Utility

- Ideal view for leaflet morphology
- Coaptation
- Aortic regurgitation (AR) color flow Doppler
- Aortic stenosis (AS) planimetry.

Midesophageal Aortic Valve: Long Axis View

Long axis view is seen at:

a. Multiplane angle range 120° - 160°
b. Short axis view at 30° - 60°

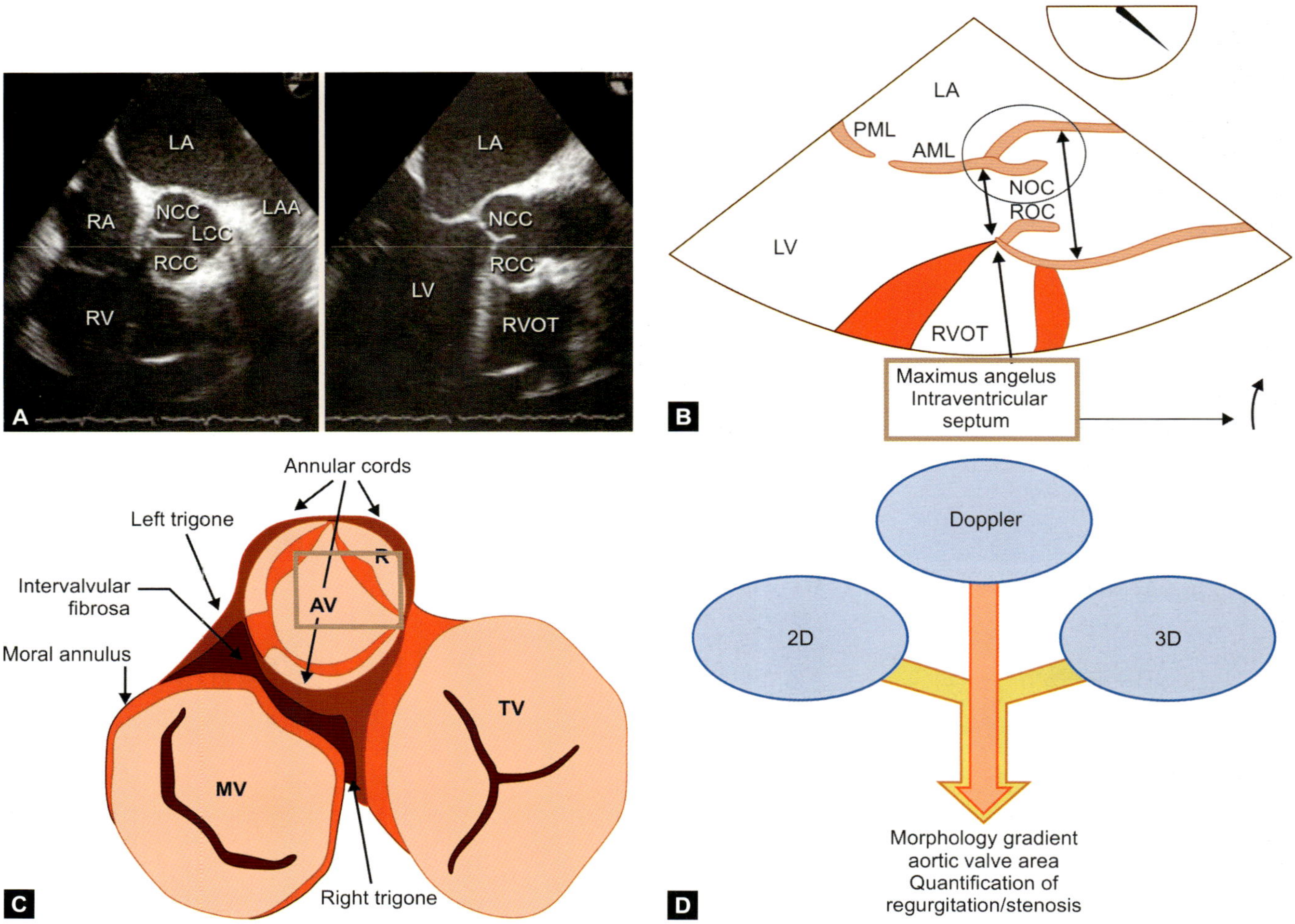

Figures 3A to D (A) The normal aortic valve; (B) The aortic root with annulus and sinotubular function diameter; (C) The aortic annulus and its "enface" relationship to mitral and tricuspid valve; (D) The aortic valve disease

Abbreviations: RA, right atrium; RV, right ventricle; LV, left ventricle; RVOT, right ventricular outflow tract; NCC, noncoronary cusp; RCC, right coronary cusp; LCC, left coronary cusp; LA, left atrium

Midesophageal Aortic Valve: Short and Long Axis View

These are obtained at a multiplane angle 30°–60° **(Figures 4A to D)** short axis view and 120°–180° **(Figures 5A and B)** long axis view.

Clinical Utility for Aortic Valve Disease

- Dimensions of aortic valve annulus, sinotubular junction (STJ)
- Impaired leaflet opening
- Leaflet prolapse
- Best view for colour flow Doppler for AR
- Ascending aorta pathology (atherosclerosis, aneurysm, dissection)
- Best view for continuous wave (CW) Doppler for aortic regurgitation
- Ascending aorta pathology (atherosclerosis, aneurysm, dissection).

Transgastric: Long Axis View (Figures 6A and B)

Multiplane angle range—90°–120°.

Clinical Utility

- Evaluation of aortic valve outflow tract
- Best view for continuous wave (CW) Doppler.

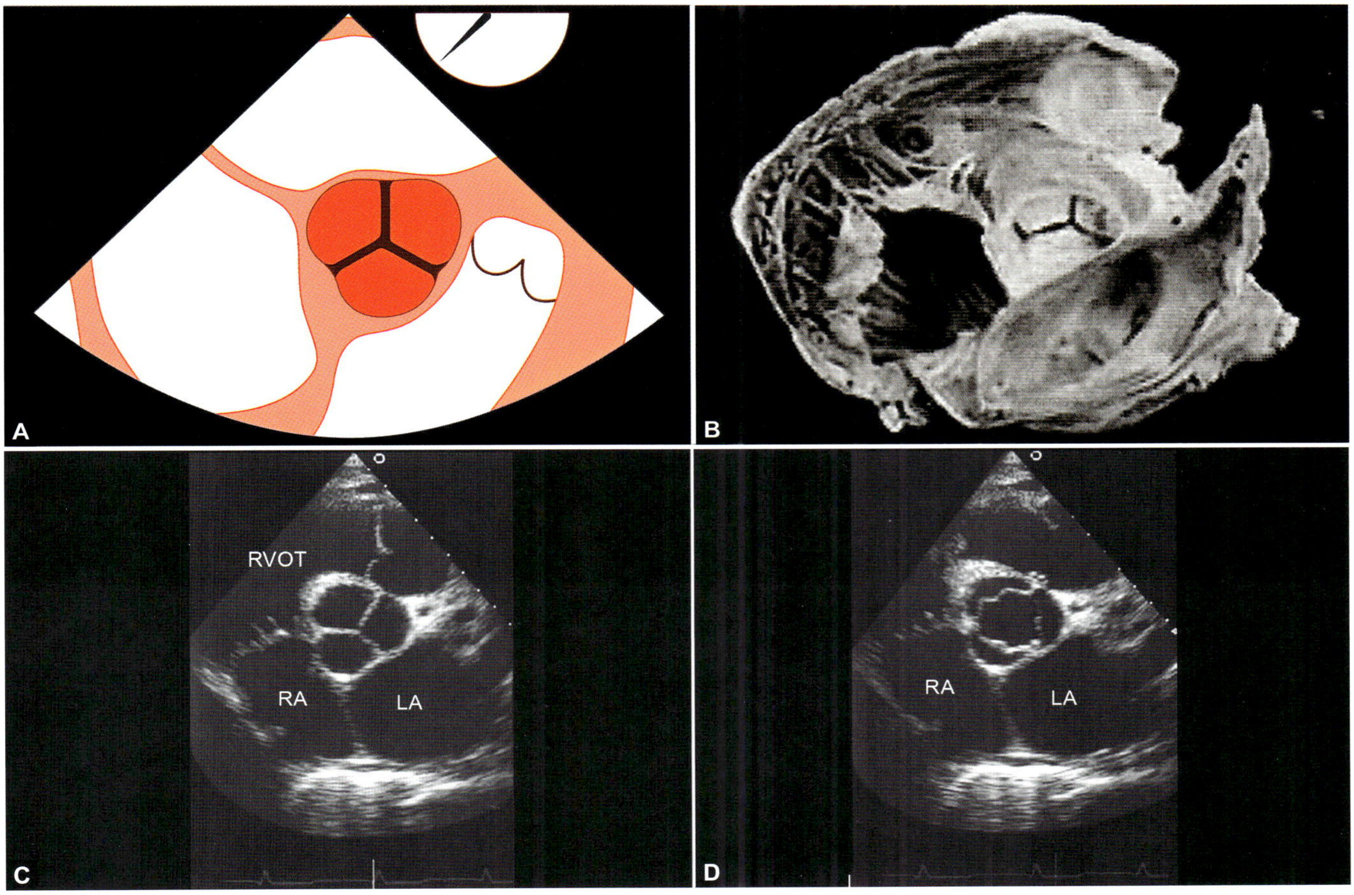

Figures 4A to D The midesophageal aortic valve short axis view
Abbreviations: RA, right artium; RVOT, right ventricular outflow tract; LA, left atrium

Flow chart 1 The lesions of aortic valve complex

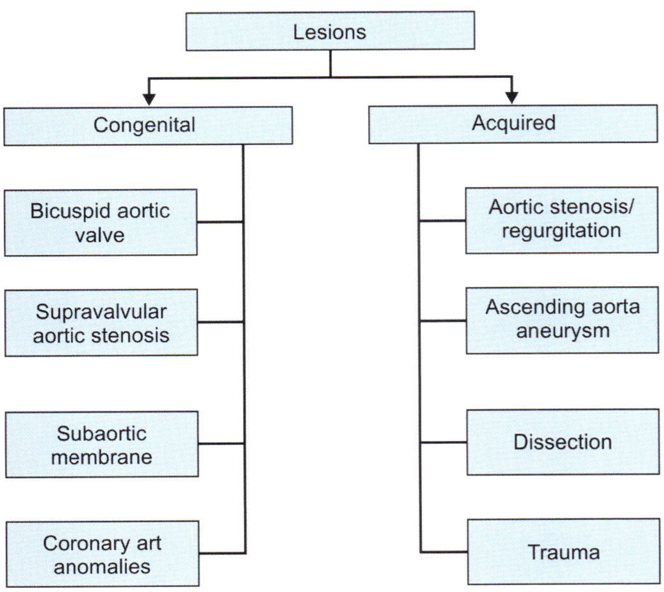

Deep Transgastric: Long Axis View (Figures 7A and B)

Multiplane angle range—0°–20°.

Clinical Utility

- Evaluation of aortic valve outflow tract.
- Best view for continuous wave Doppler.

CAUSES AND ANATOMIC PRESENTATION

Aortic Stenosis Causes

- *Most common:*
  - Bicuspid aortic valve with calcification
  - Senile or degenerative calcific AS
  - Rheumatic AS

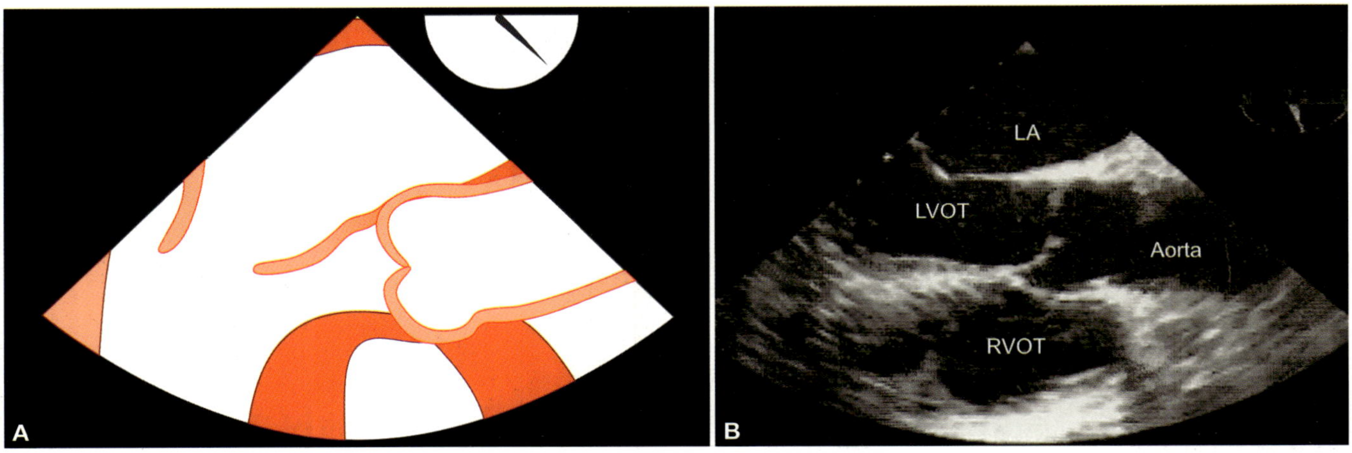

Figures 5A and B The midesophageal aortic valve long axis view
Abbreviations: LVOT, left ventricular outflow tract; RVOT, right ventricular outflow tract; LA, left atrium

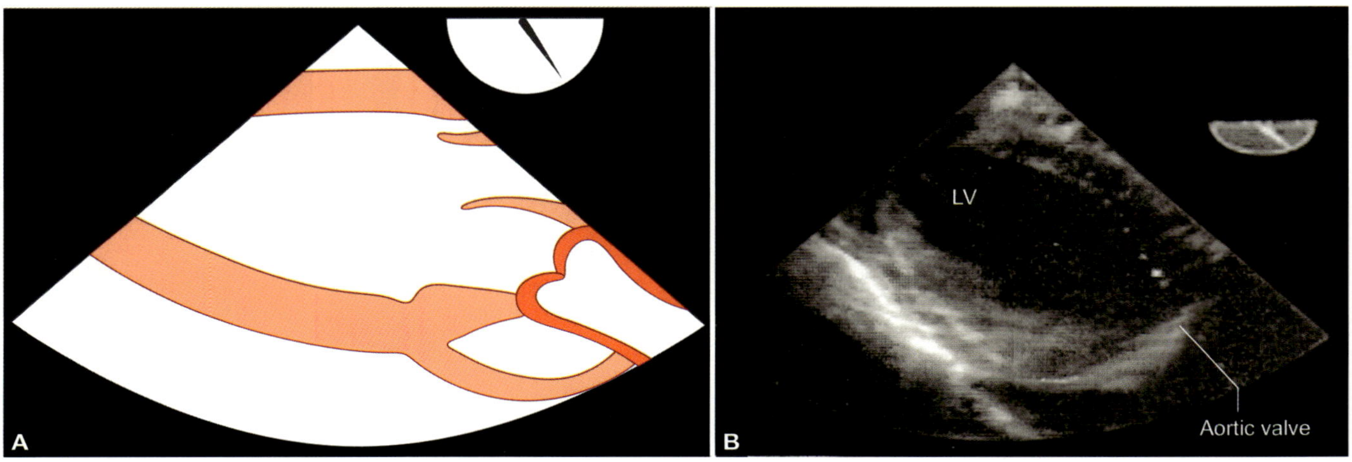

Figures 6A and B The transgastric long axis view of aortic valve

- *Less common:*
  - Congenital
  - Type 2 hyperlipoproteinemia
  - Ochronosis.

Anatomic Evaluation

Combination of short and long axis images to identify:
- Number of leaflets
- Describe leaf mobility, thickness, and calcification
- Combination of imaging and Doppler allows the determination of the level of obstruction; subvalvular, valvular, or supravalvular.
- Transesophageal echocardiography may be helpful when image quality is suboptimal.

Calcific Aortic Stenosis

- Nodular calcific masses on aortic side of cusps.
- No commissural fusion.
- Free edges of cusps are not involved.
- Stellate-shaped systolic orifice.

Calcific Aortic Stenosis (long-axis)

Midesophageal long-axis view showing echogenic and immobile aortic valve.

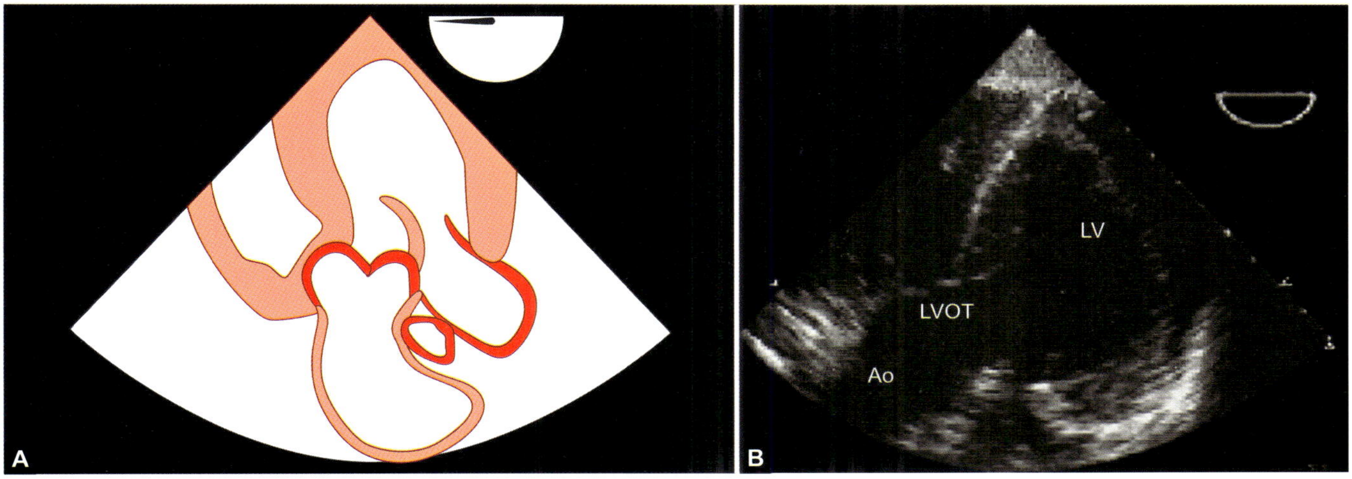

Figures 7A and B The deep transgastric long axis view of aortic valve
Abbreviations: LV, left ventricle; LVOT, left ventricular outflow tract; AO, aorta

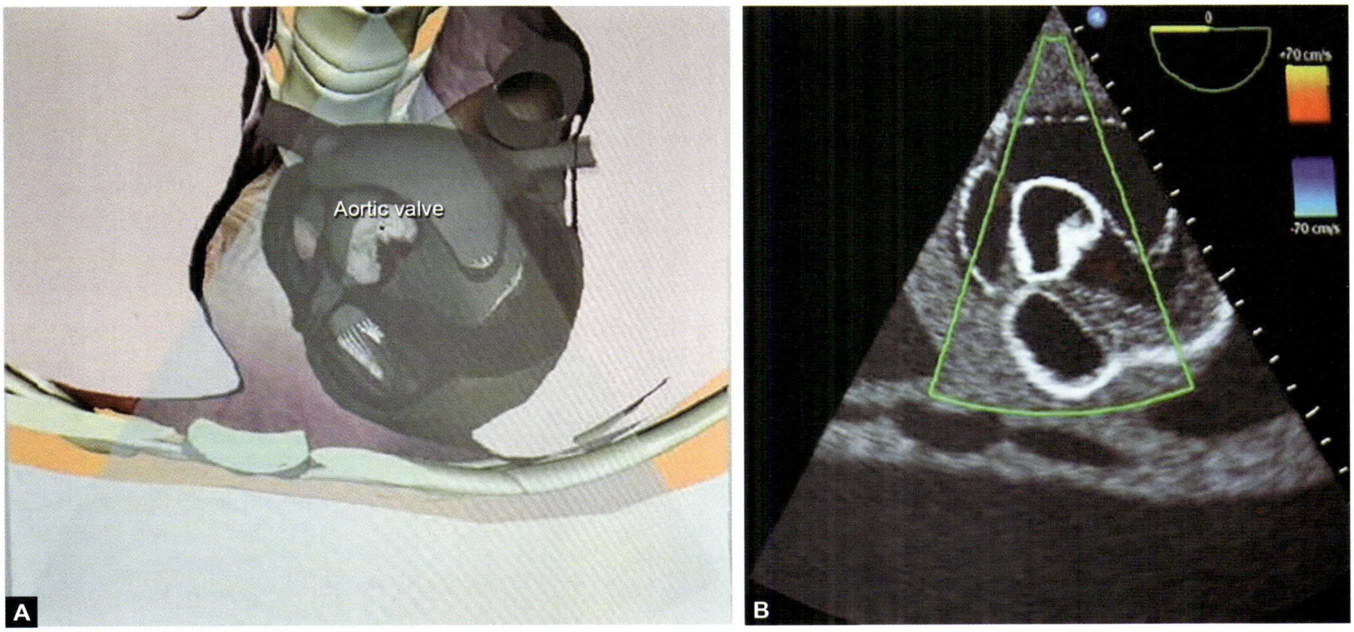

Figures 8A and B The simulation view of aortic stenosis valvular

Calcific Aortic Stenosis (Short-axis) (Figures 8A and B)

Midesophageal short-axis view showing calcified aortic valve leaflets. Immobility of the cusps results in only a slit like aortic valve orifice in systole.

Intraoperative Transesophageal Echocardiography of Aortic Valve (Table 1)

Intraoperative TEE is used to diagnose in acute critical care setting and to confirm valve anatomy, function and hemodynamics in elective surgeries. It permits

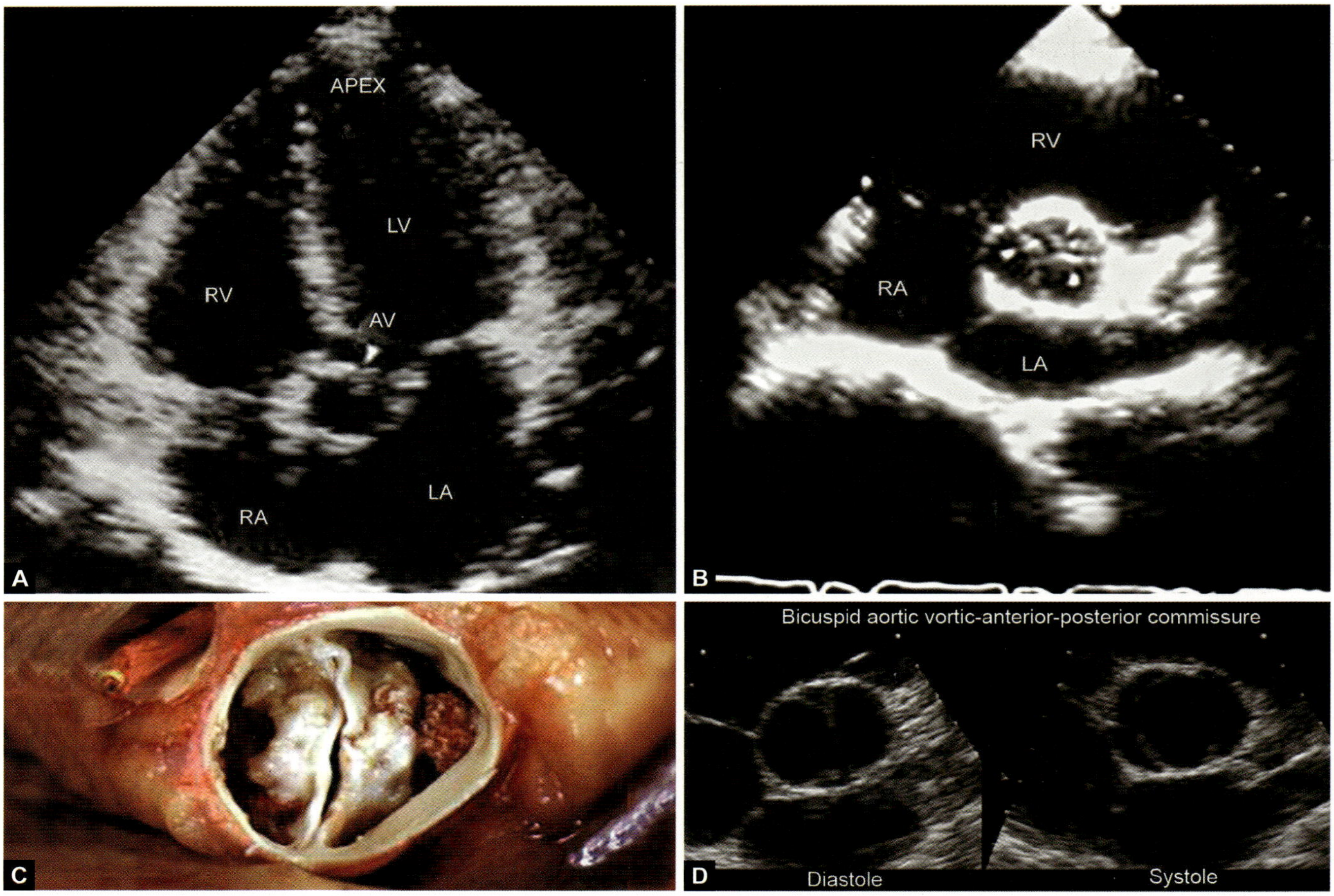

Figures 9A to D (A) 2D-apical five chamber view; (B) Severe calcific aortic stenosis in short axis view; (C) Enface view of bicuspid aortic valve; (D) Bicuspid aortic valve aortic, anterior and posterior commissure view showing diastole and systole
Abbreviations: RA, right atrium; RV, right ventricular; LV, left ventricle; LA, left atrium; AV, aortic valve

informed decision regarding surgical intervention type of intervention (repair v/s replacement) and the need for associated valve repair.[1-5]

TABLE 1 Intraoperative transesophageal echocardiography of aortic valve

Prebypass	*Postoperatively*
• Optimizes hemodynamics • Determines LV function • Determines the size of the valve to be implanted • In ross procedure, for evaluation of pulmonary valve autograft	• Patient prosthesis mismatch • Success if repair (the degree of residual aortic insufficiency is important in valve repair) • LV function with low LV compliance in patient with long standing AS

Bicuspid Aortic Valve on Transthoracic Echo (Figures 9A to D)[6,7]

- Fusion of the right and left coronary cusps (80%).
- Fusion of the right and noncoronary cusps (20%).
- Two cusps are seen in systole with only two commissures framing an elliptical systolic orifice (the fish mouth appearance).
- Diastolic images may mimic a tricuspid valve when a raphe is present.
- Parasternal long-axis echocardiogram may show
  - An asymmetric closure line
  - Systolic doming
  - Diastolic prolapse of the cusps
- In children, valve may be stenotic
- Without extensive calcification

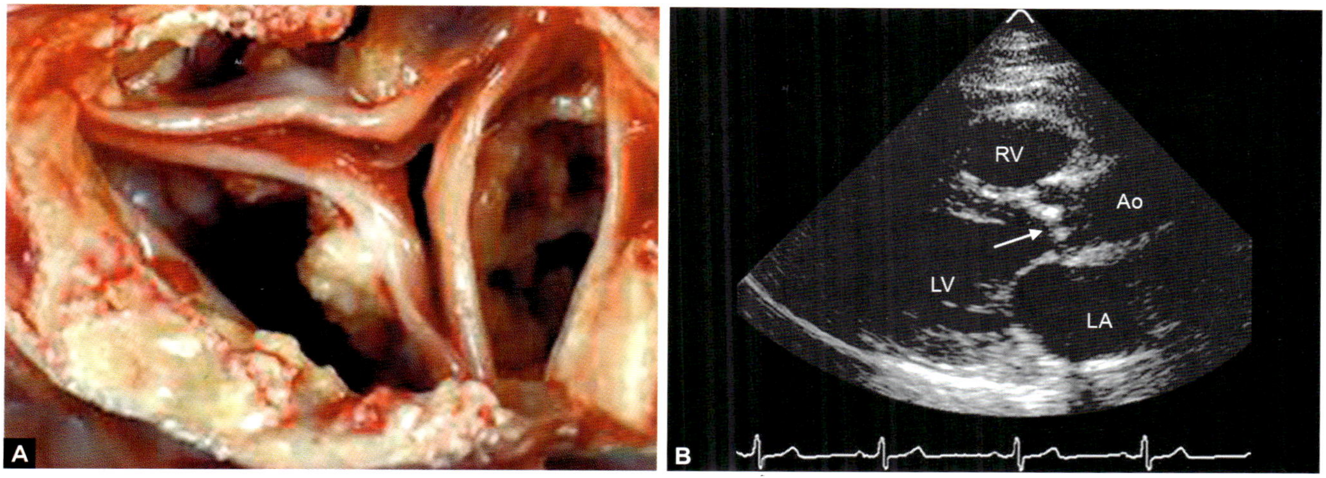

Figures 10A and B (A) Calcific aortic valve following rheumatic stenosis; (B) Calcific long axis view showing coaptation of aortic valve between the right and noncoronary cusp
Abbreviations: LV, left ventricle; LA, left atrium; RV, right ventricle; Ao, aorta

- In adults, stenosis typically is due to calcific changes, which often obscures the number of cusps, making determination of bicuspid vs. tricuspid valve difficult.

Calcific Aortic Stenosis

- Calcification of a bicuspid or tricuspid valve, the severity can be graded semiquantitatively aortic stenosis.
- The degree of valve calcification is a predictor of clinical outcome.

Aortic Sclerosis

- Thickened calcified cusps with preserved mobility.
- Typically associated with peak Doppler velocity of less than 2.5 m/sec.

Rheumatic Aortic Stenosis (Figures 10A and B)

- *Characterized by:*
  - Commissural fusion
  - Triangular systolic orifice
  - Thickening and calcification
- Accompanied by rheumatic mitral valve changes which may be sessile or mobile.
- Parasternal short-axis view showing commissural fusion, leaflet thickening and calcification, small triangular systolic orifice **(Figures 11A and B)**.

Subvalvular Aortic Stenosis

- Thin discrete membrane consisting of endocardial fold and fibrous tissue.
- A fibromuscular ridge.
- Diffuse tunnel-like narrowing of the left ventricular outflow tract (LVOT).
- Accessory or anomalous mitral valve tissue.

Supravalvular Aortic Stenosis (Figure 12)

- *Type I:* Thick, fibrous ring above the aortic valve with less mobility and has the easily identifiable 'hourglass' appearance of the aorta. Rule out aortic insufficiency along with aortic stenosis **(Figures 13A and B)**.
- *Type II:* Thin, discrete fibrous membrane located above the aortic valve.
- The membrane usually mobile and may demonstrate doming during systole.
- *Type III:* Diffuse narrowing.

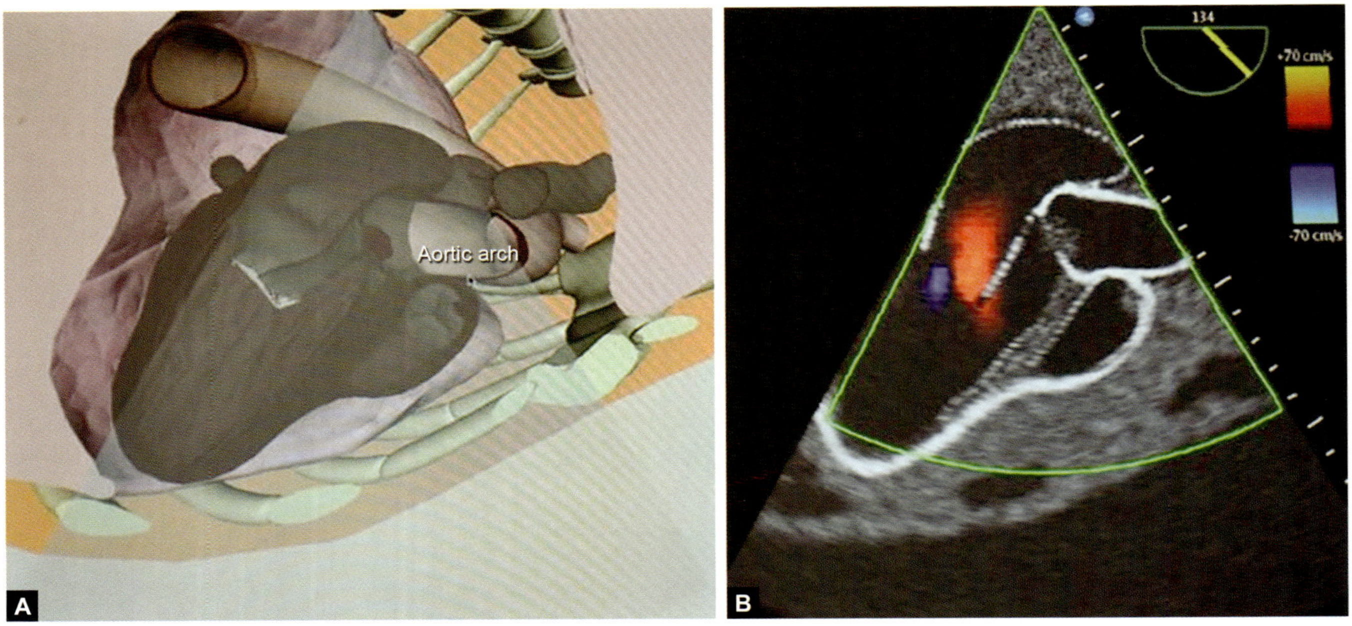

Figures 11A and B The simulation view of aortic valve infective endocarditis

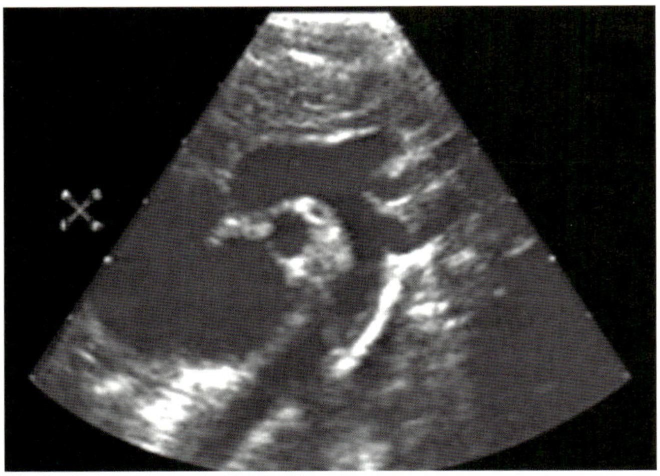

Figure 12 2D-suprasternal view of aortic valve

HOW TO ASSESS AORTIC STENOSIS?

Doppler Assessment of Aortic Stenosis

The primary hemodynamic parameters recommended (EAE/ASE Recommendations for Clinical Practice 2008)

- Peak transvalvular velocity
- Mean transvalvular gradient
- Valve area by continuity equation.

Peak Transvalvular Velocity on Transthoracic Echo

- Continuous-wave Doppler ultrasound.
- Multiple acoustic windows.
- Apical and suprasternal or right parasternal most frequently yield the highest velocity **(Figures 14A and B)**
- Rarely subcostal or supraclavicular windows may be required.
- Three or more beats are averaged in sinus rhythm, with irregular rhythms at least five consecutive beats.
- Aortic stenosis jet velocity is defined as the highest velocity signal obtained from any window after a careful examination.
- Any deviation from a parallel intercept angle results in velocity underestimation.
- The degree of underestimation is 5% or less if the intercept angle is within 15° of parallel.
- Angle correction should not be used because it is likely to introduce more error given the unpredictable jet direction **(Figures 15A and B)**.

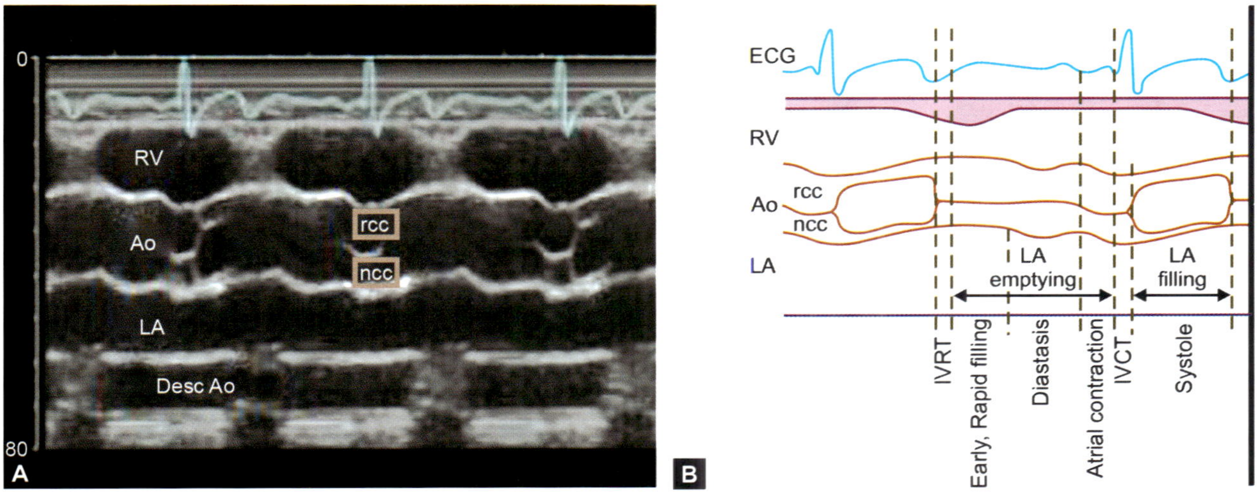

Figures 13A and B M mode-normal aortic valve

Abbreviations: RV, right ventricular; AO, aorta; LA, left atrium; Desc Ao, descending aorta; rcc; ncc, ECG, Echocardiogram; IVRT, isovolumic relaxation time; IVCT, isovolumic contraction time

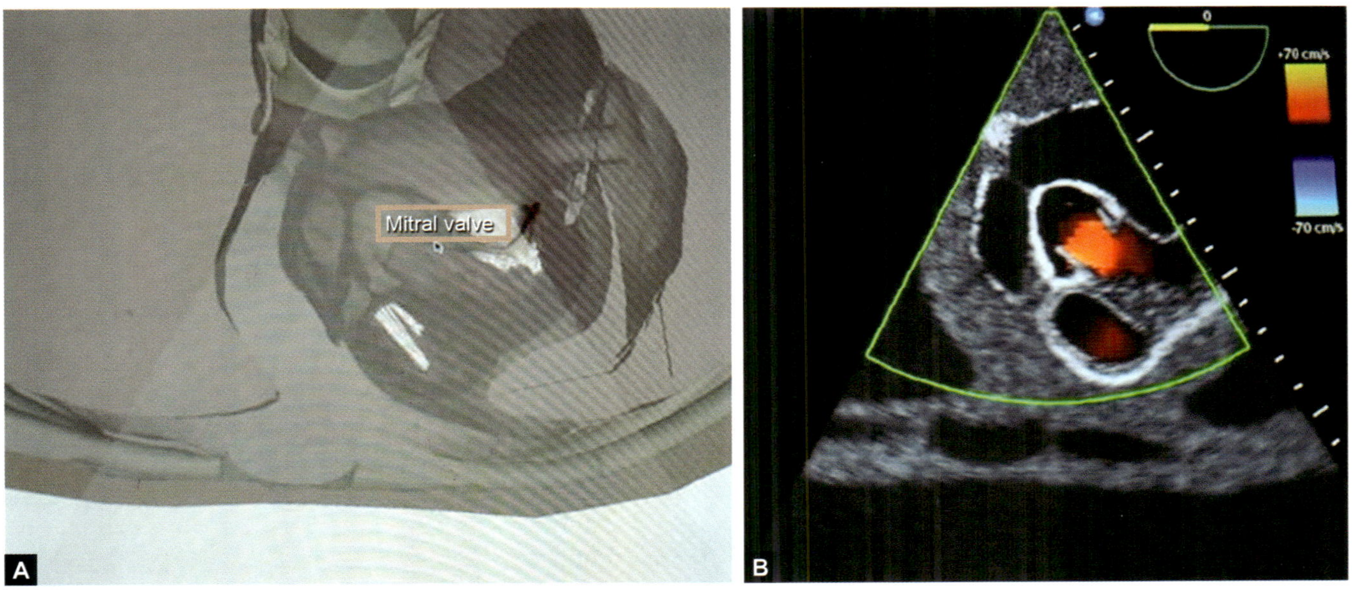

Figures 14A and B The simulation view of aortic insufficiency

- The shape of the CW Doppler velocity curve is helpful in distinguishing the level and severity of obstruction.
- With severe obstruction, maximum velocity occurs later in systole and the curve is more rounded in shape.
- With mild obstruction, the peak is in early systole with a triangular shape of the velocity curve.

Mean Transvalvular Gradient (Figures 16A to F)

- The difference in pressure between the left ventricle and aorta in systole.
- Gradients are calculated from velocity information.
- The relationship between peak and mean gradient depends on the shape of the velocity curve.

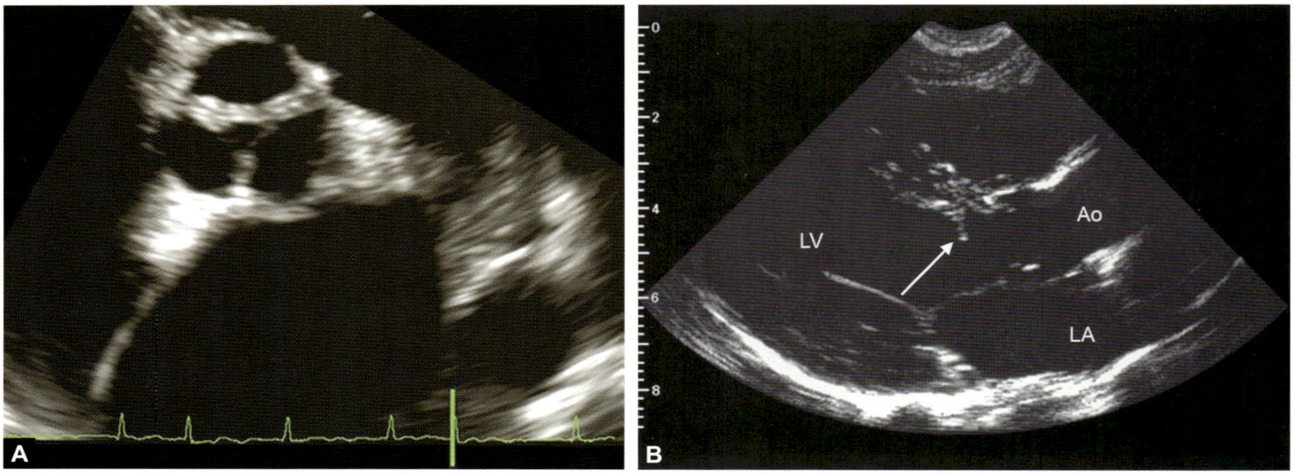

Figures 15A and B (A) Commissural fusion and leaflet thickening of aortic valve; (B) TEE in midesophageal longitudinal axis view showing a thickend noncoronary cusp of aortic valve

Abbreviations: LV, left ventricle; LA, left atrium; Ao, aorta

- Bernoulli equations $\Delta P = 4v^2$.
- The maximum gradient is calculated from maximum velocity ΔP max = $4v^2$ max.
- The mean gradient is calculated by averaging the instantaneous gradients over the ejection period.
- The simplified Bernoulli equation assumes that the proximal velocity can be ignored.
- When the proximal velocity is over 1.5 m/s or the aortic velocity is 3.0 m/s, the proximal velocity should be included in the Bernoulli equation ΔP max = 4 (v^2 max-v^2 proximal).
- Sources of error for pressure gradient calculations
- Malalignment of jet and ultrasound beam.
- Recording of MR jet.
- Neglect of an elevated proximal velocity.
- Any underestimation of aortic velocity results in an even greater underestimation in gradients, due to the squared relationship between velocity and pressure difference.
- The accuracy of the Bernoulli equation to quantify AS pressure gradients is well-established.

Pressure Recovery

- The conversion of potential energy to kinetic energy across a narrowed valve results in a high velocity and a drop in pressure.
- Distal to the orifice, flow decelerates again. Kinetic energy will be reconverted into potential energy with a corresponding increase in pressure, the so-called PR.
- Pressure recovery is greatest in stenosis with gradual distal widening.
- Aortic stenosis with its abrupt widening from the small orifice to the larger aorta has an unfavorable geometry for pressure recovery.

$$PR = 4v^2 \times 2EOA/AoA(1\text{-}EOA/AoA)$$

- Comparing pressure gradients calculated from Doppler velocities to pressures measured at cardiac catheterization.

Aortic Valve Area Continuity Equation

- The velocity time integral (VTI) is measured by tracing the dense modal velocity throughout systole.
- Left ventricular outflow tract (LVOT) diameter is measured from the inner edge to inner edge of the septal endocardium, and the anterior mitral leaflet in midsystole.

Limitations of Continuity-equation Valve Area

- Intra-and interobserver variability.
- Aortic stenosis jet and LVOT velocity 3–4%.
- LVOT diameter 5–8%.
- When subaortic flow velocities are abnormal SV calculation at this site are not accurate.

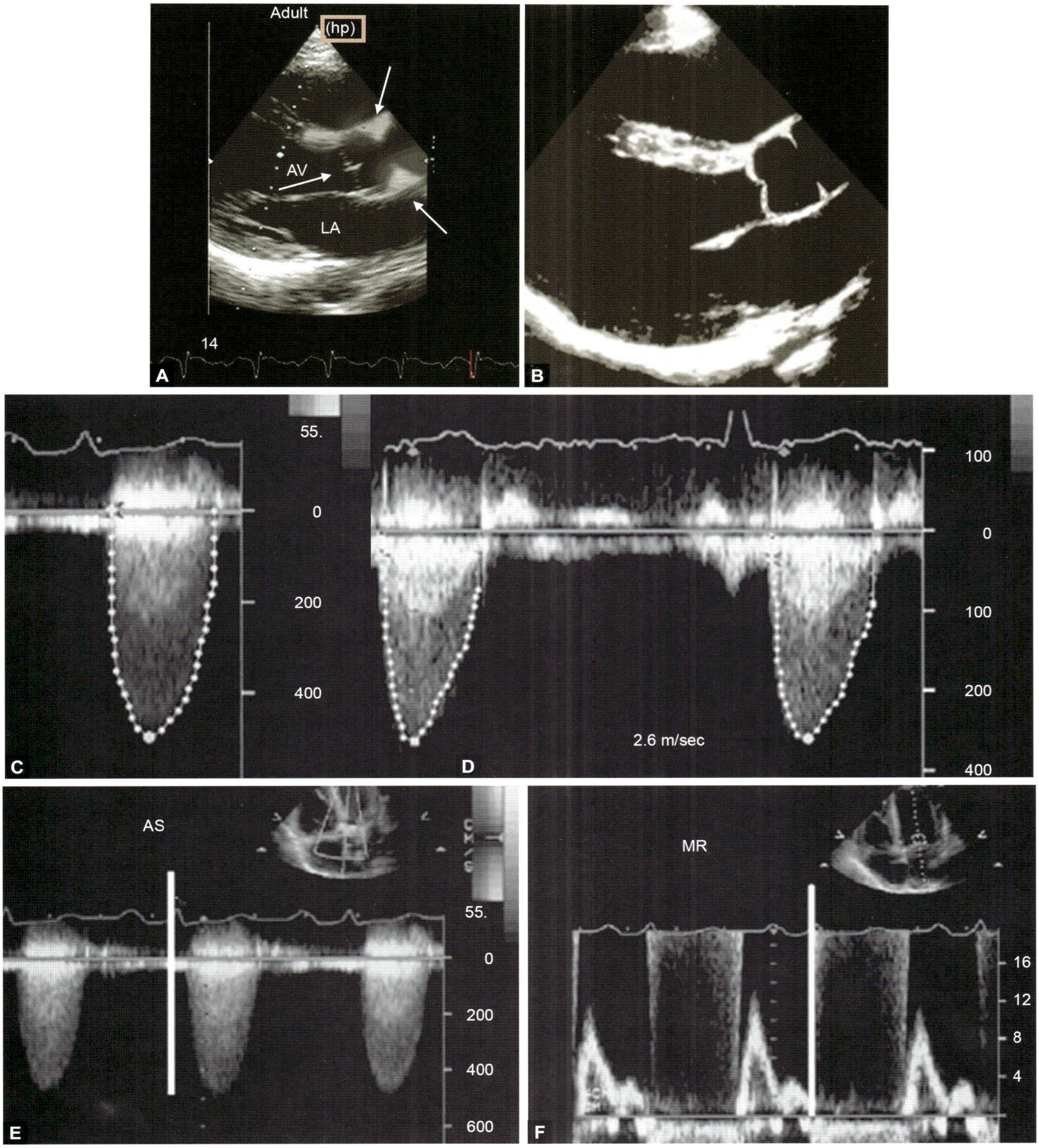

Figures 16A to F (A and B) Doming of the aortic valve in long axis view causing; (C and D) Measure transvalvular gradient; (E and F) Mean transvalvular gradient across the aortic valve

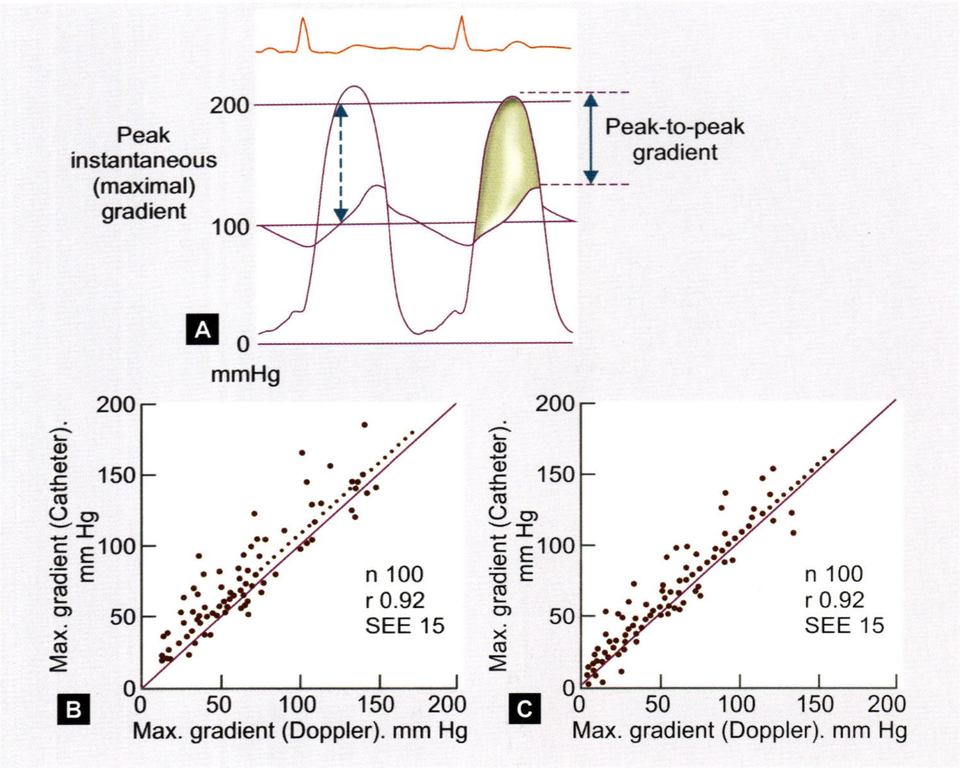

Figures 17A to C Changes in aortic velocity, mean gradient, and valve area

- Ample volume placement near to septum or anterior mitral leaflet.
- Observed changes in valve area with changes in flow rate.
- Aortic stenosis and normal LV function, the effects of flow rate are minimal.
- This effect may be significant in presence concurrent LV dysfunction.
- Low-flow low-gradient AS includes the following conditions:
  - Effective orifice area < 1.0 cm^2.
  - LV ejection fraction < 40%.
  - Mean pressure gradient < 30–40 mm Hg.
  - Severe AS and severely reduced LVEF represent 5% of AS patients.

DOBUTAMINE STRESS ECHO

- Provides information on the changes in aortic velocity, mean gradient, and valve area as flow rate increases **(Figures 17A to C)**.
- Measure of the contractile response to dobutamine.
- Helpful to differentiate two clinical situations
  - Severe AS causing LV systolic dysfunction
  - Moderate AS with another cause of LV dysfunction.

Role in decision-making in adults with AS is controversial and the findings recommend as reliable are:
Stress findings of severe stenosis.

- AVA <1 cm^2.
- Jet velocity > 4 m/s.
- Mean gradient > 40 mm of Hg.
- Lack of contractile reserve.
- Failure of LVEF to ↑ by 20% is a poor prognostic sign.
- A low dose starting at 2.5 or 5 mg/kg/min with an incremental increase in the infusion every 3–5 min to a maximum dose of 10–20 mg/kg/min.[8]
- *The infusion should be stopped as soon as:*
  - Positive result is obtained
  - Heart rate begins to rise more than 10–20 bpm over baselines or exceeds 100 bpm.

Serial Measurements

- During follow-up any significant changes in results should be checked in detail.

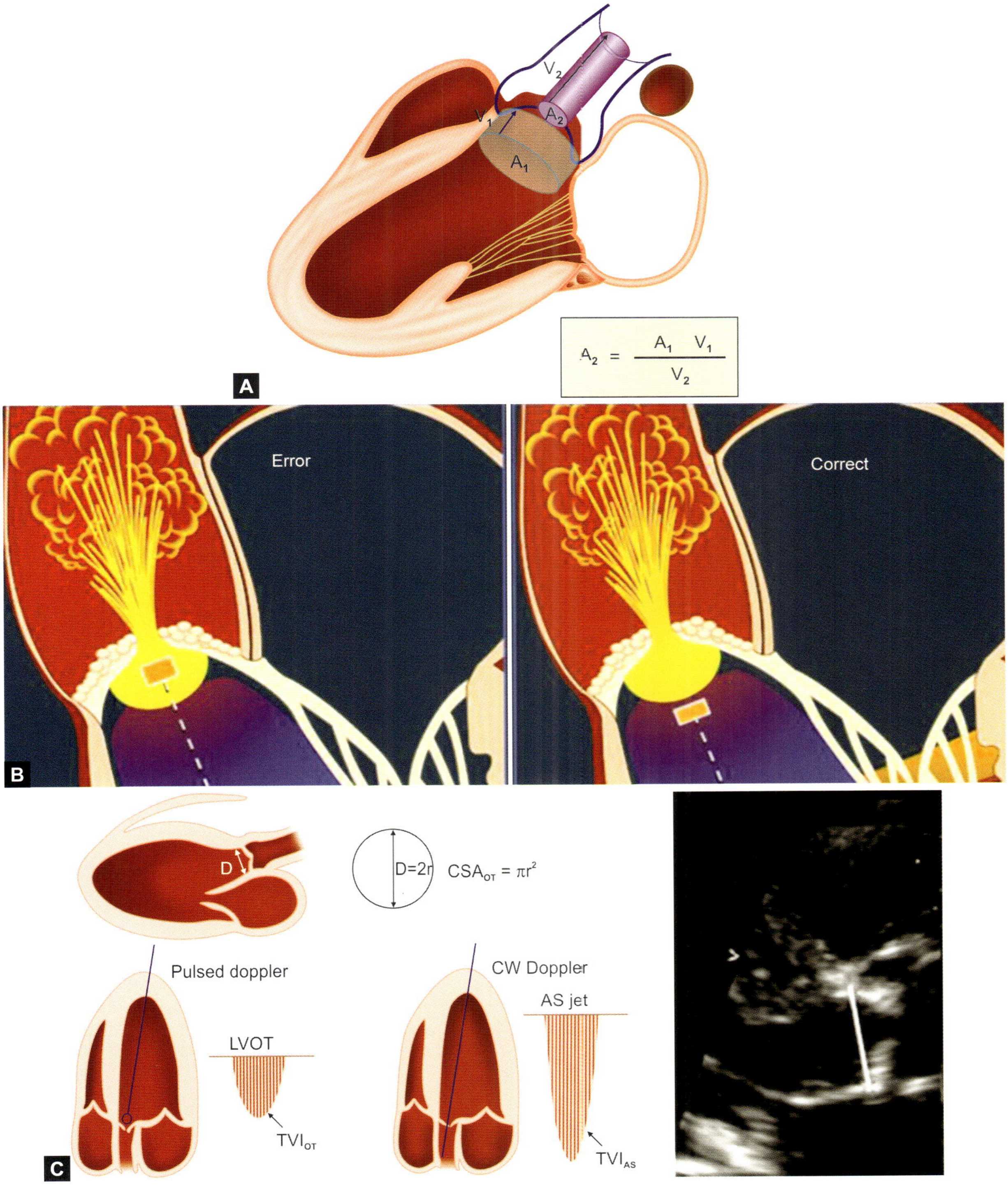

Figures 18A to C Continuity equations for aortic valve area estimation

- Make sure that aortic jet velocity is recorded from the same window with the same quality (always report the window where highest velocities can be recorded) **(Figures 18A to C)**.
- When AVA changes, look for changes in the different components incorporated in the equation.
- Left ventricular outflow tract (LVOT) size rarely changes over time in adults.

SUMMARY

The aortic root, with its characteristic morphology, has attracted the interest of researchers in both clinical and basic sciences, and the emergence of aortic root replacement surgery has further increased the significance of such studies. In addition to clinical observations, both experimental and theoretical studies have attempted to elucidate the dynamics of the aortic root; however, to date, most of these studies have dealt with simplified models of the aortic root, and are thus not readily applicable to clinical settings. Recently, 3D finite element analyses of the aortic root have been reported, in which realistic shapes of both aorta and valve leaflet were modeled. So far, however, only a few studies have taken into consideration the effect of blood flow, an essential component of aortic root dynamics, due the difficulty in computation. We have developed a computational program for fluid-structure interaction analysis based on the arbitrary Lagrangian-Eulerian finite element method, and applied it to the simulation of aortic root dynamics. The results suggest the importance of vortex formation in the sinus of Valsalva in the smooth closure of the aortic valve.

REFERENCES

1. Goertz AW, Lindner KH, Schutz W, et al. Influence of phenylephrine bolus administration on left ventricular filling dynamics in patients with coronary artery disease and patients with valvular aortic stenosis. Anesthesiology 1994;81:49-58.
2. Yang SS, Bentivoglia LG, Maranhao V, et al. Assessment of valvular regurgitation. In: Yang SS, Bentivoglia LG, Maranhao V, et al. (Eds). From cardiac catheterization data to hemodynamic parameters, 2nd edn. Philadelphia: FA Davis; 1988.pp.152-65.
3. Howie MB, Black HA, Romanelli VA, et al. A comparison of isoflurane versus fentanyl as primary anesthetics for mitral valve surgery. Anesth Analg. 1996;83:941-48.
4. Fuchs RM, Heuser RR, Yin FCP, et al. Limitations of pulmonary wedge V waves in diagnosing mitral regurgitation. Am J Cardiol. 1982;49:849-54.
5. Moore RA, Neary M, Gallagher J, et al. Determination of pulmonary capillary wedge position in patients with giant v-waves. J Cardiothorac Anesth. 1987;1:108-13.
6. Schaefer BM, et al. Am J Cardiol. 2007;99:686-90.
7. Schaefer BM, et al. Heart. 2008;94:1634-8.
8. Nishimura RA, et al. Circulation. 2002;106:809-13.

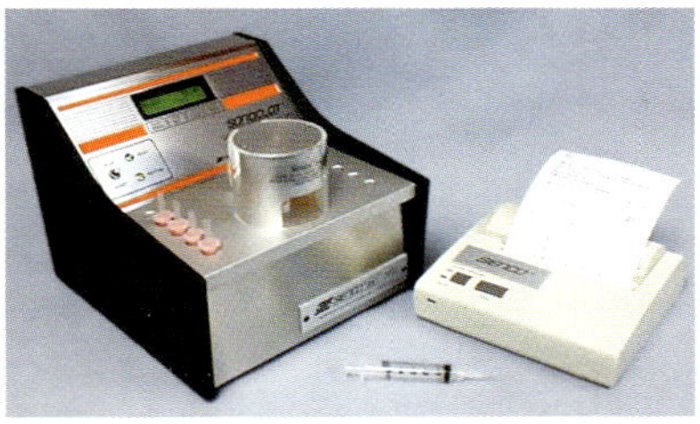

Section 4

Perioperative Bleeding in Cardiac Surgery

Section Outline

- Simulation for Perioperative Coagulation Dysfunction in Cardiac Surgery
- Simulations for Coagulation Dysfunction in Liver Disease
- Simulation for Perioperative Coagulation Dysfunction in Liver Surgery
- The Coagulation Tests are Simple to Perform and Fascinating but Difficult to Interpret
- Point-of-Care Testing of Coagulation in the Bleeding Cardiac Patients

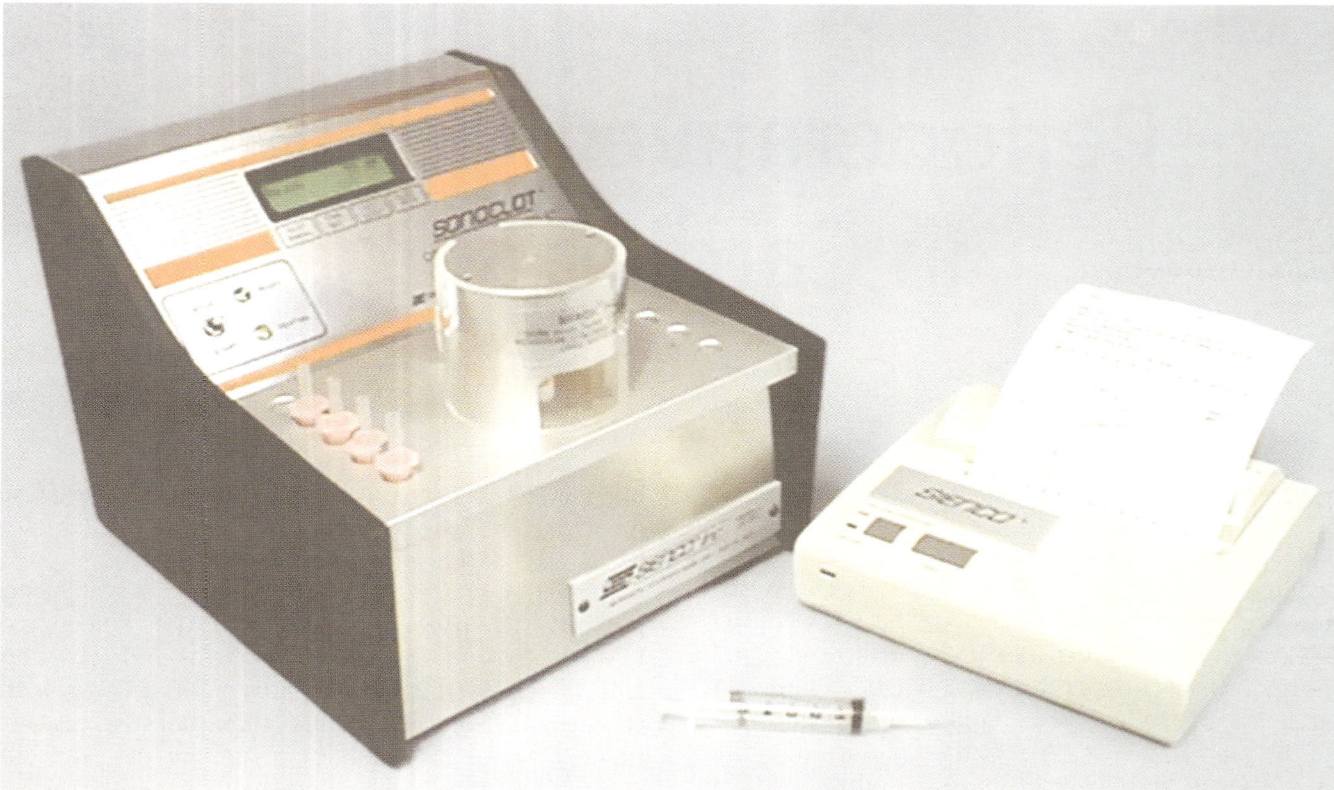
SONOCLOT

Chapter 17

Simulation for Perioperative Coagulation Dysfunction in Cardiac Surgery

Poonam Malhotra Kapoor, Sameer Taneja

Chapter Outline

- Problems of the Cardiac Surgical Patient
- Summary of Basic Signature Interpretation
- Cardiac Surgery and Postoperative Care
- Sonoclot and Cardiac Surgery

INTRODUCTION

For a normal coagulation function, cardiac surgery, when a lot of bleeding contemplated, the coagulation factor, namely I, II, III, V, VII, X and others involving both the intrinsic and the extrinsic pathway have to be within normal limits alongwith functional fibrinogen levels and also there has to be adequate quantity and quality of the platelets. A delicate shift in balance of either of the three causes postoperative hemorrhage which is a common scenario postcardiopulmonary bypass (CPB) in a cardiac patient.

During CPB, the platelets which are the center of the coagulation universe and which provide the binding surface for clotting factors and also assist in clot formation and retraction, undergo a lot of shear and stress, thereby getting damaged and preventing adequate coagulation. The standard coagulation tests being used so far, have been prothrombin time, partial thromboplast which detects mainly the extrinsic pathway and not both systems. The second phase for bleeding involves the use of elaborate laboratory tests involves those to detect fibrin polymerization, which is laborious and time consuming.

Viscoelastic tests like Sonoclot or thromboelastography (TEG), pave the pathway for instant detection of bleeding cause, there and then in the operating room or ICU. The entire gamut of signature curves in this point of care testing, tests all the steps in the bleeding cascade, namely fibrin formation, clot strength rate and clot lysis with cellular componants involved in haemostasis and also about the platelet function in the form of clot retraction. Point of care tells us about hypercoagulation states or presence of dilutional coagulopathy or increased fibrinolysis within the operating room ICU resorting to extensive battery of tests.

PROBLEMS OF THE CARDIAC SURGICAL PATIENT

The cardiac surgical patient is preoperatively on antiplatelet drugs and heparin and has underlying platelet abnormalities intrinsically and also because of CPB which leads to disturbed hemostasis. Post-CPB fibrinolysis, heparin reversal and platelet dysfunction due to surgical and foreign CPB surface persists. Hazards of blood transfusions and its effect on mortality and availability all have led to most centers resorting to point of care testing in the OR/ICU itself, which help us in:

- Managing anticoagulation
- Manage blood product usage
- Differentiate between mechanical v/s hemostatic

And also help identify hypercoagulation patients—all possible due to the principle of Microviscometry.

The thrombolytic pharmacotherapy is picked up by the POC tests like Sonoclot which otherwise remains undiagnosed and the patient continues to bleed.

Automated results of Sonoclot analyzer:

- Time until initial clot formation (activated clotting time)
- Clot formation rate.

How to Sonoclot test interpreted?
There are three straight steps:

- Time until initial clot formation
- Rate of fibrin gel formation
- Clot retraction

Step 1—Initial Clot Formation Time

Automated results: Onset Time or Activated Clotting Time

Step 2—Fibrin Gel Formation

Fibrinogen converts into a fibrin gel

- Once thrombin forms in the sample, fibrinogen quickly converts into a fibrin gel.
- The fibrinogen to fibrin reaction is affected by fibrinogen, thrombin generation, and thrombin inhibitors such as AT3 **(Figures 1 and 2)**.

Automated result: Clot Rate: The slope of the Sonoclot Signature during gel formation

- The fibrinogen to fibrin reaction is characterized by the slope during the gel formation phase **(Figure 3)**.
- This result has particular importance in evaluating the performance of thrombin inhibitors and heparin anticoagulant effect.

Step 3—Clot Retraction: Cellular Level

Clot retraction: Clot retraction causes a peak or peaks on the Sonoclot Signature **(Figures 4 and 5)**.

Quantative platelet function can be characterized by the time-to-peak.

SUMMARY OF BASIC SIGNATURE INTERPRETATION

Automated Results

Step 1: Time for initial clot formation (typically the activated clotting time) **(Figure 6)**
Step 2: Fibrin formation (Clot Rate) **(Figure 7)**

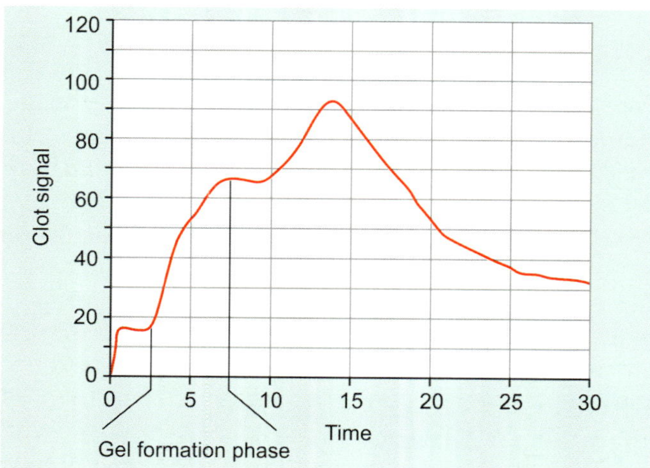

Figure 1 The rise in clot signal curve from 20 to 60 in 7 minutes is due to fbrinogen converting into fibrin gel

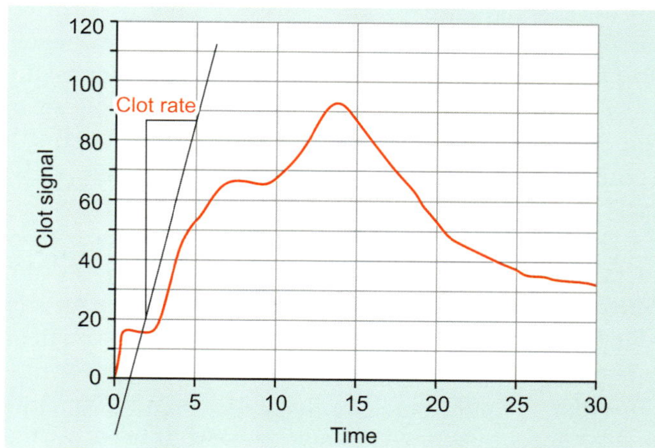

Figure 2 The peak in the curve denote clot retraction, measured as time-to-peak

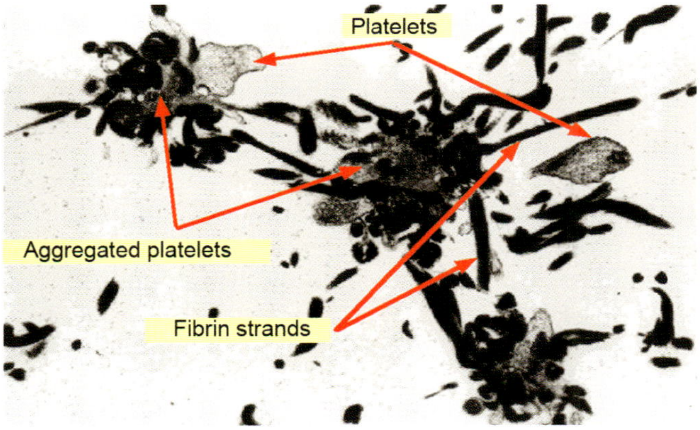

Figure 3 Platelets and fibrin interaction

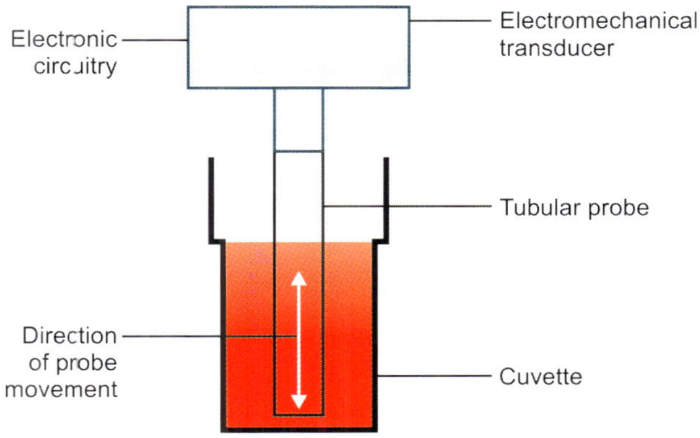

Figure 6 Principle of operation: Microviscometer

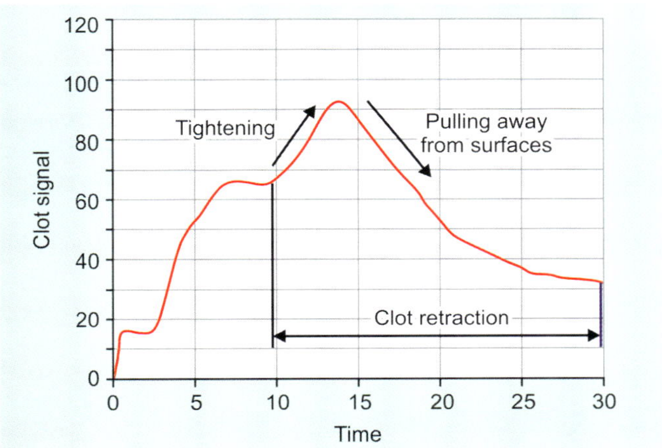

Figure 4 The clot retraction phase—causes the peak and time-to-peak

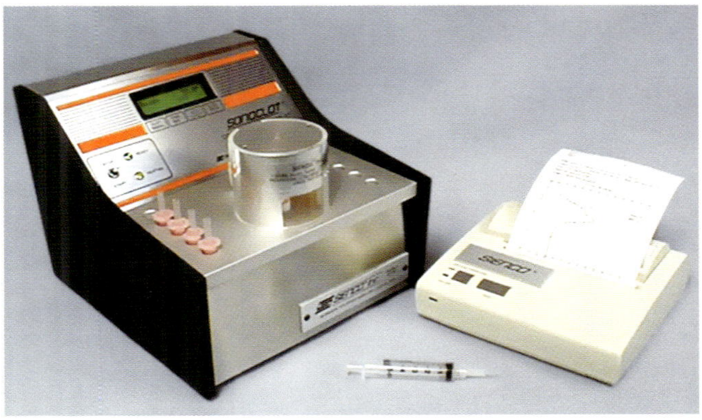

Figure 7 Sonoclot analyzer and graphics printer

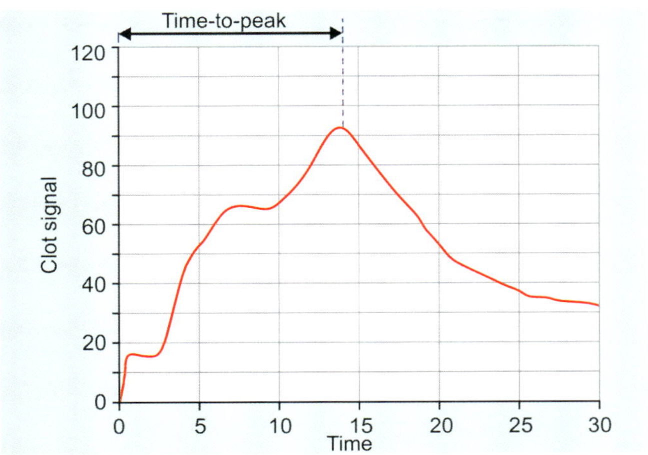

Figure 5 Time-to-peak gives a quantitative platelet function

Quantitative/Qualitative Results

Step 3: Clot retraction (Platelet function) **(Figure 8)**
Step 4: Hyperfibrinolysis **(Figure 9)**
Hyperfibrinolysis: The fibrin gel quickly dissolves back into a liquid.

Conclusion

Sonoclot helps to find the target patient population that would really benefit from an antifibrinolytic therapy after cardiac surgery. Restriction of tranexamic acid (TA) uses to a particular group of patients determined by using Sonoclot would cause its inappropriate consumption and a reduction in total hospital costs. Sonoclot-guided approach also has a high capability to differentiate

CHAPTER 17

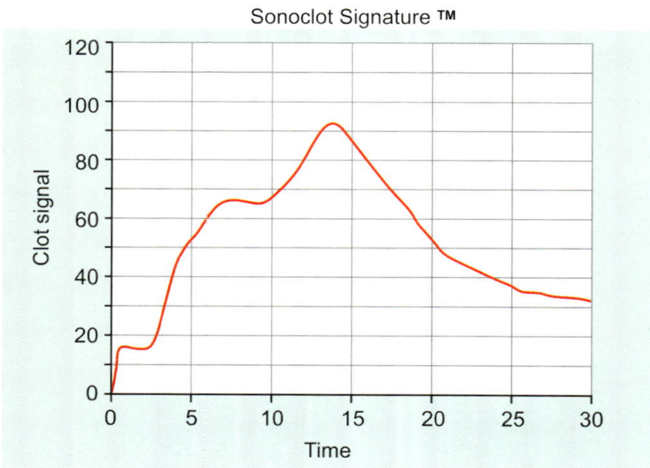

Figure 8 Interpreting a Sonoclot Signature—a normal curve

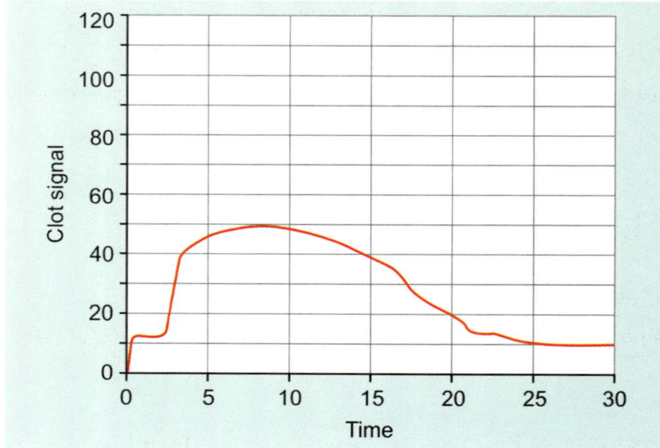

Figure 10 Atypical curve suggests no peak and decreased platelet numbers

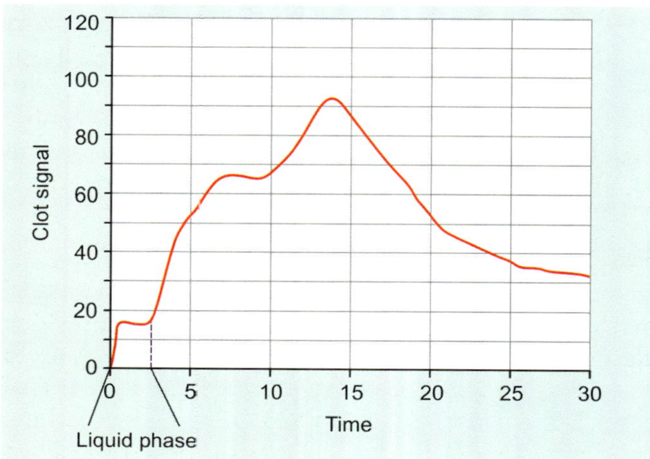

Figure 9 Interpreting a Sonoclot Signature—the liquid phase is the initial phase of clot formation

surgical bleeding from the nonsurgical one in patients with excessive postop chest drainage. Adopting of a Sonoclot containing transfusion management to the perioperative care of cardiac surgical patients, either at low or high risk for transfusion, may further decrease the morbidity and hospital costs related to perioperative transfusion and help save cost by avoiding experience hemostatic drugs.

CARDIAC SURGERY AND POSTOPERATIVE CARE

Coagulation management of patients undergoing cardiac surgery is complex because of a balance between anticoagulation for cardiopulmonary bypass (CPB) and hemostasis after CPB. Furthermore, an increasing number of patients have impaired platelet function at baseline due to administration of antiplatelet drugs. During CPB, optimal anticoagulation dictates that coagulation is antagonized and platelets are prevented from activation so that clots do not form. After surgery, coagulation abnormalities, platelet dysfunction, and fibrinolysis can occur, creating a situation whereby hemostatic integrity must be restored **(Figure 10)**.

The complex process of anticoagulation with heparin, antagonism with protamine, and postoperative hemostasis therapy can be guided by point of care (POC) tests that assess hemostatic function in a timely and accurate manner. Although studies report that viscoelastic POC coagulation devices may predict excessive bleeding after CPB, findings are not consistent and evidence supporting its usefulness as a predictor of bleeding is minimal.[2-4] Normal viscoelastic test results in a bleeding patient are unlikely due to a significant coagulopathy (high negative predictive value).[5] Therefore, viscoelastic POC tests may be useful in early identification and targeted treatment of a surgical bleeding.

The institution of transfusion algorithms based on TEG/thromboelastometry (ROTEM) parameters has been demonstrated to reduce transfusion requirements in adults and children undergoing cardiac surgery.[6-10] Furthermore, it has been recently shown that implementation of ROTEM-guided coagulation management is cost-effective.[8] To detect nonheparin related hemostatic problems in the presence of large

TABLE 1 Modified version of the TEG-based transfusion algorithm proposed by Royston and Kier[1]

TEG Parameter	*Implication*	*Treatment*
14 < r < 21 (mm)	Mild deficiency in coagulation factors	1 unit FFP
21 ≤ r < 28 (mm)	Moderate deficiency in coagulation factors	2 units FFP
r ≥ 28 (mm)	Severe deficiency in coagulation factors	4 units FFP
40 ≤ MA < 48 (mm)	Moderate deficiency in the number/function of platelets	1 unit platelets
MA < 40 (mm)	Severe deficiency in the number/function of platelets	2 units platelets
LY30 > 7.5 (%)	Exaggerated fibrinolysis	Aprotinin, Tranexamic acid

Abbreviations: TEG, thromboelastography; MA, maximum amplitude; FFP, fresh frozen plasma

amounts of heparin, tests with heparinase have been developed and one study showed that implementation of an algorithm based upon heparinase-modified TEG resulted in a significant reduction of transfusion blood products.[11]

POC coagulation analyzers measuring activated clotting time (ACT) are routinely being used in cardiac surgical patients to guide heparin-induced anticoagulation and its reversal.[12-15] Besides standard ACT machines, viscoelastic POC analyzers also provide ACT results with comparable accuracy and performance. The ACT provided by the Sonoclot analyzer is being used to guide heparin therapy, and several tests with different characteristics are commercially available. More recently, a novel assay has also been developed to measure ACT by TEG **(Table 1)**.[16]

Besides providing information on the initiation phase of coagulation, the Sonoclot Analyzer also measures the kinetics of fibrin formation and clot development, expressed as CR (the maximum slope of the Sonoclot Signature during initial fibrin polymerization and clot development). Furthermore, the function of the platelets is being analyzed and reported as PF (derived from the timing and quality of the clot retraction). The nominal range of values for the PF goes from 0, representing no PF (no clot retraction and flat Sonoclot Signature after fibrin formation), to approximately 5, representing strong PF (clot retraction occurs sooner and is very strong, with clearly defined, sharp peaks in the Sonoclot Signature after fibrin formation).[17]

The Sonoclot Analyzer has been criticized because its results were influenced by age, sex, and platelet count.[18] Additionally, studies showed poor reproducibility of some of the measured variables, especially clot rate (CR) and platelet function (PF).[19] However, others found the Sonoclot Analyzer to be valuable and reliable in patients undergoing cardiac surgical procedures[20] and the Sonoclot Analyzer has even demonstrated a precision close to that of thromboelastography.[21] In more recent studies, test variability of ACT values determined by Sonoclot were comparable to other established ACT analyzers (8–9% on average). Furthermore, test variability for PF determined by gbACT/and H-gbACT/ (heparinase glass-bead test) was 6–10% in a recent study assessing PF after administration of the glycoprotein IIb/IIIa (GP IIb/IIIa) antagonist tirofiban with or without heparin.

SONOCLOT AND CARDIAC SURGERY

Postoperative bleeding remains a significant cause of morbidity and mortality after cardiac surgery in which cardiopulmonary bypass has been used, resulting in re-exploration of the chest in approximately 3% of cases.[22] The cause of excessive bleeding may be failure, or a combination of both. Hemostatic failure after cardiopulmonary bypass may be caused by inadequate reversal of heparin with protamine, hemodilution causing a moderate decrease in plasma clotting factors or platelet abnormalities, including a decrease in platelet count and a decrease in platelet aggregation.[23] These changes in coagulation may be induced by use during cardiopulmonary bypass. SCT is better than routine clotting studies for predicting postoperative hemorrhage caused by coagulopathy.[24] Shenaq and Saleem[25] concluded that SCT provided predictable information on platelet function after cardiopulmonary bypass. Of 24 patients who bled after operation but had a normal SCT signature, 22 were found to have a surgical cause for the bleeding. In 25 patients with abnormal signatures associated with postoperative bleeding, the bleeding was controlled and the signature returned to normal after platelet transfusion.

CHAPTER 17

REFERENCES

1. Royston D, von Kier S. Reduced haemostatic factor transfusion using heparinase-modified thromboelastography during cardiopulmonary bypass. Br J Anaesth 2001;86:575-78.
2. Tuman KJ, Spiess BD, McCarthy RJ, Ivankovich AD. Comparison of viscoelastic measures of coagulation after cardiopulmonary bypass. Anesth Analg 1989;69:69-75.
3. Nuttall GA, Oliver WC, Ereth MH, Santrach PJ. Coagulation tests predict bleeding after cardiopulmonary bypass. J Cardiothorac Vasc Anesth 1997;11:815-23.
4. Wang JS, Lin CY, Hung WT, O'Connor MF, Thisted RA, Lee BK, Karp RB, Yang MW. Thromboelastogram fails to predict postoperative hemorrhage in cardiac patients. Ann Thorac Surg 1992;53:435-9.
5. Cammerer U, Dietrich W, Rampf T, Braun SL, Richter JA. The predictive value of modified computerized thromboelastography and platelet function analysis for postoperative blood loss in routine cardiac surgery. Anesth Analg 2003;96:51-7.
6. Shore-Lesserson L, Manspeizer HE, DePerio M, Francis S, Vela-Cantos F, Ergin MA. Thromboelastography-guided transfusion algorithm reduces transfusions in complex cardiac surgery. Anesth Analg 1999;88:312-9.
7. Anderson L, Quasim I, Soutar R, Steven M, Macfie A, Korte W. An audit of red cell and blood product use after the institution of thromboelastometry in a cardiac intensive care unit. Transfus Med 2006;16:31-9.
8. Spalding GJ, Hartrumpf M, Sierig T, Oesberg N, Kirschke CG, Albes JM. Cost reduction of perioperative coagulation management in cardiac surgery: value of 'bedside' thrombelastography (ROTEM). Eur J Cardiothorac Surg 2007;31:1052-7.
9. Avidan MS, Alcock EL, Da FJ, Ponte J, Desai JB, Despotis GJ, Hunt BJ. Comparison of structured use of routine laboratory tests or near-patient assessment with clinical judgement in the management of bleeding after cardiac surgery. Br J Anaesth 2004;92:178-86.
10. Miller BE, Guzzetta NA, Tosone SR, Levy JH. Rapid evaluation of coagulopathies after cardiopulmonary bypass in children using modified thromboelastography. Anesth Analg 2000;90:1324-30.
11. Royston D, von Kier S. Reduced haemostatic factor transfusion using heparinase-modified thrombelastography during cardiopulmonary bypass. Br J Anaesth 2001;86:575-8.
12. Bull MH, Huse WM, Bull BS. Evaluation of tests used to monitor heparin therapy during extracorporeal circulation. Anesthesiology 1975;43:346-53.
13. Despotis GJ, Gravlee G, Filos K, Levy J. Anticoagulation monitoring during cardiac surgery: a review of current and emerging techniques. Anesthesiology 1999;91:1122-51.
14. Prisco D, Paniccia R. Point-of-Care Testing of Hemostasis in Cardiac Surgery. Thromb J 2003;1:1.
15. Shore-Lesserson L. Monitoring anticoagulation and hemostasis in cardiac surgery. Anesthesiol Clin North Am 2003;21:511-26.
16. Chavez JJ, Foley DE, Snider CC, Howell JC, Cohen E, Muenchen RA, Carroll RC. A novel thrombelastograph tissue factor/kaolin assay of activated clotting times for monitoring heparin anticoagulation during cardiopulmonary bypass. Anesth Analg 2004;99:1290-4.
17. Tucci MA, Ganter MT, Hamiel CR, Klaghofer R, Zollinger A, Hofer CK. Platelet function monitoring with the Sonoclot analyzer after in vitro tirofiban and heparin administration. J Thorac Cardiovasc Surg 2006;131:1314-22.
18. Horlocker TT, Schroeder DR. Effect of age, gender, and platelet count on Sonoclot coagulation analysis in patients undergoing orthopedic operations. Mayo Clin Proc 1997;72:214-9.
19. Ekback G, Carlsson O, Schott U. Sonoclot coagulation analysis: a study of test variability. J Cardiothorac Vasc Anesth 1999;13:393-7.
20. Saleem A, Blifeld C, Saleh SA, Yawn DH, Mace ML, Schwartz M, Crawford ES. Viscoelastic measurement of clot formation: a new test of platelet function. Ann Clin Lab Sci 1983;13:115-24.
21. Forestier F, Belisle S, Contant C, Harel F, Janvier G, Hardy JF. [Reproducibility and interchangeability of the Thromboelastograph, Sonoclot and Hemochron-activated coagulation time in cardiac surgery]. Can J Anaesth 2001;48:902-10.
22. Salzman WE, Weinsten MJ, Weintraub RM, Ware JA, thurer RL, et al. Treatment with desmopressin acetate to reduce blood loss after cardiac surgery. New England Journal of Medicine 1986;314:1402-06.
23. Harker LA, Malpass TW, Branson HE, Hassel EA et al. Mechanism of abnormal bleeding in patients undergoing cardiopulmonary bypass: Aquired transient platelet dysfunction associated with selective granule release. Blood 1980;56:924-7.
24. Tuman KJ, Spiess BD, McCarthy RJ, Ivaankovich AD et al. comparison of viscoelastic measures of coagulation after cardiopulmonary bypass. Anaesthesia and analgesia 1989; 69: 69-75.
25. Shenaq SA, Saleem A. Viscoelastic measurement of clot formation: the sonoclot. In: Ellison N, Jobes DR, (Eds). Effective Hemostasis in cardiac surgery. Philadelphia: WB Saunders; 1988.pp.183-9.

Chapter 18

Simulations for Coagulation Dysfunction in Liver Disease

Priyanka Saxena

Chapter Outline

- Hemostatic Profiles in Patients with Liver Disease
- Laboratory Evaluation of Hemostatic Disturbances in Chronic Liver Disease
- Clinical Scenarios

INTRODUCTION

Liver plays an essential role in the coagulation pathways and is involved in both primary as well as secondary hemostasis. Liver is seat of synthesis of all coagulation factors as well as inhibitors (except von Willebrand factor). Any impairment in liver function leads to severe hemostatic disturbances.

Contrary to popular beliefs, that chronic liver disease leads to a hypocoagulable state, patients with liver disease suffer from complex hemostatic defects. It is increasingly being recognized that these patients not only have bleeding tendencies but may develop thrombotic complications also. The recent hypothesis on hemostasis in liver disease states that patients with liver disease are in a state of rebalanced hemostasis which is much more delicate and unstable than in healthy individuals **(Figure 1)**. This delicate balance may tilt to either side by any inciting agent or evidence. The patients with chronic liver disease may present with several coagulation abnormalities as outlined here.

HEMOSTATIC PROFILES IN PATIENTS WITH LIVER DISEASE

1. Thrombocytopenia.
2. Reduced levels of coagulation factors.
3. Reduced levels of inhibitors of coagulation.
4. Reduced levels of fibrinolytic proteins.
5. Increased plasma levels of factor VIII and von Willebrand factor.

LABORATORY EVALUATION OF HEMOSTATIC DISTURBANCES IN CHRONIC LIVER DISEASE

Several testing modalities are available for evaluation of coagulation disturbances in liver disease. The most commonly employed includes prothrombin time-international normalized ratio (PT-INR). The INR values are employed by the clinicians all over the world to detect abnormalities of coagulation pathway in these

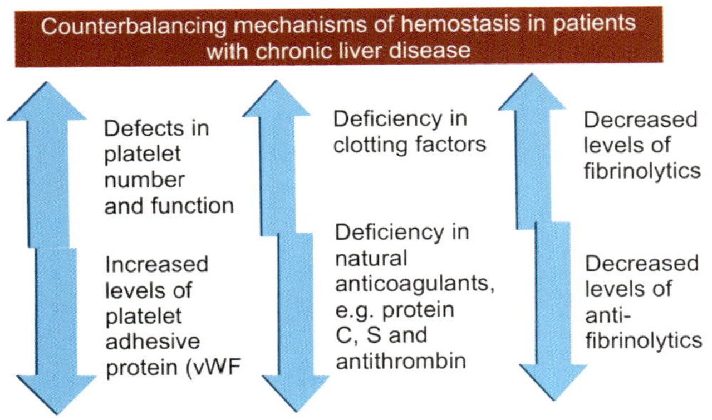

Figure 1 Hemostatic mechanisms showing rebalanced state in patients with liver disease

patients. However, in this context it is important to note that INR values in liver disease give wide interlaboratory variability. Also they are capable of detecting only a small part of coagulation process (i.e. the extrinsic pathway only), thereby giving incomplete information about the clotting process at large. In comparison, the global coagulation assays like the Sonoclot analyzer give an accurate assessment of the entire coagulation pathway and may be more helpful in the overall management of hemostatic defects in these patients. **Table 1** outlines the common laboratory tests and their advantages in management of patients with chronic liver disease.

In view of the above-mentioned hemostatic intricacies in patients with liver disease we will discuss some case scenarios pertaining to coagulation dysfunction in patients with liver disease.

CLINICAL SCENARIOS

Five clinical scenarios pertaining to coagulation abnormalities in patients with chronic liver disease have been described. The diagnosis, investigation and management of these cases has been discussed.

Case 1: A 55 Years Old Female Presented to ILBS with Chief Complaints

- Progressively worsening abdominal distension × 15 days
- Reduced urine output × 3 days
- Loss of appetite and worsening lethargy × 3 days

On Examination

- Pallor+, jaundice+
- Central nervous system (CNS): Altered sensorium
- *P/A:* Soft, nontender, ascites ++.

Diagnosis

Nonalcoholic steatohepatitis (NASH) induced chronic liver disease. Decompensated with ascites, spontaneous bacterial peritonitis and hepatic encephalopathy grade 4.

Disseminated Koch's (abdominal and pulmonary).

Clinical Review

On the basis of deteriorating clinical condition, patient was admitted in liver coma intensive care unit (ICU) and shifted on ventilator.

One week after admission in ICU a tracheostomy was planned.

Subsequently patient had oral mucosal ooze.

The following investigations were carried out:

- *Platelet count:* 16×10^9/L
- *PT-INR:* 2.24

TABLE 1 Common laboratory tests for coagulation assessment in liver disease

Test	*Advantages*	*Disadvantages*
PT-INR	• Quick and inexpensive • Correlates with severity of liver disease	• Interlaboratory variation • Does not predict bleeding risk
APTT	Quick and inexpensive	Measures only intrinsic pathway
Platelet count	Quick and inexpensive	Gives no information about platelet function
Platelet function assays	Gives information about platelet dysfunction	Not widely available
Fibrinogen	Gives accurate quantification of fibrinogen levels	• Acute phase reactant • Does not predict bleeding risk
Factor assays	Give idea about individual factor levels	• Interlaboratory variation • Affected by other disease processes as well
Global coagulation assays	Give an idea about the entire coagulation process	Not widely available

SECTION 4

- *Fibrinogen:* 193.4 mg/dL.
- *Hb:* 9.0g/dL

In response to mucosal bleeds and severe thrombocytopenia, Sonoclot analysis was done prior to tracheostomy **(Figure 2)**.

The Sonoclot parameters obtained were as follows:

- *ACT:* 253s
- *CR:* 12.6 clot signal units/min
- *PF:* 0.2

In view of the deranged Sonoclot parameters and intermittent mucosal oozing tracheostomy was deferred and blood products were transfused.

Patient was transfused with:

- 3 units fresh frozen plasma
- 6 units of cryoprecipitate
- 6 units of random donor platelet concentrate
- 2 units of packed RBCs
- The condition of the patient improved with the transfused blood products.

Two days later a repeat Sonoclot was performed **(Figure 3)**.

The corrected Sonoclot parameters obtained were as follows:

- *ACT:* 190s
- *CR:* 23 clot signal units/min
- *PF:* 3.7

Results

- Sonoclot parameters improved dramatically after transfusions.

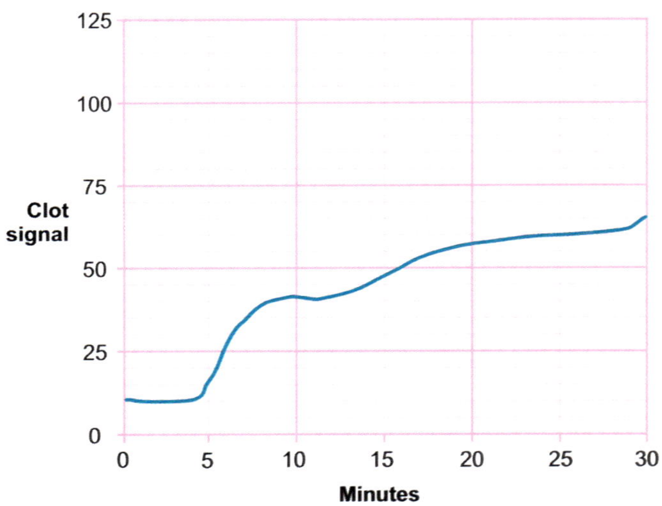

Figure 2 Abnormal Sonoclot signature in patient with mucosal ooze (Case 1)

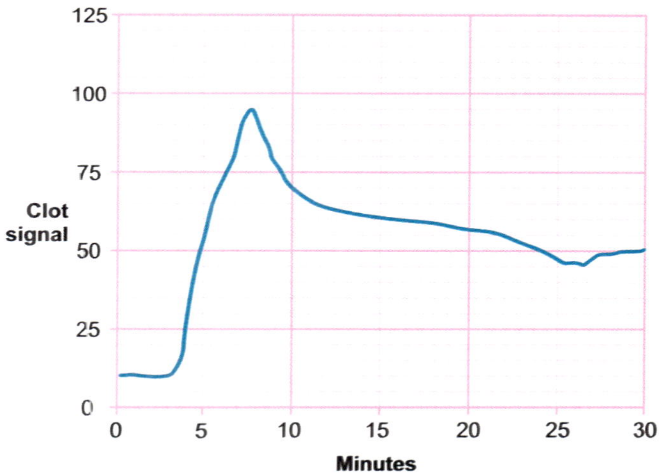

Figure 3 Corrected Sonoclot signature in patient with mucosal ooze, post-transfusion (Case 1)

- Mucosal oozing stopped completely.
- On the basis of corrected Sonoclot parameters tracheostomy was carried out successfully under antibiotic cover.
- Patient remained hemodynamically stable after the procedure.

Discussion

Q.1. Why were fresh frozen plasma (FFP), cryoprecipitate and platelet concentrate, all transfused in this patient?

Ans. The decision for type of blood component to be used for transfusion is taken on the basis of Sonoclot parameters. ACT, which is suggestive of coagulation factors levels (until thrombin generation), is grossly prolonged in this case. These factor deficiencies can be replenished by the use of FFP. Clot rate, which relates to the rate of clot polymerization is dependent on the concentration as well as activity of fibrinogen. Though the fibrinogen levels in this patient are reported to be normal, the low clot rate may correspond to dysfibrinogenemia, which is very common in patients with advanced liver disease. On this basis, the patient was transfused with cryoprecipitate which is a fibrinogen rich blood product.

The low platelet function value in this patient corresponds to the severe thrombocytopenia reported in this patient. Hence, the decision to transfuse random donor platelet concentrate was taken.

Q.2. How is the FFP dose to be transfused decided?

Ans. The dose of FFP is 10–15 mL/kg body weight, every 12–24 hours (The bag volume was 150 mL). Accordingly,

CHAPTER 18

the dose calculated was three units initially. The patient responded well and no further FFP transfusion was required.

Q.3. How is the cryoprecipitate dose decided?
Ans. The dose of cryoprecipitate in cases of hypofibrinogenemia/dysfibrinogenemia (as in this case) is 1–2 units/10 kg. Accordingly, the dose was calculated to be six units of cryoprecipitate in this case. (1 unit of cryo-contains 150–250 mg fibrinogen).

Q.4. On what basis was 6 units random donor platelet concentrate (RDPC) given to the patient?
Ans. The standard dose of RDPC to be transfused in adults is 5–6 units. Accordingly, 6 units of RDPC were transfused.One unit raises the platelet count by 3,000–4,000/uL.

Debriefing

A fifty-five years old female with nonalcoholic steatohepatitis (NASH) induced cirrhosis and severe hepatic coagulopathy on mechanical ventilator had grossly deranged Sonoclot parameters. The Sonoclot analysis demonstrated severe reduction in clotting factor levels, abnormal clot polymerization and severe thrombocytopenia. Clinically, the patient had to be taken up for tracheostomy, which could not be done in the face of severe mucosal bleeds. Adequate blood products were transfused. The patient responded well. Sonoclot parameters returned to almost normal. Clinically, the mucosal bleeds stopped completely.

Case 2: 32 Years Male Presented to ILBS with Chief Complaints

- Fever × 2 days
- Altered sensorium × 1 day
- Decreased urine output × 1 day

On Examination

- Pallor +, Icterus +
- *CNS:* Altered sensorium
- *P/A:* Hepatosplenomegaly+, free fluid+

Diagnosis

Acute on chronic liver failure (ACLF): Alcoholic with hepatitis B reactivation.

Decompensated with ascites and jaundice, HE grade IV.

Sepsis and B/L pneumonia.

CTP (Child-pugh score)—13/15.

Clinical Review

On the basis of deteriorating clinical condition and progressive hepatic encephalopathy, patient was admitted in liver coma ICU and shifted on ventilator.

On 3rd day of admission, patient developed spontaneous, diffuse mucocutanoeus bleeds from oral cavity and nasal cavity.

The following investigations were carried out:

- *Platelet count:* 65 × 10^9/L
- *PT-INR:* 10
- *Fibrinogen:* 122 mg/dL
- *Hb:* 9.0 g/dL
- In response severe bleeding, prolonged PT-INR and thrombocytopenia Sonoclot analysis was done **(Figure 4)**.

The Sonoclot parameters obtained were as follows:

- *ACT:* 352s
- *CR:* 14.1 clot signal units/min
- *PF:* 0.0

The Sonoclot parameters were grossly deranged. PF value of 0.0 with a platelet count of 65 × 10^9/L demonstrated the possibility of severe platelet dysfunction.

Patient was transfused with several blood products to correct the hemodynamic instability.

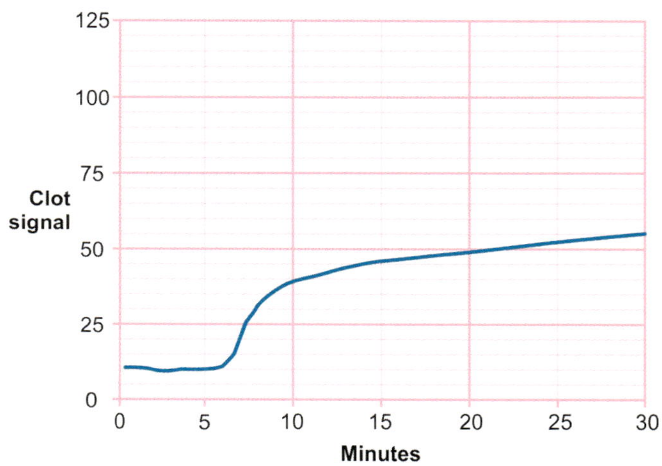

Figure 4 Abnormal Sonoclot signature in patient with diffuse mucocutaneous bleeds (Case 2)

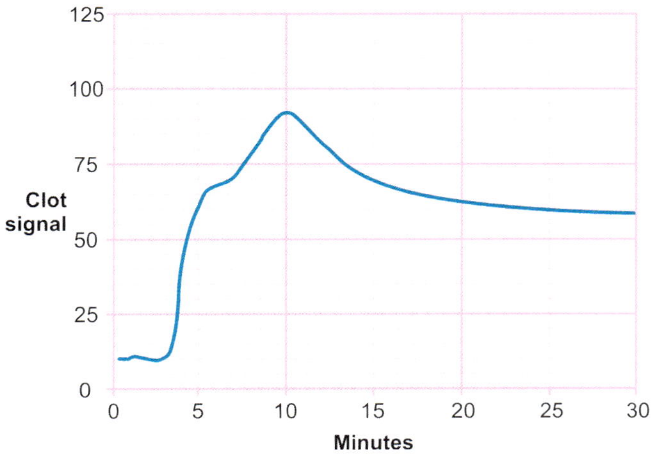

Figure 5 Corrected Sonoclot signature in patient with diffuse mucocutaneous bleeds, post-transfusion (Case 2)

Patient was transfused with:

- 6 units fresh frozen plasma
- 6 units cryoprecipitate
- 6 units of random donor platelet concentrate
- 2 units of packed rate blood cells (PRBC)

The condition of the patient improved with the transfused blood products.

A twenty-four hours later a repeat Sonoclot was performed **(Figure 5)**.

The corrected Sonoclot parameters obtained were as follows:

- *ACT:* 182 s
- *CR:* 26 clot signal units/min
- *PF:* 2.3

Results

- There was dramatic improvement in Sonoclot parameters after transfusion of blood products.
- Mucocutaneous bleeds stopped altogether.
- Patient was hemodynamically stable.

Discussion

Q.1. Why were six units RDPC transfused in this patient when the platelet counts were not dangerously low?

Ans. Though the platelet counts were 65 × 10^9/L, (which would not require transfusion of platelet concentrates in any other scenario), it is to be noted that the Sonoclot value for platelet function was 0.0. This means that no platelet activity was recorded. This could be due to platelet dysfunction which is very common in patients with advanced liver disease and may be one of the major contributors of spontaneous bleeds in this patient. Hence, it was mandatory to transfuse the platelet concentrate in this case.

Q.2. How much hemoglobin is raised per unit of PRBC transfusion?

Ans. One unit of PRBC raises hemoglobin by 1 g/dL in an adult and hematocrit by 3%.

Q.3. What is the frequency of checking the patient vitals during transfusion of various blood products?

Ans. Vitals are to be checked 15 minutes and then every half hour thereafter up to half an hour after transfusion.

Q.4. Why cannot we give whole blood instead of transfusing all the components separately in this case?

Ans. The use of whole blood in clinical settings has declined considerably in recent years. The most important reason for this is that the storage requirement of every component is different. While FFP should be stored at –30°C for maximal efficiency, the platelet concentrates are stored at 22+/–2°C with constant agitation. In contrast the whole blood is stored at 4°C which causes continuous loss of the various components, thereby compromising the efficacy of the blood product. Hence, the components are much more efficient than whole blood.

Debriefing

A thirty-five years old male patient with acute on chronic liver failure due to alcohol and hepatitis B reactivation was admitted to liver coma ICU. The patient had diffuse spontaneous bleeds with grossly deranged Sonoclot parameters. The platelet function value was recorded as nil on the analyzer. Adequate blood products were transfused and the patient responded optimally. Platelet function improved to normal values and the bleeding stopped altogether. Hemodynamic stability was restored.

Case 3: A 34 Years Old Male Presented to Our Institute with Chief Complaints

- Jaundice × 2 months
- Abdominal distension × 10 days
- Bluish discoloration (hematoma) on abdominal wall × 10 days

CHAPTER 18

On Examination

- Pallor –, Icterus ++
- *P/A:* Abdomen distended, ecchymosis +
- *Liver and spleen:* Not palpable due to distension
- Scrotal swelling +

Diagnosis

Chronic liver disease: Ethanol-related with portal hypertension.

Decompensated with jaundice, ascites, coagulopathy and presence of rectus sheath hematoma.

CTP (Child-Pugh score)—13/15.

Clinical Review

The patient was admitted in the private ward of our institute for the above mentioned clinical condition. In view of the increasing size of rectus sheath hematoma the following investigations were carried out:

- *Hb:* 5.2 g/dL
- *PCV:* 15.8%
- *Platelet count:* 180 × 10^9/L
- *PT-INR:* 1.4
- *APTT:* 29.2 (control 28.0)

The above investigations revealed severe anemia (due to hematoma formation). Surprisingly, the platelet count and PT-INR were within normal limits.

To diagnose the cause of hematoma formation in the rectus sheath, Sonoclot analysis was performed **(Figure 6)**.

The Sonoclot parameters obtained were as follows:
- *ACT:* 161s
- *CR:* 29 clot signal units/min
- *PF:* 0.9

Sonoclot parameters revealed abnormal PF value inspite of normal platelet counts. This indicated presence of possible platelet dysfunction in this patient.

Patient was transfused with:
- 3 units PRBCs
- 1 unit SDPC

2 days later a repeat Sonoclot was performed **(Figure 7)**.

The corrected Sonoclot parameters obtained were as follows:
- *ACT:* 156 s
- *CR:* 32 clot signal units/min
- *PF:* 1.5

Results

- Improvement was seen in Sonoclot parameters post-transfusion. Platelet function corrected to normal.
- The size of hematoma stopped increasing and gradually started resolving.
- Patient was managed conservatively and discharged in stable state.

Discussion

Q.1. Why was this patient given only single donor platelet concentrates (SDPC) and not any other blood product?

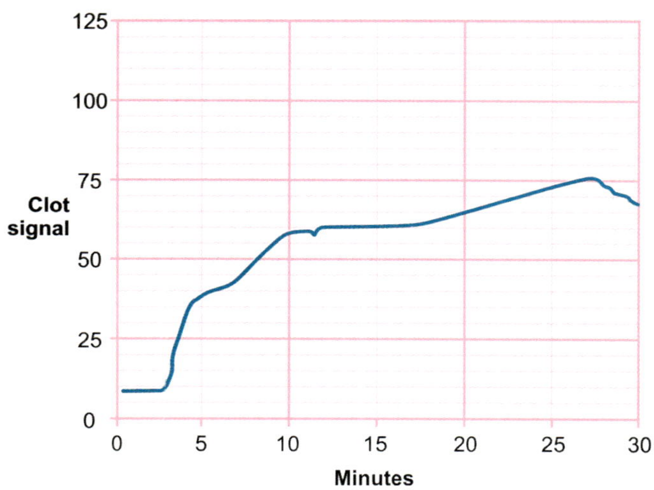

Figure 6 Abnormal Sonoclot signature in patient with rectus sheath hematoma (Case 3)

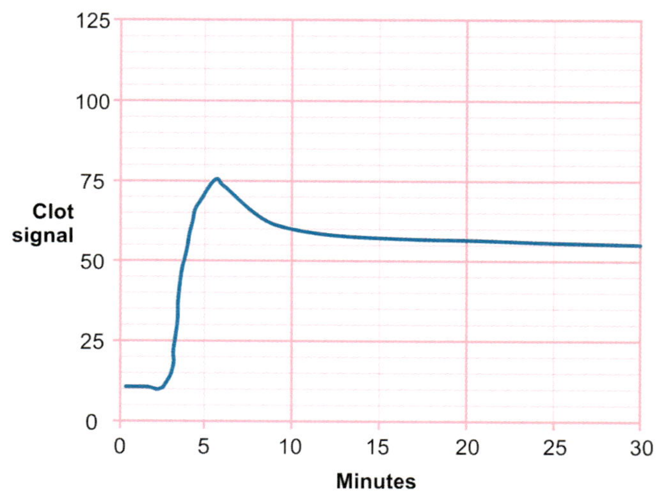

Figure 7 Corrected Sonoclot signature in patient with rectus sheath hematoma, post-transfusion (Case 3)

SECTION 4

Ans. All the Sonoclot parameters of this patient except for platelet function were normal. Other investigations including PT-INR and platelet counts were also normal. Hence, this patient demonstrates the classic case of bleeding due to platelet dysfunction in the setting of liver disease. The only treatment in this condition is transfusion of platelet concentrates. Plasma and cryoprecipitate transfusions were not required.

Q.2. How long should it take to transfuse platelets?
Ans. Platelets should be transfused over a period of 20 minutes to one hour.

Q.3. What is the standard dose for SDPC? What is the correlation between SDPC and RDPC?
Ans. The standard dose of SDPC in adults is one unit. One unit of SDPC raises the platelet count by approximately 40 × 10^9/L. One unit of SDPC is roughly equivalent to 5–6 units of RDPC.

Debriefing

A thirty-four years old male patient with alcohol related chronic liver disease and portal hypertension got admitted for evaluation of progressively increasing abdominal wall hematoma. The routine laboratory investigations showed normal platelet counts, normal PT-INR and normal APTT values. The hemoglobin levels were low owing to the increasing hematoma. The Sonoclot parameters were also normal except for gross derangement of platelet function value. This decline in platelet function value indicated the inability to form clot inspite of normal platelet counts of the patient. For correction of this platelet dysfunction, the patient was transfused with one unit of SDPC. The Sonoclot parameters subsequently corrected to normal. Also, the hematoma stopped increasing in size and resolved gradually.

Case 4: A 35 Years Old Male Patient Presented to ILBS with Chief Complaints

- Yellowish discoloration of urine and sclera × 2 weeks
- Loss of appetite and weakness × 2 weeks
- Passage of black colored stools × 4–5 days

On Examination

- Pallor–, Icterus ++
- *P/A:* Hepatosplenomegaly+, free fluid+

Diagnosis

- *Chronic liver disease:* Hepatitis C-related
- Decompensated with jaundice, ascites and GI bleed.
- Acute kidney injury.
- CTP (Child-pugh score)—12/15.

Clinical Review

The patient was admitted for treatment of above mentioned complaints. In view of the history of malena the following investigations were carried out:

- *PT-INR:* 2.68
- *Platelet count:* 150 × 10^9/L
- *Fibrinogen:* 200.8 mg/dL
- *Hemoglobin:* 10 g/dL

PT-INR was increased while platelet count and fibrinogen were within normal limits.

To determine the exact cause of coagulopathy in this patient, Sonoclot analysis was performed **(Figure 8)**.

The Sonoclot parameters obtained were as follows:

- *ACT:* 361s
- *CR:* 6.0 clot signal units/min
- *PF:* 2.5

Sonoclot parameters revealed prolonged ACT and severely low clot rate with good platelet functions.

On the basis of the Sonoclot parameters blood products were transfused.

Patient was transfused with:

- 3 units of FFP
- 4 units of cryoprecipitate.

Next day a repeat Sonoclot was performed **(Figure 9)**.

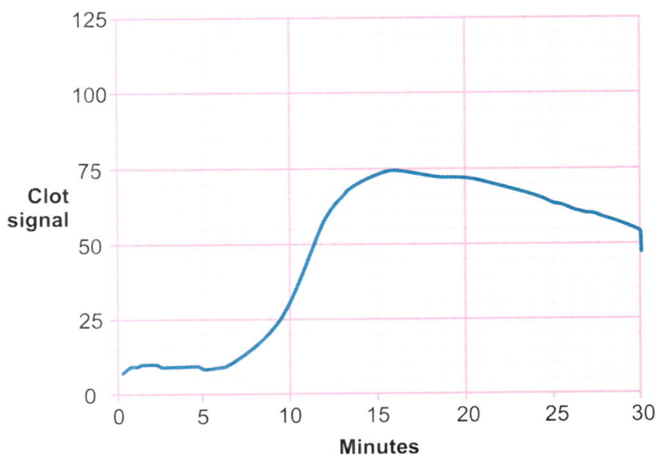

Figure 8 Abnormal Sonoclot signature in patient with malena (Case 4)

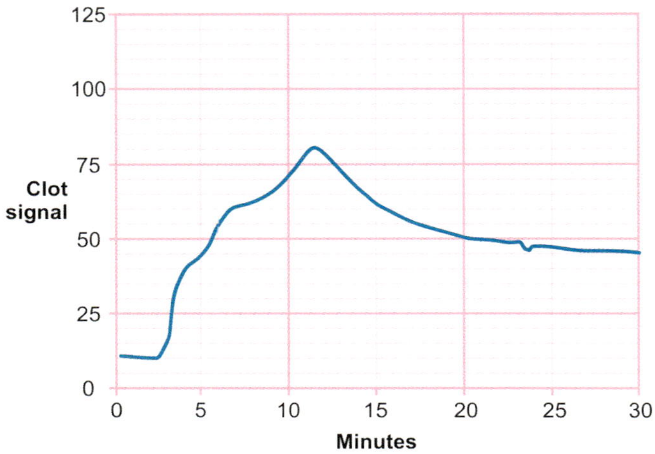

Figure 9 Corrected Sonoclot signature in patient with malena, post-transfusion (Case 4)

The corrected Sonoclot parameters obtained were as follows:

- *ACT:* 157 s
- *CR:* 32 clot signal units/min
- *PF:* 2.2

Results

- There was substantial improvement in Sonoclot parameters post-transfusion. The ACT and clot rate returned to normal levels.
- The bleeding stopped.
- Patient was being managed conservatively in the ward for other issues.

Discussion

Q.1. Why was cryoprecipitate given in this patient when fibrinogen levels were normal?

Ans. The decision to give cryoprecipitate was based on abnormal Sonoclot parameters. The abnormal clot rate which gives the rate of clot polymerization can be corrected by giving cryo ppt. Though fibrinogen concentration in this patient is normal, there is presence of abnormal fibrinogen molecule which is functionally inactive. This state of dysfibrinogenemia, which has also been described in case no. 2 previously is characteristic of patients with chronic liver diseases. The only way to correct this abnormality is to give fibrinogen rich blood products.

Q.2. Fresh frozen plasma also contains fair amount of fibrinogen. Why was cryo ppt administered additionally?

Ans. Though FFP contains some amount of fibrinogen, cryo ppt is considered to be fibrinogen rich. Also, where as one unit of FFP is around 200 mL, one unit of cryo ppt is only about 10–15 mL and contains 150–250 mg of fibrinogen. Hence, small volumes of cryo ppt correct fibrinogen adequately without the risk of fluid overload. An important point to note here is that patients with liver disease already suffer from edema and ascites and so are more prone to fluid overload. Hence, in patients with chronic liver disease one has to be very accurate and specific while administering blood products and cryoprecipitate is the product of choice in such conditions.

Q.3. What are the transfusion reactions one must look for while transfusing blood products?

Ans. It is mandatory to monitor the patient for signs and symptoms of transfusion reactions such as fever, chills, sudden hypotension, chest tightness, allergic skin rashes, etc. All observations should be duly recorded and followed up.

Debriefing

A thirty-five years old male with hepatitis C related chronic liver disease, malena and acute renal injury was admitted in general ward. The coagulation work-up for malena revealed increased PT-INR and normal fibrinogen and platelet counts. The Sonoclot parameters showed highly anomalous values of ACT and clot rate, while the platelet function was normal. These values reflected the probable presence of a functionally abnormal fibrinogen molecule (severely low clot rate and normal fibrinogen concentration). On the basis of these Sonoclot values the patient was promptly transfused with FFP and cryoprecipitate. The patient responded very well to the above transfusions. Sonoclot parameters returned to normal. Also the patient improved hemodynamically.

Case 5: A 43 Years Old Male Presented to ILBS with Chief Complaints

- Progressive jaundice × 1 and ½ months
- Abdominal pain × 15 days

On Examination

- Pallor -, Icterus ++
- *P/A:* Soft, tender, mild hepatomegaly

Doppler Study

Occlusive thrombus portal vein and SMV-likely acute onset.

Diagnosis

- *Chronic liver disease:* Ethanol-related decompensated with jaundice.
- Portal vein thrombosis
- Acute kidney injury.
- CTP(Child-Pugh score)—13/15

Clinical Review

The patient was admitted for the management of acute onset portal vein thrombosis. In view of the above mentioned clinical condition the following investigations were carried out:

- *PT-INR:* 1.7
- *Platelet count:* 120×10^9/L
- *Fibrinogen:* 244 mg/dL

The PT-INR values were prolonged and platelet counts were borderline while fibrinogen levels were absolutely normal. In view of the radiological findings and laboratory parameters, Sonoclot analysis was performed **(Figure 10)**:

The Sonoclot parameters obtained were as follows:

- *ACT:* 182s
- *CR:* 56 clot signal units/min
- *PF:* 4.0

Increased clot rate and good platelet functions in this case showed evidence of prothrombotic state.

Contrast enhanced computerized tomography (CECT) abdomen was done to confirm the presence of thrombus.

Contrast Enhanced Computerized Tomography

Extensive acute and sub-acute thrombosis of SMV and hepatic portal vein.

Management

Patient underwent intravascular thrombolysis and transluminal thrombectomy followed by heparin and urokinase infusions. No bleed was observed. Later patient was maintained on acitrom 2 mg daily on an INR of 2.5.

Two weeks later:

Patient visited the outpatient department. A repeat Sonoclot was performed to assess the prothrombotic vs coagulopathic state.

The corrected Sonoclot parameters obtained were as follows **(Figure 11)**:

- *ACT:* 200s
- *CR:* 21 clot signal units/min
- *PF:* 2.2

Result

Clot rate showed improvement. There was no evidence of hypercoagulability on Sonoclot analysis.

Repeat PT-INR: 2.5.

Patient was completely asymptomatic. He was kept under follow-up.

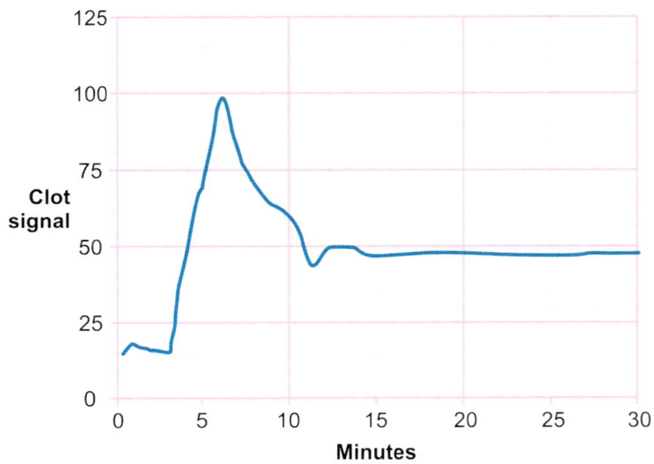

Figure 10 Abnormal Sonoclot signature in patient with occlusive portal vein thrombus (Case 5)

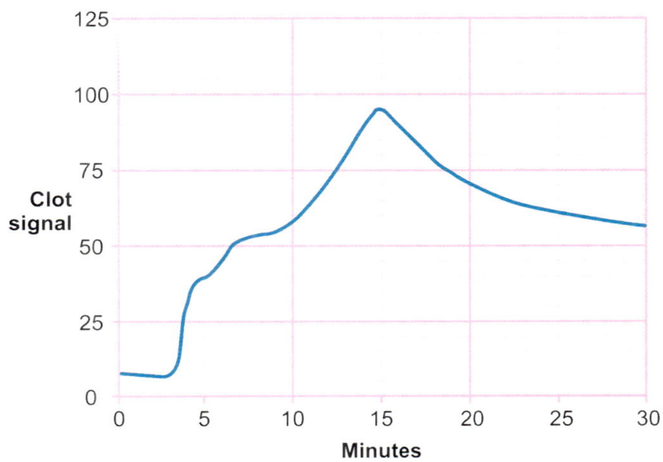

Figure 11 Corrected Sonoclot signature in patient with occlusive portal vein thrombus, post-thrombolysis (Case 5)

Discussion

Q.1. Why are patients with chronic liver disease prone to develop thrombus?

Ans. Patients with chronic liver disease are in a state of rebalanced hemostasis **(Figure 1)** as has been described in the introductory section of this chapter. This state is highly unstable and is prone to tilt either in favor of bleed or thrombosis, depending in the clinical condition of the patient. In case the balance tilts towards thrombosis, such complications result.

Q.2. Inspite of raised PT-INR in this case, why was the patient not transfused?

Ans. As has already been explained, the patients with chronic liver disease have a higher threshold of bleeding as compared to normal individuals. The counteracting mechanisms of hemostasis and thrombosis operating in these patients prevent them from bleeding even at higher PT-INR values. Hence, any amounts of unnecessary transfusions in these patients will only add up to the fluid overload, adding to additional problems and complicating the clinical picture.

Q.3. What parameters of Sonoclot reliably predict prothrombotic state?

Ans. It is difficult to state exactly what Sonoclot parameters would accurately represent prothrombotic state. A low ACT and high clot rate would definitely indicate hypercoagulability. In our case the ACT was on the higher side of normal. Only clot rate was the accurate predictor. It was because of the complexity of hemostatic defects found in patients with chronic liver disease. Hence in chronic liver disease patients, clot rate might act as the most accurate predictor of hypercoagulable state.

Debriefing

Forty-three years old male was admitted for evaluation and management of portal vein thrombus. Though the PT-INR values of the patient were on the higher side and platelet counts on the lower side, the Sonoclot parameters accurately synchronized with the clinical picture of the patient. The clot rate was much higher than normal. This patient was taken up for thrombolysis and subsequent thrombectomy and put on oral anticoagulants. The post-management Sonoclot parameters were within the normal range (though the PT-INR values were raised due to anticoagulation). Clinically, there was no evidence of either bleeding or thrombosis. The patient responded very well to the treatment and is currently under follow-up.

BIBLIOGRAPHY

1. Caldwell HS, Northup PG. Coagulation in liver disease: A guide for the clinician. Clinical Gastroenterology and Hepatology. 2013;11:1064-74.
2. Lisman T, Caldwell SH, Burroughs AK, et al. Hemostasis and thrombosis in patients with liver disease: the ups and downs. Journal of Hepatology. 2010;53(2):362-71.
3. Lisman T, Porte J. Rebalanced hemostasis in patients with liver disease: evidence and clinical consequences. Blood. 2010.
4. Saxena P, Bihari C, Rastogi A, et al. Sonoclot signature analysis in patients with liver disease and its correlation with conventional coagulation studies. Advances in Hematology, 2013; Article ID 237351.
5. Saxena P, Bihari C, Rastogi A, et al. Sonoclot signature analysis in patients with liver disease and its correlation with conventional coagulation studies. Adv Hemato 2013, 2013;(10):237351.
6. Senzolo M, Burra P, Cholongitas E, et al. New insights into the coagulopathy of liver disease and liver transplantation. World Journal of Gastroenterology. 2006;12(48):7725-36.

SECTION 4

Chapter 19

Simulation for Perioperative Coagulation Dysfunction in Liver Surgery

S Mohan

Chapter Outline

To simulate: Imitate/produce a computer model of/ pretend to feel—Oxford English Mini Dictionary.

Till recently in the developed world and to a large extent in the rest of the world medical training followed the apprentice model, where medical graduates learn the art of treating and diagnosing under the watchful eye of experienced clinicians. This goes on till the mentor decides that the mentee has acquired sufficient skills to practice the art on his own. This decision can either be subjective or objective via examinations and so forth. The ethical dilemma is of course how long can this situation be allowed in this art whereas the rest of the world have shifted to much better systems of training, e.g. aviation, astronomy, etc. Moreover medical field has started seeing the potential in teaching using computer simulations which have led to an increase in the quality of training and safety in other fields.

Anesthesia has been at the forefront among the medical specialties in absorbing this new technology. For more than a decade, simulation-based training and assessment of competencies have existed in Europe, and particularly in United Kingdom. Simulation can be used to learn and provide positive feedback in a controlled manner with no negative effects in term of patient care. Certainly, it will be helpful to have had a simulation drill rather than to face a terrible situation of having to deal with anaphylaxis or malignant hyperthermia in real life for the first time. Simulation also in the future will be helpful in evaluating the competencies learned during residency programs.

PROBLEMS IN LIVER SURGERY AND TRANSPLANTATION

In the field of liver surgery and transplantation where the expertise is available at very few places, not every anesthesia provider has the opportunity to deal first hand with coagulopathy in the operative environment. This has created a heterogeneous clinical experience for residents in anesthesia for liver transplant training. Simulation courses provid a standardized in-depth exposure to clinical issues involved in the perioperative care of liver transplant patients. Agarwal et al. found that anesthesia residents undergoing a preplacement simulation course in anesthesia for liver transplant could improve their performance by up to 92 % from a basal 75%.

ROLE OF SIMULATORS

Simulators can come in handy to train the average anesthesia provider with the necessary skills, especially when having to face scenarios with polytrauma which may involve the solid abdominal organs as well. Coagulopathy and massive blood transfusion along with other problems have been found to be the most altered physiology in patients with liver disease needing better care.

In the area of liver transplantation where the coagulation balance is so delicate and individualized that no two patients behave in the same way under the same operating scenarios, simulators can help immensely in training programs and for evaluation as well. Anesthetic management practices for liver transplantation vary across different institutes both within and across countries. The use of cell salvage, transesophageal echocardiography, thromboelastography, and ultrasound guidance for catheter placement vary among institutions. Coagulation parameter monitoring like activated clotting time, prothrombin time, international normalized ratio (INR), fibrinogen, platelet function, and thromboelastography vary considerably among centers even in developed countries. Atleast a quarter of the surveyed institutes in the US do not seem to use point of care coagulation monitoring devices leading to varied transfusion practices and may be the consequences out of them.

SECTION 4

ROLE OF ANTIFIBRINOLYTICS

Administration of antifibrinolytics and more expensive coagulation adjuncts like activated factor VII do not seem to be done on a scientific basis across the world. A relationship between case volume, anesthetic technique, and outcomes in surgical procedures other than liver transplantation has been described in the literature. Simulation can be a valuable strategy to elucidate latent conditions, for which simulation interventions can then be designed. Simulation can also be used to standardize practice in the field of liver transplantation, coagulation and transfusion medicine which might improve quality across geographic locations. This will also help introduce tested technologies like point of care devices like coagulation analyzers, glucose management, etc. which will go a long way in improving care for these clinical scenarios. Designing simulation-based strategies could help standardize treatment algorithms across centres. Presumed benefits might include a reduced need for blood products and, therefore, a lower transfusion-related cost. Studies have shown patients receiving over 6 red blood cell units intraoperatively displayed reduced survival. Convincing evidence has been provided by Hevesi et al. when standardized teams used set protocols, especially intraoperative transfusion practices to influence mortality rates in a beneficial manner. Ozier has collected data to show marked interinstitutional differences in blood use. Differences in transfusion practices probably account for a substantial part of the variability. Recent data also have demonstrated ongoing controversy relating to volume replacement therapy and its impact on blood loss.

Simulation can be either web/computer based or based on virtual reality. Initial simulation courses were developed based on resuscitation stimulators. Immersive virtual reality simulators seem to be the mostly used model in anesthesia training. For the purpose of developing transfusion policies, credentialing and most importantly on going certification virtual reality based simulators seem to be the preferred choice.

BIBLIOGRAPHY

1. Abbas R, et al. Blood transfusion requirement during liver transplantation is an important risk factor for mortality. J Am Coll Surg. 2013;216(5):902-7.
2. Agarwal S, et al. Simulation: A teaching tool for liver transplantation anesthesiology. Clin Transplant. 2012; 26:564–70.
3. Boin IF, et al. Intraoperative massive transfusion decreases survival after liver transplantation. Transplant Proc. 2008;40:789.
4. Boin IF. Intraoperative massive transfusion decreases survival after liver transplantation. Transplant Proc. 2008;40(3):789-91.
5. Christing SP. Simulation and quality improvement in anaesthesiology. Anesthesiology Clin. 2011;29:13-28.
6. Dalmau A, Sabate´ A, Aparicio I. Hemostasis and coagulation monitoring and management during liver transplantation. Curr Opin Organ Transplant. 2009;14:286.
7. Hevesi ZG. Designated liver transplant anesthesia team reduces blood transfusion, need for mechanical ventilation, and duration of intensive care. Liver Transpl . 2009;15(5):460-5.
8. Ozier Y. Changing trends in transfusion practice in liver transplantation. Curr Opin Organ Transplant. 2008; 13(3):304-9.
9. Roman S, et al. Anesthesia for liver transplantation in United States academic centers: intraoperative practice. Journal of Clinical Anesthesia. 2013;25:542-50.

Chapter 20

The Coagulation Tests are Simple to Perform and Fascinating but Difficult to Interpret

Vilash Hiremath, Sanketh Hiremath, Arun Kumar

Chapter Outline

BLEEDING PATIENT: LABORATORY EVALUATION

In all bleeding cases the first evaluation to start with bleeding time, platelet count, prothrombin time, activated partial thromboplastin time and thrombin time. If the cause of bleeding is not evident, then second series of tests for fibrinolysis and fibrin polymerization detected by urea clot solubility/factor XIII chromogenic assay.[1]

Global hemostasis test/clot viscoelastic test by Sonoclot coagulation and platelet function analyzer **(Figures 1 and 2)**: Sonoclot almost exclusively used in open heart surgery and liver transplant procedures to access coagulation process particularly in trauma. Entire process includes fibrin formation, clot strength/rate and clot lysis with cellular composition leading to hemostasis providing graphical and numerical presentation. Interestingly these tests does not obey classic coagulation cascade model with intrinsic and extrinsic pathways. Sonoclot gives additional information on clot retraction depends on the platelet function. Citrated or native whole blood, platelet-rich plasma (PRP) and percutaneous pericardio-peritoneal shunt (PPP) can be used with or without activators. These instruments can be used for predicting tool for hypercoagulation which depends on the high thrombin generation, for instance **(Figures 3A and B)**.

Thalassemia patient with splenectomy have normal thrombin generation still have hypercoagulation state will be important diagnostic. Decreased activated clotting time (ACT) and normal/increased clot strength will be suggestive of hypercoagulation. Plasma based assay like prothrombin time (PT), activated partial thromboplastin time (APTT) abnormality in liver disease will not detect hypercoagulation in spite of clear evidence of increasing bleeding tendency.

Hyperfibrinolysis is neglected test in coagulation lab due to insufficient predicting tool for hyperfibrinolysis. It can be easily detected by Sonoclot viscoelastic test to differentiate primary or secondary fibrinolysis. Massive bleeding is major cause in trauma, primary

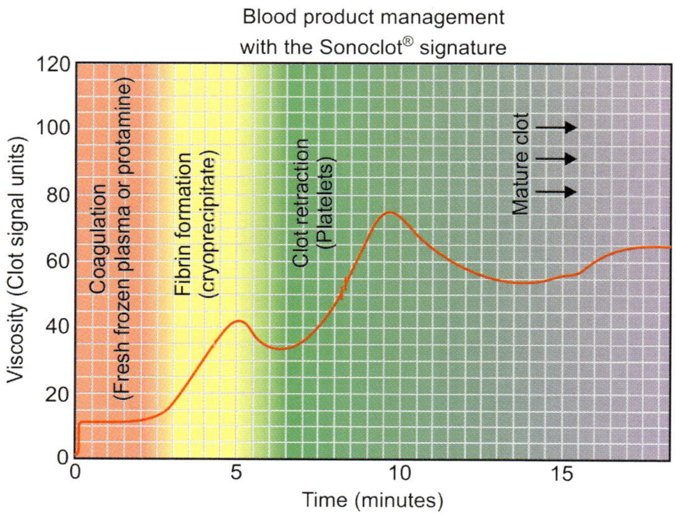

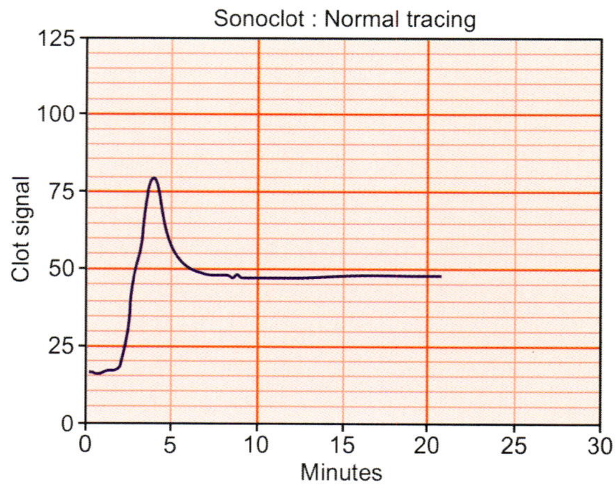

Style	Time	Test	Application	Result	Range
	9:33:32	gbACT+	Normal range	ACT = 119	100.C–180.0
				Clot Rate = 42	(9.0–45.0)
				Platelet function =4.2	(> 1.5)

Figure 1 Sonoclot tracing showing fibrin formation to mature clot process

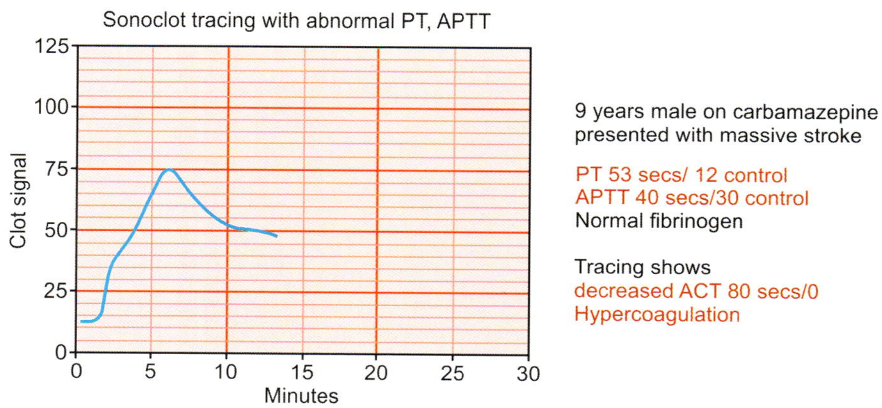

Style	Time	Patient	Test	Result	Range
	3:32:22 PM		gbACT+	ACT = 80 ✓	100.0–155.0
				Clot Rate = 33	(11.0–35.0)
				Platelet function = 2.8	(> 1.5)

Figure 2 Hypercoagulation detection in liver disease

Abbreviations: ACT, activated clotting time; PT, prothrombin time, APTT, activated partial thromboplastin time

pulmonary hypertension (PPH) and dengue shock syndrome prostate cancer, target pharmacotherapy of thrombolytic which is under diagnosed.[2]

Factor XIII deficiency: Most under diagnosed, unawareness at clinical side and incorrect diagnostic test in the lab contribute to this problem. Clinical symptoms may or may not suggestive of factor XIII deficiency still need to do traditional clot solubility test used to screen factor XIII deficiency is qualitative and detect severe cases only. Prothrombin time (PT), activated partial thromboplastin time (APTT), thrombin time (TT) do not show prolongation, if possible Factor XIII chromogenic assay is recommended which measure ammonia released during the transglutaminase reaction. Factor XIII deficiency is frequently associated

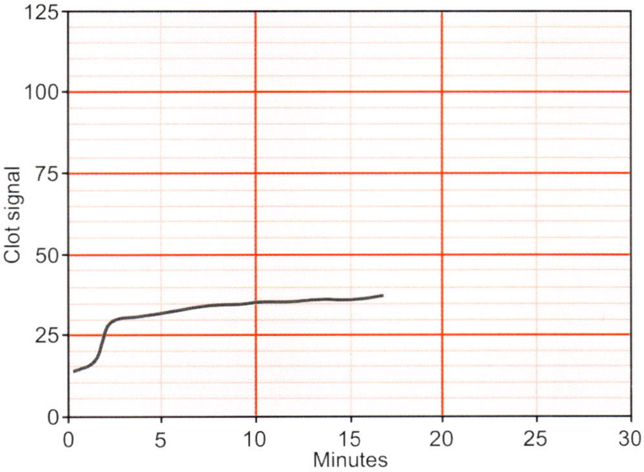

Test	Result	Range
gbACT+	ACT = 93	(100.0–155.0)
	Clot Rate = 20	(9.0–35.0)
	Platelet Function = 0.1	(> 1.5)

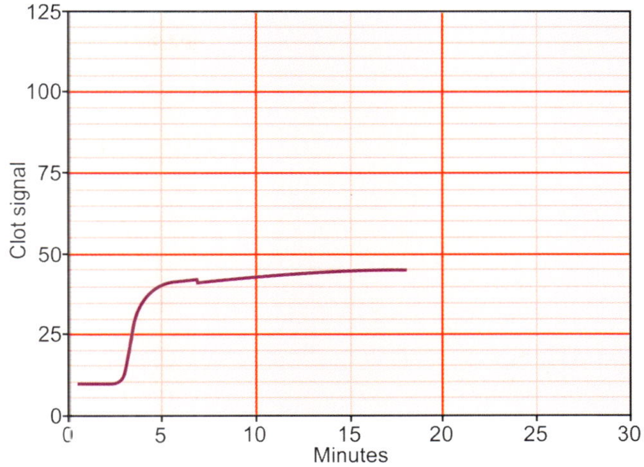

Test	Result	Range
gbACT+	ACT = 158	(100.0–180.0)
	Clot Rate = 35	(11.0–45.0)
	Platelet Function = 0.0	(> 1.5)

- Bleeding disorder work-up: Epistaxis
- Sonoclot PF shows 0.1 and 0.0, suggestive platelet dysfunction
- Platelet aggregation shows decreased aggregation to ADP, AA, Collagen and normal response to ristocetin suggestive of thrombasthenia (Platelet count should be normal)

Chnl	Reag	Lot No.	Reag. Conc.	Units	PPP	PRP
1	Adenosine diphosphate		20	uM	0.074	0.949
2	Arachidonic acid		500	ug/mL	0.071	0.838
3	Collagen		10	ug/mL	0.069	0.959
4	Ristocetin		1	mg/mL	0.065	0.744

Chnl	Curve No.	Max %	TMax	Slope	Slope 2	Lag	% Area under curve
1 ADP	842	2.2	1	3.4		596.5	
2 ADP	843	2.1	295	11.0		12.3	
3 COL	844	8.0	328	10.9		23.9	
4 RISTO	845	35.0	50	54.2		2.7	

Chnl	Date and Time	Comment
1	4/8/2014 3:30:53 PM	
2	4/8/2014 3:31:24 PM	
3	4/8/2014 3:31:31 PM	
4	4/8/2014 3:31:38 PM	

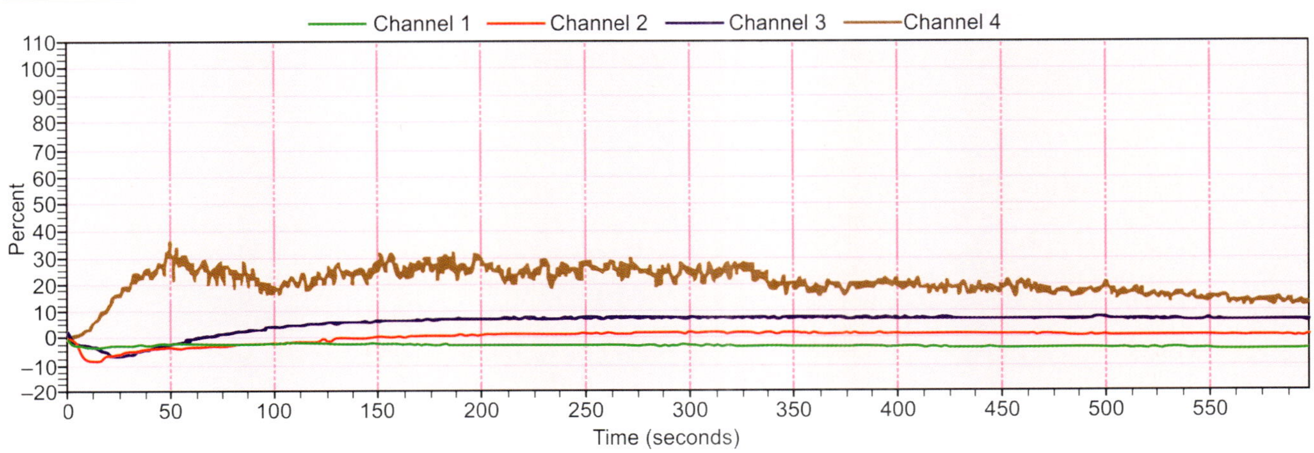

Figure 3A Sonoclot and platelet aggregation work-up in a case of epistaxis

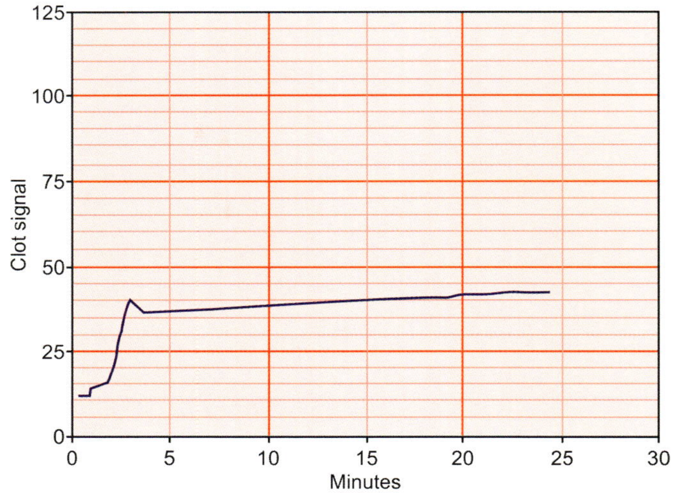

Test	Result	Range
gbACT+	ACT = 104	(100.0–180.0)
✓	Clot Rate = 28	(11.0–45.0)
	Platelet Function = 0.7	(> 1.5)

- Bleeding disorder work-up: Epistaxis
- Sonoclot PF shows 0.7, suggestive platelet dysfunction
- Platelet aggregation shows decreased aggregation to ADP, AA, collagen and Ristocetin suggestion of thrombasthenia (Platelet count should be normal)

Chnl		Reag	Lot No.	Reag. Conc.	Units	PPP	PRP
1	✓	Adencsine diphosphate		20	uM	0.1	0.359
2	✓	Arachidonic acid		500	ug/mL	0.102	0.357
3	✓	Collagen		10	ug/mL	0.098	0.365
4	✓	Ristocetin		1	mg/mL	0.095	0.323

Chnl	Curve No.	Max %	TMax	Slope	Slope 2	Lag	% Area under curve
1	825 ✓	2.0	60	4.7		582.4	
2	826 ✓	5.3	39	10.8		597	
3	827 ✓	3.0	20	16.9		595.9	
4	828 ✓	1.3	6	14.4		454.6	

Chnl	Date and Time	Comment
1	3/28/2014 1:23:16 PM	
2	3/28/2014 1:23:25 PM	
3	3/28/2014 1:23:31 PM	
4	3/28/2014 1:23:37 PM	

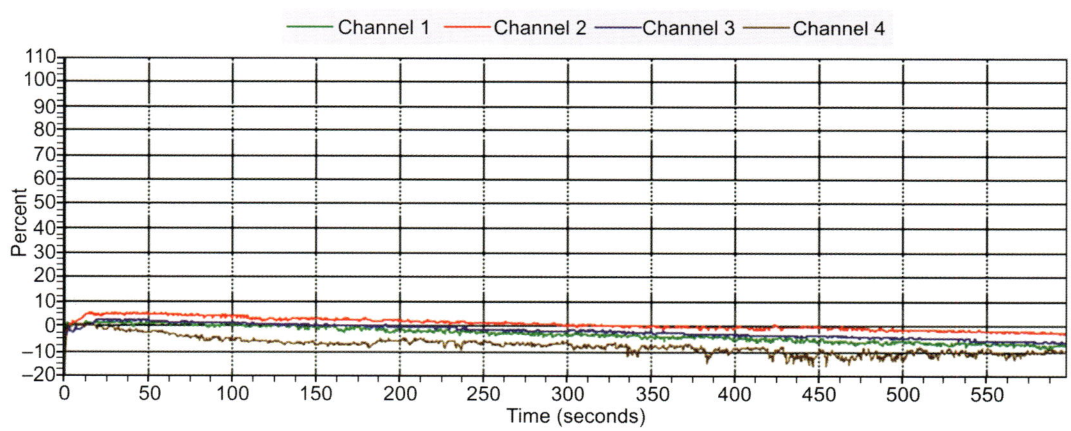

Figure 3B Case of thrombasthenia

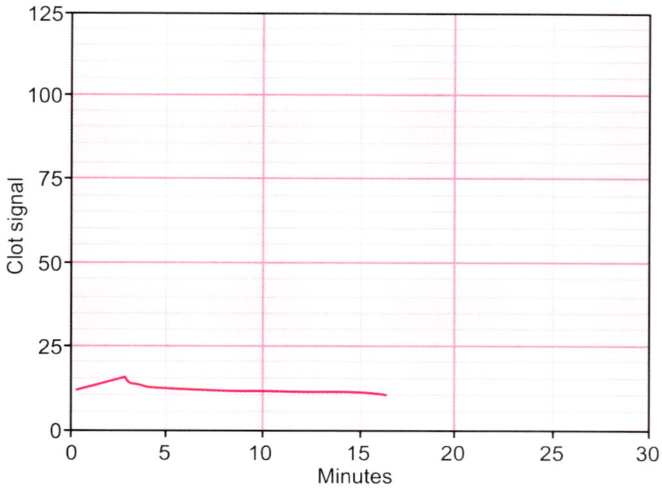

Test	Result	Range
gbACT+	ACT = ? > 980	(100.0–180.0)
	Clot Rate = ?	(9.0–35.0)
	Platelet Function = ?	(> 1.5)

- **2 years old boy bleeding disorder work-up**:
- Pro onged ACT due to nonavailability of fibrinogen
- Fibrinogen level < 1%
- No thrombin generation also can be seen in factor deficiency

Figure 4 Case of afibrinoçenemia

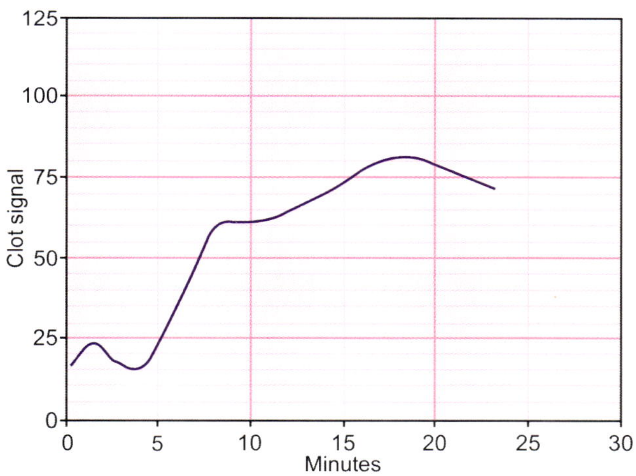

Test	Result	Range
gbACT+	ACT = 254	(100.0–180.0)
	Clot Rate = 13.8	(9.0–35.0)
	Platelet Function = 1.8	(> 1.5)

Figure 5 Case of direct thrombin inhibitors (DTI) monitoring

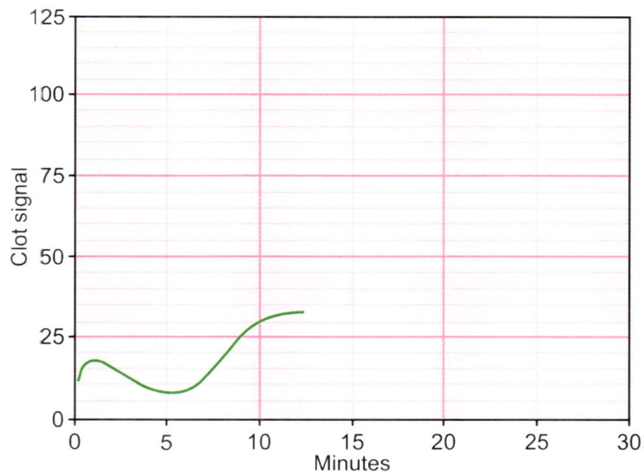

Test	Result	Range
gbACT+	ACT = 369	(100.0–155.0)
	Clot Rate = 7.7	(9.0–35.0)
	Platelet Function = ?	(> 1.5)

Figure 6 Case of low molecular weight heparin (LMWH) monitoring

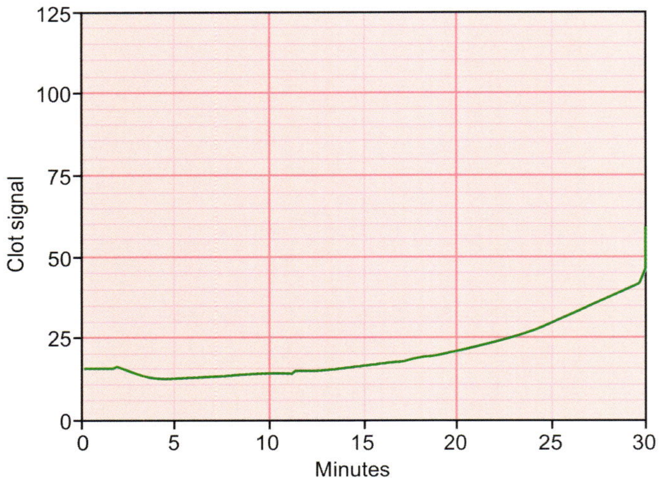

- 10 years boy, scrotum swelling, postoperative bleeding
- Factor VIII < 1%
- PF 0.1, not due to platelet dysfunction (no thrombin generation)

Test	Result	Range
gbACT+	ACT = 711 ✓	(100.0–155.0)
	Clot Rate = 1.0	(9.0–35.0)
	Platelet Function = 0.1	(> 1.5)

Figure 7 Case of hemophilia A

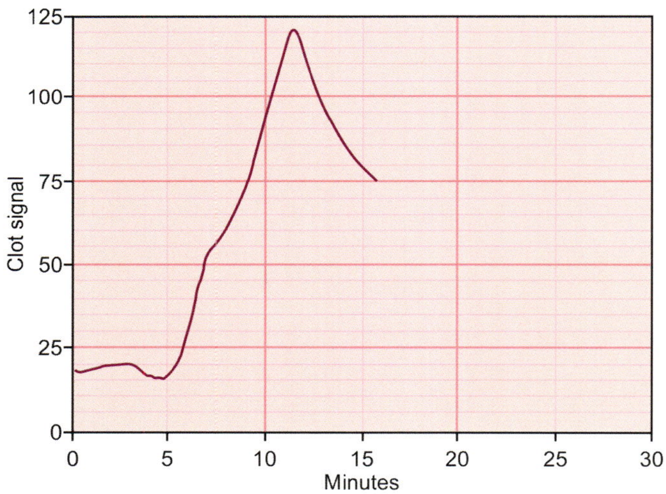

- 54 years male, skin bleeding over thigh and back
- ACT increased due to factor X deficiency (< 1%)
- Differential diagnosis—acquired hemophilia

Test	Result	Range
gbACT+	ACT = 303 ✓	(100.0–180.0)
	Clot Rate = 20	(9.0–45.0)
	Platelet Function = 4.5	(> 1.5)

Figure 8 Case of amyloidosis

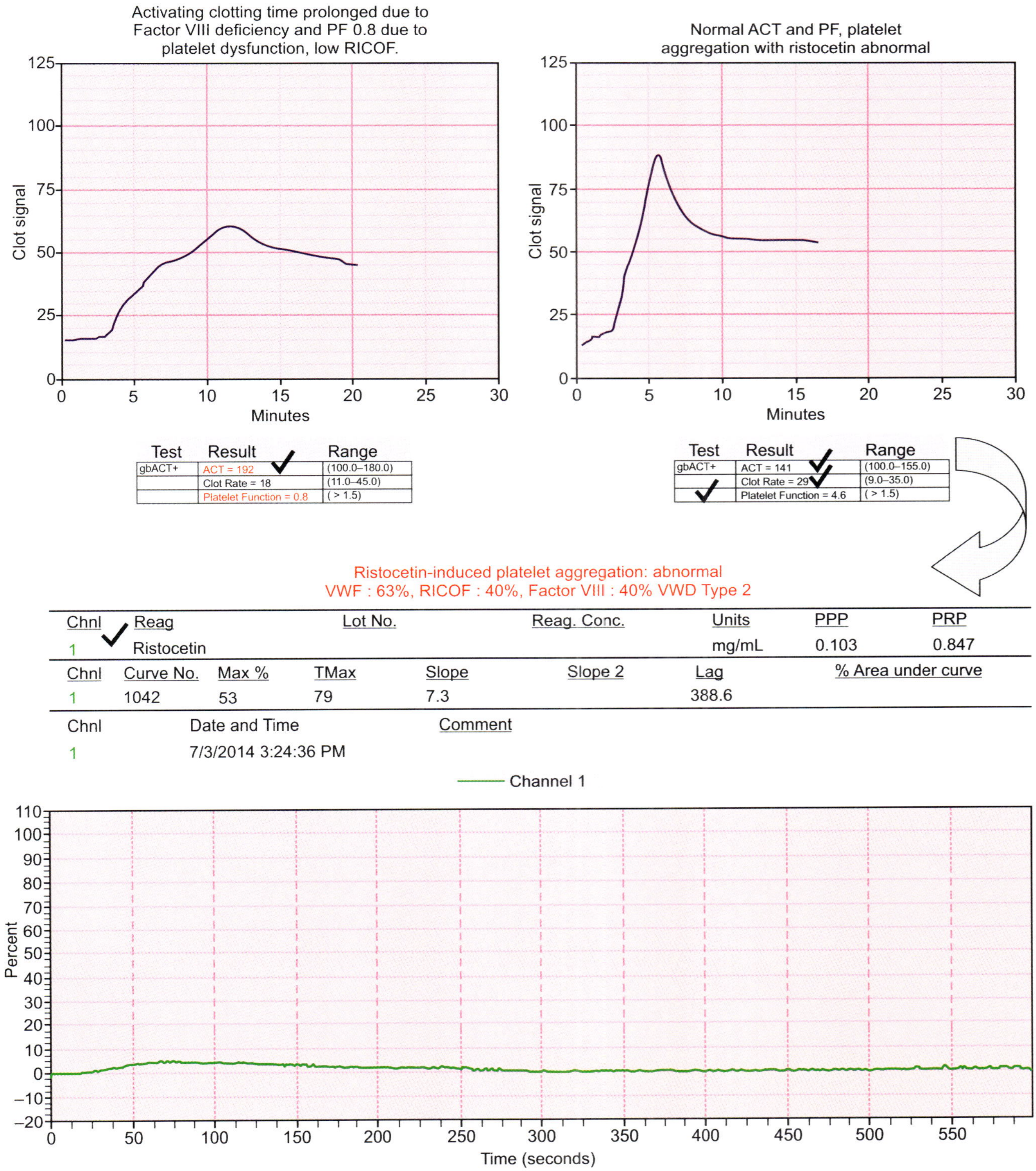

Figure 9 von Willebrand disease: Activating clotting time (ACT) prolonged due to factor VIII deficiency and PF 0.8 due to platelet dysfunction, low ristocetin cofactor activity (RiCOf)

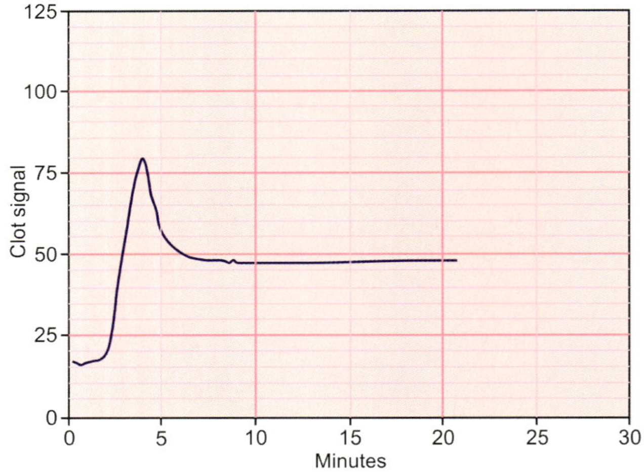

Test	Result	Range
gbACT+	ACT = 119	(100.0–180.0)
	Clot Rate = 42	(9.0–45.0)
	Platelet Function = 4.2	(> 1.5)

Ristocetin aggregation abnormal, VWF normal, Abs to GPIbα (Platelet antibody)

Chnl	Reag	Lot No.	Reag. Conc.	Units	PPP	PRP
1 ✓	Adenosine diphosphate		20	uM	0.054	0.83
2 ✓	Arachidonic acid		500	ug/mL	0.072	0.803
3 ✓	Collagen		10	ug/mL	0.037	0.77
4 ✓	Ristocetin		1	mg/mL	0.027	0.729

Chnl	Curve No.	Max %	TMax	Slope	Slope 2	Lag	% Area under curve
1	1100 ADP	88.5	469	128.7		5.2	
2	1101 AA	91.1	307	128.0		8.3	
3	1102 COL	89.3	373	150.8		29.6	
4	1103 RISTO	2.1	600	3.1		150.7	

Chnl	Date and Time	Comment
1	7/16/2014 10:03:32 AM	
2	7/16/2014 10:04:00 AM	
3	7/16/2014 10:04:12 AM	
4	7/16/2014 10:04:20 AM	

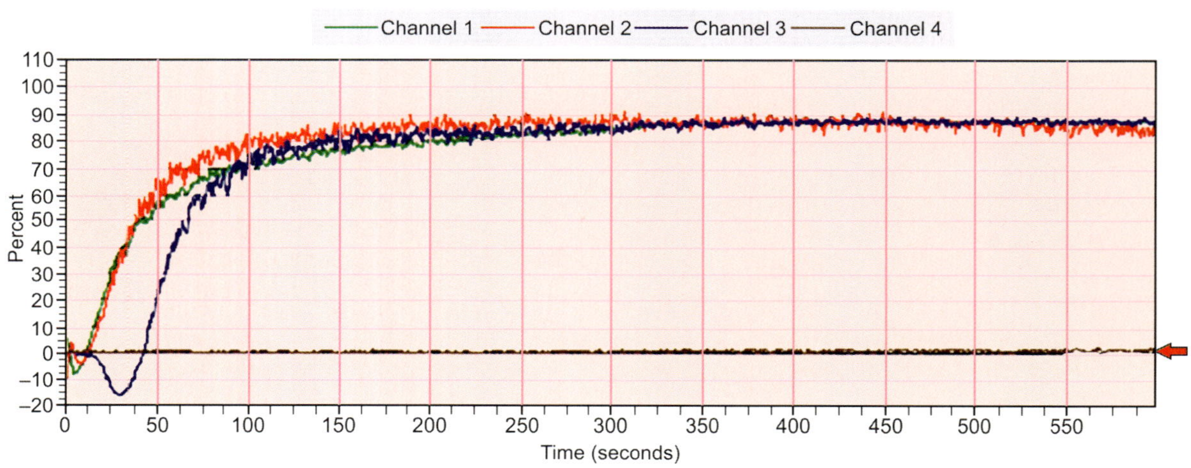

Figure 10 Case of cutaneous vasculitis

with impaired wound healing and leads to abortion in pregnant women.

Sonoclot does not detect platelet adhesion in some cases hence not sensitive to von Willebrand's disease (VWD). However, it can detect platelet dysfunction due to GPIIb/IIIa receptor which depends on thrombin generation. This test is good for monitoring of bypassing agent, factor replacement in hemophilia, afibrinogenemia and guides transfusion.[3]

VON WILLEBRAND DISEASE

von Willebrand disease (VWD) may not present like textbook fashion, under diagnosed because of heterogeneous disorder with varying mucocutaneous bleeding phenotype caused by von Willebrand factor (VWF) deficiency or abnormality and may be mistakenly identified as Shaken baby syndrome (SBS) in infants. Normal APTT, factor VIII, VWF antigen does not exclude VWD, additional tests like ristocetin-induced platelet aggregation (RIPA), von Willebrand factor (VWF) ristocetin cofactor activity (RiCOf) require to diagnose. People with blood group O generally will have lower levels than non-O blood group. All puberty menorrhagia case should evaluate for VWD/GT. Acquired VWD is very common.

Factor VIII Clot-based Assay

One stage clot based assay is the most generally used for technical simplicity. Mild factor deficiency is missed hence Factor VIII by chromogenic assay will be preferred choice. This test is alone not sufficient to identify, diagnose and exclude VWD. Normal level will not always exclude and an abnormal level will not necessarily define, nor give information on the subtypes. However, Factor VIII chromogenic assay preferred in postoperative bleeding due to acute phase reactant and Hemophilia monitoring.

Ristocetin-induced platelet aggregation requires rapid testing of freshly collected blood samples to evaluate qualitative defects from type 2B, however latex immunoassay uses gain of function GP1b∝ to bind VWF cannot be used. This test requires VWF and platelet both to be from patient.

RIPA and RiCOf cannot be replaced for each other, both test should be done.

RIPA abnormal can be seen in Bernard-Soulier syndrome (BSS), VWD and antibody to GP1bα due to autoimmune specifically cutaneous purpura.[4]

Impaired platelet function test includes aggregations assay using light transmittance aggregometry on platelet rich plasma and whole blood impedance method for thrombocytopenic samples it is good to start with Ristocetin (RIPA) to evaluate BSS, VWD type 2B and antibody to GP1b∝. When there is impaired aggregation with all agonist except Ristocetin with or without thrombocytopenia Glanzmann thrombasthenia to be considered. Acquired GT is common in multiple myeloma, Evan syndrome, lymphoproliferative disorder **(Figures 4 to 10)**.

Thrombin Time

One of the most common problem in hospital lab is heparin contamination, if prolongation is not due to heparin possible cause of generalized bleeding is highly suggestive of disseminated intravascular coagulation (DIC). No single test is sensitive or specific for DIC, FDP-D-Dimer mild positivity simply indicate fibrinolysis, Sonoclot based clot viscoelastic test will best tool detect primary/secondary fibrinolysis.

Activated partial thromboplastin time (APTT) prolongation will be due to factor deficiency in bleeding, lupus anticoagulant (LA) due to antiphospholipid antibody syndrome (APLA), contact factor deficiency and LA in pregnancy, Factor VIII inhibitor in hemophilia and liver disease. Few thrombotic patients presented with bleeding, prolonged APTT due LA with hypoprothrombinemia.

THROMBOTIC PATIENT: LABORATORY EVALUATION (SUMMARY)

As Shakespeare wrote "what's in a name that which we call rose by any other word would smell as sweet". May be roses do not have an "image problem" **(Figure 11)** but same cannot be said for the most famous or infamous, misnomers in thrombosis called lupus anticoagulant and antiphospholipid syndrome.

Antiphospholipid antibodies (APLA) detection should be optimal, reproducible and unfortunately these tests are poorly standardized, test to includes LA, ACA beta 2 GPI. These tests are here to study, till better ones replace them.

Lupus anticoagulant: It is generally a prolonged APTT that prompts an evaluation for LA, APTT reagent composition can vary widely. Normal APTT does not exclude LA, acute phase reactant and pregnancy will shorten APTT mask weak LA.

CHAPTER 20

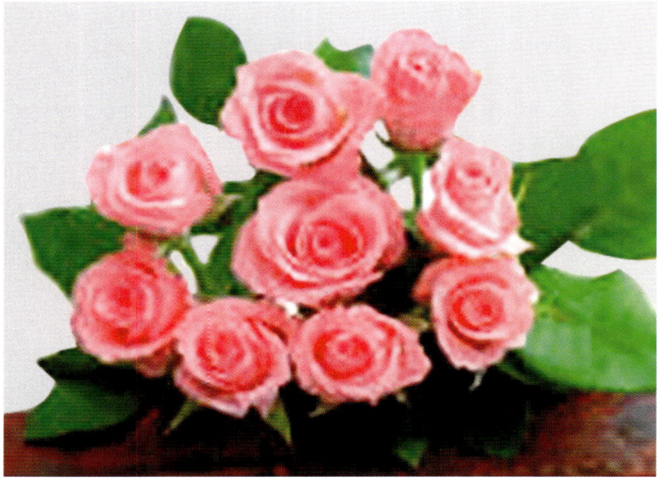

Figure 11 Roses have no image bleeding problem

Dilute Russell's viper venom time (DRVVT): Russell viper venom contains an enzyme that directly activates Factor X. LA mixing study is still (debatable) can help to eliminates cause other than LA, however mixing study cannot be over emphasized.

Lupus anticoagulant (LA) is more strongly associated with thrombosis than anticardiolipin antibodies (ACA) and positive beta 2 GPI is more strongly associated with thrombosis than anticardiolipin (ACA).

Antiphospholipid antibodies (APLA) panel should include fibrinogen assay and TT to rule out dysfibrinogenemia

Antiphospholipid antibodies (APLA) heterogeneity and reagent variation have prevented for generation of reference material as gold standard assay.

REFERENCES

1. Quick AJ, Hussey CV, Geppert MT. Prothrombin: analytical and clinical comparison of the one and two stage methods. Am J Med Sci. 1963;246:517-26. [PubMed]
2. Ratnoff OD. Why do people bleed? In: Wintrobe MM, ed. Blood, pure and eloquent. New York: McGraw Hill, 1980; 601-42.
3. Fish R, Pinney J, Jain P, et al. The incidence of major hemorrhagic complications after renal biopsies in patients with monoclonal gammopathies. Clin J Am Soc Nephrol. 2010;2010:1977-80.
4. Soares SM, Fervenza FC, Lager DJ, et al. Bleeding complications after transcutaneous kidney biopsy in patients with systemic amyloidosis: single center experience in 101 patients. Am J Kidney Dis. 2008;52: 1079-83.

Chapter 21

Point-of-Care Testing of Coagulation in the Bleeding Cardiac Patients

Poonam Malhotra Kapoor, Klaus Gorlinger, Vandana Bhardwaj

Chapter Outline

INTRODUCTION

Nowadays, point of care (POC) devices like thromboelastography (TEG), Sonoclot analyzer and the newly FDA approved rotational thromboelastometry (ROTEM) with faster results to assess coagulopathies are available on bedside of patients. These viscoelastic POC devices are used to measure the time until clot formation, the dynamics of clot formation, and the stability of clots over time.[1] The TEG device has the limitation of inability to distinguish hypofibrinogenemia from thrombocytopenia. However, ROTEM is more suitable as fibrin-specific clot formation (FIBTEM) can be analyzed by inhibiting PLT-fibrinogen interaction using cytochalasin D. However, point-of-care testing (POC) devices such as thromboelastogram (TEG), rotational thromboelastometry (ROTEM), Sonoclot and others provide *in vitro* assessment of global coagulation, starting from clot formation and continuing through maximal clot amplitude, retraction, and clot lysis.

Coagulopathy in critically-ill patients undergoing major surgeries is common and of multifactorial origin. The bleeding associated with coagulopahy and transfusion of blood products is a concerned cause of morbidity and mortality.[2,3] The management of these patients was earlier guided by conventional laboratory coagulations tests like platelet count, prothrombin time, activated partial thromboplastin time and serum fibrinogen levels.[5] The lengthy turnaround time of these laboratory tests was a cause of undue delay and improper treatment.[4] The standard laboratory tests, such as prothrombin time (PT) and activated partial thromboplastin time (aPTT), fail to incorporate cellular elements and analyze isolated component of the coagulation cascade. These laboratory tests overlook essential factors such as rate of clot formation, maximal clot strength, and degree of clot dissolution.

Viscoelastic POC techniques (ROTEM®, TEG®) are based on thromboelastography, which was described decades ago by Hartert.[5] These tests are used to measure the time until clot formation begins, the dynamics of clot formation, and the solidity and stability of clots over time are measured. They enable parallel measurements to be performed on a single blood sample after clotting has been activated using a variety of agonists. A special advantage of viscoelastic techniques is that they can directly detect hyperfibrinolysis. Aggregometric tests combined with viscoelastic methods yield a far broader diagnostic spectrum than do conventional laboratory testing of coagulation.

POSTOPERATIVE BLEEDING AND TRANSFUSION REQUIREMENTS

Postoperative bleeding is a common problem following surgery for cardiac patients **(Figure 1)**. This increased incidence of bleeding has been attributed to pre-existing hematological abnormalities.[6] Particularly, in the cyanotic patient, an association between thrombocytopenia and high hematocrit as well as decreased fibrinogen levels has been demonstrated.[7] Systemic heparinisation and exposure to cardiopulmonary bypass (CPB) during surgery further increases the risk of bleeding exponentially.[8] Presently, postoperative bleeding in these patients is managed by transfusion of blood and blood products based primarily on repeated measurements of activated clotting time (ACT) and guided by drain output as well as hematocrit readings. The choice of blood product to be transfused remains arbitrary as the routine laboratory evaluation of platelet count, platelet function, prothrombin time (PT), activated partial thromboplastin time (aPTT), fibrinogen assay, etc. This empirical transfusion of blood products often results in malutilization of limited resources, additional cost and the risk of acquiring blood-borne diseases and transfusion-related immunological reactions.

TRANSFUSION ASSOCIATED CIRCULATORY OVERLOAD

Transfusion associated circulatory overload (TACO) is an established, but grossly underdiagnosed and underreported complication of blood transfusion. TACO leads to a prolonged hospital stay and morbidity in the patients developing this complication[9] **(Figures 2 and 3)** in the form of a circulatory overload.

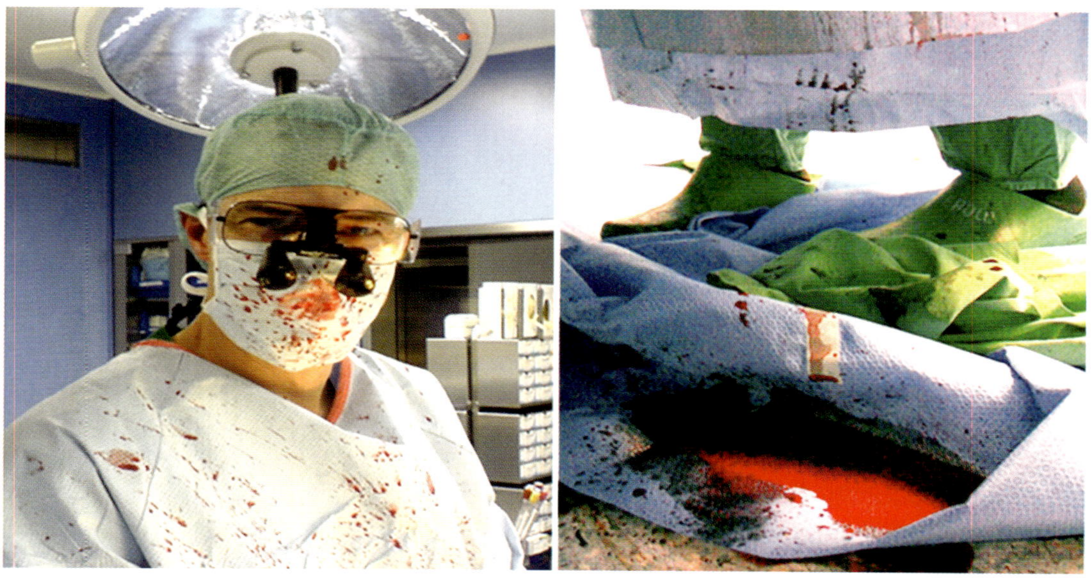

Figure 1 The cardiac surgical patient bleeds

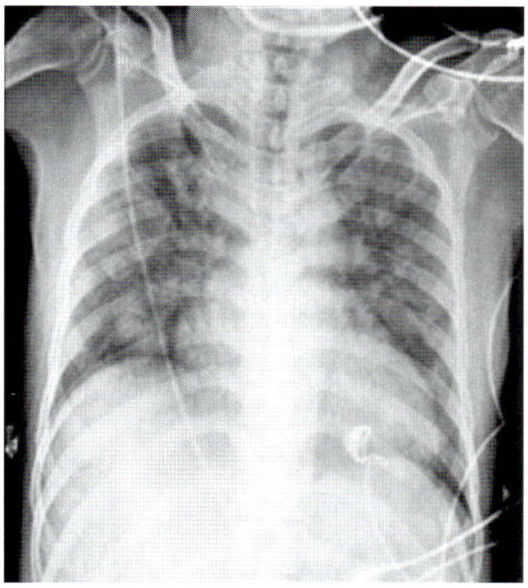

Figure 2 Chest X-ray after transfusion associated circulatory overload

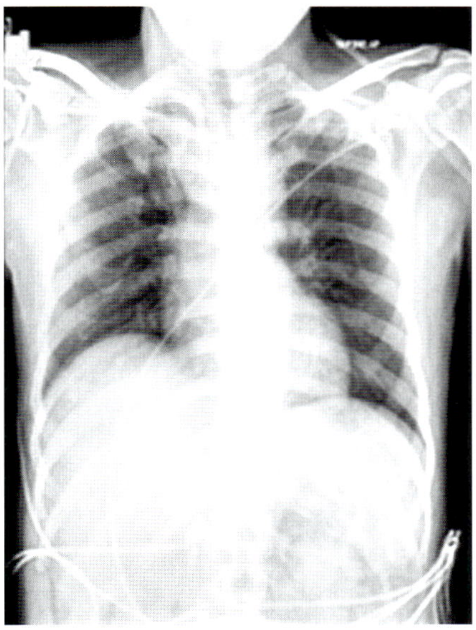

Figure 3 Resolved transfusions associated circulatory overload

COAGULATION TESTING IN THE PERIOPERATIVE PERIOD

Coagulation testing in the perioperative period remains unsatisfactory with ACT alone. There is high dilemma and priority attached to the exact parameter to decide the final transfusion types.

Platelet function in particular is of interestedly in cardiac surgery as cardiopulmonary bypass itself creates known platelet dysfunction, but also because more and more patients are on antiplatelet agents due to coronary stent procedures. Viscoelastic point-of-care tests like Sonoclot Analysis (Sienco Inc., Arvada, Colo), thromboelastography and rapid thromboelastometry gives complete functional assessment of different aspects of the entire coagulation cascade as well as that of the platelets and is cheaper, quicker and can be performed at the patient's bedside. They come in handy in such a scenario as they give minute to minute changes in platelet function with a typical signature curve for each machine.

MANAGEMENT OF BLEEDING PATIENT

The evolving role of the blood bank in the management of the bleeding patient is now well described in literature. The impact of TEG as an early diagnostic predictor for bleeding is known. Even in both TEG and ROTEM are usually thought to be POC instruments, there are some technical differences between the two instruments. In the ROTEM, the torsion wire rotates into the cup **(Figure 4)**. This gives a great stability to the instrument, regardless of disturbances the environment, and that makes it suitable as a POC instrument in the emergency room. In the TEG instrument, the cup rotates into the torsion wire and as a consequence, vibrations and other kind of physical disturbances near the instrument

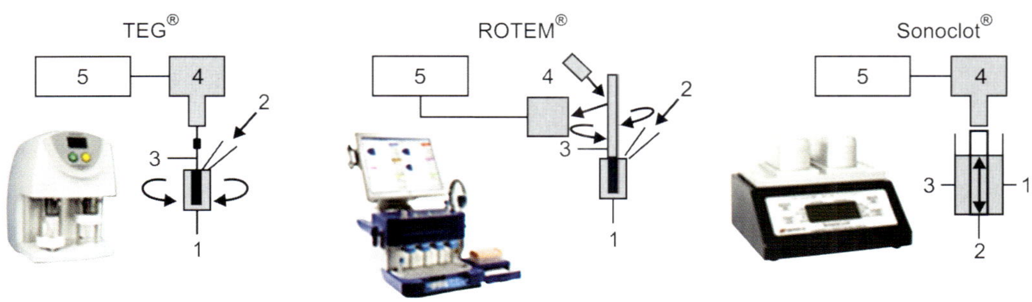

Figure 4 Biomechanical working principles behind the three viscoelastic coagulation monitoring devices: (1) Blood sample in rotating cup for TEG® and in cuvette for ROTEM® and Sonoclot®, (2) Coagulation activator, (3) pin and torsion wire for TEG®, pin and rotating axis for ROTEM® and disposable plastic probe for Sonoclot®, (4) electromechanical signal transducer/signal detector, (5) data processor

may affect the results. The TEG instrument requires daily calibration and routine quality controls, as well as standardization in its use to ensure the optimal performance and reliable results. These demands can hardly be accomplished by busy emergency room personnel.

INTERPRETING A SONOCLOT SIGNATURE

How Does The Sonoclot Analyzer Work? (Figure 5)

As soon as the sample is added the instrument starts analyzing the sample and analysis is also reflected on the attached computer in real time.

This graph illustrates how the Sonoclot Signature is used to monitor different phases of hemostasis, from coagulation through fibrin formation and clot retraction to the formation of a mature clot **(Figure 6)**.

Step 1: Activated Clotting Time (ACT) (Figure 7)

This is the period from the beginning of the test when the sample is still a liquid until the point where fibrinogen begins to convert into a fibrin gel, thus increasing the viscosity of the sample. The Sonoclot Analyzer produces an automated result as the Onset or Activated Clotting Time. This is the point where the viscosity measurement rises by 1.0 Clot Signal unit on the Sonoclot Signature.

Step 2: Fibrin Gel Formation (Figure 8)

This is the period during which fibrinogen forms a fibrin gel and is represented by the first rise in the Sonoclot Signature. The Sonoclot Analyzer produces an automated result called the Clot Rate. The Clot Rate is the maximum slope of the Sonoclot Signature during initial gel formation.

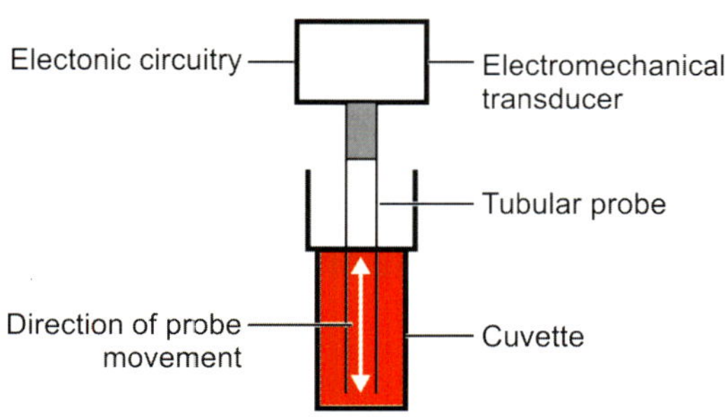

Figure 5 Individual parts of a Sonoclot analyzer machine

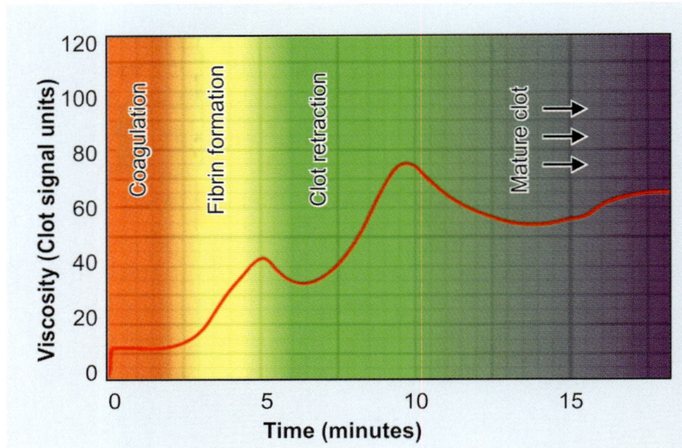

Figure 6 Hemostatic phases of the Sonoclot signature

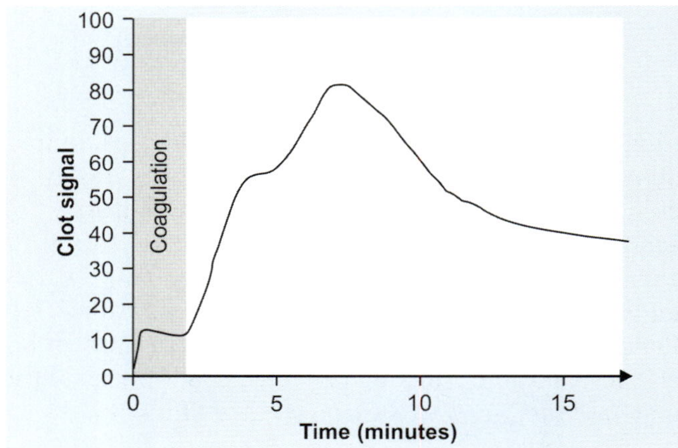

Figure 7 Activated clotting time (ACT) measurements

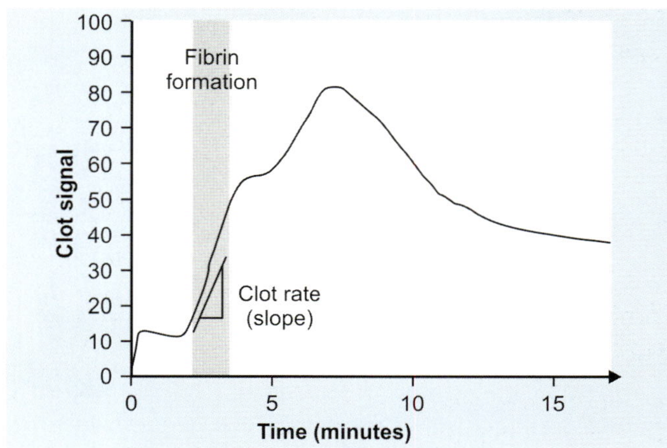

Figure 8 Fibrin gel formations stage

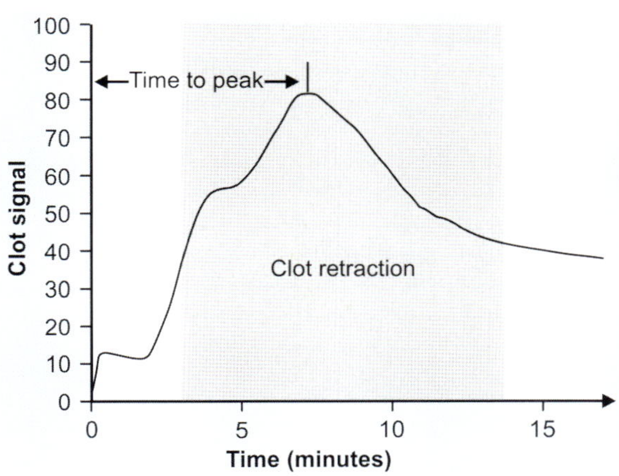

Figure 9 Clot retraction phase

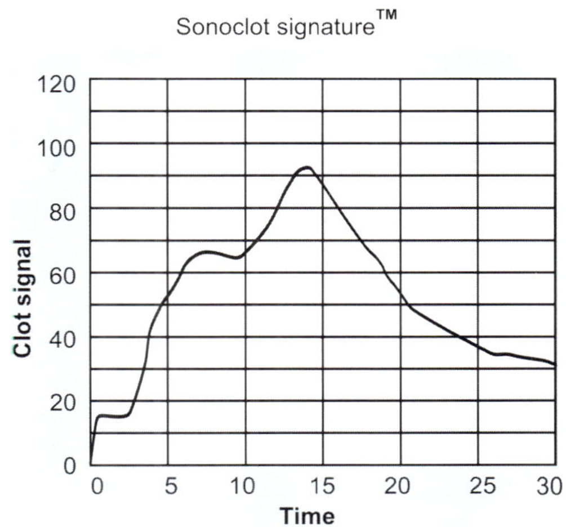

Figure 10 Complete sonoclot signature

Step 3: Clot Retraction (Figure 9)

Clot retraction causes a peak or peaks on the Sonoclot Signature. Historically, platelet function has been characterized by several graphical indicators such as the Time-to-Peak. Now the Sonoclot Analyzer, when run using Signature Viewer Software, produces an automated result called "Platelet Function." The Platelet Function number quantifies the quality of the clot retraction. Results will have values between 0 (no platelet function) and 5 (strong platelet function).

WHAT CAN FUNCTIONAL HEMOSTASIS MONITORING PROVIDE THE SURGICAL TEAM?

Quick hemostasis performance answers to:

- Management of anticoagulation
- Management of blood product usage
- Differentiate mechanical versus hemostatic bleeders
- Identify Hypercoagulable Patients

WHAT DOES THE SONOCLOT ANALYZER PRODUCE? (FIGURE 10)

- Automated results
- Time until initial
- Clot formation
- Activated clotting time
- Clot formation rate

DIFFERENT STEPS TO PERFORM SONOCLOT ANALYSIS

Figure 11 shows different steps to perform sonoclot analysis.

ROTATIONAL THROMBOELASTOMETRY (ROTEM) (FIGURES 12A AND B)

Rotational Thromboelastometer (ROTEM)

ROTEM is an advancement of TEG and differs in the way of analyzing the coagulation process: in the TEG, the cup is slowly oscillated and changes in viscoelasticity are measured by a pin attached to a suspended torsion wire; whereas, in ROTEM, the cup remains fixed while, the pin is oscillated. Moreover, the improved design of ROTEM allows it to be used as a portable device at bed-side of patient. The ROTEM device has four independent analyzer channels which enable the simultaneous independent tests of all parameters **(Figure 13)**. The various systems of ROTEM are available by use of different activated reagents:

- **INTEM:** Coagulation is activated by contact phase to monitor the coagulation via the intrinsic pathway (e.g. factor VIII).

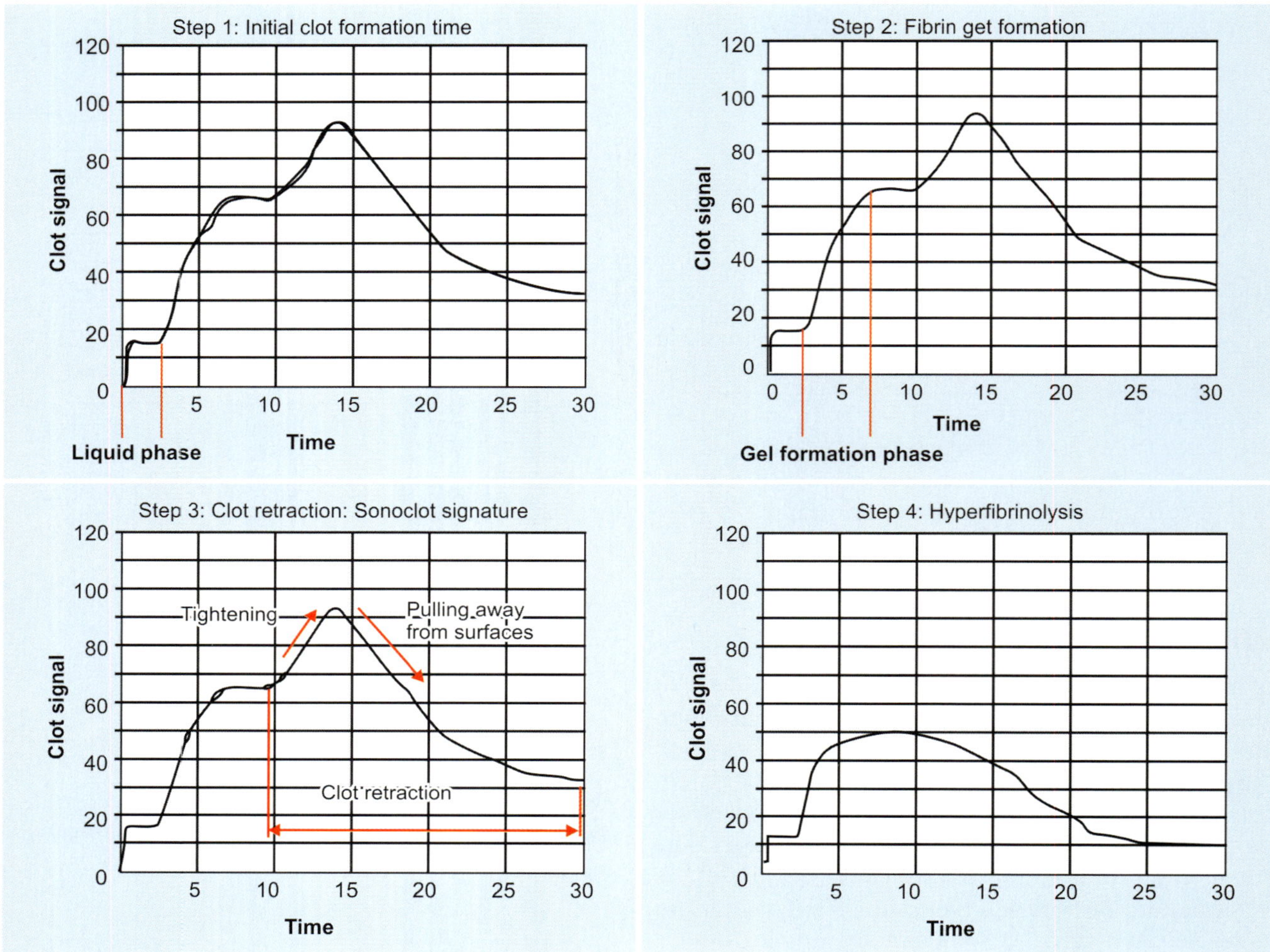

Figure 11 Different steps to perform sonoclot analysis

- **EXTEM:** Coagulation is activated by a small amount of tissue factor to monitor the coagulation via the extrinsic pathway.
- **HEPTEM:** Coagulation is activated as in INTEM, in the presence of heparin. The comparison of HEPTEM with INTEM parameters can help in detection of heparin-related coagulation disturbances.
- **FIBTEM:** Coagulation is activated as in EXTEM to monitor the clot firmness after neglecting platelet contribution to the clot firmness. FIBTEM is always used in conjunction with EXTEM, so that the clot formation is only dependent on fibrin.
- **APTEM:** Coagulation is activated as in EXTEM to monitor the clot firmness after blocking hyperfibrinolysis by aprotinin. APTEM is always used in conjunction with EXTEM so as to rapidly detect fibrinolysis.
- **ECATEM:** To measure direct thrombin inhibitor (DTI) effects.

ROTEM AND HEMOSTATIC MANAGEMENT

The rotational thromboelastometer has been used for POC management in various clinical settings.[10, 11] Weber CF and Gorlinger K et al. demonstrated that the hemostatic management based on POC devices (ROTEM) can reduce the patient exposure to blood products and provides significant benefits with respect

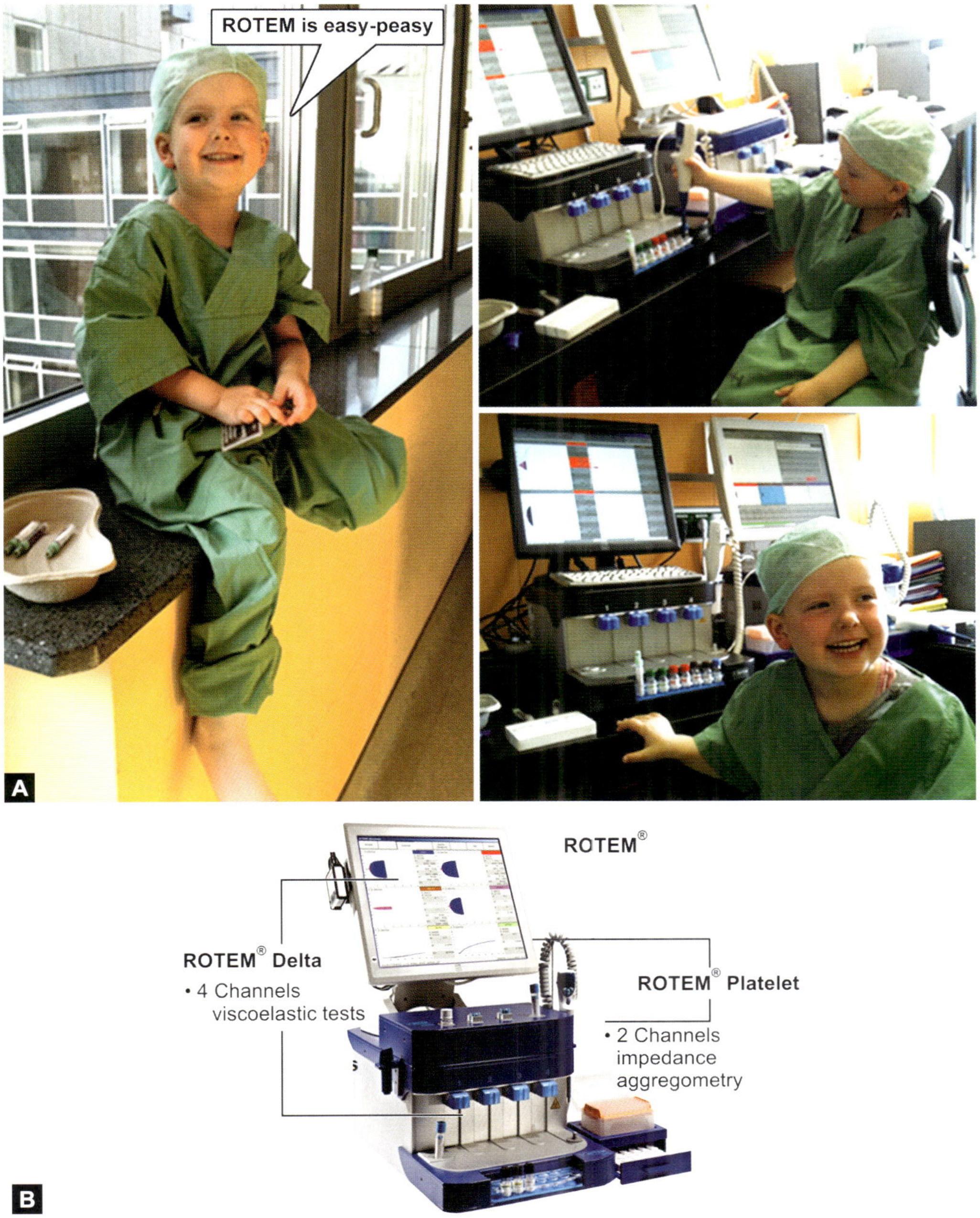

Figures 12A and B Rotational thromboelastometry (ROTEM)

to clinical outcomes in cardiac surgery patients.[12] Similarly, Fayed M, Mourad W and Gorlinger K et al. observed that ROTEM is able to predict preoperative transfusion requirements in adult living donor transplant recipients, which may allow better preparation and less cross-matching prior to surgery.[13]

ROTEM and Conventional Laboratory Tests

The ability of ROTEM to predict thrombocytopenia and hypofibrinogenemia has been tested. Engberink et al. evaluated the ROTEM device to predict

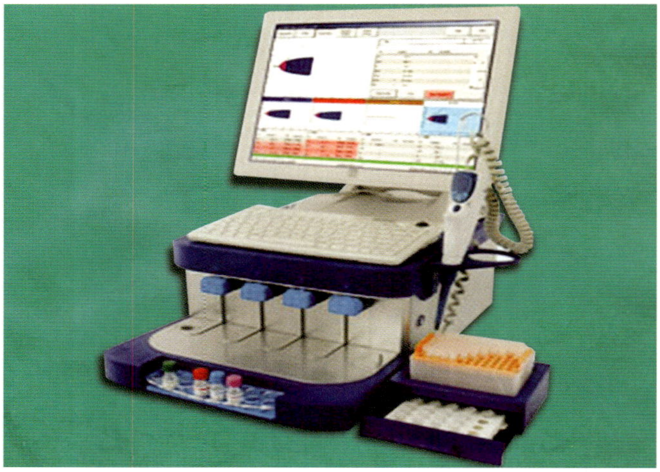

Figure 13 Rotational thromboelastometry (ROTEM) machine

thrombocytopenia and hypofibrinogenemia in cardiac surgery patients using the clot amplitude after 5 minutes. The authors observed that the turnaround time for ROTEM tests (12 minutes), was comparable with emergency requests for platelet count, (13 minutes) and shorter than emergency requests for fibrinogen levels (37 minutes).[14] The ROTEM parameters have been compared and correlated with conventional laboratory coagulation tests. Ogawa et al. conducted a prospective observational study to compare different ROTEM parameters with standard coagulation tests in elective cardiac surgery patients. The author observed strong correlations between FIBTEM-amplitude at 10 minutes (A10) and fibrinogen level ($r = 0.87$; p $p<0.001$) and between EXTEM/ INTEM-A10 variables and platelet count ($r = 0.72$ and 0.67, respectively; $p<0.001$). Receiver operating characteristic analysis demonstrated that EXTEM-A10 and INTEM-A10 are predictive of thrombocytopenia below 80 X 10^9/L (area under the curve [AUC], 0.83 and 0.82, respectively), and FIBTEM-A10 was highly predictive of fibrinogen level below 200 mg/dL (AUC, 0.96).[15]

ROTEM and Postoperative Bleeding Predictability

The diagnostic ability of ROTEM to predict postoperative bleeding is a matter of controversy. Reinhofer et al. studied the value of rotational thromboelastometry to monitor disturbed hemostasis and bleeding risk in patients with cardiopulmonary bypass. The author observed that the positive predictive value and specificity of ROTEM variables like clot formation time (71%, 94%) and FIBTEM (73%, 95%) to predict postoperative bleeding was significantly higher than conventional laboratory tests like aPTT (56%, 72%) and prothrombin time (43%, 5%).[16]

Contrary to this, Davidson et al. observed that ROTEM thromboelastometry has poor positive predictive value (14.8%) to identify patients who bleed more than 200 mL/h in the early postoperative period after cardiac surgery. However, its negative predictive value was found to be good (100%). The authors realized that their study was not adequately powered to confirm its poor positive predictive value as the prevalence of bleeding in the early postoperative period was small (13.7%).[17]

UTILITY OF SONOCLOT ANALYSIS AND TRANEXAMIC ACID IN TETRALOGY OF FALLOT PATIENTS UNDERGOING INTRACARDIAC REPAIR

Utility of sonoclot analysis and tranexamic acid (TA) in tetralogy of Fallot (TOF) patients undergoing intracardiac repair has been described by Malhotra et al. in TOF patients. The authors previously studied that the sonoclot analysis is a point-of-care test to monitor the coagulation process, presenting a comprehensive evaluation of the clot formation and retraction as well as platelet function.[18] They concluded that the sonoclot analysis is an easily performed, reproducible, point-of-care method for coagulation monitoring which diagnoses the exact nature of coagulopathy including deficiency of coagulation factors or fibrinogen or defects in platelet-fibrin interaction or platelet function **(Table 1)**. The DR15 values on Sonoclot have proven to be a reliable marker of hyperfibrinolysis involving the use of TA in TOF patients undergoing intracardiac repair. However, further studies are required to validate the reference values of DR15, to initiate action in controlling the postoperative bleeding due to hyperfibrinolysis.

COMPARISON OF THREE POINT-OF-CARE TESTING DEVICES TO DETECT HEMOSTATIC CHANGES IN ADULT ELECTIVE CARDIAC SURGERY: A PROSPECTIVE OBSERVATIONAL STUDY

In a study done by Espinosa et al,[19] the authors found the significant significant changes for all TEG variables

SECTION 4

TABLE 1 Nomenclature, variable definitions and reference ranges of the TEG, ROTEM and sonoclot instruments

	TEG	*ROTEM*	*Sonoclot*
Clot time to 2 mm amplitude	R (reaction time) (4-8)	CT (clotting time) • EXTEM CT (42-74 sec) • INTEM CT (137-246 sec)	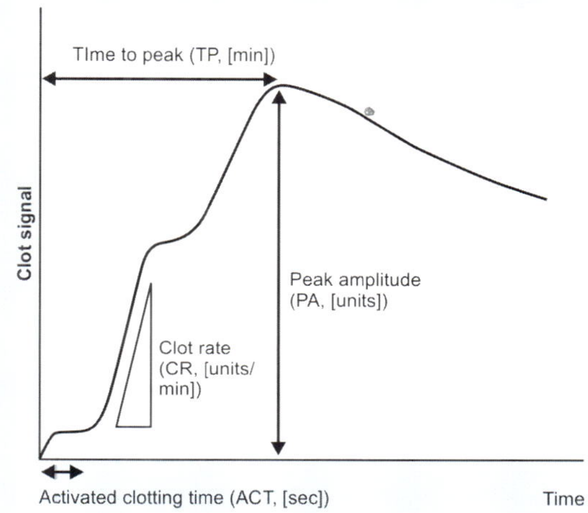
Clot kinetics Time from 2 to 20 mm Clot firmness	k (kinetics) (1-4 min)	CFT (Clot formation time) • EXTEM CFT (46–148 sec) • INTEM CFT (40–100 sec)	
Clot kinetics Alpha angle	Alpha angle (53–67°)	Alpha angle • EXTEM Angle (63–81°) • INTEM angle (71–82°)	Son Act (85–145 sec) Clot rate R1 (15–45 clot signal units/min) Peak (mm) Time to peak (540–600 sec) R_3 (>2 mm/min)
Clot strength	MA (maximum amplitude) (55–73 mm)	MCF (maximum clot firmness) • EXTEM MCF (49–71 mm) • INTEM MCF (52–72 mm) • FIBTEM MCF (9–25 mm)	
Clot elasticity	G(46–10.9 dynes/cm^2)	-	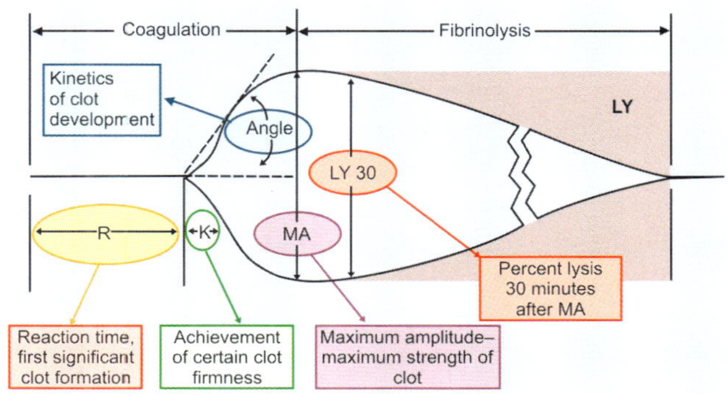
Time unit the beginning of fibrin formation	-	-	
Rate of fibrin formation	-	-	
Completion of firbin formation	-	-	
Index of fibrinogen conversion to fibrin	-	-	
Platelet-induced clot retraction	-	-	

EXTEM reagent contains tissue factor, INTEM reagent contains ellagic acid, FIBTEM reagent contains platelet inhibitor

CHAPTER 21

Flow chart 1 Algorithm for treating coagulopathy by TEG only, if patient had significant bleeding

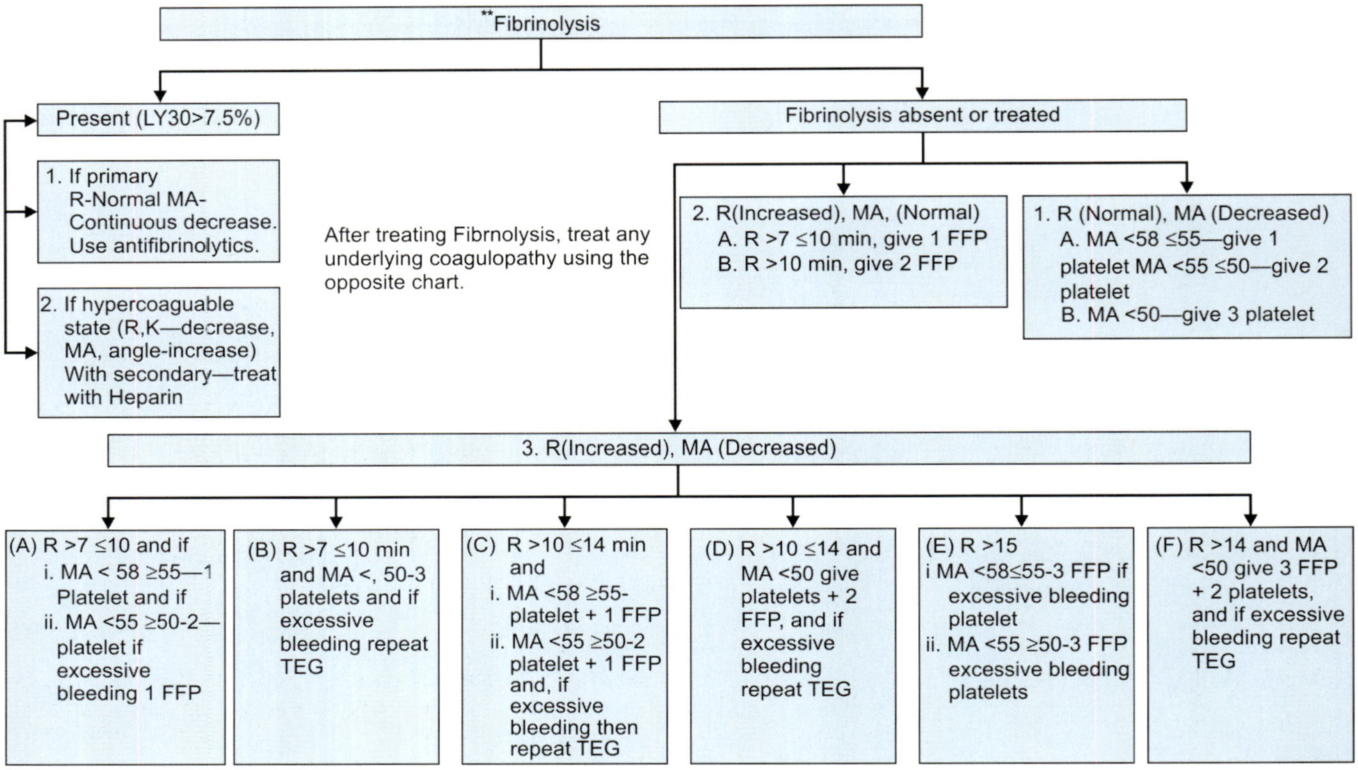

** This chart assumes that Heparin used during surgery has been completely reversed with Protamine, and that the angle is normal. If Heparin reversal is not complete, then heparin reversal must be recommended with protamine in conjunction with the treatment chart. *(Adapted with permission from S. Manikappa et al 20)*

after surgery, for three of the ROTEM variables, and for one variable from the Sonoclot. There were significant correlations postoperatively between plasma fibrinogen levels and variables from the three instruments.

They concluded that the TEG and ROTEM may be used to detect changes in hemostasis following cardiac surgery with CPB. Sonoclot seems to be less suitable to detect changes. Variables from the three instruments correlate with plasma fibrinogen and could be used to monitor treatment with fibrinogen concentrate. In their study on “The use of thromboelastograph to decipher changes in transfusion therapy in cardiac surgery, guided by the TEG.

S Manikappa et al.[20] concluded that Thromboelastograph is a useful diagnostic tool to detect coagulopathies following cardiopulmonary bypass. It helps in instituting appropriate blood and blood component therapy thereby avoiding unnecessary transfusion and associated risks. Accurate detection of coagulopathy is possible with heparinase pretreatment of the blood sample **(Flow chart 1)**.

COMPARISON OF CONVENTIONAL TEG® TECHNIQUE WITH ROTEM® TECHNIQUE

Aggregometric testing of whole-blood samples is used mainly to study platelet function.[21] In bleeding patients in whom the hematocrit is greater than 30% and the platelet count exceeds 70-100/nl, aggregometric tests can be used to screen for disorders of primary hemostasis, e.g. von Willebrand syndrome, and to quantify the effect of antiplatelet medications. The available aggregometric POC tests (Multiplate®, PFA-100®, TEG® Platelet Mapping™ Assay, VerifyNow®) differ in the agonists that are used to activate the platelets in the test cells, such as collagen, adenosine phosphate, epinephrine, arachidonic acid, and thrombin, and in the shearing forces that are generated in the test cells **(Figure 14)**.

SECTION 4

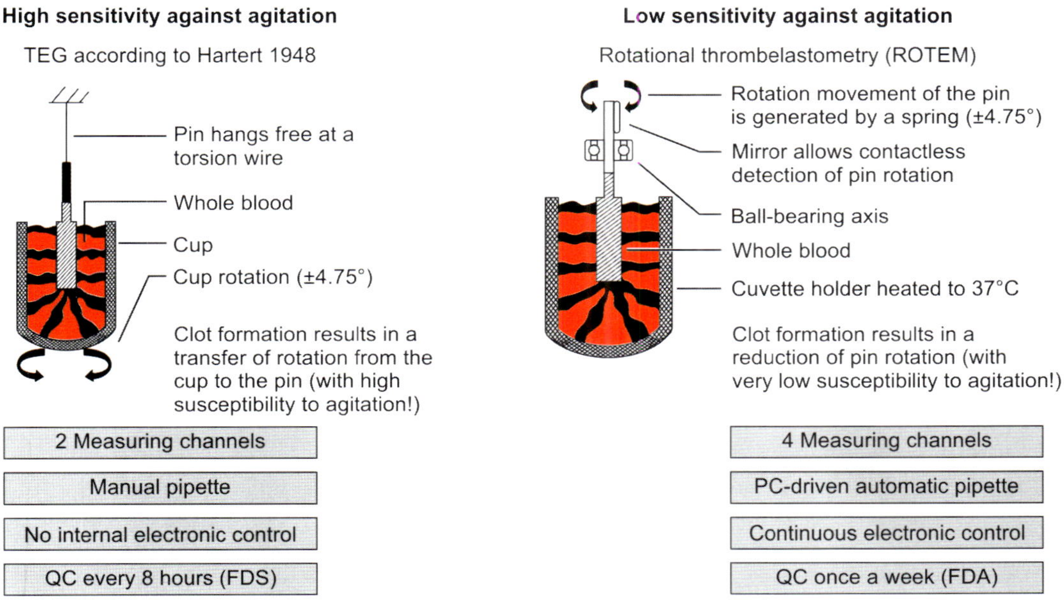

Figure 14 Comparison of conventional TEG® technique with ROTEM® technique

CONCLUSION

The viscoelastic POC tests are dynamic tests of coagulation, giving us minute to minute information on transfusions requirements. They have reasonable sensitivity and specificity as shown by various studies. Which is better of the three needs more validated studies for blood products usage judiciously these tests reduce patient exposure to unnecessary blood component therapy. Although cost may be a factor, it has to be measured against diseases transmitted by transfusion of blood and blood products.

REFERENCES

1. Meybohm P, Zacharowski K, Weber CF. Point-of-care coagulation management in intensive care medicine. Crit Care. 2013;17:218.
2. Levi M, Opal SM: Coagulation abnormalities in critically ill patients. Crit Care. 2006;10:222.
3. Murphy GJ, Reeves BC, Rogers CA, Rizvi SI, Culliford L, Angelini GD. Increased mortality, postoperative morbidity, and cost after red blood cell transfusion in patients having cardiac surgery. Circulation. 2007; 116:2544-52.
4. Avidan MS, Alcock EL, Da Fonseca J, et al. Comparison of structured used of routine laboratory tests or near-patient assessment with clinical judgment in the management of bleeding after cardiac surgery. Br J Anaesth. 2004;92:178-86.
5. Hartert H. Thrombelastography: a method for physical analysis of blood coagulation. Z Gesamte Exp Med. 1951;117:189-203.
6. Bahnson HT, Ziegler RF. A Consideration of the Causes of Death Following Operation for Congenital Heart Disease of the Cyanotic Type. Surg Gynec Obstet. 1950;90:60-76.
7. Hartmann RC. Hemorrhagic disorder occurring in patients with cyanotic congenital heart disease. Bull Hopkins Hosp. 1952;91:49-67.
8. Laffey JG, Boylan JF, Cheng DC. The systemic inflammatory response to cardiac surgery: implications for the anaesthesiologist. Anaesthesiology. 2002; 97:215-52.
9. Agnihotri N, Agnihotri A. Transfusion Associated Circulatory Overload. Indian Journal of Critical Care Medicine. 2014;18(6):396-8.
10. Haas T, Gorlinger K, Grassetto A, Agostini V, Simioni P, Nardi G. Thromboelastometry for guiding management of the critically ill patients: a systematic review of the literature. Minerva Anestesiol. 2014;80: 1320-35.
11. Gorlinger K, Lesserson LS, Dirkmann D, Hanke AA, Meyer NR, Tanaka KA. Management of haemorrhage in cardiothoracic surgery. J Cardiothorac Vasc Anesth. 2013;27(4):20-34.
12. Weber CF, Gorlinger K, Meininger D, Herrmann E, Bingold T, Moritz A, et al. Point-of-Care testing, a prospective, randomized clinical trial of efficacy in coagulopathic cardiac surgery patients. Anesthesiology. 2012;117: 531-47.

13. Fayed N, Mourad W, Yassena K, Gorlinger K. Preoperative thromboelastometry as a predictor of transfusion requirements during adult living donor liver transplantation. Transfus Med Hemother 2015;42:99-108.
14. Engberink RH, Kuiper GJ, Wetzels RJ, Nelemans PJ, Lance MD, Beckers EA et al. Rapid and correct prediction of thrombocytopenia and hypofibrinogemia with rotational thromboelastometry in cardiac surgery. J Cardiothorac Vasc Anesth. 2014; 28:210-6.
15. Ogawa S, Szlam F, Chen EP, Nishimura T, Kim H, Roback JD, et al. A comparative evaluation of rotation thromboelastometry and standard coagulation tests in hemodilution-induced coagulation changes after cardiac surgery. Transfusion. 2012;52:14-22.
16. Reinhofer M, Brauer M, Franke U, Barz D, Marx G, Lösche W. The value of rotation thromboelastometry to monitor disturbed perioperative haemostasis and bleeding risk in patients with cardiopulmonary bypass. Blood Coagul Fibrinolysis. 2008,19:212-19.
17. Davidson SJ, McGrowder D, Roughton M, Kelleher AA. Can ROTEM Thromboelastometry Predict Postoperative Bleeding After Cardiac Surgery? J Cardiothorac Vasc Anesth. 2008;22:655-61.
18. Aggarwal V, Malhotra Kapoor P, Choudhury M, Kiran U, Chowdhury U. Utility of Sonoclot analysis and tranexamic acid in tetralogy of Fallot patients undergoing intracardiac repair, 2012; 15(1):26-31.
19. Espinosa A, Stenseth R, Videm V, Pleym H. Comparison of three point-of-care testing devices to detect hemostatic changes in adult elective cardiac surgery: a prospective observational study. BMN Anaesthesiology. 2014;14:80.
20. Manikappa S, Mehta Y, Juneja R, Trehan N. Changes in transfusion therapy guided by thromboelastograph in cardiac surgery. Ann Card Anaesth. 2001;4(1): 21-7.
21. Jambor C, von Pape KW, Spannagl M, Dietrich W, Giebl A, Weisser H: Multiple electrode whole blood aggregometry, PFA-100, and in vivo bleeding time for the point-of-care assessment of aspirin-induced platelet dysfunction in the preoperative setting. Anesth Analg. 2011;113:31-39.

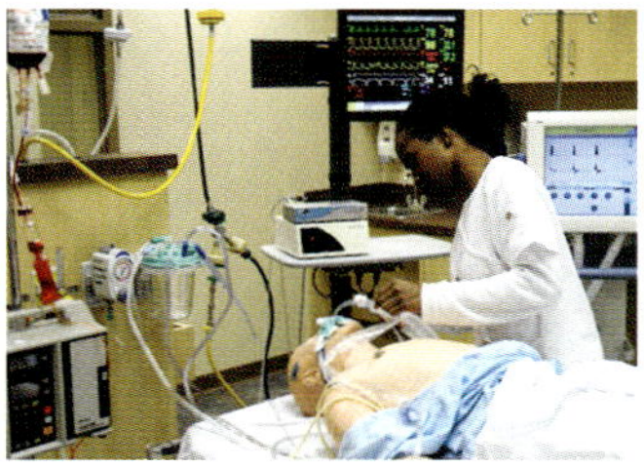

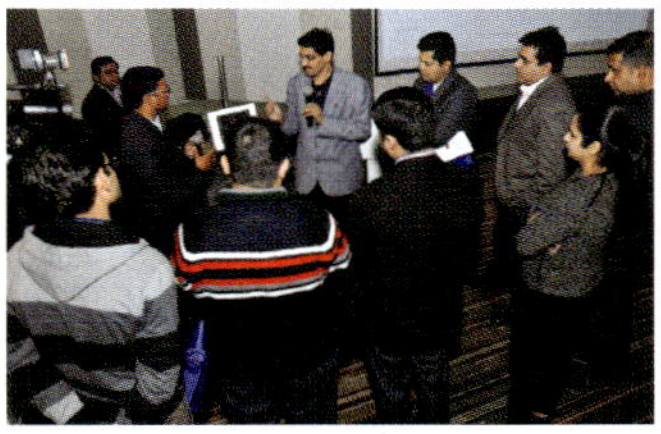

Section 5

Simulation for Hemodynamic Monitoring

Section Outline

- Simulation in Hemodynamic Monitoring
- Use of Simulation in Advanced Monitoring and Critical Care

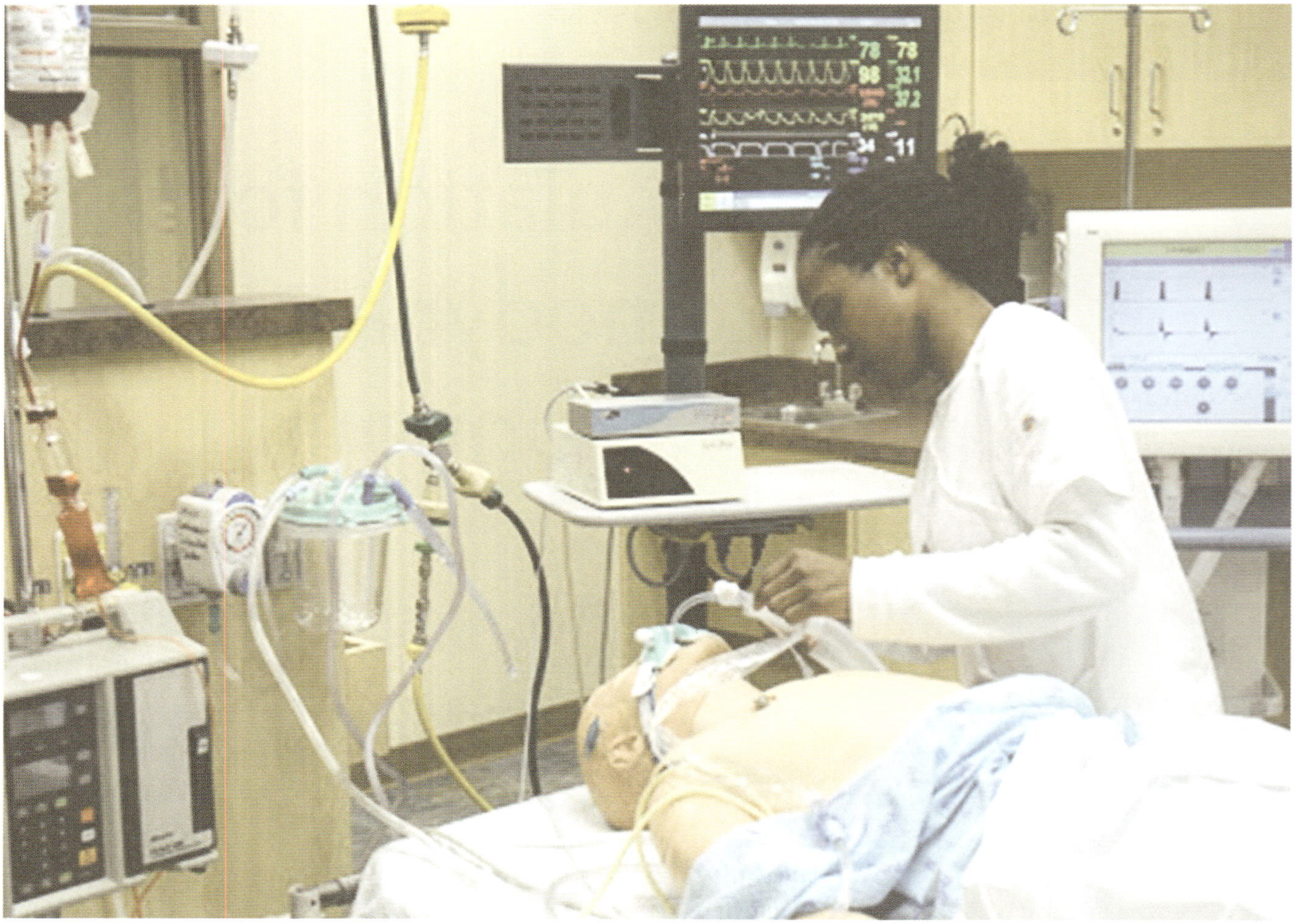

Chapter 22

Simulation in Hemodynamic Monitoring

Yatin Mehta, Richie Jain, Naman Shastri

Chapter Outline

- Types of Medical Simulators
- Role in Critical Care and Hemodynamics
- Applications of Simulation in Critical Care
- Limitations
- Future of Patient Simulation in Critical Care and Anesthesiology

I hear, and I forget
I see, and I remember
I do, and I understand.

—**Confucius**

Decisions made in critical care are often complicated, requiring an in-depth understanding of the relations between complex diseases, available interventions, and patients with a wide range of characteristics. Standard modeling techniques such as decision trees and statistical modeling have difficulty in capturing these interactions as the complexity of the problem increases. Simulation, using current technology, offers innovative and reproducible training experience. It enables standardized scenario building and reflective learning. The technology could be used very effectively for the assessment of competence too. Simulation has been used for technology development and appraisal over the years.

DEFINITION

The word "Simulate," as per Merriam-Webster's dictionary, means "to give or create the effect of, to imitate." Simulation is a technique to replace or amplify real patient experiences with guided experiences, artificially contrived, which evokes or replicates substantial aspects of real world in a fully interactive manner (as defined by David Gaba, MD of Stanford University). Replication of only a very narrowly defined sub-domain is usually referred to as a "part-task trainer." *Fidelity* refers to the accuracy with which the simulation reproduces the domain, both in the number of elements that the simulator presents, and in the faithfulness of those datastreams to their real world behavior.

TYPES OF MEDICAL SIMULATORS

Medical simulators now in use are quite varied in their characteristics and fidelity. At the lowest fidelity (and correspondingly lowest cost) are computer assisted instruction programs that represent certain portions of the anesthesiologists work environment on-screen. Higher fidelity can be achieved by designing actual physical devices or space to replicate portions of the domain. Physical simulations can range from narrowly limited part-task trainers to full scale operating suites or intensive care units. Virtual reality based simulation is still in its infancy, but this exciting approach uses a virtual, computer generated space with multiple sensory feedback mechanisms to simulate the work environment of the anesthesiologist with the potential for very high fidelity, low operating costs and a broader range of datastreams than is possible with physical simulators.

Screen-based Simulations

Screen based simulators typically use a standard personal computer (PC) to represent selected visual and auditory components of the environment, usually providing dynamic clinical data in real-time from physiologic and pharmacologic models. The predominant advantage of such a system is the widespread availability of the platform, and the low cost associated with distributing software once developed. Examples include SLEEPER and BODY Simulation, Anesthesia Simulator™ etc.

Virtual Reality Simulations

Virtual reality (VR) describes a technique whereby a computer generated space and objects within it are presented to the user in a three dimensional representation with multiple sensory feedback cues. Visual data can be presented via goggles or a computer screen, and auditory information is presented via earphones. Often tactile, or "haptic" feedback is delivered to allow the realistic manipulation of objects and devices within the virtual environment. The computing power necessary is at the leading edge of available graphic workstations. The wide range of VR systems currently being developed are spread along a continuum of cost vs. realism in the input/output and modalities. VR could theoretically be used in a hybrid simulator, with a VR patient "laid over" a real clinical environment.

Mannequin-based Simulators (Realistic Simulators)

Currently, full-size mannequin patients are used in most simulation centers—Sim Man® from Leardal, Human Patient Simulator-HPS II from METI®, Comprehensive Anesthesia Simulation Environment (CASE) series—to name a few. They are backed by complex software-based physiology. The person operating this software can make the mannequin as realistic as a real patient. The mannequin has mechanical internal structures similar to the human body. It has functional airway and lungs. The heart and circulatory systems are imitated by a compressor and a network of tubes, such that there will be heart beat and palpable pulses. Various organ systems can be made even more realistic by using coloured fluids—red fluid circulating as blood and yellowish fluid to fill the urinary bladder.

ROLE IN CRITICAL CARE AND HEMODYNAMICS

In acute care specialties, we work in multidisciplinary teams to manage patients. But, we rarely practice training exercises as teams. The aviation industry has well-structured teamwork training programs like Crew Resource Management. D Gaba and his team at Stanford realized the potential of simulation-based team training. They adopted this to develop the Anesthesia Crisis Resource Management (ACRM) Programme. It teaches the principles of team behavior in crisis situations and assesses decision making, interpersonal communication and team management. The CRM model is applicable in other acute medical specialties like emergency medicine, intensive care and neonatology. In the ACRM, an individual is exposed to a patient care scenario that escalates in a full-blown crisis (e.g. an anesthetized patient developing severe arrhythmia over a period of a few minutes). In this situation, the anesthetist is expected to play a leader's role. He/she should guide the whole theater team to resolve the crisis. However, successfully resolving the arrhythmia is not the only task. In a scenario, he/she should not get fixed to a certain aspect of physiology, but should look at the rapidly evolving clinical situation, review and refocus appropriately.

APPLICATIONS OF SIMULATION IN CRITICAL CARE

- Development of regular technical skills such as endotracheal intubation, central venous cannulation, arterial cannulation, tracheostomy, etc.
- Rare procedures such as cricothyrotomy and chest tube insertion can be rehearsed and be appropriately used at critical clinical junctures.
- Simulation can be used for assessment of clinical competencies. Simulation-based scenarios, when used to assess various skills and competencies, need to be validated as the assessment tools. For e.g. objective structured clinical examination (OSCE) has been used to assess the technical skills and theoretical aspects in various clinical specialties.
- Development and testing the efficacy of newer hemodynamic monitors.
- Research.
- Decreasing or limiting "ERRORS" in clinical practice.

LIMITATIONS

- One of the criticisms is the extent to which a simulator can reproduce the real-life situations. In the healthcare set-up, we should be aware of the differences between simulated and real patient anatomy to maximally utilize the benefit of such training.
- Simulator fidelity may be inadequate to probe specific errors.
- Subjects know they are being evaluated, may exhibit artifactual behaviors such as hypervigilance or cavalier attitudes.
- Cost involved in simulation exercise is quite high.

FUTURE OF PATIENT SIMULATION IN CRITICAL CARE AND ANESTHESIOLOGY

The use of patient simulators has now grown beyond its initial phase as a purely experimental technology and modality to enter a new period of growth and consolidation. Although many questions remain unanswered about the impact of the technology there now seems little question that simulation will be a significant technique for education, training, and research within anesthesiology and in many other domains in health care. At the level of basic health care education, simulators have already begun to make their mark in applications aimed at professional students (e.g. medicine and nursing).[3] The expansion of clinical training beyond anesthesiology, for resident physicians and for experienced clinicians (physicians, nurses, and combined teams) has been an important development. Not only has this brought the benefits of simulation-based training to these other health care settings, it has also brought anesthesiologists to the forefront of issues related to education, training, and performance assessment.[4] As the profession of anesthesiology has sought to redefine its role within health care, the emergence of anesthesiologists both as experts in the use of simulation and as experts in the cognitive skills of complex dynamic decision making has added another important role for the profession. It is likely that simulation-based training, lead largely by anesthesiologists, will become a routine part of the initial and recurrent training of all clinicians who work in settings involving high complexity and dynamism. The early 21st century will probably see VR simulations take over from computer screen and realistic simulations.

REFERENCES

1. Gaba DM. The future vision of simulation in healthcare. Qual Saf Health Care. 2004;13:i2-10.
2. Burt DE. Virtual reality in anaesthesia. Br J Anaesth. 1995;75:472-80.
3. Cumin D, Merry AF. Simulators for use in anaesthesia. Anaesthesia. 2007;62:151-62.
4. Cumin D, Weller J, Henderson K, Merry AF. Standards for simulation in anaesthesia: Creating confidence in tools. Br J Anaesth. 2010; 105: 45-51.

Chapter 23

Use of Simulation in Advanced Monitoring and Critical Care

Poonam Malhotra Kapoor, Yatin Mehta, Naman Shastri

Chapter Outline

- Teaching the Management of Hemodynamic Parameter
- Model-driven Simulators
- Instructor-driven Simulators
- Virtual Reality Simulators
- Task Specific Models
- Case Scenarios

INTRODUCTION

The expansion of Internet has caused a growing interest in developing databases and software related to biomedical research. Such databases permit access to data for developing and testing new computer models and algorithms. Keeping the vital parameters in optimal values for the cardiac work and arterial pressure is a very complex process. Great progress has been made in modeling techniques of cardiovascular system, that help to better diagnose the cardiovascular diseases, which are the number one cause of deaths in the world. There are several computer models that simulate the cardiovascular system ranging from microlevel (e.g. cells) to macrolevel (e.g. organs) and up to system level.

Critical care physicians maintain certain patient state variables within an acceptable operating range by infusing several drugs. For example, in the case of patients with congestive heart failure, measured variables such as mean arterial pressure (MAP) and cardiac output (CO) are of primary importance and are maintained using sodium nitroprusside (SNP) and dopamine (DPM). In addition, they may be required to administer anesthetics and monitor the depth of anesthesia (DOA) during surgical procedures. Research in simulation and educational innovations look towards new ways of training the professionals to improve patient care, reduce the amount of time to knowledge acquisition and mastery difficult skills.[1]

TEACHING THE MANAGEMENT OF HEMODYNAMIC PARAMETER

There is hope that research into models of the cardiovascular system will clarify understanding about these conditions, leading ultimately to improvements in treatment. The cardiovascular system is a distributed system, composed of blood with varying nonlinear viscous and inertial properties interacting with vessels of complex morphology, nonlinear elastic walls, and multiple levels of homeostatic system controlling many distributed properties. A completed description of this system would be incredibly complex and could not be accomplished in close form.

However, the use of linear approximations and lumped parameters allows a much simplified description in terms of linear ordinary differential equation. Many such models have been use to explain various aspects of the cardiovascular system. Such models provide a concrete, analytical framework as a basis for understanding the full system.

Any model to teach hemodynamics should be sophisticated enough to embody the behavior which is being taught, but it should not be so complicated that it cannot be understood in and of itself. Although every model will depart from reality to the extent that the assumptions made when constructing it are false, it is important that the model paint a valid picture of the real world. All model assumptions should be presented in a straightforward manner, so that students do not accept the model's version of the reality, but maintain a separate understanding of the model and of the real system that the model is meant to describe.

Such a computer simulation of hemodynamics would provide correct results for simulated physiology experiments, but would not be so complicated that it is viewed as an incomprehensible jumble of constituents and relations **(Figure 1)**.

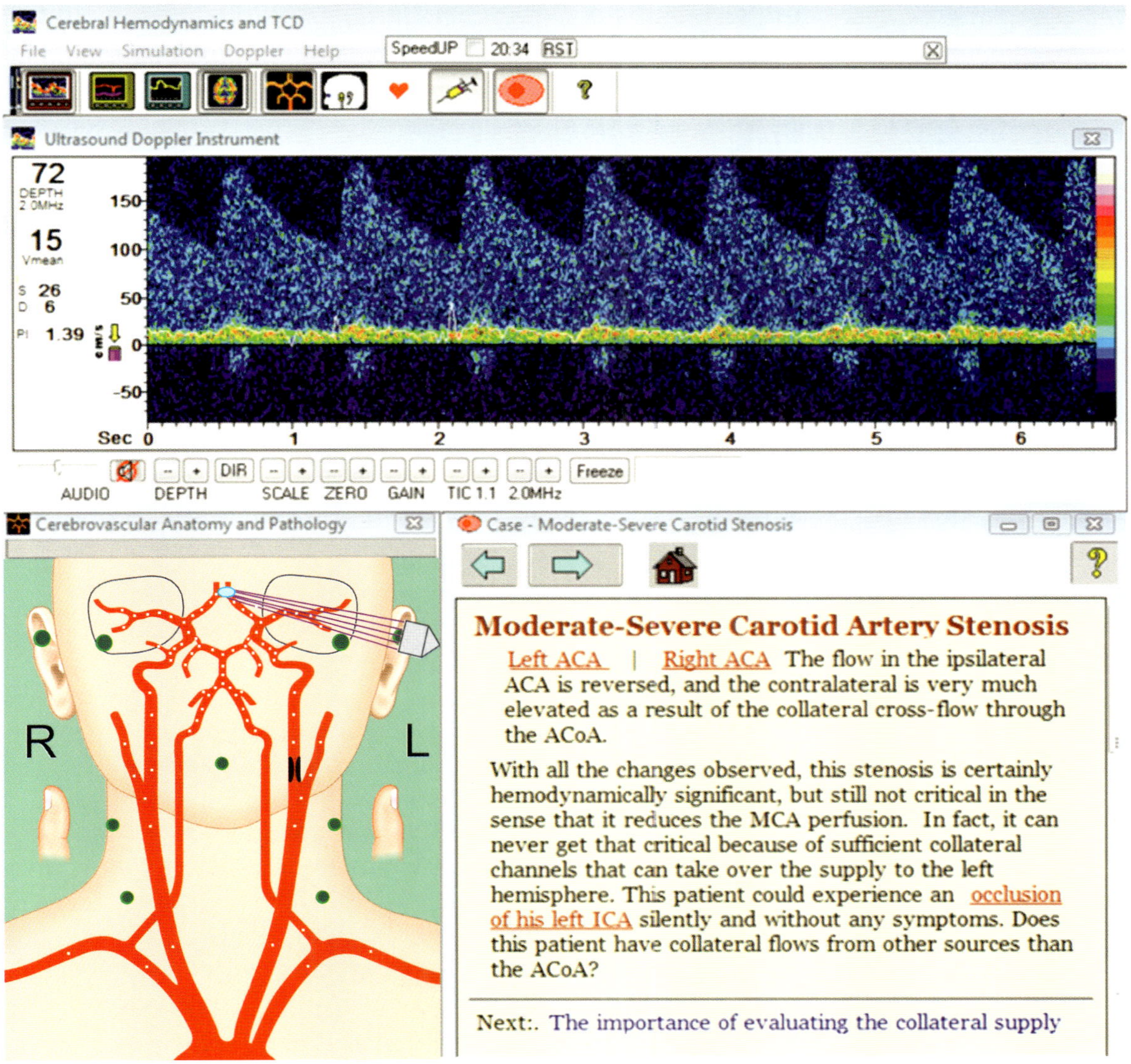

Figure 1 Computer simulation of hemodynamics

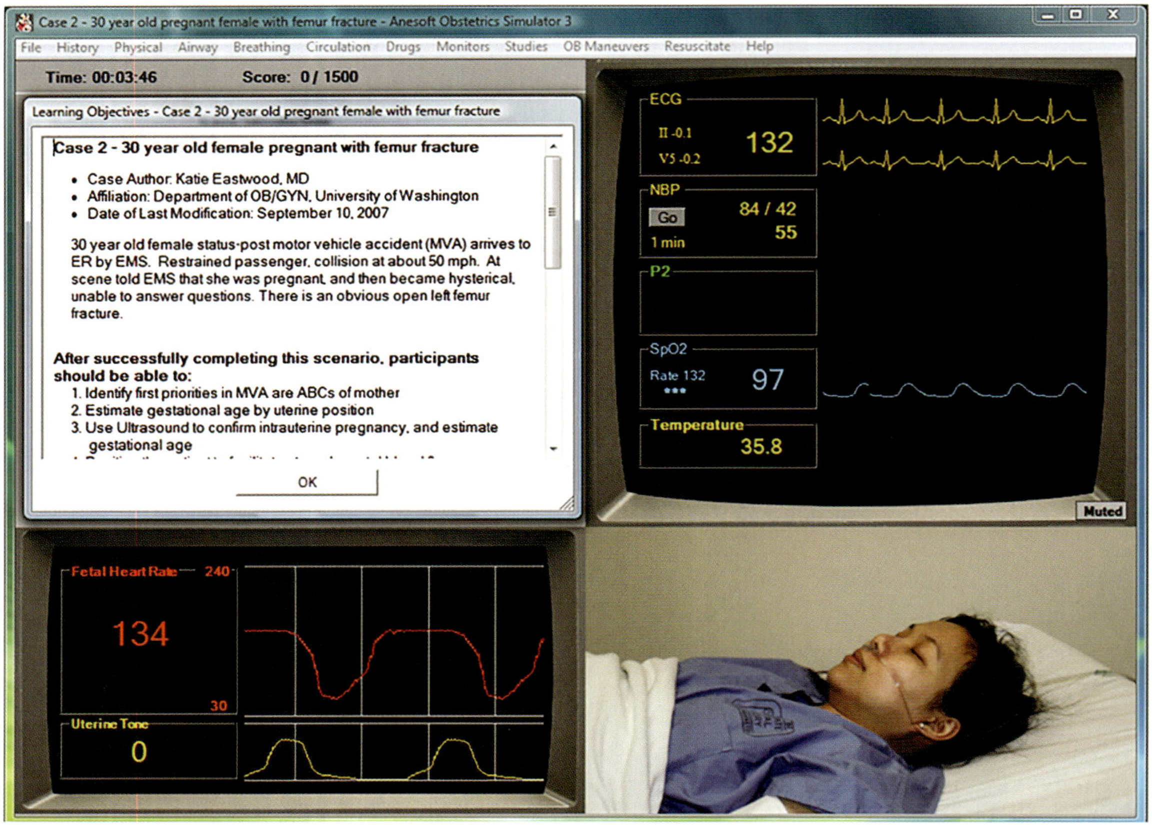

Figure 2 Screen-based simulations

Screen-based simulations provide a powerful mean to analyze and understand the cardiovascular system by simulating situations that are impossible to carry out in a laboratory **(Figure 2)**. Visualization is a tool to create attractive environment for time dependent physiological processes to enable an effective teaching/learning process, while eliminating the risk to the patient's life.

The most commonly used approach for teaching human physiology are the theoretical lessons, supplemented with some simple low budget practical classes, resulting in a lack of interest and passive attitude. The laboratory practices that demonstrate how the cardiovascular system works, offer opportunities for interactive learning and better understanding of theoretical concepts.[2]

Another classic approach mostly used for training a medical personnel is the use of clinical settings, but the learning process is very limited by the patient's clinical conditions which seldom are critical.

During the last few decades, new teaching methods have been implemented. Teaching with animal experiments is almost replaced with the use of educational audiovisual aids, human subjects, and recently by computer-aided learning.[3]

Computer simulations of mathematical models of physiological processes were initially used as biomedical research tools, and later were rapidly developed for teaching purposes.

Most contain an interactive patient vital sign screen which responds to user interventions. Computer-based simulations are generally much less expensive than other types of simulators, and are easily portable. However, physical skills and tasks cannot be taught on them. Educational content is mainly focused on learning facts, using the information learned to make treatment decisions, and evaluating the effectiveness of that treatment.

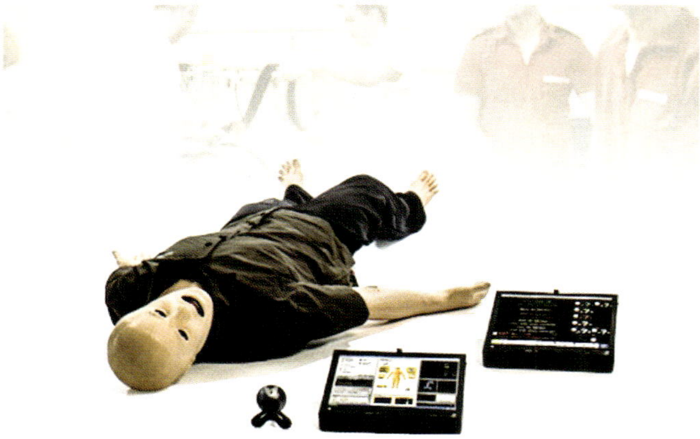

Figure 3 Model-driven simulators

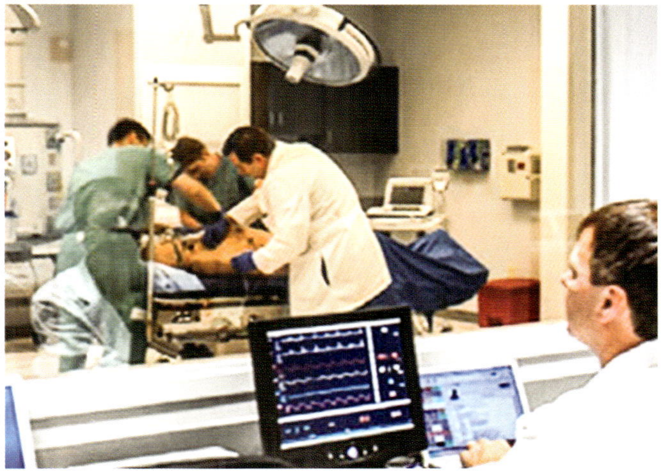

Figure 4 Instructor-driven simulators

MODEL-DRIVEN SIMULATORS

Model-driven simulators (MDS), also called high fidelity simulators, are those that use a manikin body or part of a body to physically represent the patient, and have physiologic and pharmacologic models that direct real time autonomous reactions to interventions and therapies **(Figure 3)**. These types of simulators generally integrate multiple system models to produce a realistic patient response. Suspension of disbelief is not only possible, but easy for the majority of users due to the life-like reactions.

These systems can be used to teach normal and abnormal physiology and pharmacology, equipment usage, patient and provider safety, resource management, crisis management, and many other areas. They can teach at many different educational levels, depending on how the patient is programmed.

While this style of simulator is top of the line, it can also be relatively expensive to set up, depending on the model chosen. The simulator is usually sold by itself, so monitors and ancillary equipment must often be purchased separately to create a realistic setting. The more time and money that are spent to outfit the simulation area, the more realistic is the experience. Each individual must decide how important interaction and realism are to the educational goals of the session.

INSTRUCTOR-DRIVEN SIMULATORS

Instructor-driven simulators (IDS), also called intermediate fidelity simulators, use a partial or full body manikin as a physical presence on which to practice interventions **(Figure 4)**. The simulators may interact with the user in limited ways, but the bulk of responses are created by the instructor. They often use real interventional equipment (probes, IV lines, ventilators, etc.), and may or may not use real monitoring equipment. The output signals to their displays are consistent with the patient anatomy and condition being presented and are changed by the instructor to reflect real-time changes in patient condition.

The simulators are often set up to teach more than one topic or area. Since they are not programmed to be reactive to the user, an instructor/operator will adjust the relevant vital signs to accurately reflect patient responses. Unlike static part task trainers, however, these systems can give some performance feedback. The user is presented with a much closer approximation to an actual patient and environment than with static part task trainers. Because the instructor determines what response (if any) the patient should show, it may be easier in some cases to bring out a teaching point, especially if the point is regarding a patient whose parameters are out of the normal range.

There is significantly more realism and versatility of training topics than with part task trainers, but less than with model driven simulators. Commensurate with the realism and versatility, the start-up price is also somewhere between part task trainers and the high-end model driven systems. It is up to the trainer to determine how much realism is required for an application. It is also trainer-intensive, because the trainer must teach and, at the same time, create a patient response. An alternative is to have two trainers.

CHAPTER 23

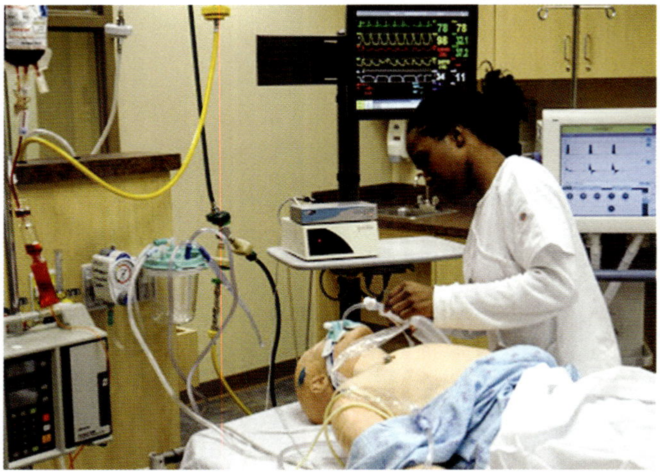

Figure 5 Virtual reality simulators

VIRTUAL REALITY SIMULATORS

Virtual reality (VR) simulators use computer modeling and complex programs to cause the user to believe that they are interacting with a patient, when in reality, they are interacting only with the "imagination" of the computer **(Figure 5)**. The simulator has some type of physical representation with sensing instruments that inform the computer of the user's movements. The program then computes the changes that should take place within the model and projects the correct response onto the screen. Systems may include some sort of three-dimensional (3D) imaging to make the environment more realistic and intuitive.

If the model has haptic (touch) feedback, it will also create the illusion that the user is coming into physical contact with the model, and the user will "feel" the patient as well as see it.

Since a VR training system is necessarily run on a computer, there is always the opportunity to collect information on trainee performance. This is a distinct advantage over non-computer-based models. User data can also be used to create critiques and to generate an individual's learning curve overtime as well as to compare an individual to a cohort of peers.

Virtual reality models have one distinct drawback. It is necessary to have a computer programmer create new modules or make significant adjustments to the current modules. These simulators are always limited by the number of programs that have already been written and tested.

TASK SPECIFIC MODELS

Task specific models are designed to teach a specific task, procedure, or anatomic region. They often resemble anatomic sections of the body, but this is not necessary. Some are automated, but there is no adjustment based on the user's actions. One benefit of task specific models is their relatively low startup and maintenance cost. The anatomic models are usually affordable enough to allow each center to have many duplicates of many models. This allows concurrent teaching of a large class, broken down into small groups, to increase the hands-on time for each trainee.

CONCLUSION

Computational models are proved to be powerful instruments in both processes of research and teaching of physiology and Pathophysiology. Simulations' advantages in comparison with the animal experiments consist on features that models poses such as timesaving, repeatability, less expensive, noninvasive on humans, etc. The complete description of the cardiovascular system as a whole is a very complicated task. However, nowadays such models become more complex and accurate. Even though most of these models are limited to simulate the normal behavior.

CASE SCENARIOS

Case 1

Chief Complaint: Chest pain and shortness of breathe times, 5 days.

HPI: 45-year-old female with chest pain and shortness of breath times, 5 days. The patient reports intermittent chest pain that lasted a couple of minutes that would resolve spontaneously until today.

Today the pain has become much worse occurring at rest every hour lasting up to 10 minutes.

Associated symptoms include shortness of breath and nausea but no vomiting. Patient denies radiation of pain, fever, cough, abdominal pain, or leg pain.

PMH:

- Hypertension

Family History:

- Hypertension
- Mother with AMI @ 50

Medications:
- None

Examination: (presentation to emergency department):
Vital Signs:
- Temp 37.6°C
- HR 90
- BP 123/79
- RR 20
- SpO_2 95% on 2L NC

Physical Examination:
- Alert and oriented, diaphoretic
- Regular rate and rhythm, no murmur/rub
- Lungs clear to auscultation.
- Abdomen round soft, nontender, active bowel sounds
- No edema, pulses intact
- No reproducible pain with palpation of chest.

Labs:
- Na 140 Hgb 11.5 INR 0.9
- K 3.8 Hct 34 PTT 37
- Cl 106 WBC 9.5 Trop I 2.5
- CO_2 24 PLT 215 CKMB 14.5
- BUN 25 CK Total 315
- Cr 0.4 BNP 240
- Gluc 120 D-dimer 0.2

Studies:
- *Chest X-ray (PA/Lat):* Significant for enlarged heart shadow
- *ECG:* Sinus rhythm with inverted T-waves in anterior leads, no ST elevations.

Hospital Course

After presentation to the emergency department, the patient received ASA, metoprolol PO, and started on heparin drip. The patient was seen by cardiology and medical management was chosen over cardiac catheterization. The patient was then transferred to the CCU for closer observation. After transfer to the CCU, the patient decompensated becoming hypotensive (80/40), tachypneic (RR 30), hypoxic (SpO_2 89%) despite increased O_2. The patient was intubated and a PreSep® catheter with $ScvO_2$ monitoring capability and an arterial line with a FloTrac Sensor® capable of continuous cardiac output monitoring were inserted. A repeat chest X-ray post-intubation revealed pulmonary edema.

Discussion (Flow chart 1)

Cardiogenic shock is an emergency requiring immediate resuscitative therapy before shock irreversibly damages vital organs. The key to a good outcome in patients with cardiogenic shock is an organized approach, with rapid diagnosis and prompt initiation of pharmacologic therapy to maintain blood pressure and cardiac output.

All patients require admission to an intensive care setting, which may involve emergent transfer to the cardiac catheterization suite, critical care transport to a tertiary care center, or internal transfer to the intensive care unit (ICU).

Early and definitive restoration of coronary blood flow is the most important intervention for achieving an improved survival rate. At present, it represents standard therapy for patients with cardiogenic shock due to myocardial ischemia.

Correction of electrolyte and acid-base abnormalities, such as hypokalemia, hypomagnesemia, and acidosis, is essential in cardiogenic shock.

Cardiogenic shock may be prevented with early revascularization in patients with myocardial infarction (MI) and with required intervention in patients with structural heart disease.

Immediate Resuscitation Measures

The goal is to prevent devastating end organ injury while the patient is being transported for definitive treatment. Maintenance of adequate mean arterial pressure to prevent adverse neurologic and renal sequelae is vital. Dopamine or noradrenaline (norepinephrine), depending on the degree of hypotension, should be initiated promptly to raise mean arterial pressure and be maintained at the minimum dose required. Dobutamine may be combined with dopamine at moderate doses or used alone for a low output state without frank hypotension. Intra-aortic balloon counterpulsation should be initiated before transportation when facilities are available. Arterial blood gas and oxygen saturation should be monitored with early institution of continuous positive airway pressure or mechanical ventilation as needed. The ECG should be monitored continuously, and defibrillating equipment, intravenous amiodarone, and lidocaine should be readily available. Transcutaneous pacing electrodes as well as provisions for temporary transvenous pacing should be placed at the patient's bedside. Aspirin and full dose

Flow chart 1 Pattern recognition for different types of shock

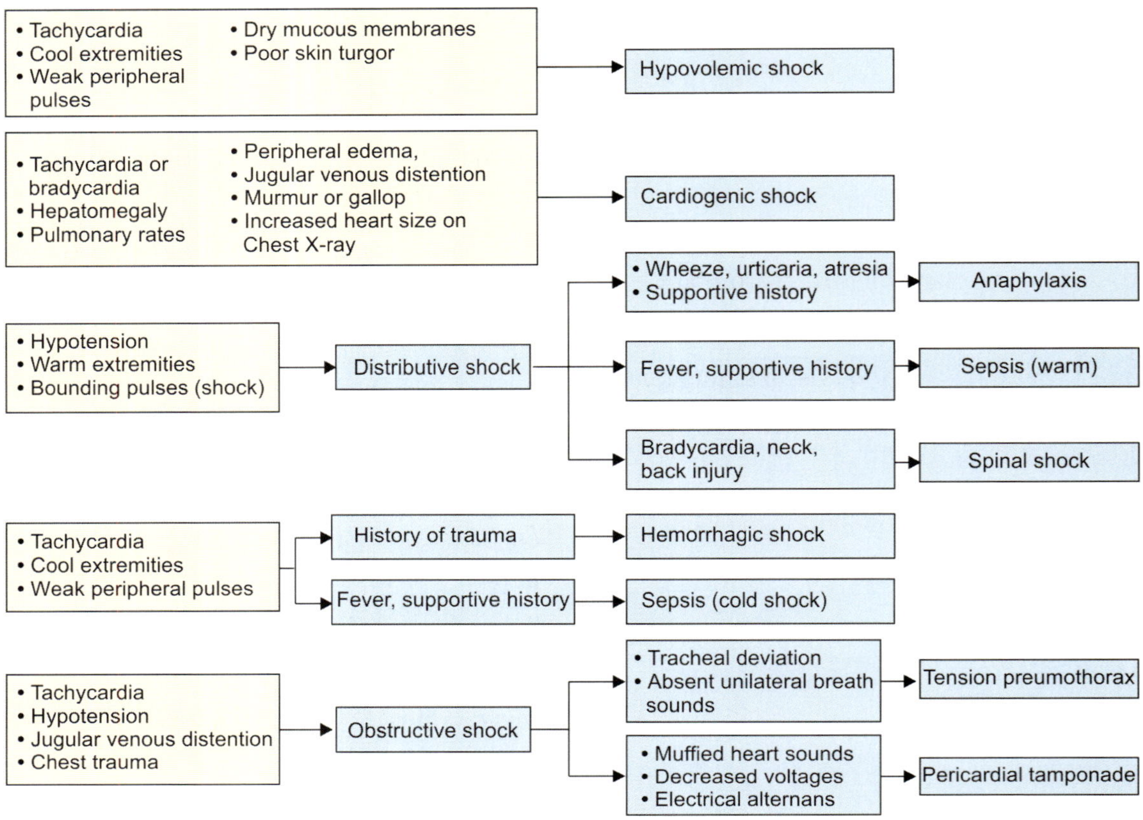

heparin should be administered. For ST elevation MI requiring transfer for angiography, intra-aortic balloon pump (IABP) placement is recommended at the local hospital when possible. A fibrinolytic agent should be initiated in patients with ST elevation MI, if the anticipated delay to angiography is more than two hours. Augmentation of blood pressure with an IABP in this situation may facilitate thrombolysis by increasing coronary perfusion pressure. Similarly, raising blood pressure (to 130 mm Hg systole) by using vasopressor support has also shown synergism in experimental models, but this increase is difficult to achieve in patients in shock. For non-ST elevation MI cardiogenic shock awaiting catheterisation, a glycoprotein IIb/IIIa inhibitor should be initiated.

Case 2

Chief Complaint: Bright red blood per rectum.

HPI: A 67-year-old male with complaint of bright red blood. Patient reports multiple episodes over the past day with a small amount of blood each time. Associated symptoms include lower abdominal pain and mild lightheadedness when changing positions. Patient denies fever, nausea or vomiting, loss of consciousness, chest pain, SOB, or dysuria.

PMH:
- Mitral valve replacement
- Diabetes mellitus
- Hypertension
- Chronic Obstructive Pulmonary Disease (COPD)
- History of UTI 5 days ago treated with TMP-SMX

Medications:
- Warfarin 5 mg PO daily
- Lisinopril 10 mg PO daily
- Insulin glargine 20 units SC daily
- TMP-SMX DS 1 tablet PO BID × 5 days (finished course yesterday)

Examination: (presentation to emergency department):
Vital Signs:
- Temp 37.8°C
- HR 110
- BP 115/70
- RR 18
- SpO_2 95%

Physical Examination:
- Awake but lethargic. Pale.
- Tachycardic, regular rhythm, no murmur/rub, positive click.
- Lungs clear to auscultation.
- Abdomen round soft, mild tenderness to palpation, no rebound tenderness, active bowel sounds.
- Weak pulses × 4, capillary refill >4 seconds.

Labs:
- Na 136 Hgb 6.5 INR 5.4
- K 4.1 Hct 19.3 PTT 35
- Cl 100 WBC 11.8
- CO2 20 PLT 215
- BUN 25
- Cr 1.4
- Gluc 187

Studies:
CT Abdomen/Pelvis: Significant for multiple diverticuli.

Hospital Course

After presentation to the emergency department, the patient rapidly decompensated becoming more tachycardic, hypotensive, and decreased level of conciousness. The patient was intubated and received 2 units PRBC, 2 units FFP, and 1L NS. A PreSep® catheter with $ScvO_2$ monitoring capability and an arterial line with a FloTrac Sensor® capable of continuous cardiac output monitoring were inserted. The patient was then transferred to the MICU. Currently, the patient is 100% mechanically ventilated without any spontaneous breaths.

Discussion

Rapid volume repletion is indicated in patients with severe hypovolemia (i.e. decreased peripheral perfusion, as indicated by delayed capillary refill and cool-mottled extremities) or hypovolemic shock (i.e. severe hypovolemia plus hypotension). Delayed therapy

TABLE 1 Stages of shock

	Stage 1	*Stage 2*	*Stage 3*	*Stage 4*
Blood volume loss	<15% (< 750 mL)	15–30% (750–1,500 mL)	30–40% (1,500–2,000 mL)	>40% (>2,000 mL) (immediately life-threatening)
Cardiac output	Compensated by constriction of vascular bed	Lower	Lower	Lower
Systolic blood pressure	Normal	Normal	<100 mm Hg	<70 mm Hg
Diastolic blood pressure	Normal	Increased		Often not detectable due to narrow gap between systolic and diastolic BP
Respiratory rate	Normal	Increased (tachypnea)	>30/min	Pronounced tachypnea
Heart rate	Slightly increased but <100/min	>100/min	>120/min	>140/min
Pulse	Normal	Weak	Weak	Weak or absent
Capillary refill	Normal (<2 sec)	Delayed (>2 sec)	Delayed (>2 sec)	Absent
Urine output	Normal (>30 mL/hour)	20–30 mL/hour	20 mL/hour	Negligible
Skin	Pale	Pale, sweaty	Cool, pale, sweaty	Cool, extremely pale, sweaty
Mental status	Normal, slight anxiousness	Slight anxiety, restlessness	Confusion, agitation	Lethargy, coma

can lead to ischemic injury and possibly to irreversible shock and multiorgan system failure. Three issues generally need to be considered in this setting: the rate of fluid replacement; the type of fluid infused; and the role for buffer therapy in patients with concurrent lactic acidosis. Vasopressors (e.g. norepinephrine) generally should not be administered, since they do not correct the primary problem and tend to further reduce tissue perfusion **(Table 1)**.

Fluid Deficit Replacement

Fluid deficit replacement can start during transport. The following fluids can be used:

Crystalloids (3 liters are needed to restore 1 liter of lost blood):

- Isotonic saline (0.9% NaCl)
- Ringer lactate

Colloids (1 liter is needed to restore 1 liter of lost blood):

- Hetastarch
- Pentastarch
- Albumin
- Dextran

Blood products (when 2,000 mL crystalloids does not help):

- Fresh-frozen plasma (FFP)
- Packed red blood cells (PRBCs)
- Whole blood transfusion

Vasopressors are not indicated in the initial treatment of hypovolemic shock but may be needed, if after fluid resuscitation systolic blood pressure <90 mm Hg. Start dopamina IV titrated up from lower dose 5 μg/kg/min to 20 μg/kg/min. Careful monitoring to assess the patient's response to dopamine is required.

REFERENCES

1. Araham WT, Adamson PB, Bourge RC, Aron MF, et al. Wireless Pulmonary artery haemodynamic monitoring in chronic heart failure: a randomized controlled trial; the Lancet 2011 - Elsevier.
2. Raven CA, et al. Simulation as a teaching strategy for nursing education and orientation in cardiac surgery, Critical Care Nurse, 2004, AACN.
3. Good ML. Patient simulation for training basic and advanced clinical skills : Medical Education 2003 - Wiley Online Liberary.

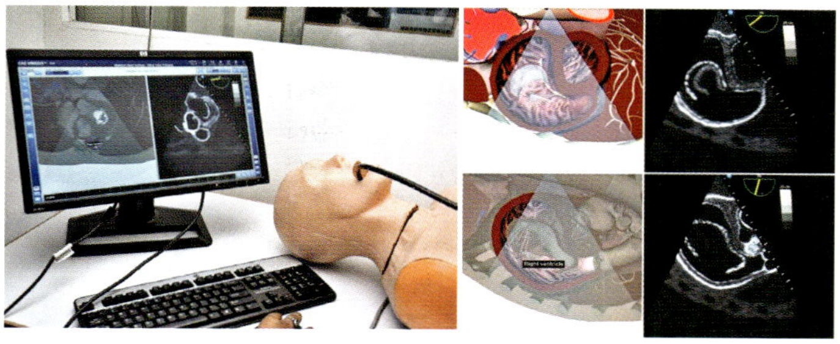

Section 6

Transesophageal Echocardiography in the Cardiac Intensive Care Unit

Section Outline

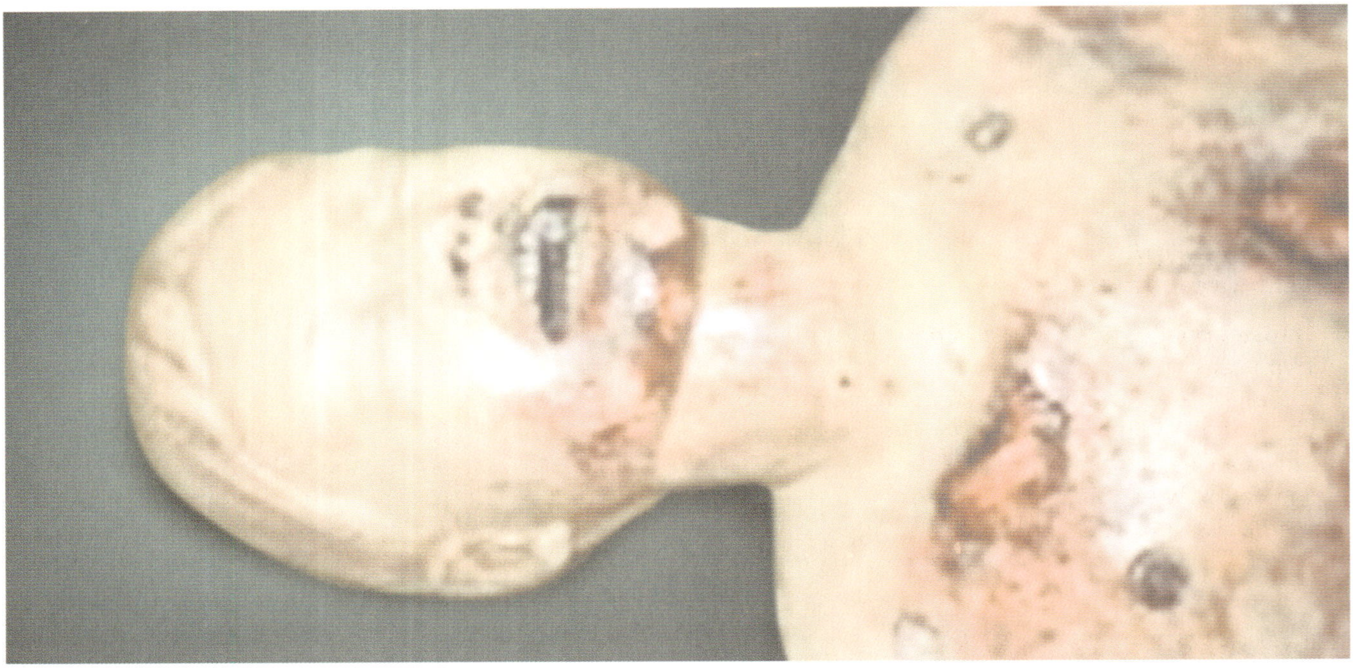

Chapter 24

Simulation for Cardiac Critical Care

Poonam Malhotra Kapoor, Mahesh Vakamudi

Chapter Outline

TRANSESOPHAGEAL ECHO OF PULMONARY ARTERY HYPERTENSION

To date, five echocardiographic parameters have been described in the literature as associated with mortality in pulmonary arterial hypertension (PAH)—degree of pericardial effusion,[1-3] right atrial area indexed to body surface area, end-diastolic eccentricity index,[6] right ventricular (RV) Tei index,[4] and tricuspid annular plane systolic excursion (TAPSE).[5] Other clinical, biological, hemodynamic, and MRI parameters have also been described.[6-11]

Preoperative TEE Assessment of Pulmonary Artery Hypertension

- Two-dimensional (2D) echocardiography shows features of long-standing RV pressure overload. Most patients present with enlarged right-side chambers, RV hypertrophy, increased interventricular septal thickness and an **abnormal interventricular septum/posterior left ventricular (LV) wall ratio (>1), inferior vena cava (IVC) diameter >20 mm, enlarged main pulmonary artery trunk and reduced global RV systolic function**.
- The abnormal pressure gradient between the left and right ventricles results in shape distortion and motion of the interventricular septum ("flattening"), which persists throughout the cardiac cycle.
- The left ventricle thus appears D-shaped, with reduced diastolic and systolic volumes but preserved global systolic function. Small pericardial effusion may be seen secondary to impaired venous and lymphatic drainage due to elevated right atrial pressure (RAP).
- LV diastolic dysfunction may occur due to altered RV-LV interaction characterized by a marked dependence of LV filling on atrial contraction.

DEFINITION AND SEVERITY OF PULMONARY HYPERTENSION

Pulmonary hypertension (PH) is a hemodynamic and pathophysiologic condition defined as an increase in mean pulmonary artery pressure (MPAP) of > 25 mm at rest as assessed by right-heart catheterization.
Mild PH: 30–40 mm hg
Moderate PH: 40–70 mm Hg
Severe PH: > 70 mm Hg.

CALCULATION OF PULMONARY HYPERTENSION USING TRICUSPID REGURGITATION JET VELOCITY

Right ventricle systolic pressure is equal to systolic pulmonary artery pressure (SPAP) in the absence of pulmonary flow obstruction. The measurement of tricuspid regurgitation (TR) jet velocity (V) and application of modified Bernoulli equation give pressure difference between RA and RV **(Table 1)**.

Adding the estimated RAP to this value give RV and PA systolic pressure **(Figure 1)**.
$SPAP = 4X\ TRV^2 + RAP$
Mean (MPAP) and diastolic PA (DPAP) pressure can also be calculated from peak diastolic (V) and end-diastolic (ED) Velocities of pulmonary regurgitation (PR), respectively.
$MPAP = 4\ X\ PRV2 + RAP$
$DPAP = 4\ X\ PRV_{ED}{}^2 + RAP$

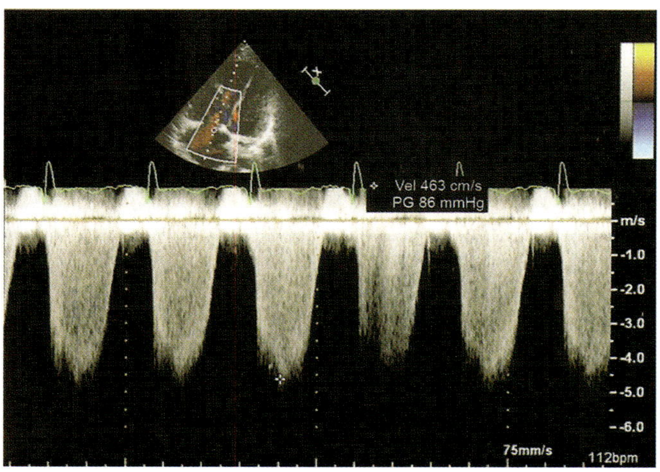

Figure 1 Tricuspid regurgitation peak velocity (TRV = 4.63 M/S)

TABLE 1 Estimation of right atrial pressure (RAP) from TR jet velocity

RAP (MM Hg)	*RA size*	*TR*	*TRV*	*IVC*
5	Normal	Less than or equal to mild	≤2.5 m/s	Normal
10	↑	Moderate	2.6–4 m/s	Dilated
15	↑↑	Severe	>4 m/s	Dilated, no respiratory variation

Limitations of using TR Jet Velocity for Measuring

Underestimation can be due to variations in Doppler angle of interrogation, underestimation of RAP (especially when it is very elevated), the presence of severe TR, or a poor TR signal. Overestimation of SPAP is less common and often is due to overestimation of RAP; it can also results from overestimating the TR signal peak velocity, as well as mistakenly using the TV closing spike due to TV closure for the tricuspid maximal velocity.

Measurement of TR velocity to estimate SPAP gives a false result in the presence of pulmonary valve (PV) stenosis. While this pressure gradient helps to estimate RV systolic pressure, transpulmonary gradient must be taken into account to estimate pulmonary artery pressure.
$SPAP = (4\ X\ TRV^2) + RAP - PSV^2$

Systolic PA pressure estimation from TR velocity may be underestimated in the presence of significant RV dysfunction. Errors in estimation of SPAP have also occurred in patients with congenital or acquired LV-RA shunt (Gerbode defect) **(Figures 2A and B)**.

Different Methods to Diagnose Pulmonary Hypertension

Pulmonary flow acceleration time is an alternative, less widely used method for screening patients for the presence of PH. Pulmonary flow acceleration time is the interval between the onsets of forward flow in the PA to its peak velocity. Values of <100 ms are associated

SECTION 6

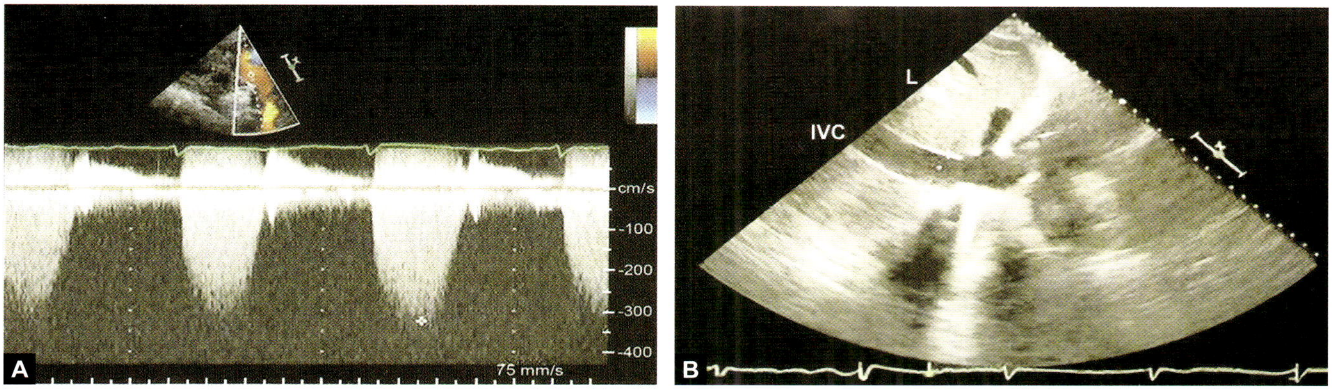

Figures 2A and B Underestimation of systolic pulmonary artery pressure (SPAP). In this patient the estimated tricuspid regurgitation (TR) gradient was 42 mm Hg. The estimated right atrial pressure (RAP) using inferior vena cava (IVC) diameter of 2.78 cm and absence of respiratory collapse (bottom) was 15 mm Hg, giving an estimated SPAP of 57 mm Hg. However, the actual pulmonary artery catheter reading for SPAP was 84 mm Hg. This underestimation was due to underestimation of the RAP, which was measured invasively as 40 mm Hg (L: Liver)

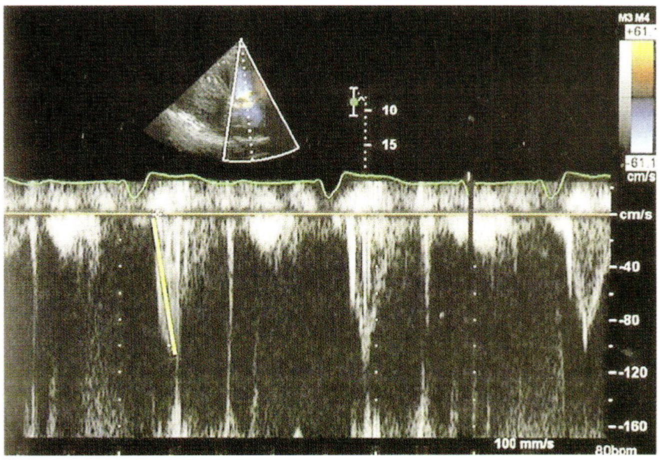

Figure 3 Evaluation of systolic pulmonary artery pressure (SPAP) using PA acceleration time (PAcT), which is the interval between the onsets of the forward flow in the PA to its peak velocity (yellow line). A value <100 ms is associated with an elevated PAP. In this patient the PAcT is 63 ms, consistent with an elevated SPAP

with PH. However, it does not provide a quantitative estimation of SPAP (**Figure 3**).

Calculation of PVR from Echo/Doppler Method

Pulmonary vascular resistance is directly proportional to the pressure gradient across the entire lungs and inversely correlates with pulmonary flow. Pulmonary vascular resistance is a hemodynamic variable, which contributes to the management of patients with advanced cardiovascular and pulmonary disease. It can be calculated by cardiac catheterization as follows:

PVR: (MPAP – mean PCWP) X 80/Cardiac output

Normal Values range between 20 and 130 dynes/s/m/cm^{-5}, which equals 0.25 – 1.6 Wood units (WU).

Pulmonary vascular resistance can also be estimated by echo/Doppler by dividing peak TR velocity (m/s) with velocity time integral (VTI) of RV outflow tract (RVOT) (cm).

PVR (WU) = TRVel X 10/RVOT VTI + 0.16

Presence of TR in Pulmonary Hypertension

No. Although TR is present to a mild degree even in normal individuals as mentioned above, in some patients with PH including those with systemic level PH, it may be completely absent or so minimal that the TR Doppler waveform is incomplete or poor in quality precluding assessment of SPAP. This presents a challenge to the echocardiographer. Occasionally, a bubble study helps as it may enhance the TR signals resulting in a complete TR waveform suitable for measuring the peak velocity. Other echo/Doppler methods including measurement of RV wall thickness (best measured using the subcostal approach taking care to exclude any adjacent trabeculations) and pulmonary acceleration time are helpful in making a diagnosis of PH but do not provide quantitative assessment of SPAP. Knowledge of SPAP may assist evaluation of a patient with dyspnea and decrease the need for invasive techniques.

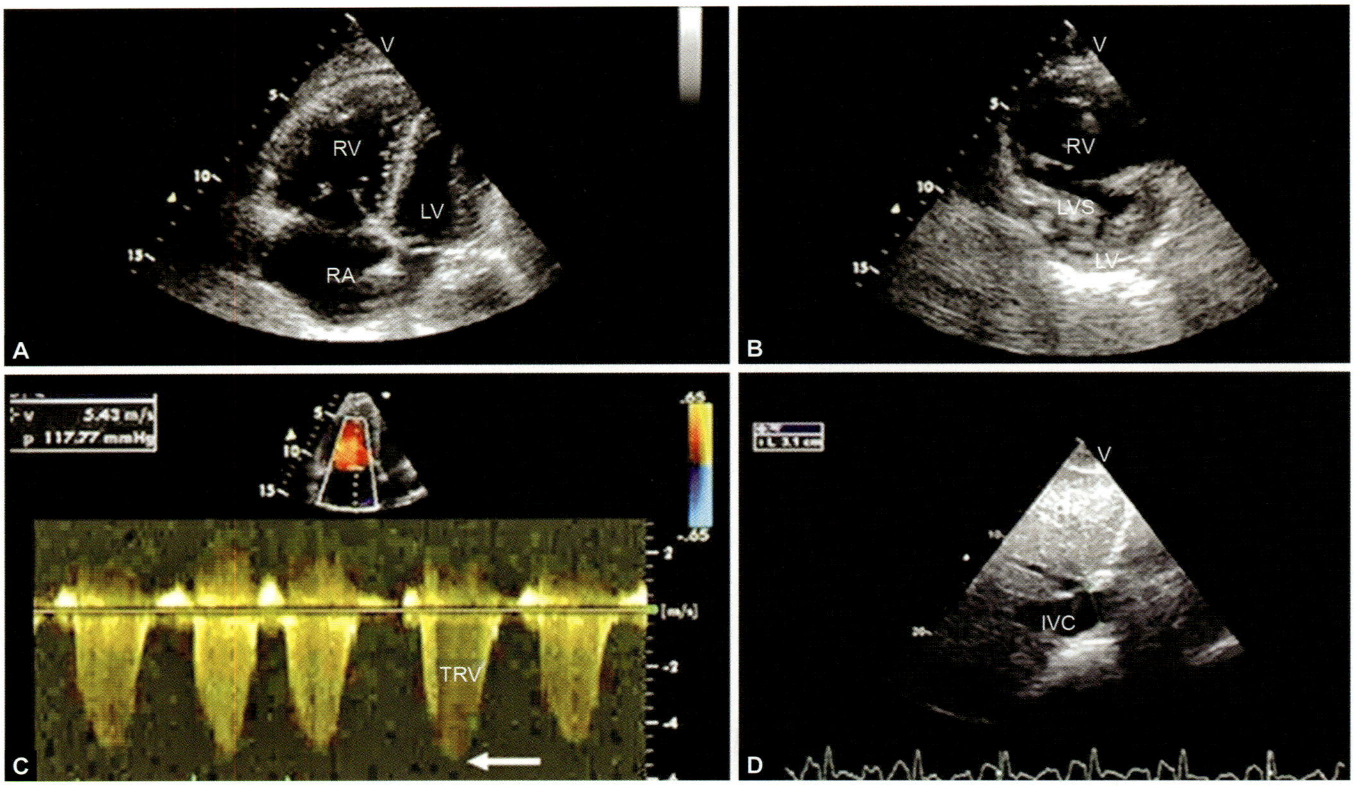

Figures 4A to D A young patient with IPAH. (A and B) Apical four-chamber and parasternal short-axis views, showing severe right ventricular enlargement and dislocation of the interventricular septum (IVS) towards the left ventricle (LV). (C) Doppler tracing of TR, showing severe PH (TRV >5 m/sec) (arrow). (D) Dilated inferior vena cava (IVC) from the subcostal view

Abbreviations: RA, Right atrium; RV, right ventricle; LV, left ventricle; IPAH, idiopathic pulmonary arterial hypertension; TR, tricuspid regurgitation; TRV, tricuspid regurgitant velocity.

EVALUATION WITH COLOR FLOW DOPPLER (FIGURES 4A TO D)

- Significant tricuspid and pulmonary valve regurgitation commonly seen in pulmonary artery hypertension **(Figure 5)**.
- Tricuspid regurgitation (TR) seen is usually caused by tricuspid annular dilatation, altered RV geometry, and apical displacement of the tricuspid leaflets.

Estimation of PVR

Pulmonary vascular resistance (PVR) may be estimated by dividing TR peak velocity (in meters per second) by the time-velocity integral of the RV outflow tract (in centimeters).

CARDIAC TAMPONADE

Cardiac tamponade is a cause of obstructive shock. It is defined by an acute circulatory failure secondary to compression of the heart chambers by a pericardial effusion.

Occult Cardiac Tamponade Detected by Transesophageal Echocardiography

Transesophageal echocardiography (TEE) is a safe, minimally invasive procedure that should be considered when the diagnosis of cardiac tamponade is a possibility and when conventional methods fail to provide conclusive diagnostic information.

TEE Findings in Cardiac Tamponade (Figure 6A to C)

Cardiac tamponade leading to circulatory arrest is easily detected by transthoracic echocardiography (TTE). Depending on the aggressiveness of treatment protocols for cardiac tamponade, it might be necessary to define the cause of the tamponade, and TEE may

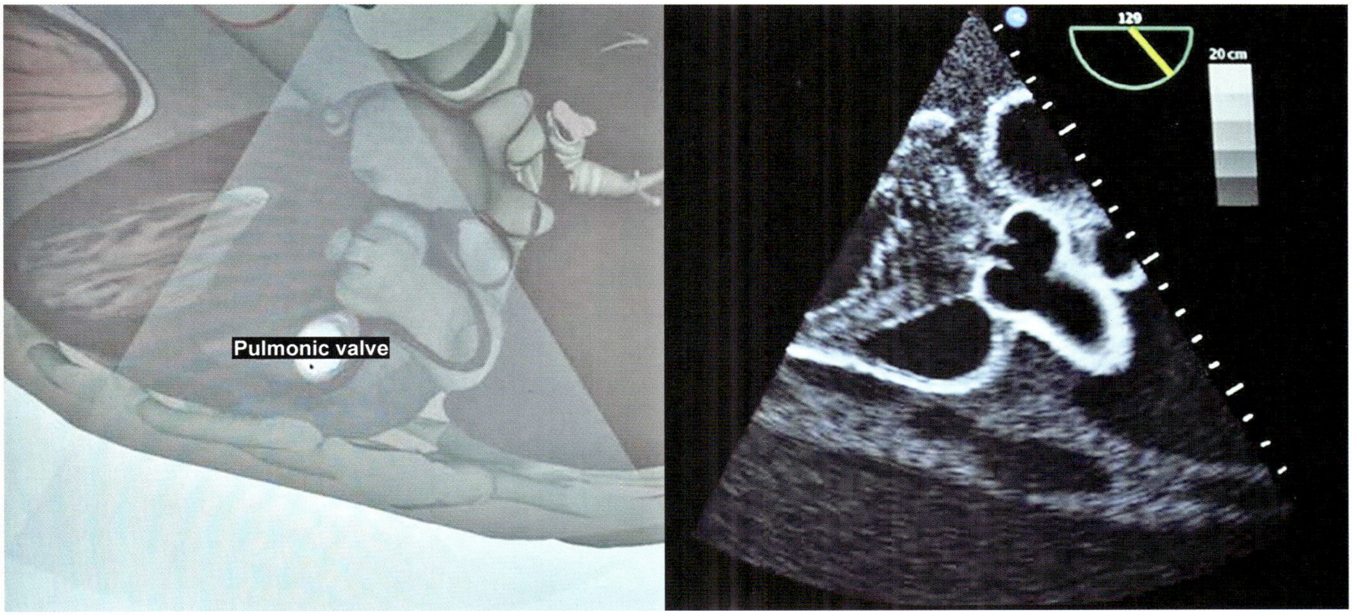

Figure 5 Simulation view of transesophageal echo (TEE) in pulmonary artery hypertension

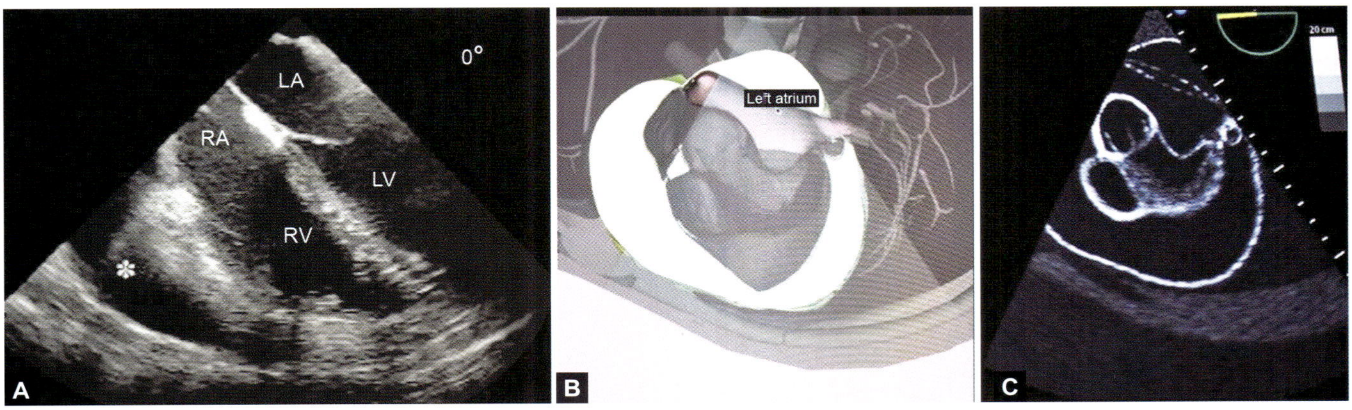

Figures 6A to C (A) Additional findings of tamponade include 25% respiratory variation of mitral valve and tricuspid valve inflow; (B and C) Simulation views of TEE in cardiac tamponade showing the dilated RA and LA

be helpful in defining causes like aortic dissection, endocarditis or myocardial free wall rupture.

The upstream position of the right ventricle renders its pump function sensitive to changes in intrathoracic pressure and lung volume. During spontaneous inspiration, venous return, filling of the right heart, early and late diastolic filling velocities, RV stroke volume, all increase. In it ejection fraction is observed. The respiratory variation in transtricuspid flow velocity (early [E] and late [A] waves) during quiet breathing is in the range 17%, whereas excessive variation tamponade.[12] Opposite changes occur during mechanical ventilation. The intrathoracic pressure increase associated with the mechanical inspiration impairs venous return, reduces RV filling (E and A velocities), PA flow, and RV stroke volume. This inspiratory decrease in RV preload can combine with an increase RV afterload (by compression of the pulmonary vascular bed due to high inspiratory pressures and/or additional positive end-expiratory pressure) to impair RV ejection.[13]

Figure 6 shows the additional findings of tamponade include 25% respiratory variation of mitral valve and tricuspid valve inflow.

PERICARDIAL EFFUSION

Echocardiographically, a pericardial effusion appears as an echolucent signal immediately adjacent to the epicardium. General guidelines on pericardial effusion size and fluid distribution patterns are presented in **Table 2**.[14] Caution is warranted when diagnosing a pericardial effusion to rule out the presence of epicardial fat which can appear similar to a pericardial fluid collection at first glance. Close observation of epicardial fat demonstrates a weak echogenic signal compared to the more echolucent signal of a pericardial fluid collection.

TABLE 2 Pericardial effusion characteristics

Severity	*Width by Echo*	*Volume (mL)*	*Localization Region*
Small	<10 mm	<100	Behind posterior LV wall
Moderate	10–15 mm	100–150	Expand laterally and apically
Large	>15 mm	>500	Evenly distributed around the heart

Echocardiographic Assessment of Pericardial Effusion (Figures 7 and 8)

TEE usually overcomes many of the imaging constraints of TTE echocardiography: the surgical site may preclude use of the optimal transthoracic window, chest tubes

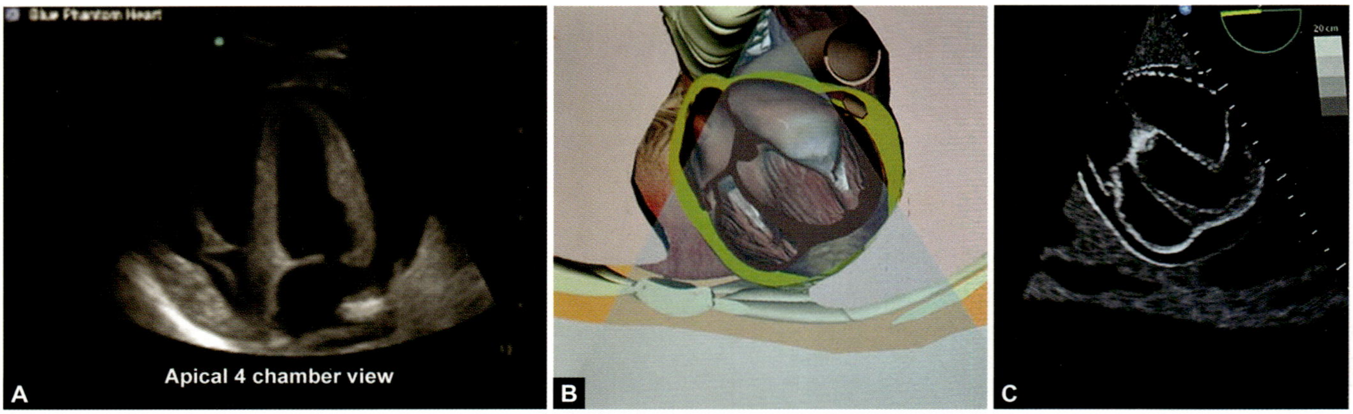

Figures 7A to C Apical four-chamber view acquired during fast trauma sonography showing pericardial effusion and right atrial collapse; Simulation view of TEE in myocardial infarction with pericardial effusion

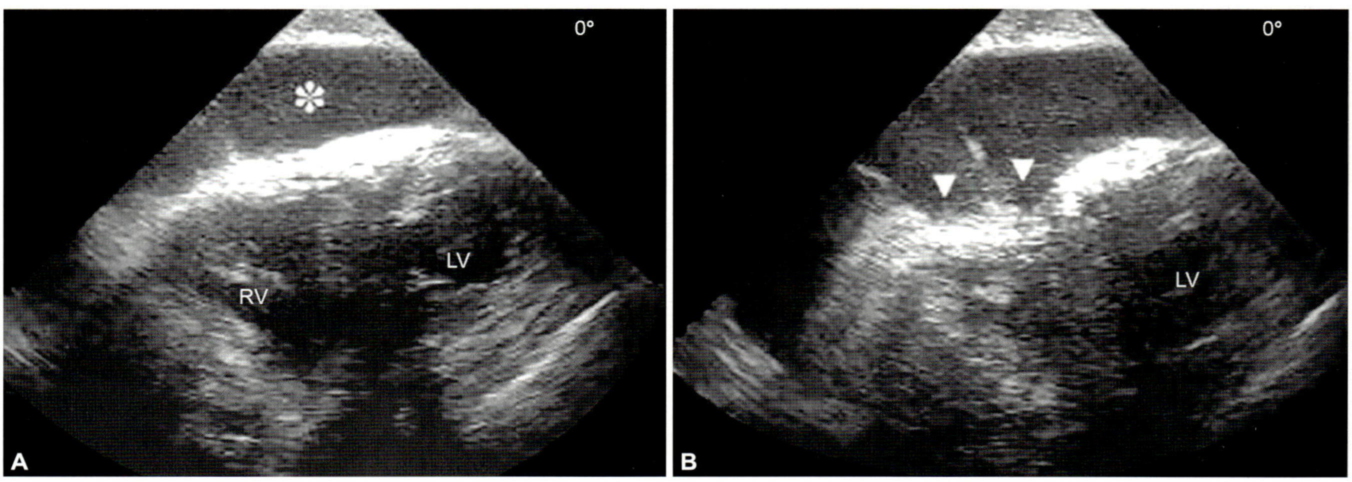

Figures 8A and B The key element of the differential diagnosis is to identify that the patient has a moderate-to-large pericardial effusion as shown in the arrows

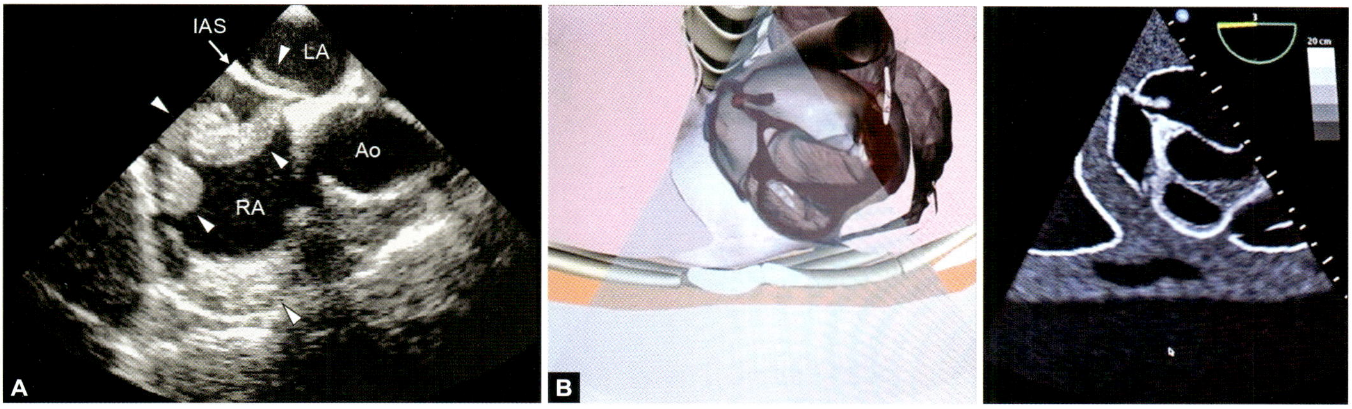

Figures 9A and B (A) Multiplane TEE (60°). Thrombus (arrowheads) makes its way through patent foramen ovale; (B) Simulation view of TEE in thrombus with PFO

can affect imaging and proper positioning of the patient, compression of the chest wall with the probe may worsen incisional pain, while some loculated effusions may be difficult to image.[8] Pericardial effusion is graded as small if the visceral and parietal pericardial layers are separated by less than 0.5 cm, moderate by 0.5–2 cm, and large when greater than 2 cm.[9] When the effusion is significant, ventricular function can be normal or depressed, particularly, if the pericardial pressure overwhelms ventricular diastolic pressures adding to resistance to myocardial and endocardial blood flow. Of note, absence of pericardial contents around the LV should not necessary exclude the absence of pericardial collection around other heart structures, such as the RV or atria.

THROMBUS WITH PATENT FORAMEN OVALE

A 36-year-old woman with a 3-week history of shortness of breath was admitted to the hospital after having suffered syncope. She also complained of left-sided leg pain. Duplex ultrasound revealed a right-sided proximal deep venous thrombosis and an occluded left popliteal artery. Echocardiography demonstrated a dilated right ventricle and tricuspid regurgitation with an estimated pulmonary systolic pressure of 80 mm Hg. Spiral CT demonstrated multiple central pulmonary emboli; cranial MRI showed multiple small infarcted zones; and transesophageal echocardiography (TEE) revealed a patent foramen ovale (PFO). After embolectomy of the left popliteal artery and a 10-day course of anticoagulation, follow-up echocardiography showed a possible thrombus in the right atrium. Therefore, TEE was performed, which revealed a thrombus '10 cm long caught in the foramen ovale on its way to the left atrium. At emergent cardiac surgery, the thrombus was extracted, the persistent foramen ovale closed, and a vena cava filter inserted. This is shown in **Figures 9 and 10**.

LEFT ATRIAL MYXOMA

Echocardiography is the most important tool to reach the definitive diagnosis rapidly and non-invasively. In addition, perioperative TEE is indispensable in planning the surgical procedure in real-time assessment of its results and for medical management in the early post-operative period.

The significance of perioperative TEE for detailed diagnosis and therapeutic guidance is underscored by:

i. Confirmation of preoperative findings with precise localization of the myxomas attachment site, which helped in surgical planning;
ii. Documentation of complete tumor removal;
iii. Evaluation of mitral valve repair; and
iv. Diagnosis and grading of post-repair mitral valve regurgitation, which led to an intraoperative change in surgical strategy, i.e. prosthetic mitral valve replacement. Furthermore, as is routine in mitral valve surgery, TEE provided to the perioperative team the functional assessment of the prosthetic mitral valve, rule-out of a paravalvular leak prior to the termination of CPB, postoperative detection of new regional wall motion abnormalities, presence of blood flow signal in the circumflex artery, assessment of left ventricular function and guidance for appropriate fluid and inotrope management.[15]

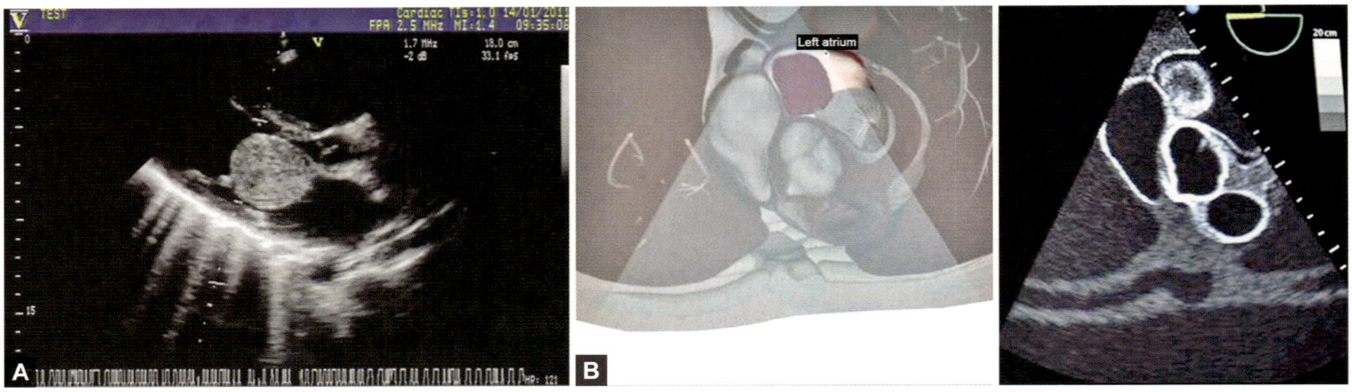

Figures 10A and B (A) Transesophageal echocardiography in left atrial myxoma; (B) Simulation view of TEE in left atrial myxoma

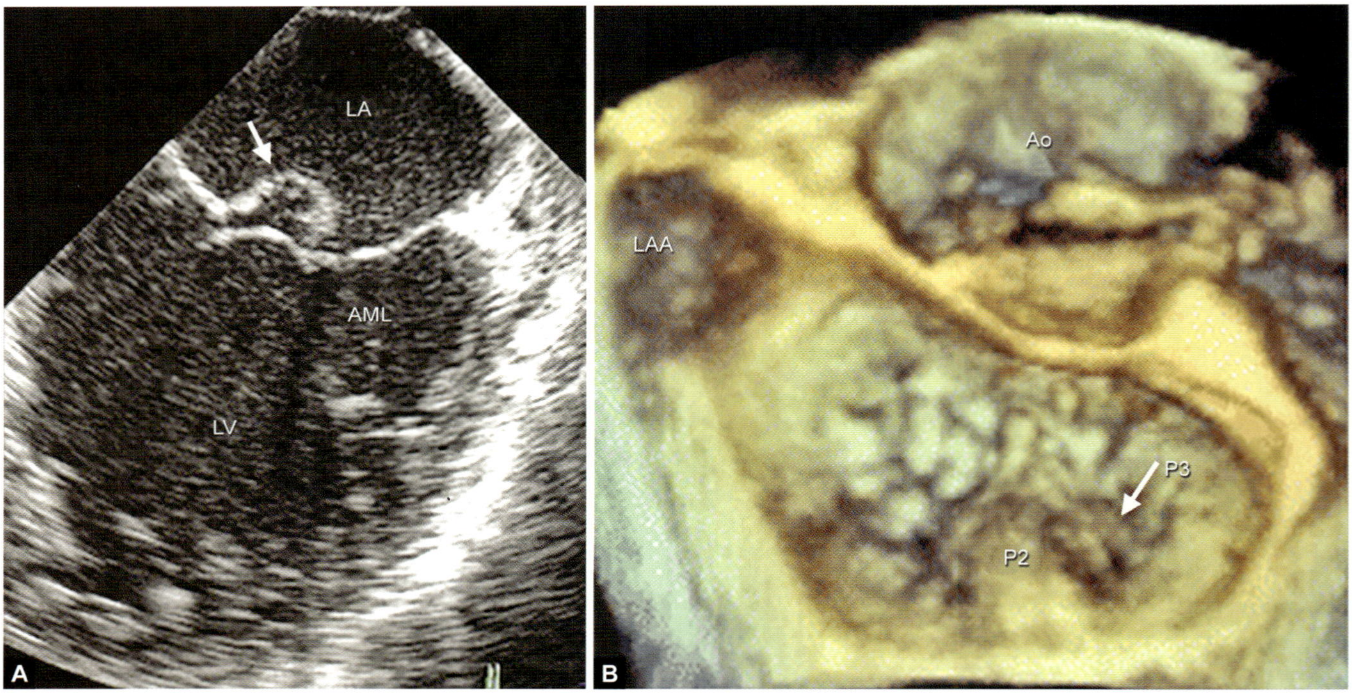

Figures 11A and B Prolapse of the posterior mitral leaflet. (A) 2D TEE showing bulging of the PML (arrow). (B) View in systole from the left atrium by live 3D TEE showing a large spoon-like leaflet in the P2 and P3 segments (arrow) but only P2 was reported by surgeon when heart was arrested and empty

Abbreviations: LA, left atrium; AML, anterior mitral leaflet; LV, left ventricle; LAA, left atrial appendage; Ao, aortic; PML, posterior mitral leaflet.

MITRAL VALVE PROLAPSE (FIGURES 11 AND 12)

Mitral valve prolapse is observed with thin leaflets or thickened degenerative myxomatous leaflets. Mitral valve prolapse is seen as an isolated condition and as a feature of disorders such as Marfan syndrome, hypertrophic cardiomyopathy, or Ehlers-Danlos syndrome. Prolapse may involve one or more of the three scallops of the posterior leaflet, the anterior leaflet, or both leaflets.

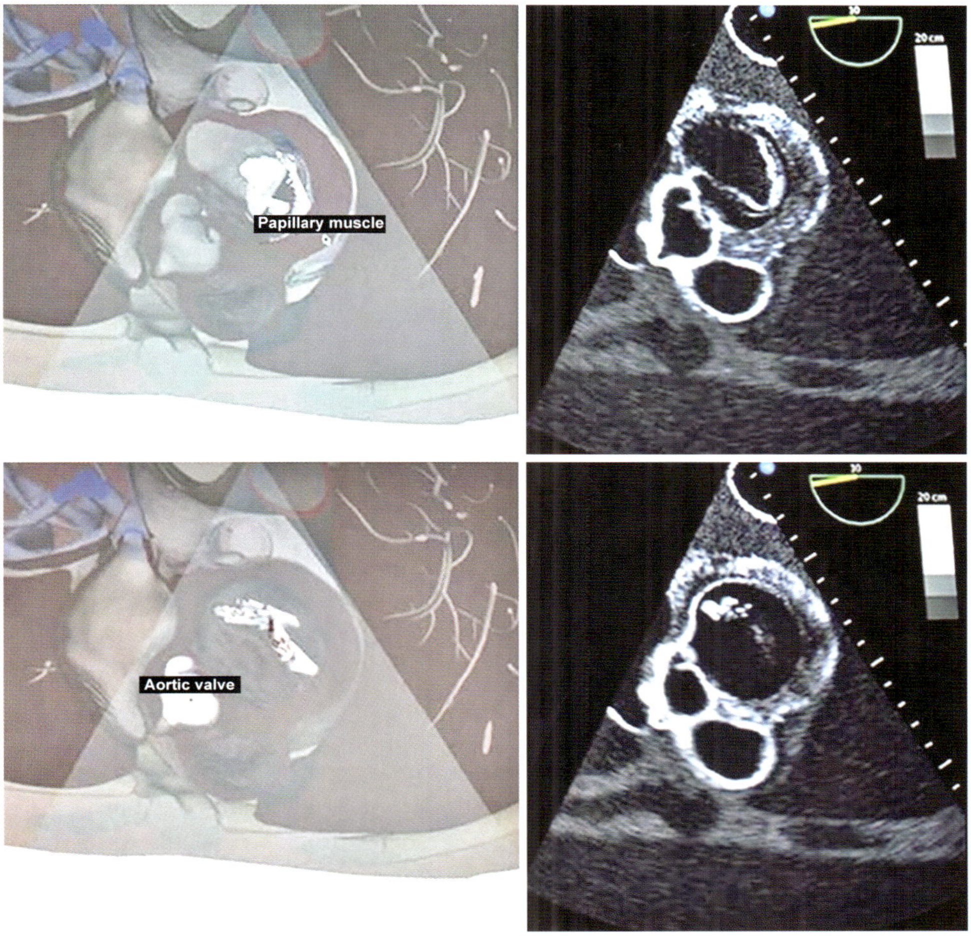

Figure 12 Simulation views of TEE in mitral valve prolapse showing the valve morphology and LV diastolic function

- While transthoracic echocardiography (TTE) is the primary diagnostic modality for evaluation of mitral disease, transesophageal echocardiography (TEE) is a helpful adjunct in selected patients.
- TEE is performed prior to percutaneous balloon valvotomy to identify atrial appendage thrombus (which is a contraindication to valvotomy) and to assess markers of thrombotic risk such as atrial spontaneous echo contrast and reduced atrial appendage ejection velocities.
- TEE is helpful during and following percutaneous mitral balloon valvotomy to guide trans-septal puncture and balloon placement and to identify complications. The residual atrial septal defect after trans-septal puncture is generally small and hemodynamically insignificant and often closes spontaneously.
- TEE is helpful when the severity and/or cause of mitral regurgitation is not well-defined on TTE.
- Intraoperative TEE is important for detecting the adequacy of mitral valve repair and the presence of paravalvular leaks after mitral valve replacement.
- The role of three-dimensional TEE is evolving in the evaluation of mitral valve morphology and assessing both mitral stenosis and mitral regurgitation.

Role of intraoperative echocardiography: Intraoperative guidance of mitral valve repair for MV prolapse in severe mitral regurgitation is an established indication for TEE and should be performed for all repairs.[16] Intraoperative TEE can enhance the success of valve repair and can reliably predict early and late mitral valve dysfunction.[17] this was confirmed in one study of 143 patients undergoing mitral valve repair, 11 patients had grade 3 or greater mitral regurgitation

CHAPTER 24

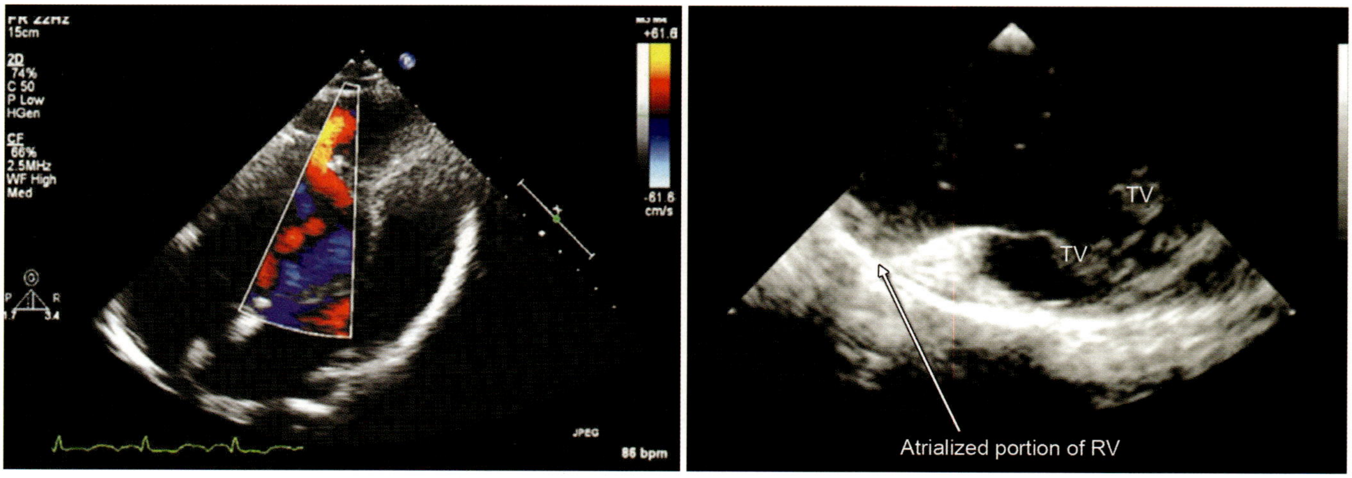

Figure 13 TEE image of a patient with Ebstein's anomaly showing apical displacement of the TV leaflet and the thin, "atrialized" portion of the affected right ventricular (RV) wall
Abbreviation: TV, tricuspid valve.

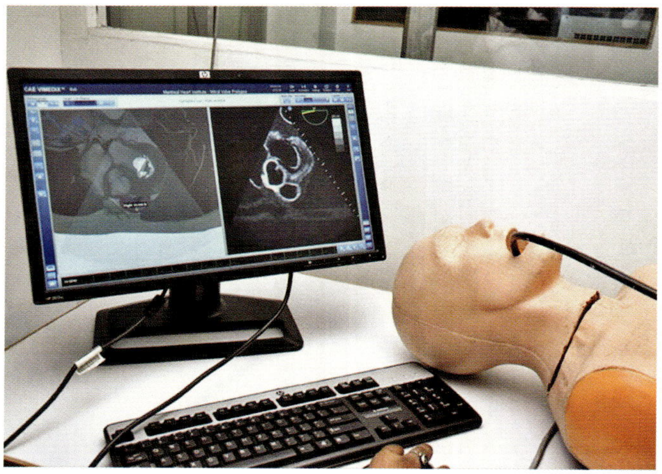

Figure 14 Ebstein's anomaly with ASD on the simulator
(*Courtesy:* Vimedix DSS)

on intraoperative TEE after discontinuation of cardiopulmonary bypass. Of these 11 patients, five underwent mitral valve replacement, five underwent revision of the mitral repair, and one was managed with observation only. A predischarge TTE was performed in 132 patients; when compared to the intraoperative TEE, there was a discrepancy of 1 grade or greater in the estimated severity of mitral regurgitation in only 17 patients (13%).

TRANSESOPHAGEAL ECHO FOR EBSTEIN'S ANOMALY (FIGURES 13 TO 15)

The diagnosis of Ebstein's anomaly by echocardiography is straightforward as inadequate delamination of the TV leaflets from the endocardium of the RV results in features that are characteristics of this anomaly, which include apical displacement of the leaflets, particularly, the septal leaflet, with associated TR and right ventricular dysfunction.

Preoperative Assessment of Ebstein Anomaly on TEE

- Midesophageal (ME) four-chamber view diagnostic:
  - Right ventricular displacement of the leaflet can be visualized.
  - Is the tricuspid valve position normal or it is displaced apically? In Ebstein's anomaly, the septal or posterior tricuspid leaflet is displaced towards the RV apex by at least 0.8 cm/m^2 (in adults, the displacement should be indexed for body surface area), in comparison with the mitral valve plane)
  - Large malformed ATL tethered to the RV wall
  - Apically displaced STL; distance from MV annulus >20 mm or >8 mm/m^2
- Dilated RA
- Dilated TV annulus - False and True should be measured

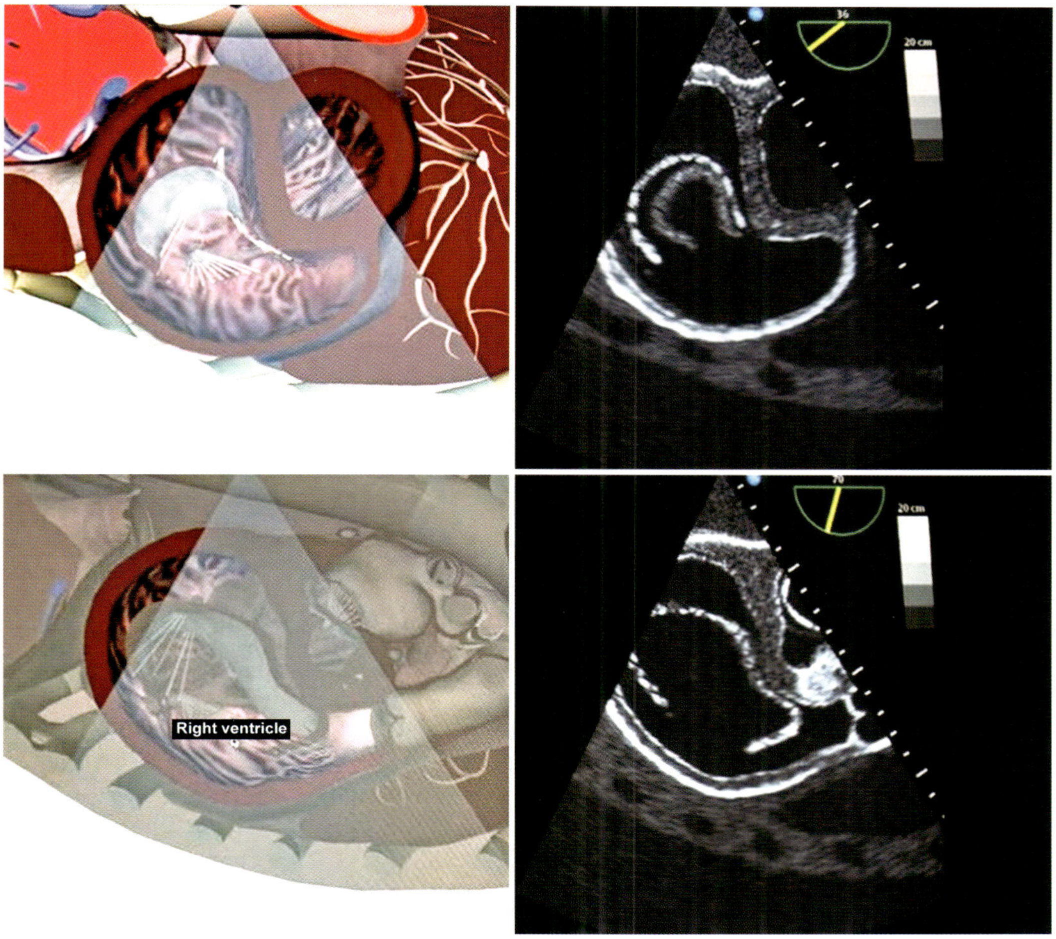

Figure 15 Simulation views of TEE in Ebstein's anomaly with ASD

- Atrialization of RV
- Small functional right ventricle or dilated right ventricle
- Right heart volume overload may be seen
- Assessment of RV and LV function.

DILATED CARDIOMYOPATHY ON TEE SIMULATION (FIGURE 16)

Dilated cardiomyopathy is associated with increased LV end-systolic and diastolic volumes. These inceased volumes result in decreased elastic recoil and reduced chamber compliance, and hence in impaired diastolic function. During the early stage of congestive heart failure, the main diastolic abnormality is slowing of LV relaxation with reduced early diastolic filling. As congestive heart failure progresses, the transmitral gradient increases with a return of mitral flow velocity to baseline, indicating a pseudonormalization of the mitral flow pattern. During a more advanced stage, the transmitral pressure gradient increases further resulting in a restrictive filling pattern.[18] This restrictive filling pattern is often seen during the decompensated stage of dilated cardiomyopathy.

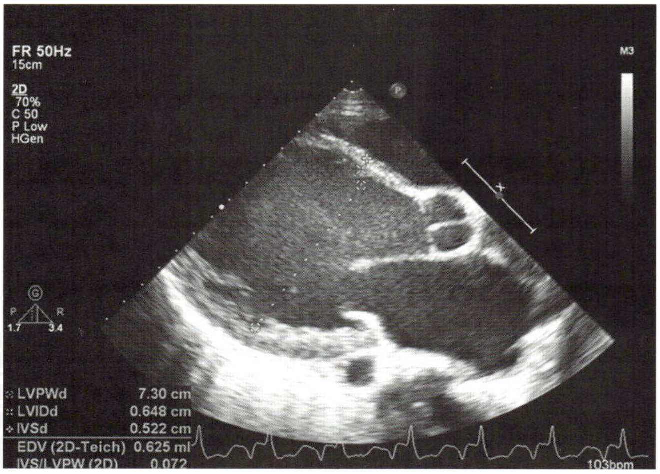

Figure 16 The left ventricle seen in this parasternal long axis view is massively dilated and poorly functioning. This degree of LV dilation tells us this is chronic process. Also note the early closure of the aortic valve from low cardiac output. Echo "smoke" can be seen within ventricle, a sign of slow-flowing blood and low cardiac output

Hypertrophic Cardiomyopathy

Hypertrophic cardiomyopathy is a genetically determined cardiac disorder that is defined by a hypertrophied, nondilated ventricle in the absence of another disease capable of producing the degree of hypertrophy noted (i.e., hypertension, aortic stenosis). LV systolic function is usually normal or hyperdynamic. Asymmetric hypertrophy affecting the interventricular septum is the most common form. However, asymmetry can affect any region including the apex, lateral, posterior, or inferior walls. A pattern of concentric hypertrophy occurs less often. About 25% of patients have a resting gradient between the left ventricular outflow tract (LVOT) and the aorta at rest. Mitral regurgitation is seen in most patients with LVOT obstruction. The LVOT gradient is nearly always associated with a forward movement of the anterior mitral valve leaflet or systolic anterior motion (SAM). The severity of this outflow tract gradient correlates with the time of onset and duration of contact between the mitral valve and the septum. This creates the midsystolic deceleration in the aortic flow profile that coincides with mitral valve-septal contact.

The patient with hypertrophic cardiomyopathy (HCM) with asymmetric septal hypertrophy and left ventricular outflow tract (LVOT) obstruction. LVOT obstruction needs to be distinguished with one from MR jet. The MR jet can be distinguished as higher velocity, with a rapid increase in velocity starting at the onset of ventricular contraction. It also extends beyond aortic valve closure. The LVOT profile is characterized by a dagger shape with a late systolic peak velocity. Diastolic dysfunction parameters are initial markers of this disease even before the appearance of hypertrophy.

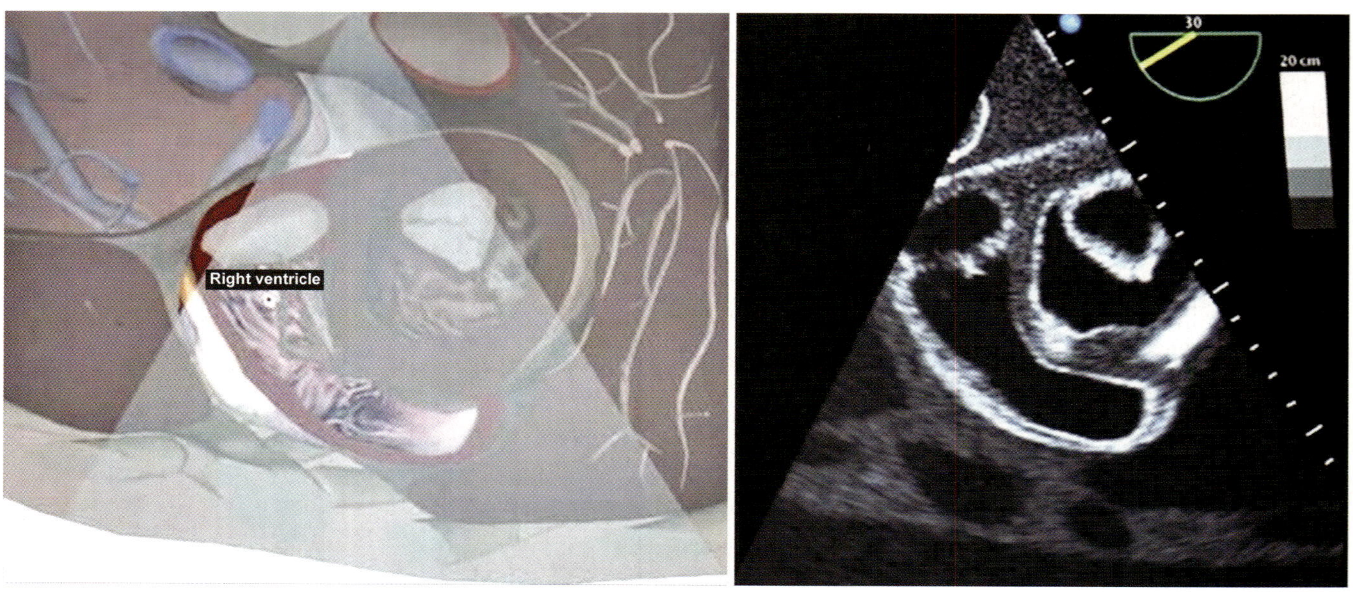

Figure 17 Simulation views of TEE in dilated cardiomyopathy in an elderly patients

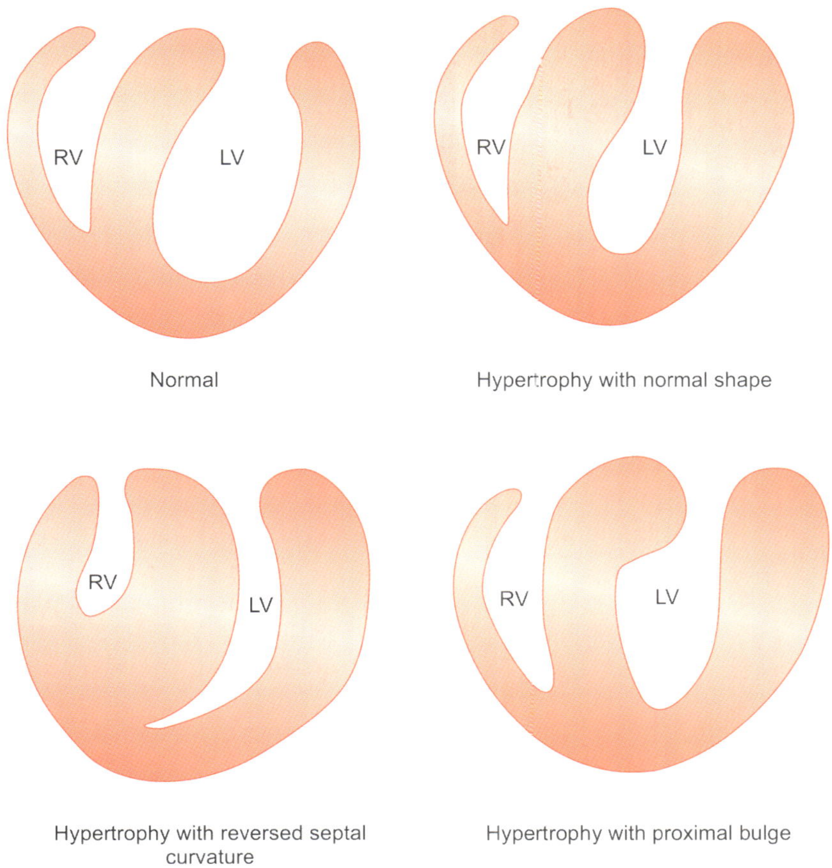

Figure 18 Hypertrophy cardiomyopathy

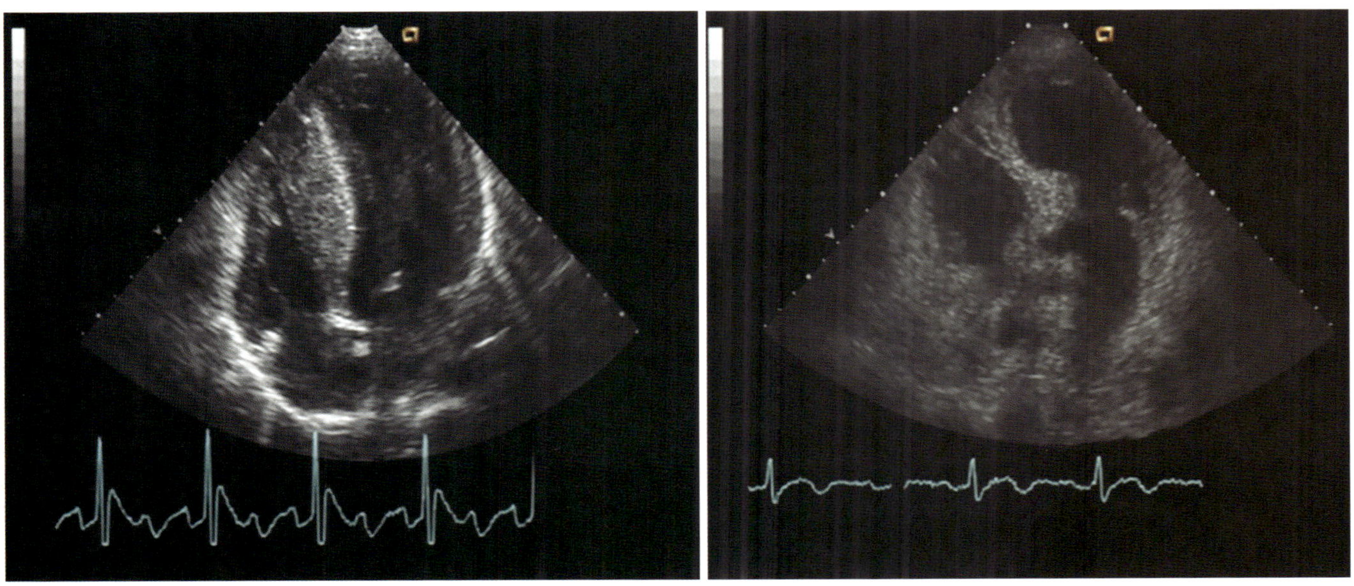

Figure 19 The deep transgastric view shows the complete septum and the two ventricles

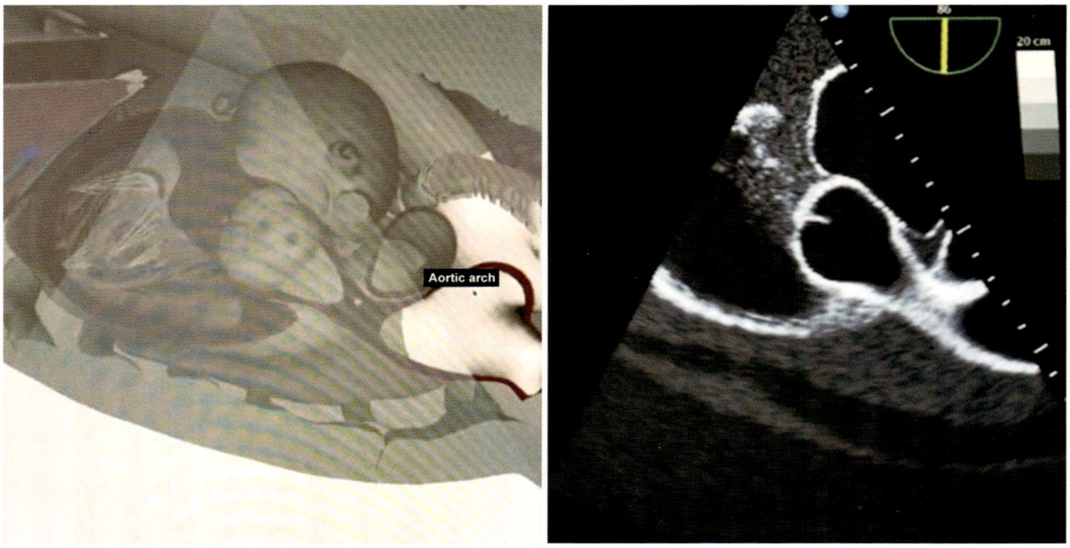

Figure 20 The left atrial appendage view at 90°

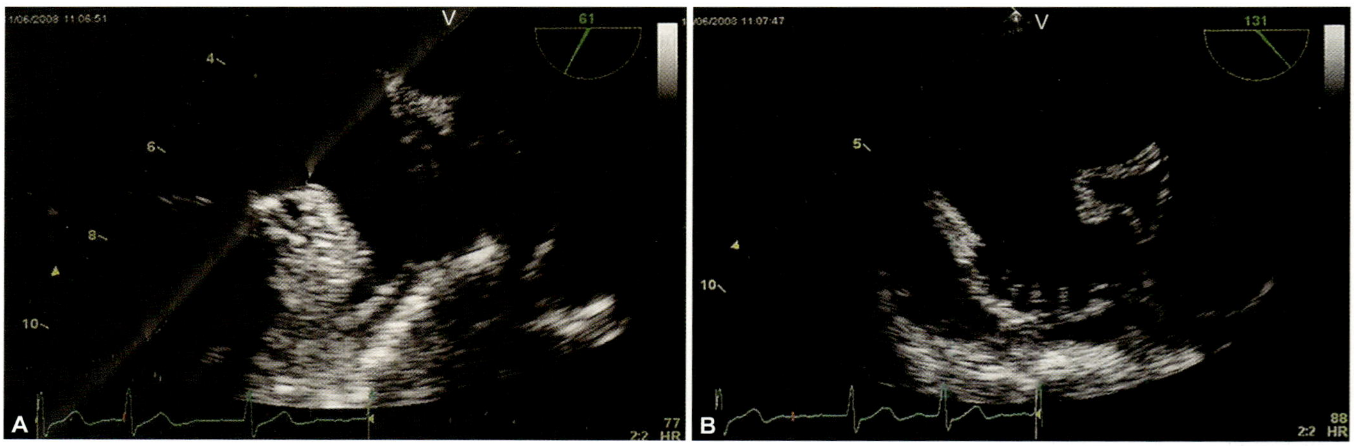

Figures 21A and B (A) Left atrial appendage imaged in 2D at 61°; (B) Left atrial appendage imaged in at 131°

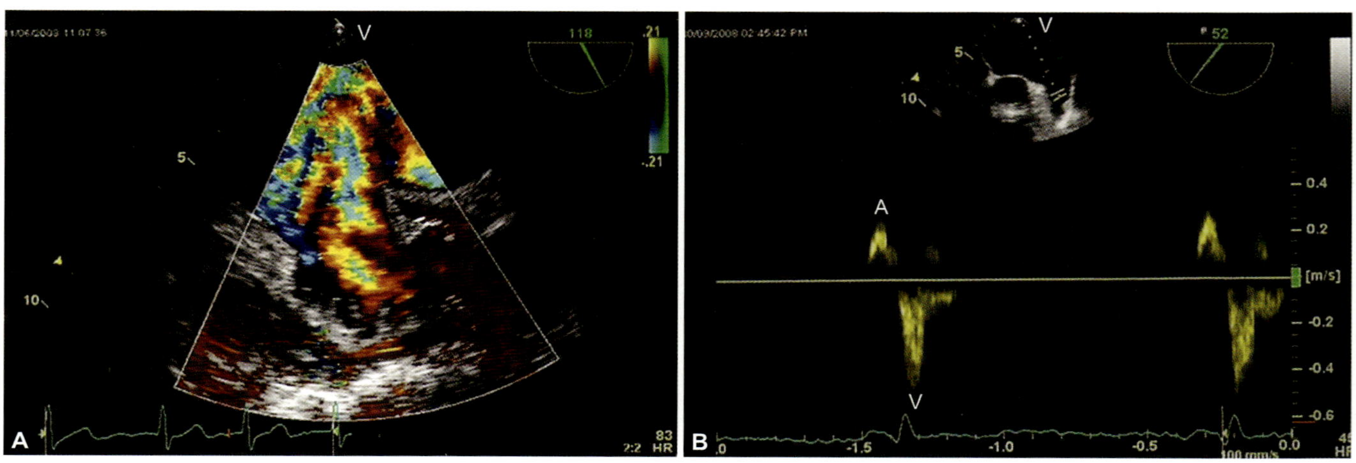

Figures 22A and B Left atrial appendage imaged in 2D with additional color Doppler at a low aliasing velocity (21 cm/s) demonstrating good flow in all areas; (B) Pulse wave Doppler of left atrial appendage blood flow demonstrating emptying (A) and filling (V) velocities

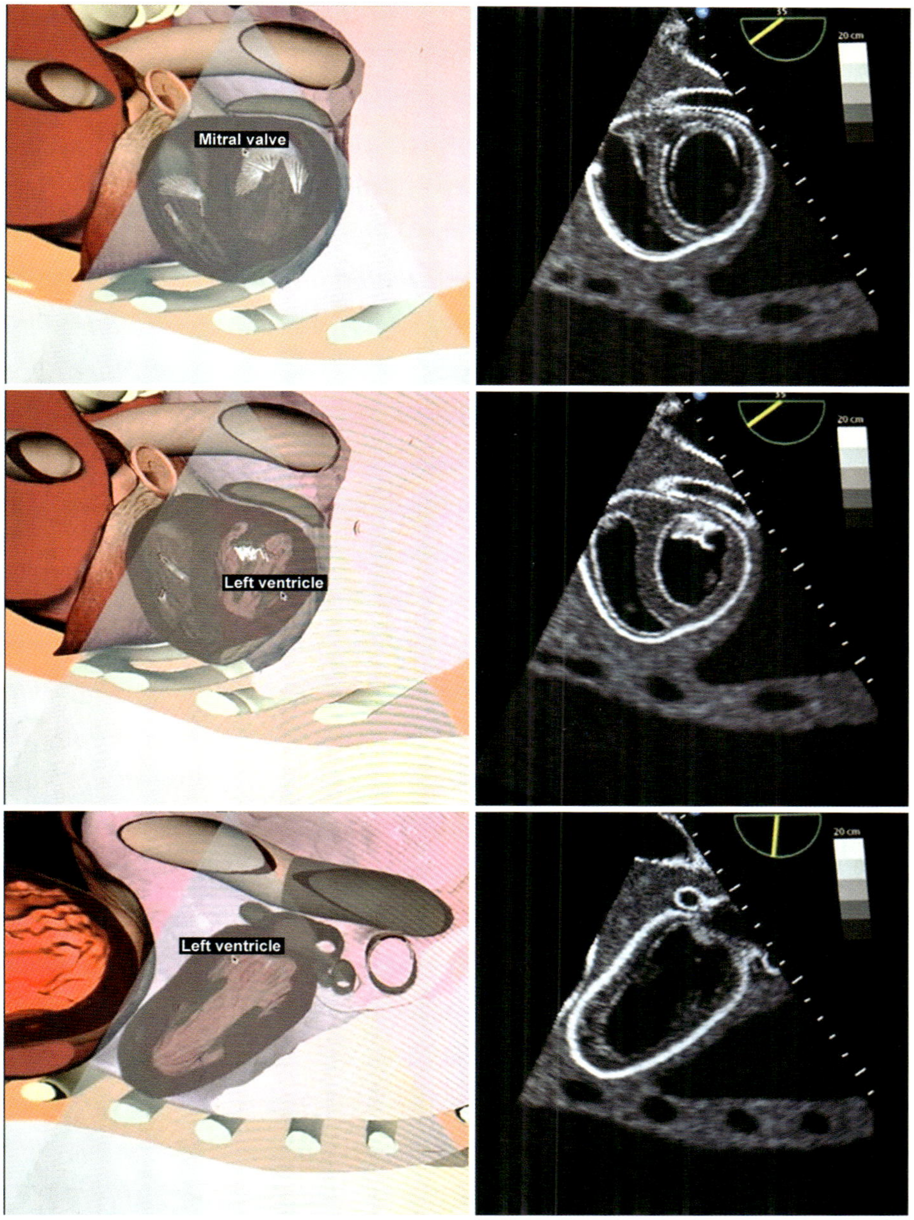

Figure 23 Simulation views of TEE in left atrial appendage

Therefore, diastolic dysfunction would be seen in this patient. With SAM of the mitral valve and LVOT obstruction, premature closure of the aortic valve is expected.

The elderly form of HCM as seen in **Figure 17** is commonly associated with LVOT obstruction, obstruction with acute symptoms, and sudden cardiac death.

Simulation views of TEE in hypertrophic cardiomyopathy (Figures 18 and 19)

Figure 18 shows different views of the hypertrophic cardiomyopathy patient.

LEFT ATRIAL APPENDAGE THROMBUS (FIGURES 20 TO 23)

The purpose of the left atrial appendage (LAA) is not fully understood. One hypothesis is that the LAA acts as a capacitance chamber allowing sudden changes in LA volume to be accommodated without marked increases in left atrial pressure (LAP). From a practical perspective, however, the LAA acts as a cul-de-sac with a high incidence of thrombus especially in the presence of atrial fibrillation (AF). It is shaped like an old fashioned money purse with a thin neck and somewhat bulbous body. The orifice of the neck of the appendage curves around the lateral aspect of the LA between the left upper pulmonary vein (LUPV) (posteriorly) and the junction of the LA and pulmonary trunk (Anteriorly). Both its shape and position relative to the esophagus demonstrate marked inter-individual variability, and so a complete assessment of the LAA imaging, I usually start at the midesophageal 4 chambers view and then withdraw the probe slightly (not quite as far as the upper esophageal window). The probe is then maximally ante-flexed and the image plane angle rotated until the appendage is seen. The LAA should be interrogated in at least 3 planes with the first 2D image usually acquired at somewhere between 0° and 60°, the second between 60° and 120°, and the final image acquired between 120° and 180°. In order to obtain the clearest image (and properly assess one of the most topographically complex cardiac structures) in each plane it is often necessary to adjust the probe depth and manually rotate the probe (clockwise or anti-clockwise). Further 2D image optimization is achieved by reducing the image sector depth and width (or zoom function used) to improve spatial and temporal resolution. Assessment of the LAA in each view should be done without lateral flexion then repeated with the use of right (± left) lateral flexion. After 2D evaluation blood flow within the LAA should be assessed (especially when there are multiple trabeculations of diverticulae/outpouching are present) using color Doppler with a low aliasing velocity (20–25 cm/s) to ensure that there is reasonable flow in all areas. Finally the global contractile function of the LAA is evaluated using pulse wave Doppler, and by measuring the peak emptying velocity. **Normal peak LAA emptying velocity is >25 cm/s**.

Because of the challenges of good appendage interrogation, the authors believe, it is important that the operators take some time to visualize normal appendages so that they understand the variations of normality that exist, and are thus able to accurately risk stratify in pre-cardioversion and stroke cases.

SECTION 6

REFERENCES

1. Eysmann SB, Palevsky HI, Reichek N, et al. Two-dimensional and Doppler-echocardiographic and cardiac catheterization correlates of survival in primary pulmonary hypertension. Circulation. 1989;80:353-60.
2. Hinderliter AL, Willis PWt, Long W, Clarke WR, Ralph D, Caldwell EJ, et al. Frequency and prognostic significance of pericardial effusion in primary pulmonary hypertension. PPH Study Group. Primary pulmonary hypertension. Am J Cardiol. 1999;84:481-4, A410.
3. Raymond RJ, Hinderliter AL, Willis PW, Ralph D, Caldwell EJ, Williams W, et al. Echocardiographic predictors of adverse outcomes in primary pulmonary hypertension. J Am Coll Cardiol. 2002;39:1214-9.
4. Yeo TC, Dujardin KS, Tei C, Mahoney DW, McGoon MD, Seward JB. Value of a Doppler-derived index combining systolic and diastolic time intervals in predicting outcome in primary pulmonary hypertension. Am J Cardiol. 1998;81:1157-61.
5. Forfia PR, Fisher MR, Mathai SC, Housten-Harris T, Hemnes AR, Borlaug BA, et al. Tricuspid annular displacement predicts survival in pulmonary hypertension. Am J Respir Crit Care Med. 2006;174:1034-41.
6. McLaughlin VV, Presberg KW, Doyle RL, Abman SH, McCrory DC, Fortin T, et al. Prognosis of pulmonary arterial hypertension: ACCP evidence-based clinical practice guidelines. Chest. 2004;126:78S-92S.
7. McLaughlin VV, Shillington A, Rich S. Survival in primary pulmonary hypertension: the impact of epoprostenol therapy. Circulation. 2002;106:1477-82.
8. Miyamoto S, Nagaya N, Satoh T, Kyotani S, Sakamaki F, Fujita M, et al. Clinical correlates and prognostic significance of six-minute walk test in patients with primary pulmonary hypertension. Comparison with cardiopulmonary exercise testing. Am J Respir Crit Care Med. 2000;161:487-92.
9. Paciocco G, Martinez FJ, Bossone E, Pielsticker E, Gillespie B, Rubenfire M. Oxygen desaturation on the six-minute walk test and mortality in untreated primary pulmonary hypertension. Eur Respir J. 2001;17:647-52.
10. Wensel R, Opitz CF, Anker SD, Winkler J, Hoffken G, Kleber FX, et al. Assessment of survival in patients with primary pulmonary hypertension: importance of cardiopulmonary exercise testing. Circulation. 2002;106:319-24.
11. Van Wolferen SA, Marcus JT, Boonstra A, Marques KM, Bronzwaer JG, Spreeuwenberg MD, et al. Prognostic value of right ventricular mass, volume, and function in idiopathic pulmonary arterial hypertension. Eur Heart J. 2007;28:1250-7.
12. Weyman AE. Principles and practice of echocardiography, 2nd edn. Philadelphia: Lea & Febiger, 1994, 829.

13. Poelaert JI, Visser CA, Everraert JA, De Deyne CS, Decruyenaere J, Colardyn FA. Doppler evaluation of right ventricular outflow impedance during positive-pressure ventilation. J Cardiothorac Vasc Anesth 1994;8: 392-7.
14. Avery EG, Shernan SK. Pericardial Disease. In Comprehensive Perioperative Transesophageal Echocardiography. 2 edn. Savage RM, Aronson S, Shernan SK (Eds). Lippincott, Williams and Wilkins. Chapter 39. 2010.
15. Gabor Erdoes, David Reineke, Reto Basciani, Thierry Carre, and Balthasar Eberl1 et al. Left atrial myxoma attached to the anterior mitral leaflet with symptoms suggestive of infective endocarditis. European Journal of Echocardiography (2010) 11, E8
16. Maurer G, Siegel RJ, Czer LS. The use of color flow mapping for intraoperative assessment of valve repair. Circulation 1991;84:1250.
17. Saiki Y, Kasegawa H, Kawase M, et al. Intraoperative TEE during mitral valve repair: does it predict early and late postoperative mitral valve dysfunction? Ann Thorac Surg 1998; 66:1277.
18. Ohno M, Cheng CP, Little WC. Mechanism of altered filling patterns of left ventricular filling during the development of congestive heart failure. Circulation 1994; 89:2241-50.

Chapter 25

Simulation for Trauma and Basic Life Support

Sanjeev Bhoi, Amit Gupta, Poonam Malhotra Kapoor

Chapter Outline

INTRODUCTION

Medical education and training has changed dramatically in the 21st century because of a dynamic shift in the attitudes of our patients and learners, as well as the creation of information technology.[1] When training health care professionals, these expectations are best met through hands-on practice in immersive-simulated medical environments **(Figure 1)**.

Patient simulation has been suggested as an ideal tool for teaching in this new generation of learners, allowing them to engage actively in their learning process while doing no harm to the patients.

- ***"In general, medical simulations aim to imitate real patients, anatomic regions, or clinical tasks, or to mirror real-life situations in which medical services are rendered."***
- "Simulation refers broadly to any device or set of conditions that attempts to present patient problems authentically, whereas a simulator, more narrowly defined, is a simulation device."

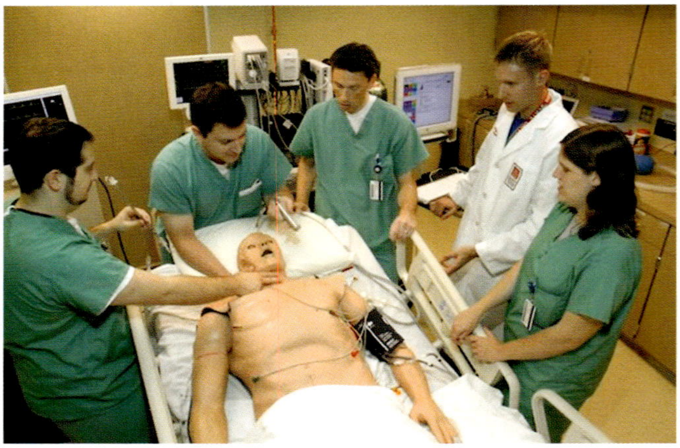

Figure 1 Simulated medical environment

By definition, simulation-based training involves immersion of a trainee in a realistic situation (scenario) created within a physical space (simulator) that replicates the real environment with

fidelity sufficient to achieve suspension of disbelief on the part of the trainee. Such training has been adopted as the standard in professions characterized by highly technical, complex, dynamic environments in which crises evolve rapidly and the risk to human life is high.

ADVANTAGES OF SIMULATION TRAINING IN TRAUMA

Trauma care is a subject neglected by the medical curriculum planners. A number of studies recently have addressed this issue and worldwide steps are being taken to impart training to medical students prior to internship through courses like the emergency trauma training course (ETTC).[2]

Simulation-based methodologies were used initially in the medical field in the 1980s for training in the management of critically ill patients in the operating room.[3] Simulation-based training has many advantages. ***It provides trainees with increased clinical experience because rare but devastating events can be simulated and practiced many times. It is convenient; trainees can schedule simulation sessions at times that fit into their schedules. It decreases the use of hospital resources by reducing the time spent teaching in expensive clinical environments. It is also much safer to train on patient simulators than on real patients.*** Simulation offers the field of trauma training multiple opportunities to enhance the effectiveness of the education provided in this challenging domain.

Trauma training aims at providing the essential information and skills that the doctor may then apply to identify and treat life threatening or potentially life threatening injuries. The ABCDE approach of advanced trauma life support (ATLS) course clearly emphasizes that injury kill in reproducible time frames. Loss of airway kills quicker than difficulty in breathing. Loss of circulating volume kills earlier than an expanding intracranial hematoma.

Trauma life support course: ATLS today is accepted as a standard of first hour trauma care the world over. ATLS aims to prepare doctors and paramedics so trained to exercise a quantum of basic knowledge and skills to save lives, reduce morbidity and avoid unnecessary harm. The overriding principle is *primumnon nocere,* that is first doing no harm. Implementation of ATLS protocols and training of doctors worldwide has led to a significant decrease in mortality and morbidity. The use of regionalized trauma centers too has been shown to decrease trauma-related morbidity and mortality.

FORMS OF SIMULATION IN TRAUMA

Life support courses such as basic and advanced cardiac life support (BCLS and ACLS, respectively), as well as basic and advanced trauma life support (BTLS and ATLS, respectively), utilize simulation techniques and principles for learning and testing.

The skills requirement which can be enhanced with the use of simulation include:[4]

- Technical and functional expertise training
- Problem-solving and decision-making skills
- Interpersonal and communications skills or team-based competencies.

All of these share a common thread in that they require active listening and collaboration besides possession of the basic knowledge and skills. With every training program, it is best to have feedback and debriefing sessions that follow. Feedback must be linked to learning outcomes and there must be effective debriefing protocols following all simulation exercises. Studies have shown that simulation improves learning.

The different forms of medical simulation technology training that can be considered for the center would include:

- *Human patient simulators*: The centerpiece is usually a full sized patient simulator that blinks, breathes, and has heartbeat, pulse, and respiratory sounds. This mannequin can be very technologically advanced **(Figure 2)**. For example, it may "interact" with learners through computer-guided teaching programs. Attached monitors can display vital signs and this can provide virtual simulation of almost every major bodily function. This simulator can be used for scenarios from simple physical examination to interdisciplinary major trauma management. Some simulators can even recognize injected medications via a laser bar-code reader and then respond with appropriate vital sign changes.
- *Simulated clinical environment*: An intensive care unit, emergency room cubicle, or operating room is prepared with all the equipment and the crash cart **(Figure 3)**. The setup is as realistic as the actual facility. Trainees can familiarize themselves with the setup and arrangements.
- *Virtual procedure stations*: Various stations can be set up, depending on what the focus is. These stations

CHAPTER 25

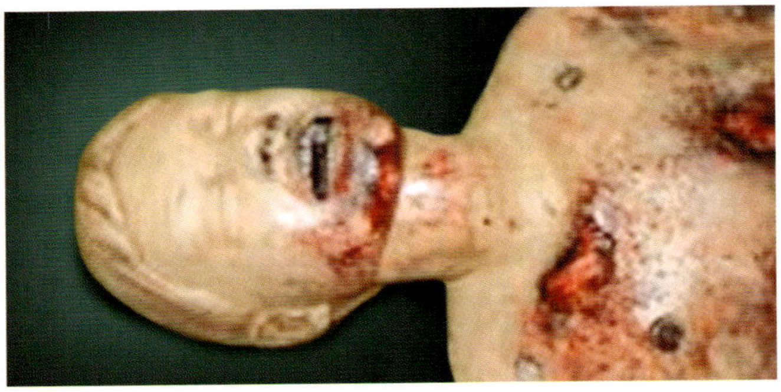

Figure 2 Human patient simulators

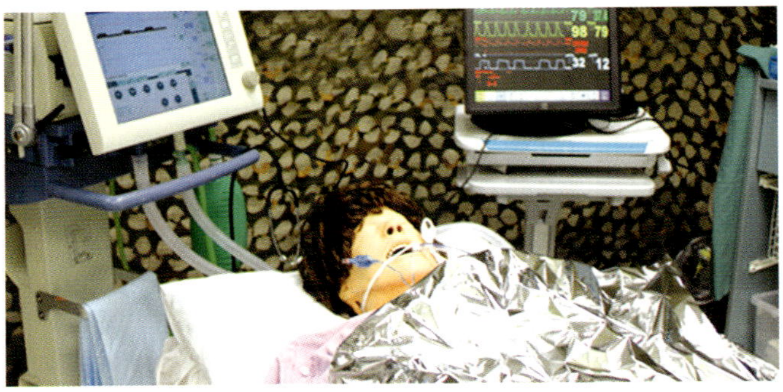

Figure 3 Simulated clinical environment

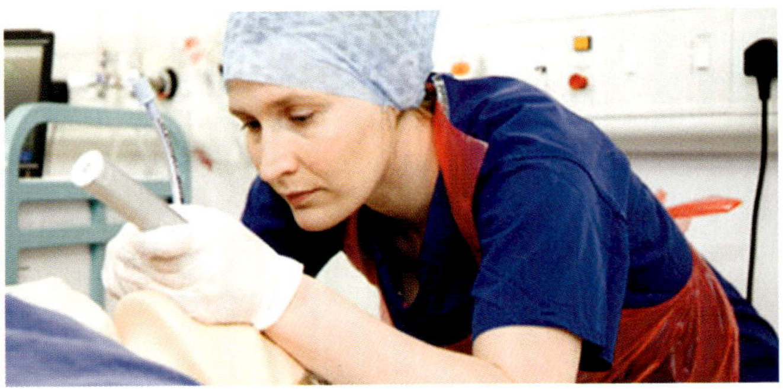

Figure 4 Virtual procedure stations

will have all the relevant equipment and setup for the procedure to be carried out, e.g. bronchoscopy, colonoscopy, intubation **(Figure 4)**. The simulators can present a variety of different scenarios and pathologies and the trainee can practice until he/she masters the technique(s).

- *Electronic medical records*: As more health care institutions adopt electronic medical records to track and manage patients, this can also be a station setup in the center **(Figure 5)**. The system utilized will have fictitious patients with their histories, notes, and lab results. There may also be system integration, such as the link between records and the laboratory as well as the radiology results (digitalized radiographs). Simulator is the best learning tool for practicing clinical skills for the trauma patients **(Figures 6A and B)**.

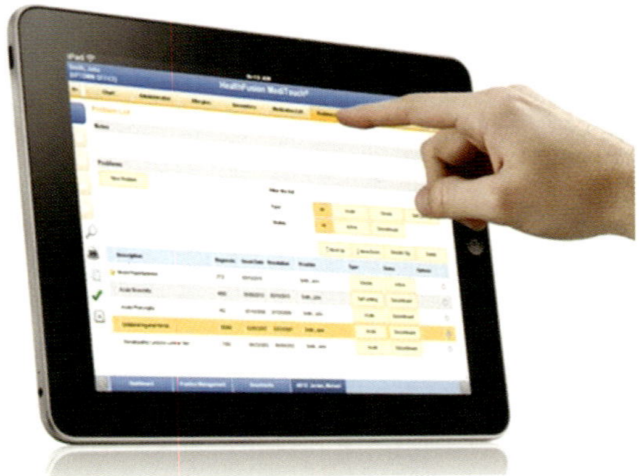

Figure 5 Electronic medical records

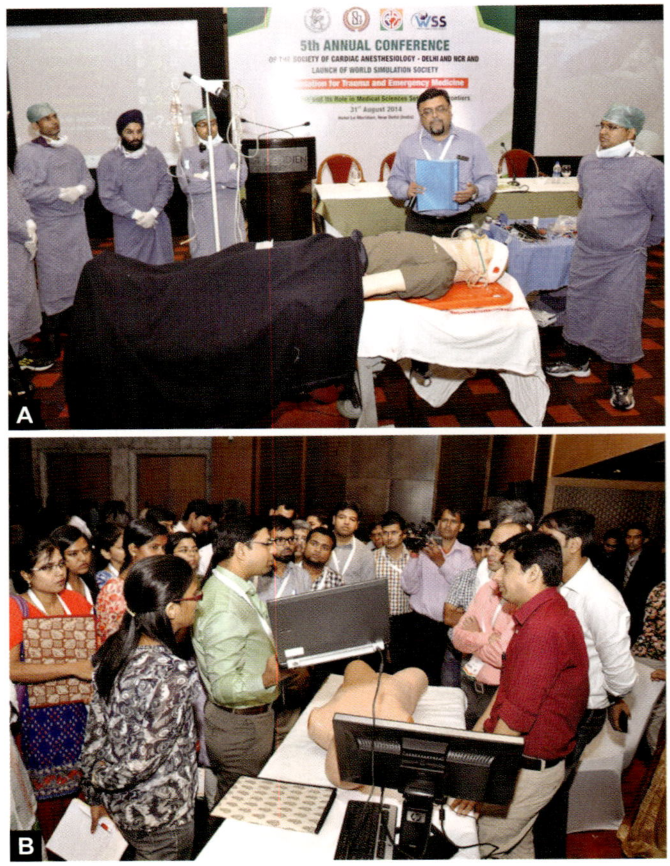

Figures 6A and B (A) Simulating a situation for teaching trauma and basic life support, is an essential emergency, done on a simulator; (B) Simulation—low and high fidelity for basic life support, a group with scenarios on the computer which are enacted on the simulator. The combination works best for simulation based teaching

The educational benefits of simulation include the following:
- Deliberate practice with feedback
- Exposure to uncommon events
- Reproducibility
- Opportunity for assessment of learners
- The absence of risks to patients.

Usual procedure simulations include:
- Cricothyroidotomy
- Chest tube insertion
- Pericardiocentesis
- Needle decompression
- Percutaneous tracheostomy
- Diagnostic peritoneal lavage
- IV cutdown
- Suturing, incisions.

The FAST diagnostic ultrasound training extension allows to:
- Learn landmarks on the body used for identification of window locations for the exam.
- Read and understand the various normal and abnormal views.
- The FAST module includes five patient image and video libraries for each window (two normal and three abnormal).

CONCLUSION

Medical simulators have the potential to revolutionize medical training and certification practices. They deliver many advantages over traditional training methods. Empirical evidence is mounting that they can enhance the acquisition of procedural skills. Human healthcare needs and costs can be expected to rise for the foreseeable future. These trends demand less costly, more efficient and more rigorous methods of training, maintaining and assessing practical knowledge and psychomotor skills. By meeting these demands, simulators can benefit human healthcare.

REFERENCES

1. Sahu S, Lata I. Simulation in resuscitation teaching and training, an evidence based practice review. J Emerg Trauma Shock. 2010;3(4):378-84.
2. Gambhir RPS, Agrawal MA. Training in trauma management. MJAFI. 2010;66:354-6.
3. Allison M, Louis H. Simulation-based training in neonatal resuscitation. Neo Reviews, vol. 6, No. 11 (November), pp. 489-492.
4. Lateef F. Simulation-based learning: Just like the real thing. J Emerg Trauma Shock. 2010;3(4):348-52.

Chapter 26

Recent Advances in Cardiopulmonary Resuscitation from 2010 to 2015

Poonam Malhotra Kapoor, Mayadhar Barik, Vandana Bhardwaj, Sameer Taneja, BS Sethi

Chapter Outline

- Sudden Cardiac Death
- Resuscitation Science: Objectives
- Return of Spontaneous Circulation
- Targeted Temperature Management
- Pharmacological Agents during Targeted Temperature Monitoring
- Physiological Changes, Side Effects and Complications of Therapeutic Hypothermia
- Postresuscitation Care
- Neuroprotective Pharmacology
- Pathophysiology of Anoxic Brain Injury after Cardiac Arrest
- Cerebral Performance Category Scale
- Pediatric Cardiopulmonary Resuscitation
- Adult Cardiopulmonary Resuscitation in Three Simple Steps: Cardiopulmonary Resuscitation Sequence: C – A- B
- Controversial Issues in Cardiopulmonary Resuscitation
- Manikin Simulator Fidelity on Neonatal Resuscitation Program Learning
- High-fidelity Simulation Provides a Realistic Simulation Experience
- Hands on + Hands Free: Simulated on-call Interaction
- Evaluating Simulation-based Advanced Cardiac Life Support Education on Patient Outcomes
- Steps in Cardiopulmonary Resuscitation
- Basic Cardiopulmonary Resuscitation—The ABCD
- Precocious Defibrillation in Basic Life Support
- Oxygen via Mouth-to-Mouth Resuscitation is Adequate
- Blood Pressure Changes with Chest Compression
- Ventilatory and Circulatory Support: Are they Synergised
- Risks to the Rescuer and Victim in Basic Life Support
- Initial Rescue Breaths
- Advanced Cardiovascular Life Support
- Changes from in 2010 Guidelines to 2015 Guidelines
- Advanced Cardiovascular Life Support Cardiac Arrest Algorithm
- Guideline Changes Cont…
- Defibrillation—Electrical Therapies
- Shockable Rhythms Ventricular Fibrillation/ Ventricular Tachycardia

INTRODUCTION

Recent statistics suggest that sudden cardiac arrest is rapidly becoming the leading cause of death in the global hospitals. Once the heart ceases to function, a healthy human brain may survive without oxygen for up to four minutes without suffering any permanent damage. Unfortunately, a typical emergency medical services (EMS) response may take 6, 8 or even 10 minutes. It is during those critical minutes that cardio pulmonary resuscitation (CPR) can provide oxygenated blood to the victim's brain and the heart, dramatically increasing his chance of survival. And if properly instructed, almost anyone can learn and perform CPR.

In March 2008, the American Heart Association (AHA) published an advisory statement outlining "hands-only" or "compression-only" CPR. This statement is a clarification addendum to the 2005 AHA guidelines for CPR and emergency cardiovascular care (ECC) which dictates that lay persons who are unable or unwilling to provide rescue breaths may perform hands-only CPR. This updated recommendation does not apply to first responders and/or medical personnel with access to CPR barrier or a mechanical respirator; unwitnessed cardiac arrest, cardiac arrest in children and infants, or cardiac arrest presumed to be of noncardiac origin (drowning, trauma, airway obstruction, acute respiratory diseases, drug overdose, etc.). AHA study concedes that when performed correctly, conventional CPR continues to prove a more effective rescue method for victims of cardiac arrest and as such we will continue to educate our students in ventilation as well as compressions on the simulators. This article, reviews the 2010 and 2015 guidelines using chiefly the SimMan simulator **(Figures 1A and B)**.

TABLE 1 Evidence-based facts: predictors of survival and brain protection

- High quality CPR
- Immediate bystander CPR
- Hands-only/conventional
- Immediate defibrillation
- Therapeutic hypothermia

SUDDEN CARDIAC DEATH

80% at home, 40% unwitnessed, poor survival rates, 40% never regain consciousness and 30% of these have significant neurological deficits.

RESUSCITATION SCIENCE: OBJECTIVES

Brief review of latest AHA information, strategies to reduce morbidity and mortality in cardiac arrests and strokes, hypothermia in cardiac arrest **(Table 1, Figures 2 and 3)**.

RETURN OF SPONTANEOUS CIRCULATION

- End-tidal CO_2 is a marker of return of spontaneous circulation (ROSC) **(Figure 4)**.
- Its utility is limited by V-Q mismatch and cannot monitor cerebral oxygen delivery
- Cerebral oximetry is a possible predictor of ROSC in cardiac arrest
- $rSO_2 > 65\%$ during a 5 minutes CPR is a strong predictor of ROSC. <30% is a poor predictor.

TARGETED TEMPERATURE MANAGEMENT

Targeted temperature management (TTM) also called as therapeutic hypothermia (TH) (till 2010–2015) is

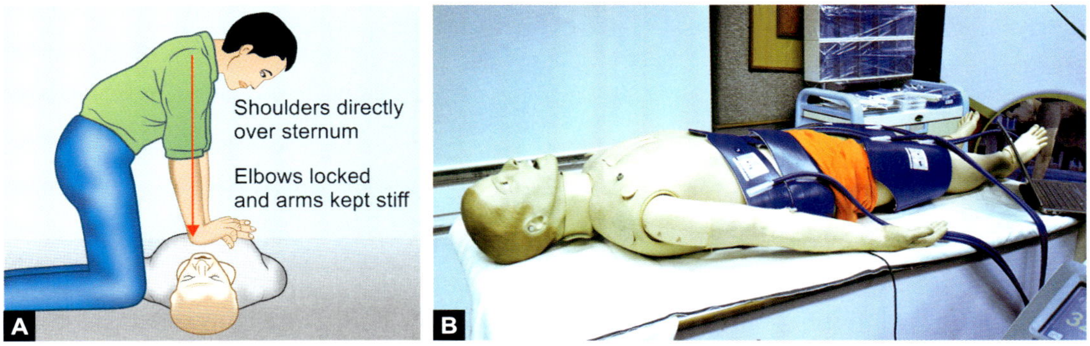

Figures 1A and B SimMan simulator

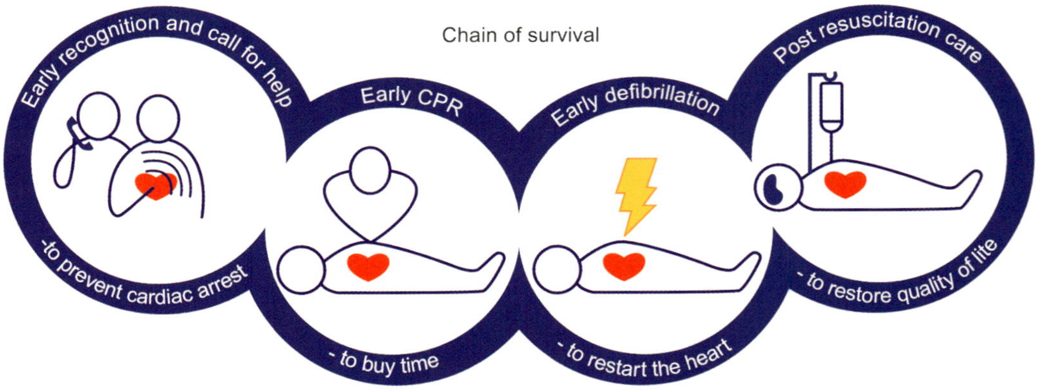

Figure 2 Chain of survival during cardiopulmonary resuscitation

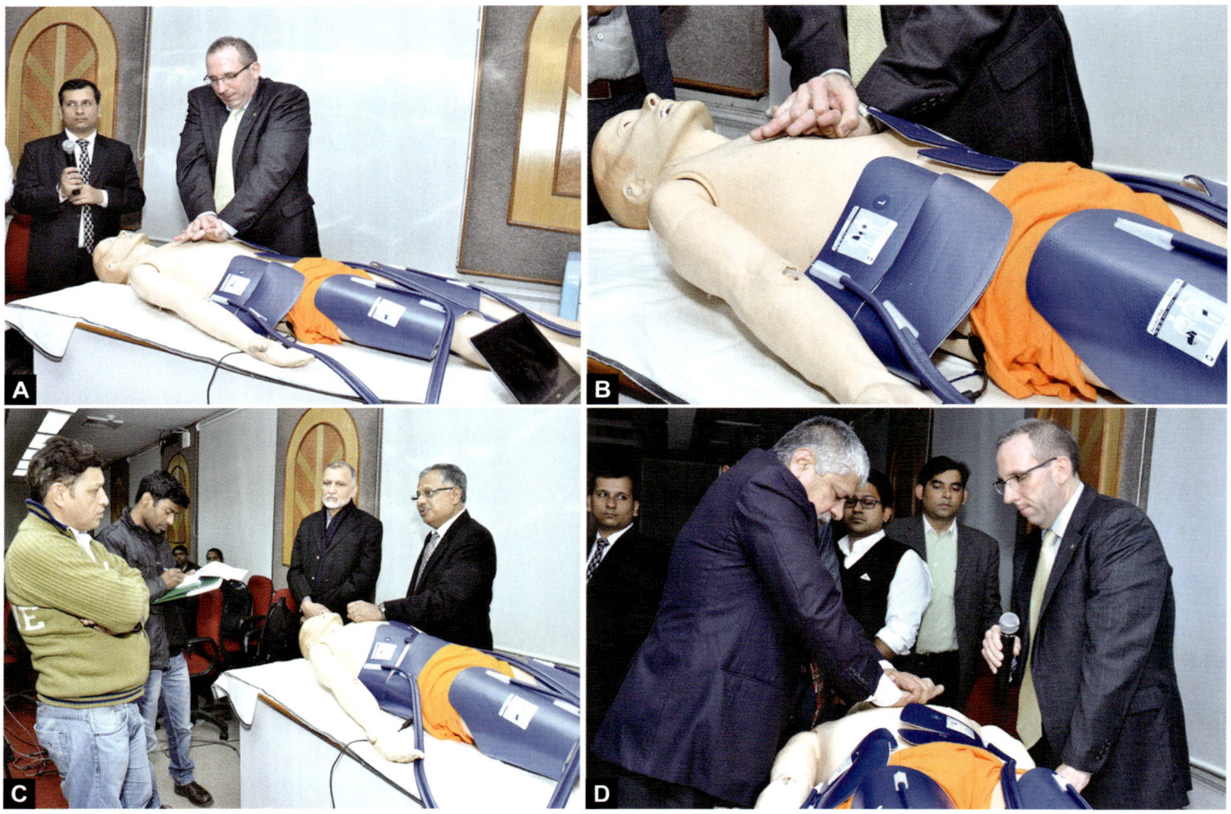

Figures 3A to D (A and B) Hands only cardiopulmonary resuscitation using the therapeutic hypothermia machine at a seminar conducted at AIIMS, in 2015; (C) Use of therapeutic hypothermia machine and simulator for resuscitation; (D) CPR compression simulation for resuscitation in a advanced cardiac life support (ACLS) workshop conducted by AHA at AIIMS

a well recommended therapeutic strategy to limit neurological injury in patients with ROSC after cardiac arrest. The beneficial effect of hypothermia comes from decrease in brain metabolism and oxygen consumption. In addition, hypothermia suppresses inflammation, oxidative stress and attenuates lipid peroxidation resulting from global cerebral ischemia.[1,2]

The therapeutic effects of hypothermia after cardiac arrest have been approved by various clinical trials. Bernard et al in 2002, studied the effect of hypothermia in 77 comatose patients who survived cardiac arrest after an initial rhythm of ventricular fibrillation (VF) or pulseless ventricular tachycardia (pVT). They randomly assigned patients to either get hypothermic

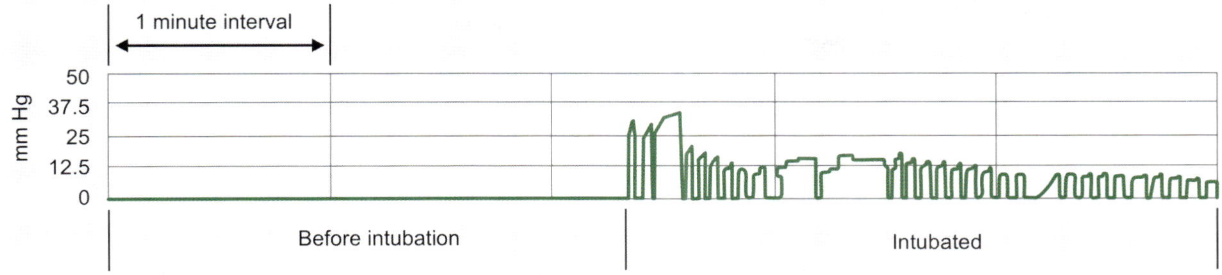

Capnography to confirm endotracheal tube placement. This capnography tracing displays the partial pressure of exhaled carbon dioxide ($PETCO_2$) in mm Hg on the vertical axis over time when intubation is performed. Once the patient is intubated, exhaled carbon dioxide is detected, confirming tracheal tube placement. The ($PETCO_2$) varies during the respiratory cycle, with highest values at end-expiration.

Figure 4 Qualitative role of capnography in resuscitation outcomes

treatment at 33 degree for 12 hours with the use of cold ice packs or standard normothermic care. The authors observed that 49% of the patients who were treated with hypothermia survived and had a favorable neurologic recovery, as compared with 26% of the patients treated with normothermia (P = 0.05).[3]

Indications and Contraindications

The use of TTM should be considered in all those comatose (Glasgow Coma Scale of less than 8) patients who get successfully resuscitated after cardiac arrest with an initial rhythm of VF or pVT and are hemodynamically stable. The therapeutic hypothermia should not be considered in patients who were comatose before cardiac arrest or whose tympanic membrane temperature is below 30°C on admission. The terminally ill patients, pregnant patients and patients with inherited coagulation disorders should also be avoided.[4]

Techniques of Cooling and Management During Hypothermia

The various cooling techniques available at present can be broadly classified into three categories:

1. Conventional cooling methods—cooled saline, ice bags are used.
2. Surface cooling methods—cold fluid or cold air is circulated through blankets, wrapped around the patient.
3. Intravascular cooling methods—cool saline is circulated through a loop of thermal regulated central venous catheters.[5]

The patient should be completely sedated and paralyzed to prevent shivering (can lead to increase oxygen consumption) and discomfort before the initiating therapeutic hypothermia. The core body temperature should be monitored during the period of TTM and blood gas analysis should be done 4–6 hourly with a target of normocarbia and sufficient oxygenation. The serum electrolytes and blood sugar should be frequently monitored and managed to prevent hypokalemia, hypomagnesemia, hypophosphatemia and hyperglycemia associated with hypothermia. In rare case, hypothermia can result in severe thrombocytopenia, blood coagulation disorders and pancreatitis. In these cases, temperature should be increased until these side effects get resolved. The rewarming is not helpful in patients who get hemodynamically deteriorated after hypothermia, as rewarming is associated with vasodilation and can further depress blood pressures.

Rewarming

The patient should be rewarmed slowly (0.3–0.5° C/h) to normal body temperature (36.5–37.5°C) after maintaining therapeutic hypothermia for 24 hours. Hyperthermia should be avoided and normal body temperature should be maintained for up to 48 hours as hyperthermia can lead to adverse outcomes.

2015 Updated AHA Guidelines Regarded TTM

In 2010 AHA guidelines, cooling the core temperature to 32–34°C was recommended for 12–24 hours in comatose patients who recovered from cardiac arrest. However, in recent 2015 AHA guidelines achieving targeted temperature between 32°C and 36°C and then maintaining it for at least 24 hours is advocated. The

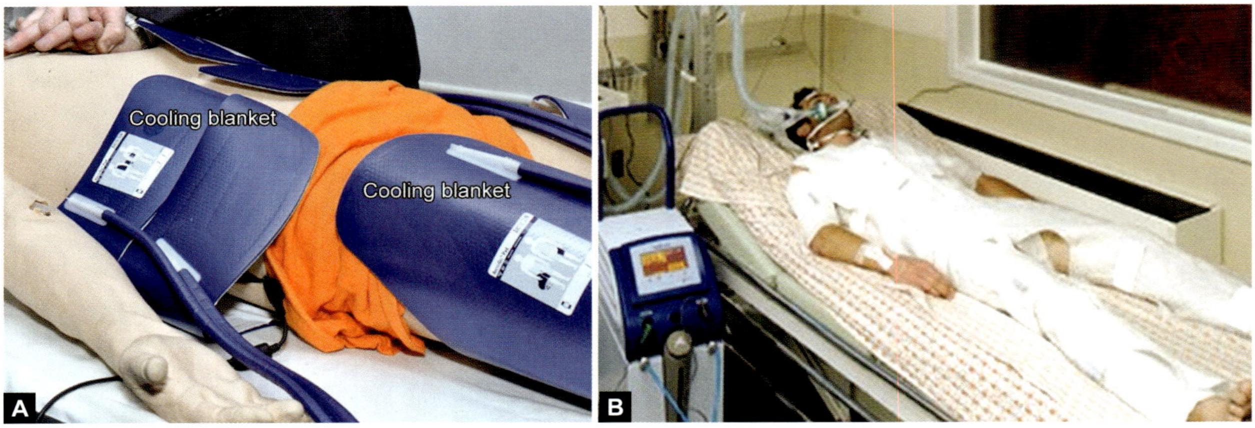

Figures 5A and B (A) Cooling blanket for therapeutic hypothermia; (B) Criticool therapy

aforementioned change resulted from some recent studies, which demonstrated similar outcomes at 33°C and 36°C. Nielson et al in 2013, randomly assigned 950 comatose patients after out-of-hospital cardiac arrest of presumed cardiac cause to TTM at either 33°C or 36°C. The author observed no significant benefit of hypothermia at 33°C temperature as compare to 36°C temperature.[6]

The 2015 guidelines have recommended actively prevention of fever after TTM as fever can worsen the neurological injury. The routine prehospital cooling has been discouraged by recent guidelines as using cold intravenous fluids in prehospital settings has potential complication and studies have failed to demonstrate any benefit of out of hospital cooling.

Cooling devices which are available are as follows **(Figures 5A and B)**:

- Commercial surface cooling devices
  - Employ heat-exchange pads that adhere to skin utilizing a hydrophilic gel that conducts heat and maintains contact between skin and pads
  - Some systems employ cooling by conduction as water circulates through pads that encircle the patient but has no direct adherence to skin
- Commercial intravascular devices for cooling.

PHARMACOLOGICAL AGENTS DURING TARGETED TEMPERATURE MONITORING

Agents for Hemodynamic Support

- Vasopressors
- Antiarrhythmics
- Muscle relaxants
- Rocuronium, vecuronium, atracurium, cis-atracurium, etc.

Others

- Sedatives and narcotics
- Lorazepam, midazolam, fentanyl, propofol, etc.

PHYSIOLOGICAL CHANGES, SIDE EFFECTS AND COMPLICATIONS OF THERAPEUTIC HYPOTHERMIA

- Shivering and cutaneous vasoconstriction
  - Causes disruption in cooling by generating heat = increase in core temperature
  - Increases O_2 consumption and demand
  - Acidosis and myocardial ischemia
  - Highest risk during induction (34–35.5°C)
  - May occur during rewarming
- Hyperglycemia (due to insulin sensitivity and pancreatic production)
  - Tight glycemic control
  - Watch for hypoglycemia during rewarming
- Cold diuresis
  - May cause hypotension, hypovolemia and hypokalemia
  - Replace fluids monitoring central venous pressure (CVP)

BP may be elevated during cooling due to vasoconstriction or decreased, secondary to diuresis

- Electrolyte changes (due to intracellular shift and tubular dysfunction)
  - K^+, Mg^{++}, phosphate during cooling
  - K^+ during rewarming
- Cardiovascular and hemodynamic changes
  - Heart rate (HR), cardiac output (CO), systemic vascular resistance (SVR)
  - QTc, PR, J wave (Osborne wave)

SECTION 6

- HR < 40 is frequent and not a cause for concern unless there is hypotension and reduced urine output
- Ventricular fibrillation unresponsive to defibrillation if overcooled
- Coagulopathies
  - Potential decrease in platelets number and function
  - May lead to increased clotting times
  - More common if core temperature < 32°C
- Ventilator related
  - Hypocapnia can cause cerebral vasoconstriction CO_2 production is decreased by 30% at a core temperature of 33°C
  - Tidal volume and rate need to be adjusted to achieve PCO_2 35–45 n and worsen brain damage
- Seizures
  - Muscle relaxants: nerve stimulator
  - Most likely secondary to global ischemic injury suffered during cardiac arrest and reperfusion
  - Rx with antiepileptics
- Decreased drug clearance
  - Need to adjust doses
- Infection
  - Risk of aspiration during resuscitation causing pneumonia
  - Impairs T cell-mediated antibodies
  - Diminished function of neutrophils
  - Impaired immune mechanisms
- Cold related skin injuries
  - Preventable with nursing care
- GI changes
  - Ileus
  - Increased amylase and lipase
  - Do not provide nutrition during therapeutic hypothermia
- Miscellaneous
  - Acute renal failure
  - Lactic acidosis.

Aggressively Manage

Hypoxia, hyper or hypocapnia, hypotension and hyperthermia.

POSTRESUSCITATION CARE

The 2015 AHA guidelines for CPR and ECC recognize the increased importance of systematic care and advancements in the multispecialty management of patients following ROSC and admission to the hospital that can affect neurologically intact survival. Part 9 of the 2015 guidelines on "postcardiac arrest care" recognizes the importance of bundled goal-oriented management and interventions to achieve optimal outcome in victims of cardiac arrest who are admitted to a hospital following ROSC. The AHA recommends that a comprehensive, structured, integrated, multidisciplinary system of care should be implemented in a consistent manner for the treatment of postcardiac arrest patients. The potential harm caused by hyperoxemia after ROSC is achieved is now recognized: once ROSC has been established and the oxygen saturation of arterial blood (SaO_2) can be monitored reliably (by pulse oximetry and/or arterial blood gas analysis), inspired oxygen is titrated to achieve a SaO_2 of 94–98%. There is much greater detail and emphasis on the treatment of the postcardiac-arrest syndrome **(Table 2)**. There is recognition that implementation of a comprehensive, structured post-resuscitation treatment protocol may improve survival in cardiac arrest victims after ROSC. There is increased emphasis on the use of primary percutaneous coronary intervention in appropriate, but comatose, patients with sustained ROSC after cardiac arrest **(Table 3)**. The recommendation for glucose control has been revised: in adults with sustained ROSC after cardiac arrest, blood glucose values >10 mmol L^{-1} should be treated but hypoglycemia must be avoided. Use of targeted temperature monitoring now includes comatose survivors of cardiac arrest associated initially with nonshockable rhythms as well as shockable rhythms. The lower level of evidence for use after cardiac arrest from nonshockable rhythms is acknowledged. It is recognized that many of the accepted predictors of

TABLE 2 Management of postcardiac arrest syndrome

- General measures
- Monitoring
- Early hemodynamic optimization
- Oxygenation
- Ventilation
- Circulatory support
- Management of acute coronary syndrome (ACS)
- Seizure control
- Glucose control
- Neuroprotective pharmacology
- Therapeutic hypothermia

poor outcome in comatose survivors of cardiac arrest are unreliable, especially if the patient has been treated with targeted temperature monitoring **(Table 4)**.

American Heart Association 2015 Update: Key Issues and Major Changes in the 2015 Guidelines[7] (Table 5)

Update recommendations for postcardiac arrest care include the following:

- Emergency coronary angiography is recommended for all patients with ST elevation and for hemodynamically or electrically unstable patients without ST elevation for whom a cardiovascular lesion is suspected.
- The targeted temperature management (TTM) recommendations have been updated with new evidence suggesting that a range of temperatures may be acceptable to target in the postcardiac arrest period **(Figures 6A and B)**.
- After targeted temperature management (TTM) is complete, fever may develop. While there are conflicting observational data about the harm of fever after TTM, the prevention of fever is considered benign and therefore is reasonable to pursue.

TABLE 3 Things to be remember during cardiopulmonary resuscitation and reversible causes

During CPR	*Reversible causes*
• Ensure high–quality CPR: rate, depth, recoil • Plan actions before interrupting CPR • Give oxygen • Consider advanced airway and capnography • Continuous chest compressions when advanced airway in place • Vascular access (intravenous, intraosseous) • Give adrenaline every 3–5 minutes • Correct reversible causes	• Hypoxia • Hypovolemia • Hypo-/hyperkalemia/metabolic • Hypothermia • Thrombosis • Tamponade–cardiac • Toxins • Tension pneumothorax

TABLE 4 Initial and later key objectives of postcardiac arrest care include

- Optimizing cardiopulmonary function and vital organ perfusion after ROSC
- Transportation to an appropriate hospital or critical-care unit with a comprehensive postcardiac arrest treatment system of care
- Identification and intervention for acute coronary syndromes (ACS)
- Temperature control to optimize neurologic recovery **(Figures 6A and B)**
- Anticipation, treatment, and prevention of multiple organ dysfunction

TABLE 5 Comparing revised and updated 2015 American Heart Association (AHA) guidelines from old 2010 guidelines

	2015 guidelines (update)	*2010*
System of care and quality improvement	**• A universal system of care with a common framework for integrated resuscitation has been added. • Separate chain of survival for IHCA and OHCA has been advised. • Use of social media like mobile phone applications to summon rescuer in nearby vicinity of OHCA has been supported. • Rapid response team (RRT) and Medical emergency team (MET) to reduce incidence of cardiac arrest in wards has been advised.**	**• No such framework in old guidelines. • Single chain of survival for IHCA and OHCA. • Use of social media was not encouraged in old guidelines. • Systematic identification of at risk patients, organized response and evaluation of outcome was recommended.**

Contd...

SECTION 6

Contd...

	2015 guidelines (update)	*2010*
Adult basic life support (BLS)	• In adult victims of cardiac arrest chest compression at a rate of 100–120/min has been recommended. • Chest compression at a depth of 2 inch (5 cm) and not greater than 2.4 inch (6 cm) is advised. • The rescuer should avoid leaning forward on chest in between chest compression to allow full chest recoil. • The use of audiovisual feedback devices for real time optimization of CPR performance is advocated. • The rescuer should provide I breadth every 10 sec (10/min) during chest compression when advanced airway is in place. • AHA 2015 guidelines recommend flexibility of activation of emergency response to better match the clinical settings. • In suspected opioid associated emergency the use of IM or intranasal naloxone should be considered.	• In adults chest compression at a rate of 100/min was recommended. • Chest compression at a depth of 2 inch (5 cm) was advised in adults. • Rescuer should allow complete chest recoil after each compression. • Feedback devices may be useful for rescuer to improve quality of CPR. • When advance airway is in place, 1 breadth every 6–8 sec (8–10/min) is advised. • — • No such recommendation.
Advanced cardiovascular life support	• The use of vasopressin does not offer any advantage over standard dose of epinephrine. • Epinephrine should be administered as soon as possible after nonshockable cardiac arrest • If after 20 min of CPR; $ETCO_2$ does not rise >10 mm Hg, it might be considered as one of the component of multimodal approach to end resuscitative efforts. • The use of extracorporeal CPR in patients with reversible illness or while awaiting cardiac transplant can be considered. • Lidocaine use can be considered after ROSC in patients with VF or pulseless VT. • Oral or IV Beta blocker can be considered after hospitalization of patient with VF or pulseless VT. • Use of impedance threshold device (ITD) as CPR adjunct is not recommended. • Use of mechanical compression device has no benefit over manual compression. However, their use can be considered when delivery of high quality manual compression is difficult (in ambulance, limited rescuer, prolonged CPR, hypothermic arrest)	• Vasopressin 40 U can replace first or second dose of epinephrine. • — • — • No such recommendation. • — • — • Use of ITD can be considered as adjunct to CPR by trained personnels. • Use of mechanical piston devices can be considered in difficult conditions like diagnostic/interventional procedures.
Postcardiac arrest care	• In comatosed patients after ROSC, targeted temperature (TTM) between 32 and 36 degree should be maintained for at least 24 hrs. • Development of fever after TTM should be actively prevented. • Routine prehospital cooling is discouraged. • Prognostication after TTM, in patients with suspected sedation or paralysis should be done after 72 hrs. • All patients who are resuscitated after cardiac arrest but progress to brain death subsequently should be considered as potential organ donor. • Patients in whom resuscitation failed or terminated should be considered as potential liver or kidney donor.	• Patients in coma after cardiac arrest and ROSC should be cooled to 32–34 degree for 12–24 hrs. • No specific recommendation about timing of prognostication. • Organ donation should be considered in patients after cardiac arrest who progress to brain death.

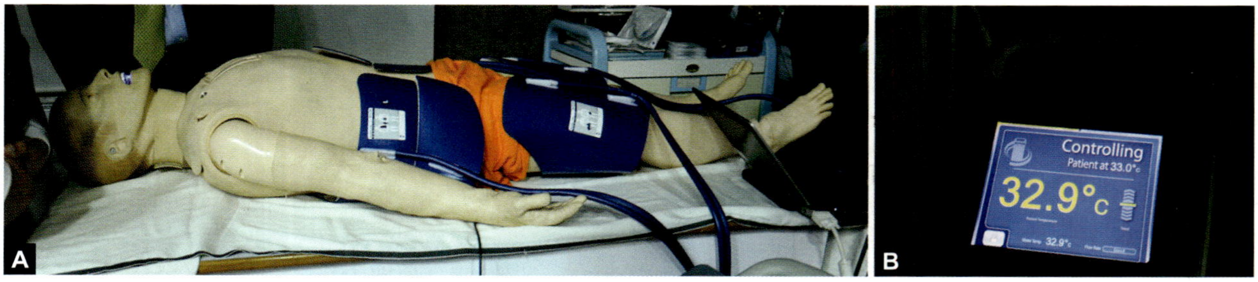

Figures 6A and B Temperature control should continue in postcardiac arrest period as well

- Identification and correction of hypotension is recommended in the immediate postcardiac arrest period.
- Prognostication is now recommended no sooner than 72 hours after the completion of TTM; for those who do not have TTM, prognostication is not recommended any sooner than 72 hours after ROSC.
- All patients who progress to brain death or circulatory death after initial cardiac arrest should be considered potential organ donors.

American Heart Association 2015 update	
Coronary angiography	Coronary angiography should be performed emergently (rather than later in the hospital stay or not at all) for out-of-hospital cardiac arrest (OHCA) patients with suspected cardiac etiology of arrest and ST elevation on ECG. Emergency coronary angiography is reasonable for select (e.g. electrically or hemodynamically unstable) adult patients who are comatose after OHCA of suspected cardiac origin but without ST elevation on ECG. Coronary angiography is reasonable in postcardiac arrest patients for whom coronary angiography is indicated, regardless of whether the patient is comatose or awake.
Targeted temperature management	All comatose (i.e. lacking meaningful response to verbal commands) adult patients with ROSC after cardiac arrest should have TTM, with a target temperature between 32°C and 36°C selected and achieved, then maintained constantly for at least 24 hours.
Hemodynamic goals after resuscitation	It may be reasonable to avoid and immediately correct hypotension (systolic blood pressure less than 90 mm Hg, mean arterial pressure less than 65 mm Hg) during postcardiac arrest care.
Prognostication after cardiac arrest	The earliest time to prognosticate a poor neurologic outcome using clinical examination in patients not treated with TTM is 72 hours after cardiac arrest, but this time can be even longer after cardiac arrest if the residual effect of sedation or paralysis is suspected to confound the clinical examination.

Postcardiac Arrest Brain Injury

Common causes of morbidity and mortality

- Brain injury is the common cause of death (60–70%) after out-of-hospital cardiac arrest (OHCA) and (20–25%) after in-hospital cardiac arrest.

NEUROPROTECTIVE PHARMACOLOGY

Multiple agents have been used in animal models like anticonvulsants, calcium and sodium, channel antagonists, immunosuppressants, protease inhibitors, magnesium, growth factors, gamma-aminobutyric acid (GABA) agonists but there is inadequate evidence to recommend any of the agents to reduce brain injury in postcardiac arrest patients.

PATHOPHYSIOLOGY OF ANOXIC BRAIN INJURY AFTER CARDIAC ARREST

Permanent (irreversible) neurological injury occurs after 5–10 minutes of complete cessation of cerebral blood flow (CBF) at normothermia.

What Happens after ROSC in a Resuscitated Patient? (Figure 7)

A wide range of destructive mechanisms is unleashed

- Excitotoxicity
- Neuroinflammation, vasospasm

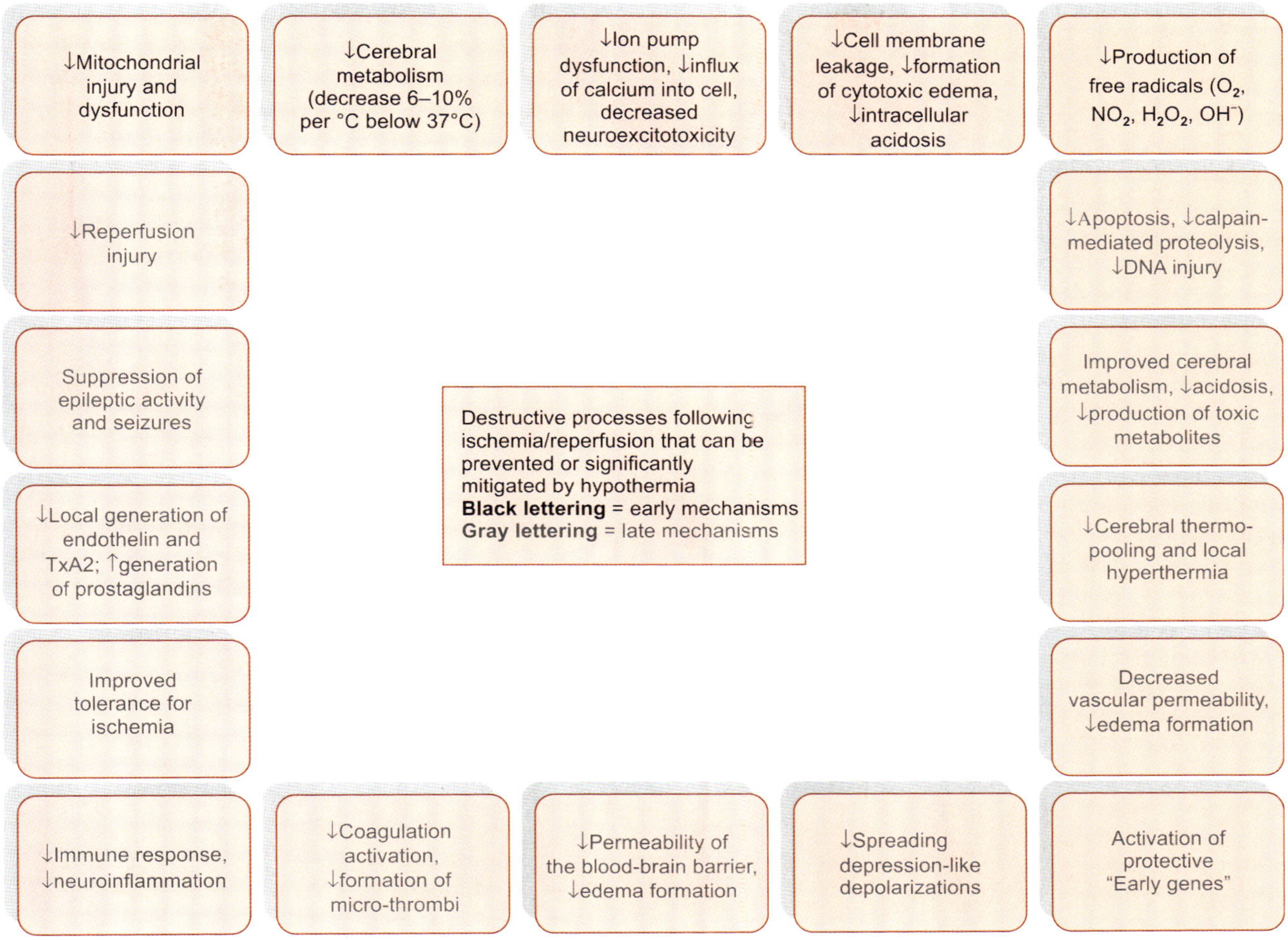

Figure 7 Phases of therapeutic hypothermia—induction phase 30–120 minutes

- Apoptosis
- Free radicals
- Seizure activity
- Disruption of blood-brain barrier (BBB)
- Blood vessel leakage, edema
- Cerebral thermopooling
- Coagulation abnormalities
- Intracranial hypertension
- Depressed cerebral function
- Neuronal death
- Irreversible brain injury.

CEREBRAL PERFORMANCE CATEGORY SCALE

- A return to normal cerebral function and normal living
- Cerebral disability but sufficient function for independent activities of daily living
- Severe disability, limited cognition, inability to carry out independent existence
- Coma
- Brain death
  - Score of 1 or 2 is considered as favorable recovery

Cerebral performance category (CPC) scale 1-5
1–2: Good outcome
3–4: Negative outcome
5: Death

PEDIATRIC CARDIOPULMONARY RESUSCITATION (FIGURES 8A AND B)

- It is an emergency procedure which is performed on person suffering cardiac or respiratory arrest

- It is a combination of rescue breathing (mouth-to-mouth resuscitation) and chest compressions
- Cardiopulmonary resuscitation (CPR) can restore circulation of oxygen-rich blood to the brain
- The *most common cause of cardiopulmonary arrest in pediatric is respiratory.*

ADULT CARDIOPULMONARY RESUSCITATION IN THREE SIMPLE STEPS: CARDIOPULMONARY RESUSCITATION SEQUENCE: C–A–B

Call: Check the victim for unresponsiveness. If there is no response, "Call 102 and get the automated external defibrillator (AED)" and return to the victim. In most locations, the emergency dispatcher can assist you with CPR instructions.

Compress chest: Begin chest compressions. Push down on the chest at about 2 inches (5 cm) 30 times right between the nipples. Pump at the rate of at least 100/minute. Allow for complete chest recoil after each compression. Minimize interruptions in chest compressions.

Airway and breathing: Tilt the head back and lift the chin. If not breathing, pinch nose and cover the yours mouth and blow until you see the chest rise. Give 2 breaths. Each breath should take 1 second **(Figures 9A and B)**.

Adult CPR: Continue with 2 breaths and 30 compressions (5 cycles) until help arrives.

Note: This ratio is for one-person and two-person CPR. In two-person CPR, the person pumping the chest stops while the other gives mouth-to-mouth breathing.

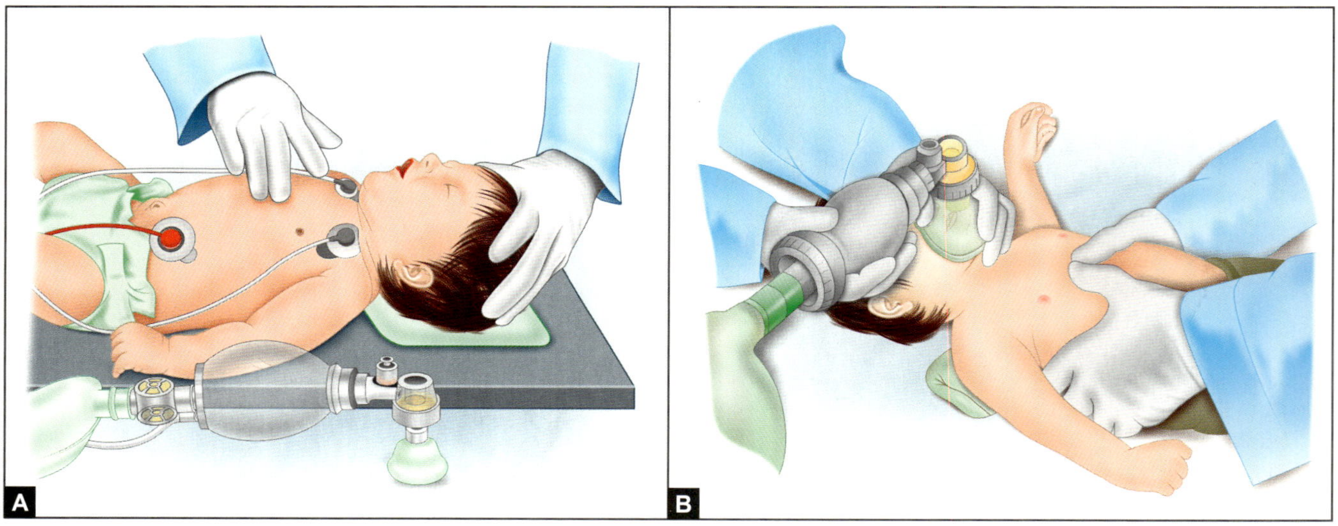

Figures 8A and B (A) Two-finger chest compression technique in infant (1 rescuer); (B) Two thumb-encircling hands chest compression in infant (2 rescuers)

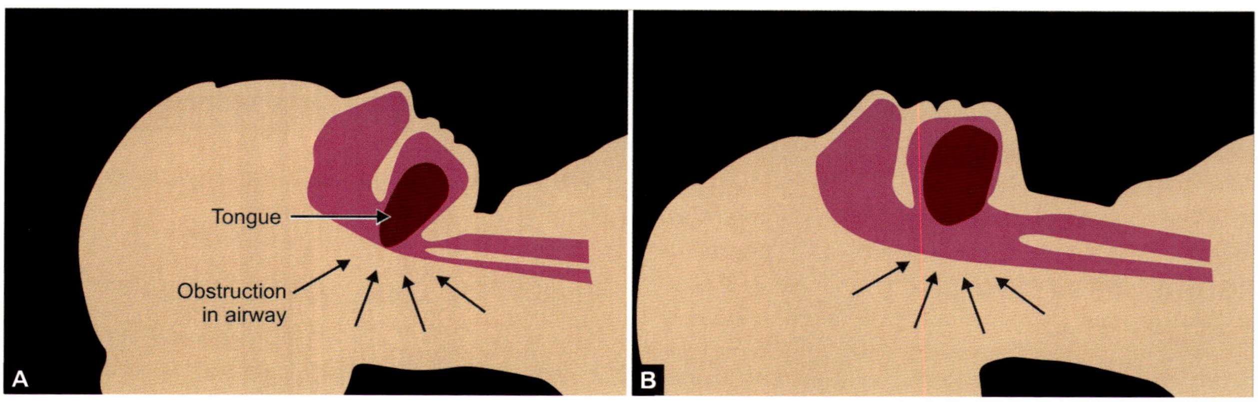

Figures 9A and B Taking care of obstruction to airway and breathing

SECTION 6

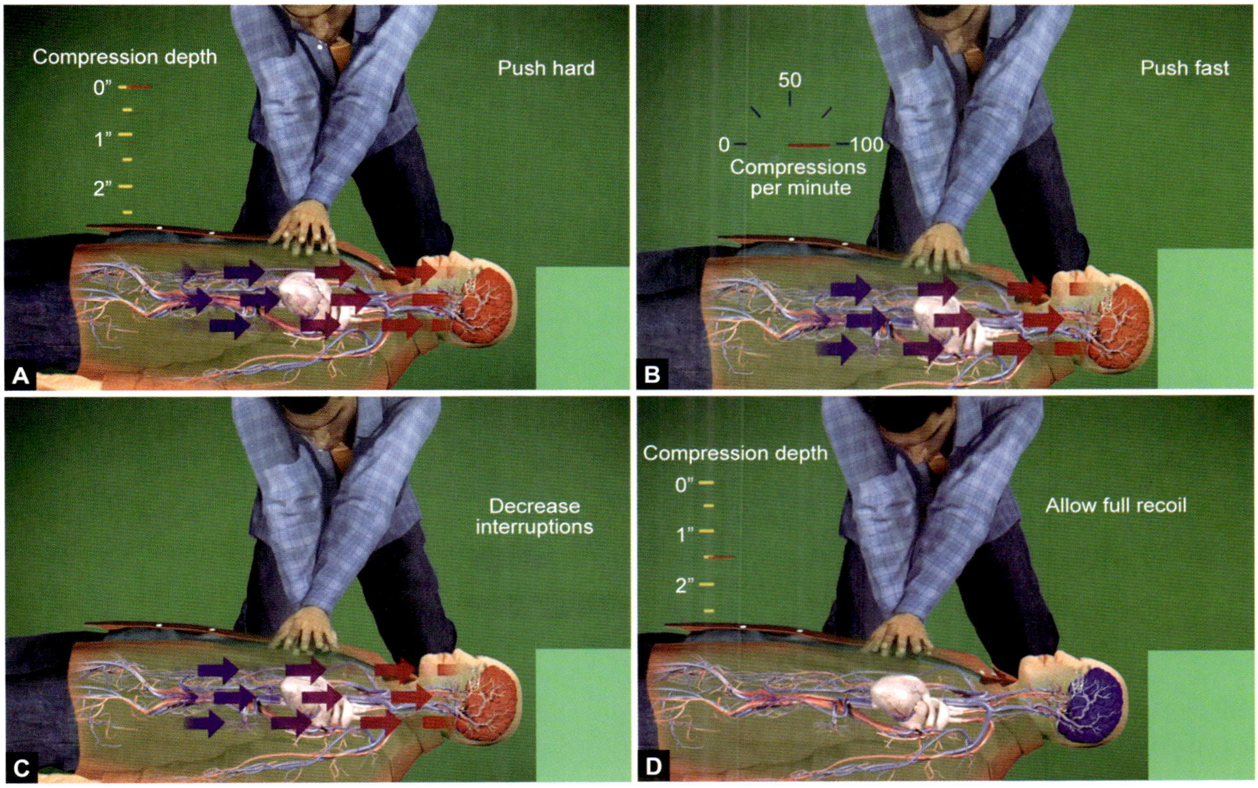

Figures 10A to D Compression for cardiopulmonary resuscitation using hands to: (A) Push hard; (B) Push fast; (C) Decrease interruptions; (D) Allow full recoil

Steps to CPR **(Figures 10A to D)**
1. Push hard
2. Push fast
3. Decrease interruptions
4. Allow full recoil

Child CPR

CPR for Children (Ages 1–8)

- CPR for children is similar to performing quick CPR for adults. There are, however, three differences.
    1. If you are alone with the child give 5 cycles (2 minutes) of CPR before calling 102.
    2. Use the heel of one hand for chest compressions. The compression rate is at least 100/minute.
    3. The compression depth is at least 1/3 of the anteroposterior diameter of the chest (about 2 inches).

Infant CPR

Give 30 Compressions

Give 30 gentle chest compressions at the rate of at least 100/minute. Position your 3rd and 4th fingers in the center of the chest half an inch below the nipples. The compression depth is at least 1/3 of the anteroposterior diameter of the chest (about 1½ inches).

Repeat

Repeat with 2 breaths and 30 compressions. After five cycles call 102 and continue the sequence.

Open the Airway

Open the airway using a head tilt lifting of chin. Do not tilt the head too far back.

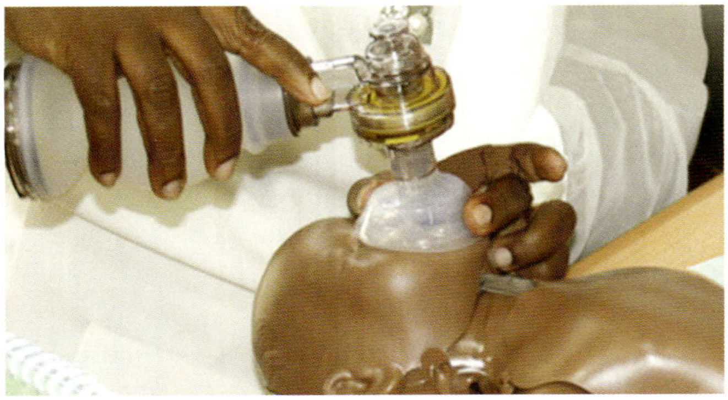

Figure 11 Laryngeal mask vs bag-mask ventilation in neonatal resuscitation

Give Two Gentle Puffs

If the baby is NOT breathing give two small gentle puffs. Cover the baby's mouth and nose with your mouth. Each breath should be one second long. You should see the baby's chest rise with each breath **(Figure 11)**.

CONTROVERSIAL ISSUES IN CARDIOPULMONARY RESUSCITATION

- There are no human studies to determine the optimal compression–ventilation ratio during CPR; a ratio of 30:2 was recommended by consensus
- There are no sufficient data to recommend CPR before defibrillation for all victims of ventricular fibrillation (VF) cardiac arrest **(Figures 12A and B)**
- The optimal energy levels (shock doses) for both monophasic and biphasic defibrillators are unknown
- The role of targeted temperature monitoring after in-hospital cardiac arrest is unknown
- There is currently insufficient evidence to support or refute the use of vasopressin as alternative to, or in combination with, epinephrine in any cardiac arrest rhythm.

MANIKIN SIMULATOR FIDELITY ON NEONATAL RESUSCITATION PROGRAM LEARNING

The neonatal resuscitation program (NRP) has been developed to educate physicians and other health care providers about newborn resuscitation and has been shown to improve neonatal resuscitation skills. Simulation-based training is recommended as an effective modality for instructing neonatal resuscitation and both low and high-fidelity manikin simulators are used **(Figure 13)**. Low and high-fidelity manikin simulators facilitate similar levels of objectively measured NRP outcomes for integrated skills station and teamwork performance.[8]

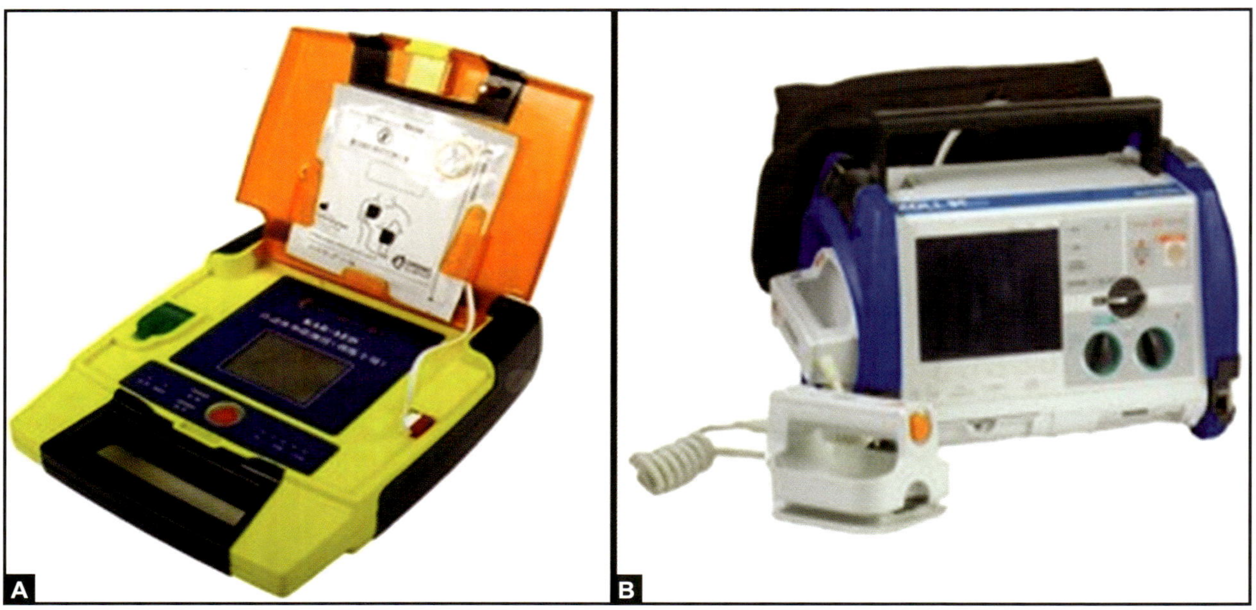

Figures 12A and B (A) AED simulation of defibrillator cardiopulmonary resuscitation simulation AED simulation defibrillator; (B) The Zoll M series has everything you need for cardiac resuscitation fast, easy to use defibrillation using synchronized cardioversion

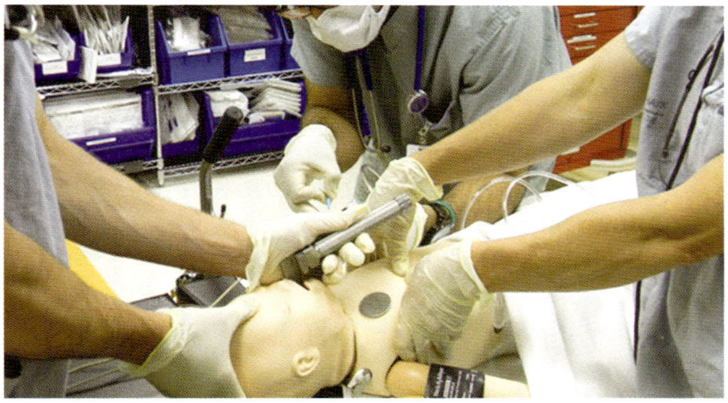

Figure 13 Anesthesia residents perform resuscitation procedures for 18-month-old patient (SimBaby)

HIGH-FIDELITY SIMULATION PROVIDES A REALISTIC SIMULATION EXPERIENCE

This is a gap in the literature regarding learning outcomes linked to the use of high-fidelity simulators compared to that of traditional teaching methods. To examine the effect of using high-fidelity simulators on knowledge and skills acquisition and retention with university students, a randomized two-arm trial using two different educational approaches on 90 nursing students assigned randomly to two groups was used at two points of time was undertaken by Robin Lewis et al[9] **(Figures 14A and B)**. The results showed significant differences in favor of the participants in the high-fidelity simulator group on both the acquisition and retention of knowledge and skills over time.[9]

However, a significant loss of cardiopulmonary resuscitation knowledge and skills occurred at three months after training in both groups. The findings of this study may assist educators in integrating high-fidelity simulators in education and training. In addition, the findings may help nursing educators to arrange additional cardiopulmonary resuscitation training sessions in order to improve cardiac arrested patients' outcomes. High-fidelity simulation (HFS) provides students with interactive learning experiences in a safe controlled environment. HFS enables teachers to implement critical clinical scenarios, such as cardiac arrest, without risk to patients. Integrating the simulation training into medical curricula will help to overcome the challenges that face many courses, specifically the shortage of clinical areas for training and the increase in numbers of nursing students.[10]

HANDS ON + HANDS FREE: SIMULATED ON-CALL INTERACTION

In hospital, doctors and nurses frequently discuss acutely unwell patients via the telephone. Telephone communication can be challenging, yet medical students receive little training in how to conduct such interactions. In a study aimed to provide a simple, innovative, simulation session to address this learning need for third-year medical students at Newcastle University.[10] Groups of students were given a pager and a supervising tutor. Students responded to a 'bleep' from a nurse practitioner in a different room, who role-played a ward nurse concerned about a patient. Speakerphones were used, allowing the entire conversation to be audible. After the call, a student-led debriefing session took place **(Figures 15A and B)**. After the debriefing another student 'held' the bleep and a different scenario

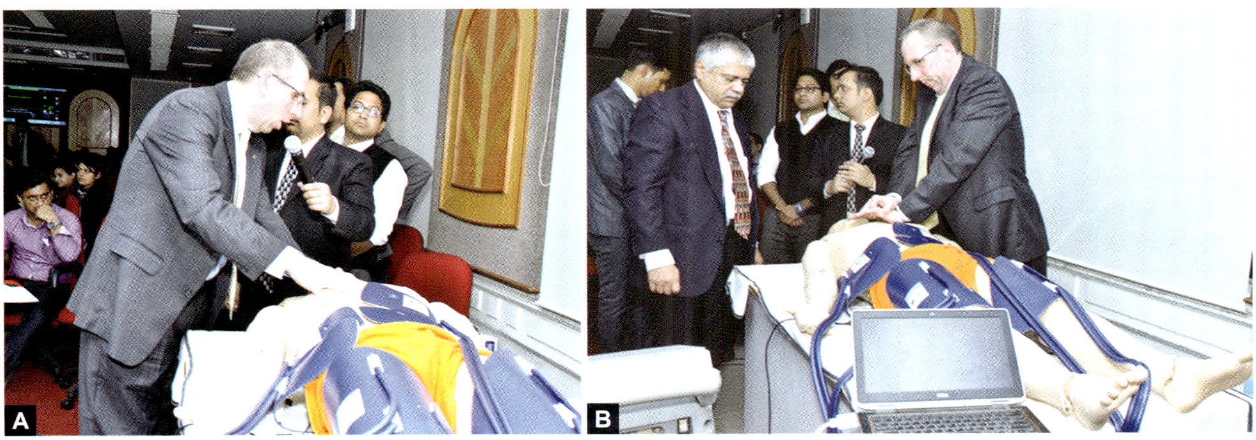

Figures 14A and B High-fidelity simulation (HFS) mannequin technology provides a realistic simulation experience

CHAPTER 26

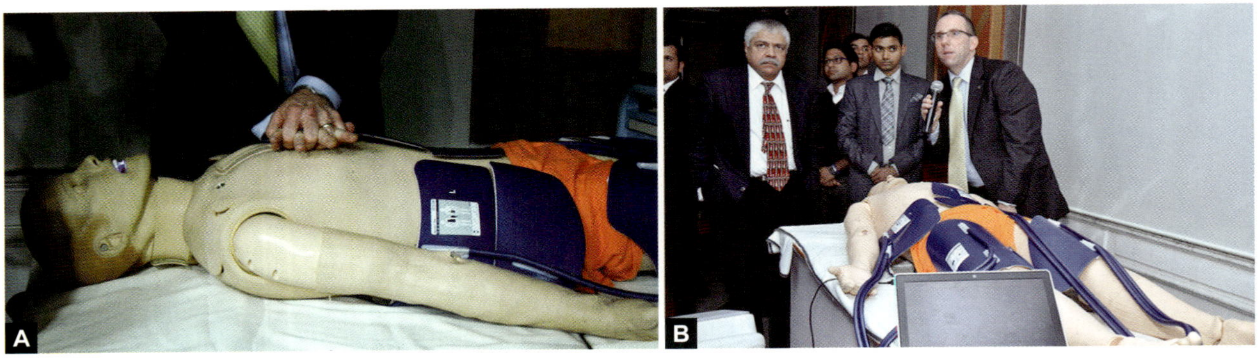

Figures 15A and B Practical application and demonstration of cardiopulmonary resuscitation

ensued. Following a resuscitation scenario, students made telephone contact with the medical registrar to hand over information pertaining to the case. Before and after the session, students rated their confidence in telephone interaction and handover using a 10-point Likert scale. Students also completed a feedback questionnaire. Fifty-four students attended the session.

A statistically significant improvement in student confidence in telephone communication and handover was seen after the session. Free-text feedback highlighted that students had not received teaching on this previously, and that they welcomed opportunities to practice such skills within a controlled, safe environment. Simulation training can be costly, but speakerphones are cheap and readily available. Given the frequency of telephone interaction in hospital, the authors believed all medical students should receive telephone communication training. Locally, our department has now incorporated these teaching methods into simulation sessions elsewhere in the curriculum. Medical students in general receive little training in how to conduct telephonic interactions.[11]

EVALUATING SIMULATION-BASED ADVANCED CARDIAC LIFE SUPPORT EDUCATION ON PATIENT OUTCOMES

Simulation training is widely accepted as an effective teaching tool, especially for dealing with high-risk situations. In a study by BMC medical education group, it was assessed whether standardized, simulation-based advanced cardiac life support (ACLS) training improved performance in managing simulated and actual cardiac arrests. A total of 103 second- and third-year internal medicine residents were randomized to two groups. The first group underwent conventional ACLS training. The second group underwent two 2 1/2-hour sessions of standardized simulation ACLS teaching. The groups were assessed by evaluators blinded to their assignment during in-hospital monthly mock codes and actual inpatient code sheets at three large academic hospitals. Primary outcomes were time to initiation of cardiopulmonary resuscitation, time to administration of first epinephrine/vasopressin, time to delivery of first defibrillation, and adherence to American Heart Association guidelines **(Figures 16A and B)**.

There were no differences in primary outcomes among the study arms and hospital sites. During 21 mock codes, the most common error was misidentification of the initial rhythm (67% [6 of 9] and 58% [7 of 12] control and simulation arms, respectively, P =.70). There were no differences in primary outcome among groups in 147 actual inpatient codes. This blinded, randomized study found no effect on primary outcomes. A notable finding was the percentage of internal medicine residents who misidentified cardiac arrest rhythms.[12]

- Medical students should receive telephonic simulation communication training
- It increases their confidence and is not costly.

STEPS IN CARDIOPULMONARY RESUSCITATION

Chest Compression Before Airway and Breath

- When cardiac arrest is recognized, the rescuer should initiate chest compressions before airway opening and rescue breathing

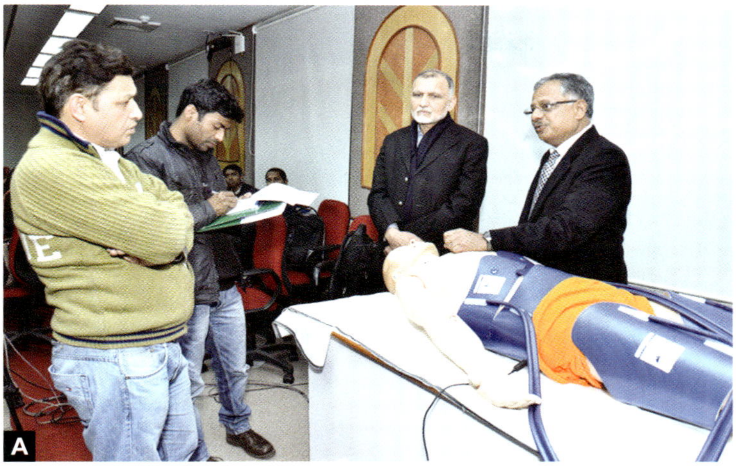

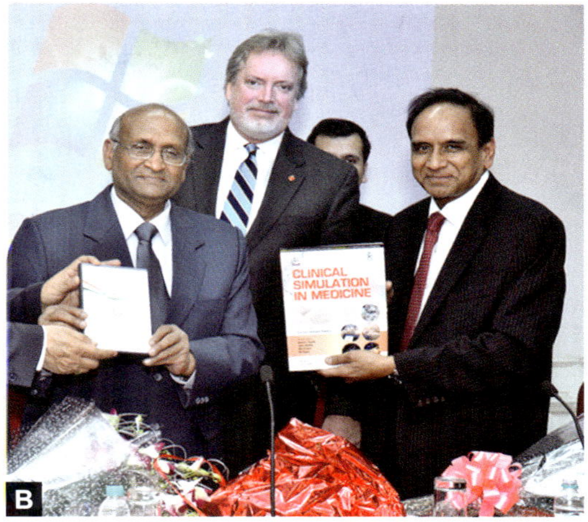

Figures 16A and B Advanced cardiac life support training and medical education on mannequin regarding cardiopulmonary resuscitation at a workshop recently held in AIIMS (New Delhi). High fidelity therapeutic hypothermia machine was used on simulator to teach of hypothermia for cardiopulmonary resuscitation

- All bystanders, trained or untrained, should provide chest compressions to the victim of cardiac arrest.
- *Compression to Ventilation Ratio of 30:2*—It is recommended that the trained rescuer provide CPR with compression to ventilation ratio of 30:2.

Type of Chest Compression

The need for high-quality CPR is once again emphasized. The rescuer should give chest compressions to a depth of at least 5 cm and at a rate of at least 100 times per minute, allow for complete chest recoil after each compression, and minimize interruptions of chest compressions.

BASIC CARDIOPULMONARY RESUSCITATION—THE ABCD

Basic cardiopulmonary resuscitation (CPR) or basic life support (BLS) (**Flow chart 1A** is for adults and **Flow chart 1B** is for pediatric population) should be started right after any health care professional inside a hospital or any professionally qualified first aid person verifies the unconsciousness of the patient **(Figure 17)**. These people should be properly trained to provide the first aid of life support, which aims to maintain adequate cerebral and heart oxygen supply until the installation of the advanced cardiovascular life support (ACLS) and reversal of the cardiac arrhythmia causing cardiopulmonary arrest (CPA) with electrical shocks, when indicated.

Basic CPR comprises not only the cardiopulmonary support measures because it begins with the verification of the unconsciousness of the patient. Once this is done, the next step is to activate the ACLS service; to put the patient in the correct position; to check the known ABCs of CPR: A (airway)—to clear airway; B (breathing) - to check breathing and the need for ventilation support; C (circulation)—to check the central pulse, if absent, begin circulatory support; and, more recently, D (defibrillation) - used in cases of ventricular fibrillation (VF) and ventricular tachycardia (VT) without pulse.

These four measures form the ABCDs of the BLS. Inclusion of defibrillation in the BLS and the activation of the ACLS (second step of the basic CPR measures) result from the observation that 80–90% of the cases of CPA have VF as the initial cardiac rhythm and its treatment requires either immediate or the most precocious possible defibrillation.

PRECOCIOUS DEFIBRILLATION IN BASIC LIFE SUPPORT (FIGURES 18A AND B)

Precocious defibrillation in basic life support (BLS) can be performed either by means of a conventional defibrillator, which requires special training of the operator for recognition of cardiac arrhythmias, or by means of an automated external defibrillator, which has the ability to recognize cardiac arrhythmias. *Defibrillation should be performed only in cases of ventricular fibrillation (VF) or ventricular tachycardia*

CHAPTER **26**

Flow chart 1A Basic life support and advanced life support in adults—flow chart as per 2010 guidelines

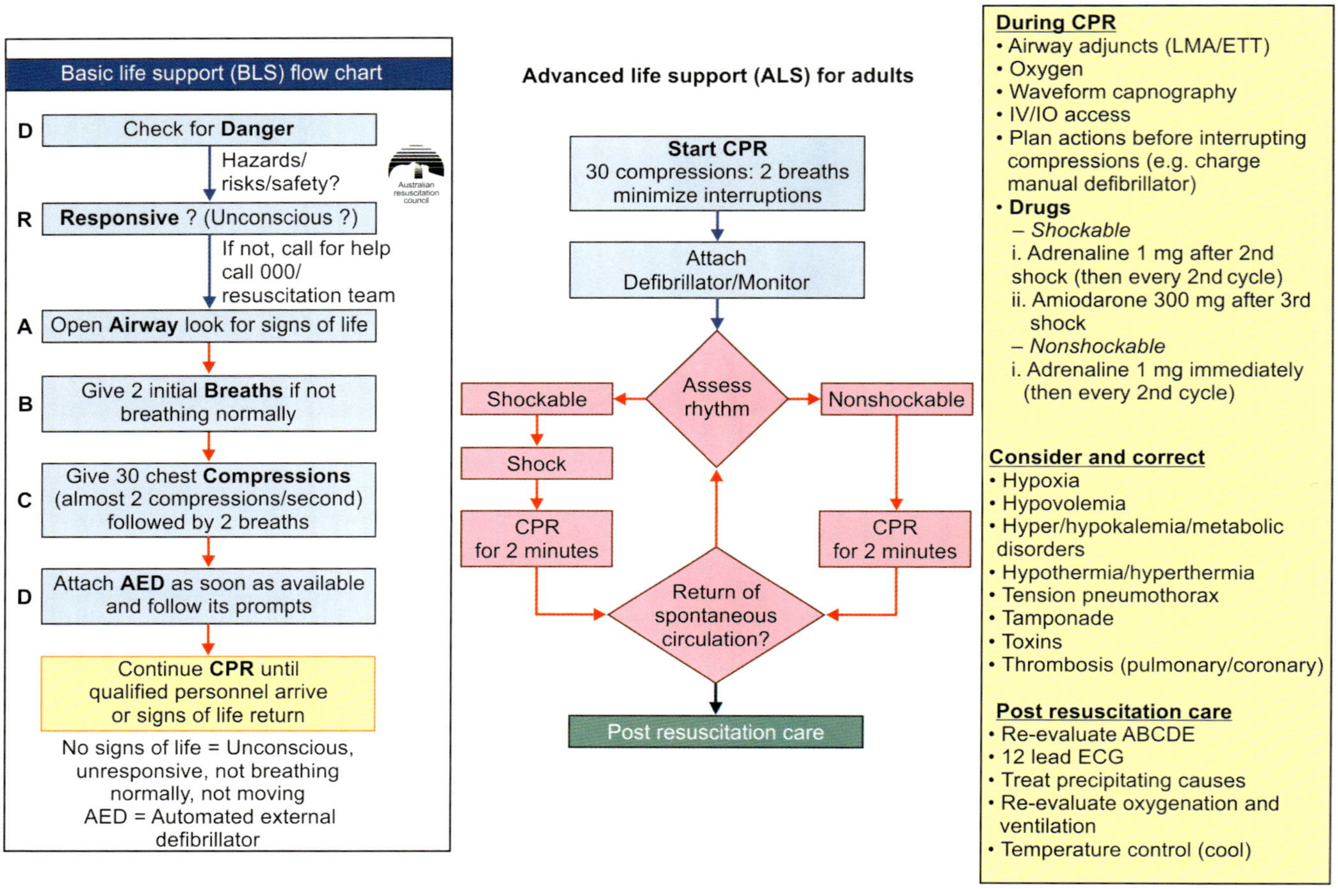

(VT) without pulse with up to three consecutive electrical shocks of progressively higher voltage. At this stage, BLS is completed and ACLS begins.[13]

In case of trauma or drowning affecting children or adults, in which pulmonary arrest precedes cardiac arrest and early ventilation is decisive for the prognosis, the basic measures of CPR should be established one minute before asking for advanced support. Recent data suggest that VF is a cardiac rhythm rarely found in individuals younger than 30 years, and therefore, the same conduct described above should be followed for this age range, in the absence of clinical and circumstantial information.[14] If more than one first aid person is available, the discussion about the activation of the ACLS is solved through the division of tasks: while one first aid person asks for the ACLS, the others begin the BLS. In case of suspected cervical damage, the patient should be very carefully positioned. If in doubt, act as if there were cervical damage, i.e. hold the patient's neck and occipital region with your hands while the victim is being moved, thus avoiding medullar compression and its harmful consequences.

OXYGEN VIA MOUTH-TO-MOUTH RESUSCITATION IS ADEQUATE

The ABCDs of CPR, when correctly performed, can provide through mouth-to-mouth ventilation air with 16–17% of oxygen, causing an alveolar tension of 80 mm Hg. This is considered adequate for the victim, in opposition to the former conception that the air expired by the first aid person would be poor in oxygen. Airway manual breathing unit (AMBU) connected to an oxygen source of 10–15 L/min allows the obtainment of inspiratory oxygen concentration of up to 90%, when coupled with a facial mask, and up to 100%, when coupled with a tracheal tube.

Flow chart 1B Basic life support healthcare provider pediatric cardiac arrest algorithm for the single rescuer—2015 update

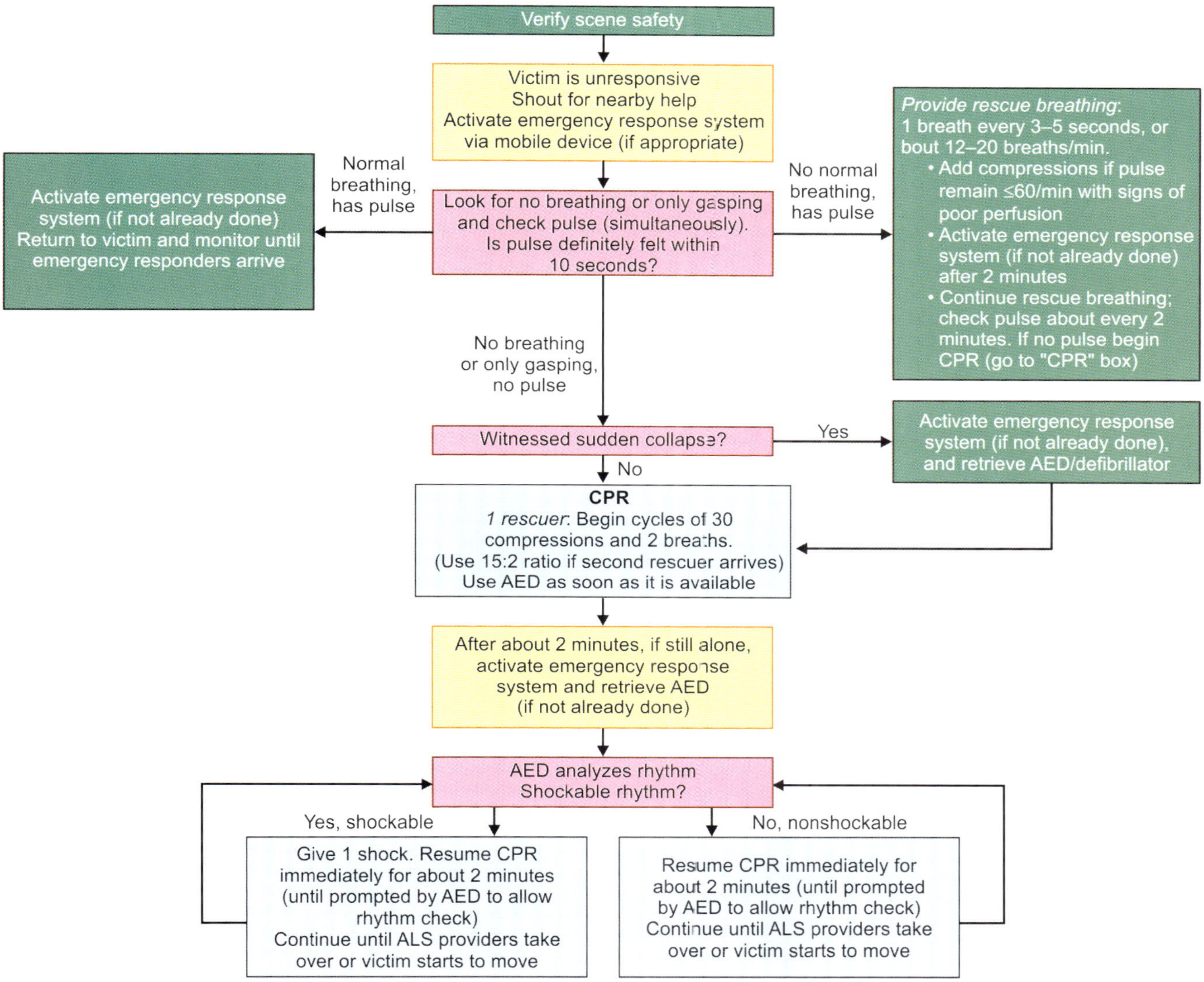

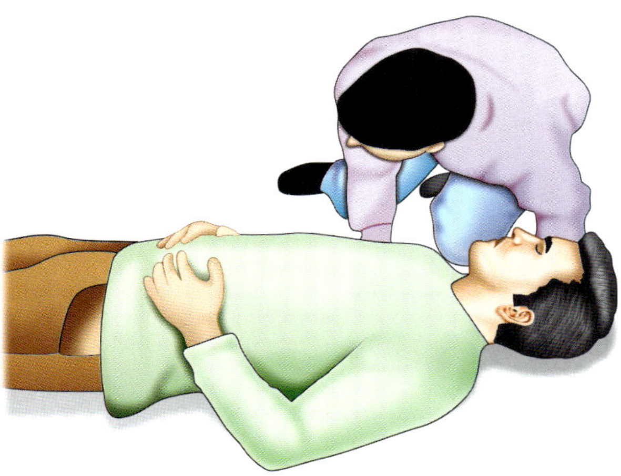

Figure 17 Basic cardiopulmonary resuscitation—The ABCD

BLOOD PRESSURE CHANGES WITH CHEST COMPRESSION

External cardiac massage by chest compression, performed according to the conventional orientation, produces systolic pressure (SP) of 60–80 mm Hg and diastolic pressure (DP) of 15–35 mm Hg. The mean carotid pressure, however, rarely exceeds 40 mm Hg. Cardiac output resulting from external chest compressions ranges from one-forth to one-third of the normal; additional studies are necessary for its better assessment.[15,16] In experimental studies, external chest compression interposed with abdominal compression revealed increase in systolic pressure (SP) and diastolic pressure (DP) in the aorta, of the coronary perfusion

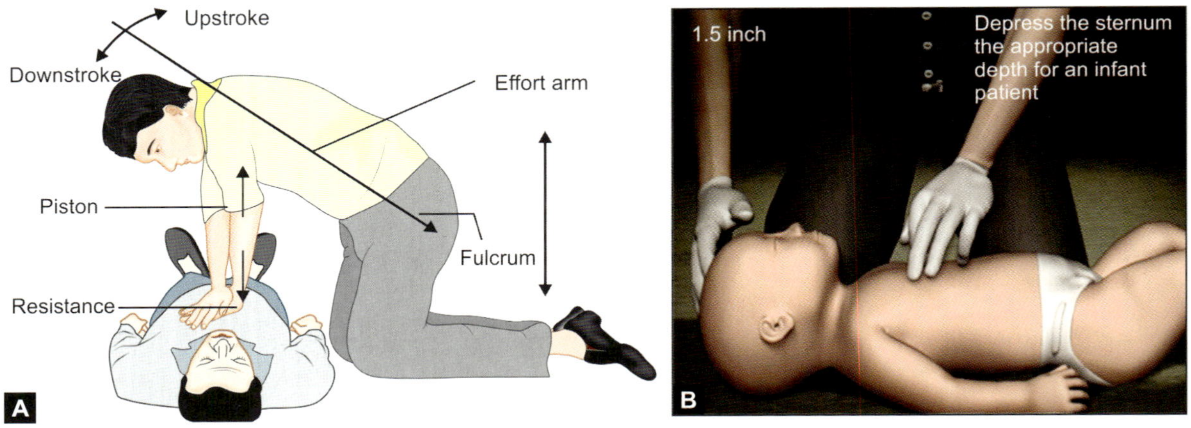

Figures 18A and B Compression before airways and breathing

Flow chart 2 Adult basic life support algorithm

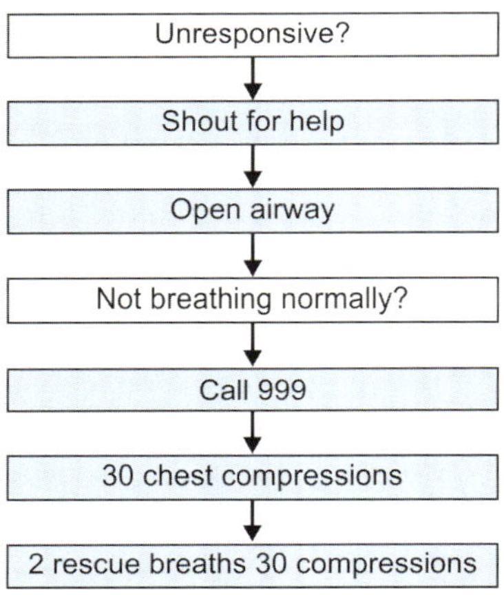

pressure (CPP) and of the venous return to the heart, resulting in the elevation of cardiac output. The success of CPR, reported in a study in pigs, was encouraging,[17] but results of CPR studies in humans were inconclusive[18] **(Flow chart 2)**.

External chest compression associated with simultaneous ventilation aims at an additional increase of the intrathoracic pressure and, therefore, of the carotid flow, when compared with isolated external chest compression. Experimental studies in animals showed an increase of the carotid flow with this technique. Clinical studies, however, showed unsatisfactory results.[19]

VENTILATORY AND CIRCULATORY SUPPORT: ARE THEY SYNERGISED?

Need for ventilatory support during the initial phase of the CPR measures was recently questioned by an experimental study in pigs,[20] stimulated by previous studies in animals. The results obtained showed similarities between the groups – ventilatory + circulatory support and isolated circulatory support, both initiated 2 minutes after CPA–in regard to survival in 24 and 48 hours and to neurological prognosis. These results, however, should not be interpreted as definitive. They do not reduce the importance of ventilatory support in the context of cardiopulmonary resuscitation, but they emphasize the importance of the re-establishment of the coronary blood flow and of the cardiac output through the measures of circulatory support.

Additional studies should be carried out to definitely clarify this question; data currently available, however, suggest that the use of isolated circulatory support is better than indifference, resulting either from ignorance of the BLS measures or from the resistance of the first aid personnel in performing mouth-to-mouth ventilation until the arrival of ACLS.

RISKS TO THE RESCUER AND VICTIM IN BASIC LIFE SUPPORT

The safety of both the rescuer and victim are paramount during a resuscitation attempt. There have been few incidents of rescuers suffering adverse effects from undertaking CPR, with only isolated reports of infections such as tuberculosis (TB) and severe acute respiratory distress syndrome (SARS). Transmission of HIV during CPR has never been reported.

Effectiveness of Barrier Devices

There have been no human studies to address the effectiveness of barrier devices during CPR; however, laboratory studies have shown that certain filters,

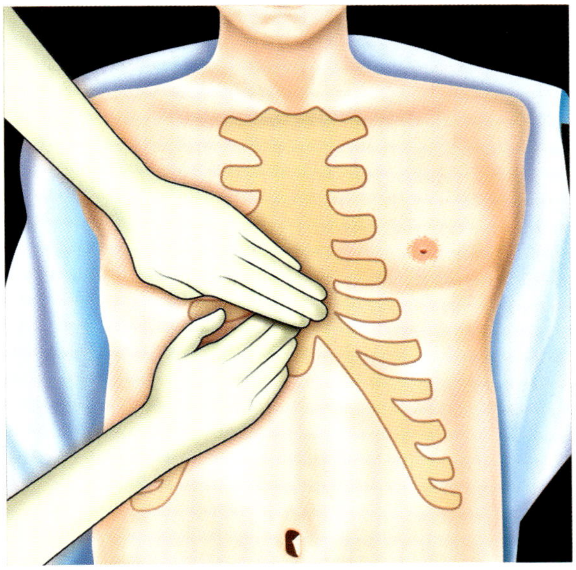

Figure 19 Risks to the rescuer and victim in basic life support

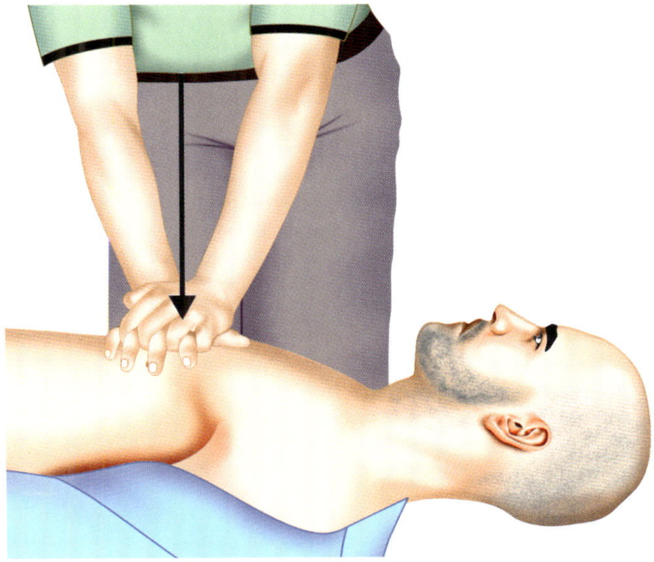

Figure 20 Initial rescue breaths

or barrier devices with one-way valves, prevent transmission of oral bacteria from the victim to the rescuer during mouth-to-mouth ventilation. Rescuers should take appropriate safety precautions where feasible, especially if the victim is known to have a serious infection such as TB or SARS. During an outbreak of a highly infectious condition (such as SARS), full protective precautions for the rescuer are essential **(Figure 19)**.

Professional Rescuer CPR

- To maintain breathing and heartbeat, perform rescue breathing and chest compressions together.
- 70% of cardiac arrest patients are in ventricular fibrillation.

INITIAL RESCUE BREATHS

During the first few minutes after nonasphyxial cardiac arrest the blood oxygen content remains high. Therefore, ventilation is less important than chest compression at this time **(Figure 20)**.

It is well recognized that skill acquisition and retention are aided by simplification of the BLS sequence of actions. It is also recognized that rescuers are frequently unwilling to carry out mouth-to-mouth ventilation for a variety of reasons, including fear of infection and distaste for the procedure. For these reasons, and to emphasize the priority of chest compressions, it is recommended that, in adults, CPR should start with chest compressions rather than initial ventilations.

ADVANCED CARDIOVASCULAR LIFE SUPPORT

The ACLS affects multiple links in the chain of survival, including interventions to prevent cardiac arrest, treat cardiac arrest, and improve outcomes of patients who achieve ROSC after cardiac arrest. The 2010 AHA guidelines for CPR and ECC continue to emphasize that the foundation of successful ACLS is good BLS, beginning with prompt high-quality CPR with minimal interruptions, and for VF/pulseless VT, attempted defibrillation within minutes of collapse. The new fifth link in the chain of survival and Part 9 of the 2015 guidelines on "postcardiac arrest care" (expanded from a subsection of the ACLS part of the 2005 AHA guidelines for CPR and ECC) emphasize the importance of comprehensive multidisciplinary care that begins with recognition of cardiac arrest and continues after ROSC through hospital discharge and beyond. Key ACLS assessments and interventions provide inessential bridge between BLS and long-term survival with good neurologic function.

CHANGES FROM IN 2010 GUIDELINES TO 2015 GUIDELINES (TABLE 5)

Airway Management

In terms of airway management, the 2010 AHA guidelines for CPR and ECC have a major new class I recommendation for adults: use of quantitative waveform capnography for confirmation and monitoring of endotracheal tube placement. In addition, the use of supraglottic advanced airways continues to be supported as an alternative to endotracheal intubation for airway management during CPR. Finally, the routine use of cricoid pressure during airway management of patients in cardiac arrest is no longer recommended.

Ventilation during CPR with an Advanced Airway 2015 (Updated)

It may be reasonable for the provider to deliver 1 breath every 6 seconds (10 breaths per minute) while continuous chest compressions are being performed (i.e. during CPR with an advanced airway).[1]

Management of Symptomatic Arrhythmias

There are several important changes in the 2010 AHA Guidelines for CPR and ECC regarding management of symptomatic arrhythmias. On the basis of new evidence of safety and potential efficacy, adenosine can now be considered for the diagnosis and treatment of stable undifferentiated wide-complex tachycardia when the rhythm is regular and the QRS waveform is monomorphic. For symptomatic or unstable bradycardia, intravenous (IV) infusion of chronotropic agents is now recommended as an equally effective alternative to external pacing when atropine is ineffective.

ADVANCED CARDIOVASCULAR LIFE SUPPORT CARDIAC ARREST ALGORITHM

For 2010 a new circular AHA ACLS cardiac arrest algorithm **(Figure 10)** has been introduced as an alternative to the traditional box-and-line format. Both algorithms represent restructured and simplified formats that focus on interventions that have the greatest impact on outcome. To that end, emphasis has been placed on delivery of high-quality CPR with minimal interruptions and defibrillation of VF/pulseless VT. Vascular access, drug delivery, and advanced airway placement, while still recommended, should not cause significant interruptions in chest compression or delay shocks. In addition, atropine is no longer recommended for routine use in the management of pulseless electrical activity (PEA)/asystole.

Real-time Monitoring and Optimization of Cardiopulmonary Resuscitation Quality

Real-time monitoring and optimization of CPR quality using either mechanical parameters (e.g. monitoring of chest compression rate and depth, adequacy of chest wall relaxation, length and duration of pauses in compression and number and depth of ventilations delivered) or, when feasible, physiologic parameters (partial pressure of end-tidal CO_2 [$PETCO_2$], arterial pressure during the relaxation phase of chest compressions, or central venous oxygen saturation [$ScvO_2$]) are encouraged. When quantitative waveform capnography is used for adults, guidelines now include recommendations for monitoring CPR quality and detecting return of spontaneous circulation (ROSC) based on $PETCO_2$ values.

New CPR prompt and feedback devices may be useful for training rescuers and as part of an overall strategy to improve the quality of CPR in actual resuscitations. Training for the complex combination of skills required to perform adequate chest compressions should focus on demonstrating mastery.

2015 (Updated): It may be reasonable to use audiovisual feedback devices during CPR for real-time optimization of CPR performance.

Finally the 2010 and 2015 AHA guidelines for CPR and ECC continue to recognize that ACLS does not end when a patient achieves return of spontaneous circulation (ROSC). Guidelines for postcardiac arrest management have been significantly expanded and now include a new early postcardiac arrest treatment algorithm **(Flow charts 3 and 4)**.

GUIDELINE CHANGES CONT...

Defibrillation

There is increased emphasis on the importance of minimally-interrupted high-quality chest compressions throughout any ALS intervention: chest compressions are paused briefly only to allow specific

Flow chart 3 Cardiac arrest algorithm as in 2015

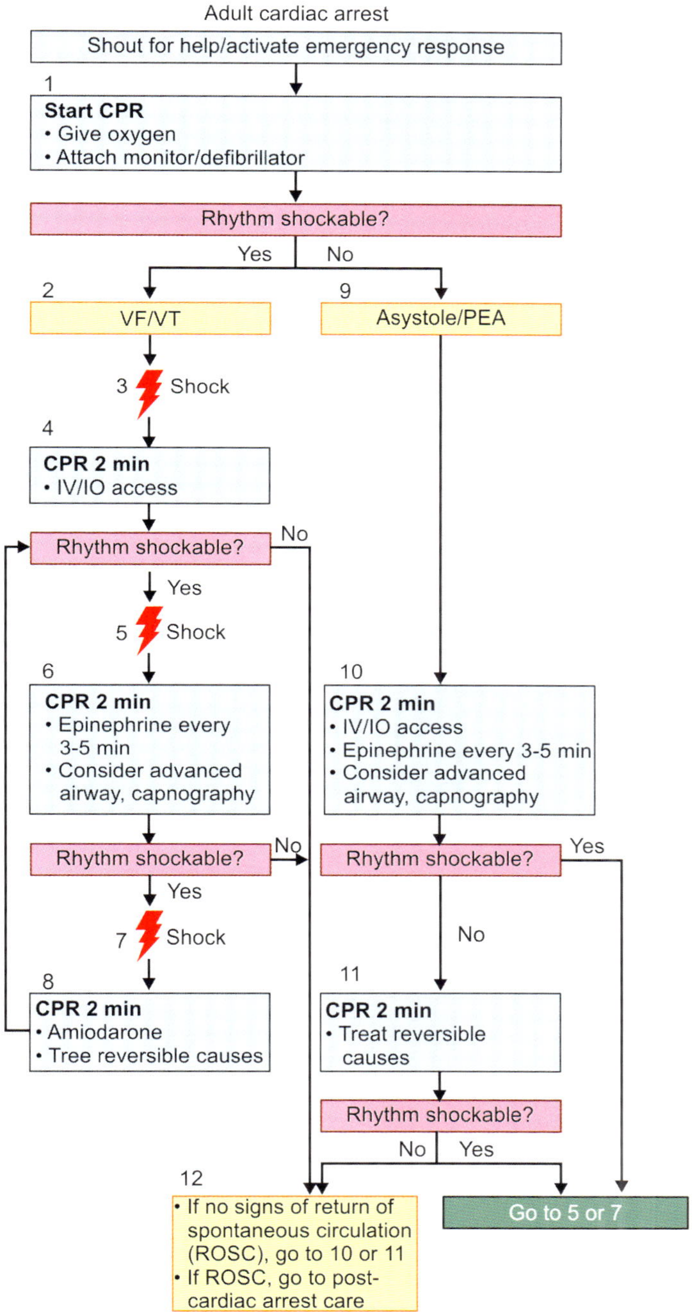

CPR Quality
- Push hard (≥2 inches [5 cm]) and fast (≥100/min) and allow complete chest recoil
- Minimize interruptions in compressions
- Avoid excessive ventilation
- Rotate compressor every 2 minutes
- If no advanced airway, 30:2 compression-ventilation ratio
- Quantitative waveform capnography
  - If $PETCO_2$ <10 mm Hg, attempt to improve CPR quality
- Intra-arterial pressure
  - If relaxation phase (diastolic) pressure <20 mm Hg, attempt to improve CPR quality

Return of spontaneous circulation (ROSC)
- Pulse and blood pressure
- Abrupt sustained increase in $PETCO_2$ (typically ≥40 mm Hg)
- Spontaneous arterial pressure waves with intra-arterial monitoring

Shock energy
- *Biphasic:* Manufacturer recommendation (eg, initial dose of 120-200 J); if unknown, use maximum available. Second and subsequent doses should be equivalent and higher doses may be considered.
- *Monophasic*: 360 J

Drug therapy
- *Epinephrine IV/IO dose*: 1 mg every 3-5 minutes
- *Vasopressin IV/IO dose*: 40 units can replace first or second dose of epinephrine
- *Amiodarone IV/IO dose*: First dose: 300 mg bolus. Second dose: 150 mg.

Advanced airway
- Supraglottic advanced airway or endotracheal intubation
- Waveform capnography to confirm and monitor ET tube placement
- 8-10 breaths per minute with continous chest compressions

Reversible causes
- Hypovolemia
- Hypoxia
- Hydrogen ion (acidosis)
- Hypo-/hyperkalemia
- Hypothermia
- Tension pneumothorax
- Tamponade, cardiac
- Toxins
- Thrombosis, pulmonary
- Thrombosis, coronary

interventions. The recommendation for a specified period of cardiopulmonary resuscitation (CPR) before out-of-hospital defibrillation, following cardiac arrest unwitnessed by the emergency medical services (EMS), has been removed. Chest compressions are now continued while a defibrillator is charged—this will minimize the preshock pause. The role of the precordial thump is de-emphasized. The use of up to three quick successive (stacked) shocks is now recommended for ventricular fibrillation/pulseless ventricular tachycardia

Flow chart 4 Cardiac arrest treatment algorithm by American Heart Association guidelines

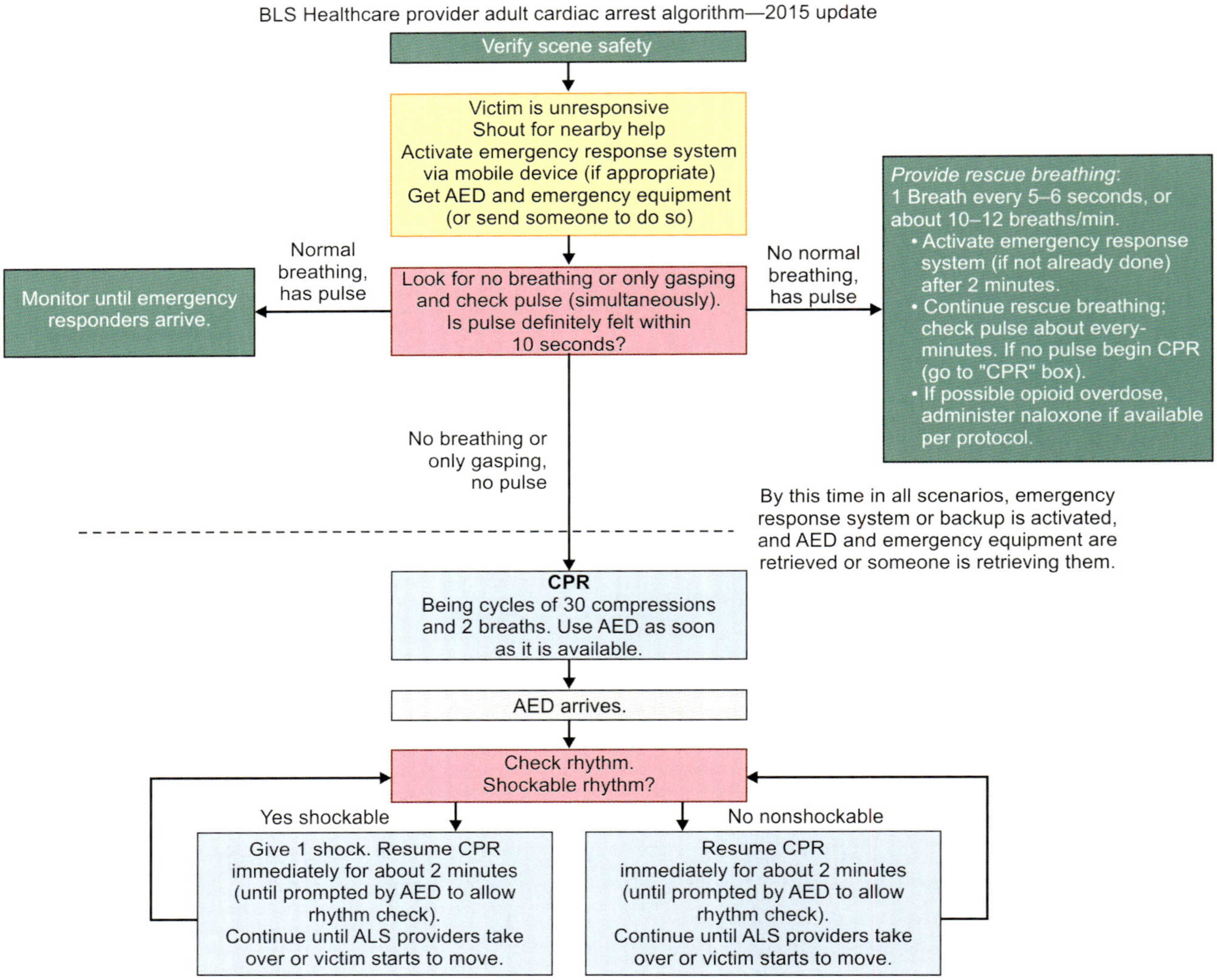

Source: American Heart Association guidelines update for CPR and ECC.

(VF/VT) occurring in the cardiac catheterization laboratory or in the immediate postoperative period following cardiac surgery.

DEFIBRILLATION—ELECTRICAL THERAPIES

The 2010 AHA guidelines for CPR and ECC have been updated to reflect new data on the use of pacing in bradycardia, and on cardioversion and defibrillation for tachycardic rhythm disturbances. Integration of AEDs into a system of care is critical in the chain of survival in public places outside of hospitals. One area of continued interest is whether delivering a longer period of CPR before defibrillation improves outcomes in cardiac arrest. In early studies, survival was improved when 1.5–3 minutes of CPR preceded defibrillation for patients with cardiac arrest of 4—5 minutes duration prior to EMS arrival.[21] However, in 2 more recent randomized controlled trials, CPR performed before defibrillation did not improve outcome. If 2 rescuers are present CPR should be performed while a defibrillator is being obtained and readied for use. Transcutaneous pacing has also been the focus of several recent trials. Pacing is not generally recommended for patients in asystolic cardiac arrest. Three randomized controlled trials[22] indicate no improvement in rate of admission to hospital or survival to hospital discharge when paramedics or physicians attempted pacing in patients with cardiac arrest due to asystole in the prehospital or hospital (ED) setting. However, it is reasonable for healthcare providers to be prepared to initiate pacing in patients with bradyarrhythmias in the event the heart rate does not respond to atropine or other chronotropic (rate-accelerating) drugs.[23] There is increased emphasis on the importance of minimally-interrupted high-quality chest compressions throughout any ALS intervention: chest compressions are paused briefly only to allow specific interventions. The recommendation for a specified period of cardiopulmonary resuscitation (CPR) before out-of-hospital defibrillation, following cardiac arrest unwitnessed by the emergency medical services (EMS), has been removed. Chest compressions are now continued while a defibrillator is charged—this will minimize the pre-shock pause. The role of the precordial thump is de-emphasized. The use of up to three quick successive (stacked) shocks is now recommended for ventricular fibrillation/pulseless ventricular tachycardia (VF/VT) occurring in the cardiac catheterization laboratory or in the immediate postoperative period following cardiac surgery.

2015 update: For witnessed adult cardiac arrest when an AED is immediately available, it is reasonable that the defibrillator be used as soon as possible. For adults with unmonitored cardiac arrest or for whom an AED is not immediately available, it is reasonable that CPR be initiated while the defibrillator equipment is being retrieved and applied and that defibrillation, if indicated, be attempted as soon as the device is ready for use.

SHOCKABLE RHYTHMS VENTRICULAR FIBRILLATION/VENTRICULAR TACHYCARDIA

The first monitored rhythm is VF/VT in approximately 25% of cardiac arrests, both in 60 or out of hospital. VF/VT will also occur at some stage during resuscitation in about 25% of cardiac arrests with an initial documented rhythm of asystole or PEA.

2015 update: For witnessed OHCA with a shockable rhythm, it may be reasonable for EMS systems with priority based, multitiered response to delay positive-pressure ventilation (PPV) by using a strategy of up to 3 cycles of 200 continuous compressions with passive oxygen insufflation and airway adjuncts.

CONCLUSION

As we mark the 50th anniversary of modern-era CPR, we must acknowledge that, despite measurable progress aimed at its prevention, cardiac arrest— both in and out of the hospital—continues to be a major public health challenge. Over these 50 years, scientific knowledge about arrest pathophysiology and resuscitation mechanisms has increased substantially. In our ongoing commitment to ensure optimal community-based care for all victims of cardiac arrest, we must continue to effectively translate the science of resuscitation into clinical care and improved resuscitation outcomes.

The primary goal of a bundled treatment strategy for the patient after cardiac arrest includes a consistently applied comprehensive therapeutic plan delivered in a multidisciplinary environment leading to the return of normal or near-normal functional status. Patients with suspected ACS should be triaged to a facility with reperfusion capabilities and a multidisciplinary team prepared to monitor patients for multi-organ dysfunction and initiate appropriate postcardiac arrest therapy, including hypothermia. Prognostic assessment in the setting of hypothermia is changing, and experts qualified in neurologic assessment in this patient population and integration of prognostic tools are essential for patients, caregivers, and families and are reviewed in detail in Part 9. As a guide to therapy, a new algorithm and a table of integrated goal therapy care were developed.

REFERENCES

1. Lanier WL. Cerebral metabolic rate and hypothermia: their relationship with ischemic neurologic injury. J Neurosurg Anesthesiol. 1995;7:216-21.
2. Maier CM, Sun GH, Cheng D, Yenari MA, Chan PH, Steinberg GK. Effects of mild hypothermia on superoxide anion production, superoxide dismutase expression, and activity following transient focal cerebral ischemia. Neurobiol Dis. 2002;11:28-42.
3. Bernard SA, Gray TW, Buist MD, et al. Treatment of comatose survivors of out-of-hospital cardiac arrest with induced hypothermia. N Engl J Med. 2002;346:557-63.
4. Holzer M. Targeted temperature management for comatose survivors of cardiac arrest. N Engl J Med. 2010;363:1256-64.

5. Vaity C, Al-Subaie N, Cecconi M. Cooling techniques for targeted temperature management post-cardiac arrest. Crit Care. 2015;19:103-9.
6. Nielsen N, Watterslev J, Cronberg T, Erlinge D, Gasche Y, Hassager C, et al. Targeted temperature management at 33°C versus 36°C after cardiac arrest. N Engl J Med. 2013;369:2197-206.
7. 2015 American Heart Association guidelines update for CPR and ECC. Circulation. 2015;132(18)Suppl 2:1-293.
8. Curran V1, Fleet L, White S, Bessell C, Deshpandey A, Drover A, Hayward M, Valcour J. A randomized controlled study of manikin simulator fidelity on neonatal resuscitation program learning outcomes. Adv Health Sci Educ Theory Pract. 2014 Jun 11. [Epub ahead of print]
9. Lewis R, Strachan A, Smith MM. Is high fidelity simulation the most effective method for the development of non-technical skills in nursing? A review of the current evidence. The Open Nursing Journal. 2012;6:82-9.
10. Fisher J, Martin R, Tate D. Hands on + hands free: simulated on-call interaction. Clin Teach. 2014;11(6):425-8.
11. Han JE, Trammell AR, Finklea JD, Udoji TN, Dressler DD, Honig EG, Abraham P, Ander DS, Cotsonis GA, Martin GS, Schulman DA. Evaluating simulation-based ACLS education on patient outcomes: a randomized, controlled pilot study. J Grad Med Educ. 2014;6(3):501-6.
12. Mahling M, Münch A, Schenk S, et al. Basic life support is effectively taught in groups of three, five and eight medical students: a prospective, randomized study. BMC Med Educ. 2014; 14:185.
13. Chugh SS, Jui J, Gunson K, et al. Current burden of sudden cardiac death: multiple source surveillance versus retrospective death certificate-based review in a large US community. J Am Coll Cardiol. 2004;44:1268–75.
14. Centers for Disease Control and Prevention. Web-based injury statistics query and reporting system (Wis QARS) (Online). Centres for Disease Control and Prevention. *www.cdc.gov/ncipc/wisqars*.
15. Guidelines for cardiopulmonary resuscitation and emergency cardiac care. Emergency Cardiac Care Committee and Subcommittees, American Heart Association. Part II. Adult basic life support. Adult Basic Life Support. JAMA. 1992;268:2184-98.
16. Paradis NA, Martin GB, Goetting MG, et al. Simultaneous aortic, jugular bulb, and right atrial pressures during cardiopulmonary resuscitation in humans. Circulation. 1989;80:361-8.
17. Lindner KH, Ahnefeld FW, Bowdler IM. Cardiopulmonary resuscitation with interposed abdominal compression after asphyxial or fibrillatory cardiac arrest in pigs. Anesthesiology. 1990;72:675-81.
18. American Heart Association. Adjuncts for artificial circulation. Textbook of Advanced Cardiac Life Support. 1994;11:1-8.
19. Krischer JP, Fine EG, Weisfeldt ML, et al. Comparison of prehospital conventional and simultaneous compression-ventilation cardiopulmonary resuscitation. Crit Care Med. 1989;17:1263-9.
20. Berg RA, Wilcoxson D, Hilwig RW, et al. The need for ventilatory support during bystander CPR. Ann Emerg Med. 1995;26:342-50.
21. Cobb LA, Fahrenbruch CE, Walsh TR, Copass MK, Olsufka M, Breskin M, Hallstrom AP. Influence of cardiopulmonary resuscitation prior to defibrillation in patients with out-of-hospital ventricular fibrillation. JAMA. 1999;281:1182–8.
22. Hedges JR, Syverud SA, Dalsey WC, Feero S, Easter R, Shultz B. Prehospital trial of emergency transcutaneous cardiac pacing. Circulation. 1987;76:1337–43.
23. Smith I, Monk TG, White PF. Comparison of transesophageal atrial pacing with anticholinergic drugs for the treatment of intraoperative bradycardia. Anesth Analg. 1994;78:245–52.

Chapter 27

Fiberoptic Bronchoscopy of a Difficult Airway

Anant Mohan, Karan Madan, Randeep Guleria

Chapter Outline

- Difficult Airways
- Causes of Difficult Intubation: Anesthesia Induced
- Patient-related Causes
- Basic Airway Evaluation in all Patients
- Management Plan of Anticipated Difficult Airway
- Indications of FFB: Intubation Elective
- Requirements for the Procedure
- Basic Equipment: Bronchoscope
- What Size to Choose?
- Anesthetizing the Airway
- Procedure Steps
- Caution Points
- Flexi-tip Tubes
- Flexi-tip Tubes/ILM Tubes
- Summary of Procedure of Bronchoscopic Intubation in a Difficult Airway

DIFFICULT AIRWAYS

Clinical situation in which a conventionally trained anesthesiologist experiences difficulty with facemask ventilation of the upper airway, difficulty with tracheal intubation, or both.

American Society of Anesthesiologists: practice guidelines for management of the difficult airway: an updated report. (February 2013), has another description, while using direct laryngoscopy, for difficulat airway which is,

- >2 attempts at intubation with the same or different blade
- or using adjuncts to direct laryngoscopy
- or using an alternative device or technique following failed intubation with direct laryngoscopy **(Figures 1A and B)**.

CAUSES OF DIFFICULT INTUBATION: ANESTHESIA INDUCED

- Inadequate preoperative assessment
- Inadequate equipment
- Poor technique
- Malfunctioning of equipment
- Inexperienced assistance.

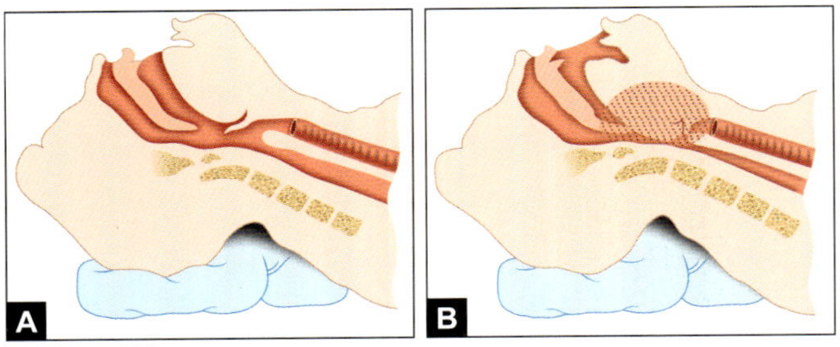

Figures 1A and B (A) Normal or (B) Difficult airway

PATIENT-RELATED CAUSES

- Pregnancy
- Inflammatory disease
- Small mouths
- Infections
- Endocrine
- Congenital
- Trauma
- Foreign body
- Tumors.

BASIC AIRWAY EVALUATION IN ALL PATIENTS

- Previous anesthetic problems
- General appearance of the neck, face, maxilla and mandible
- Jaw movements
- Head extension and movements
- The teeth and oropharynx
- The soft tissues of the neck
- Recent chest and cervical spine X-rays

Dr Binnions Lemon Law: An easy way to remember multiple tests...

- Look externally
- Evaluate the 3-3-2 rule
- Mallampati
- Obstruction?
- Neck mobility.

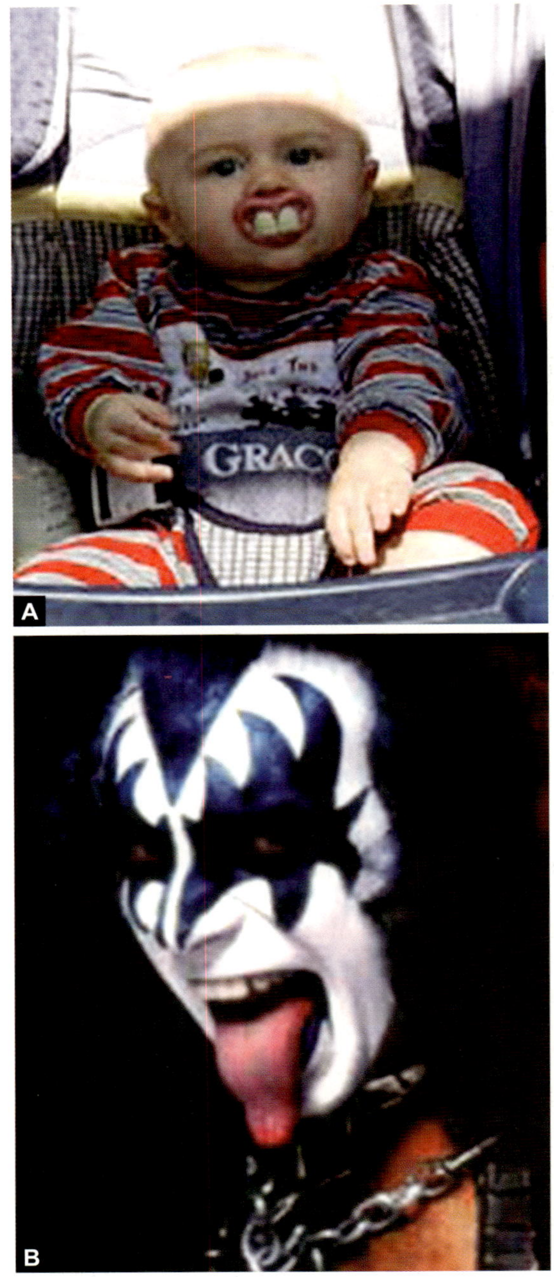

Figures 2A and B External causes of difficult intubation

L: Look Externally

- Obesity or very small
- Short muscular neck
- Prominent upper incisors (Buck teeth) **(Figure 2A)**
- Receding jaw (Dentures)

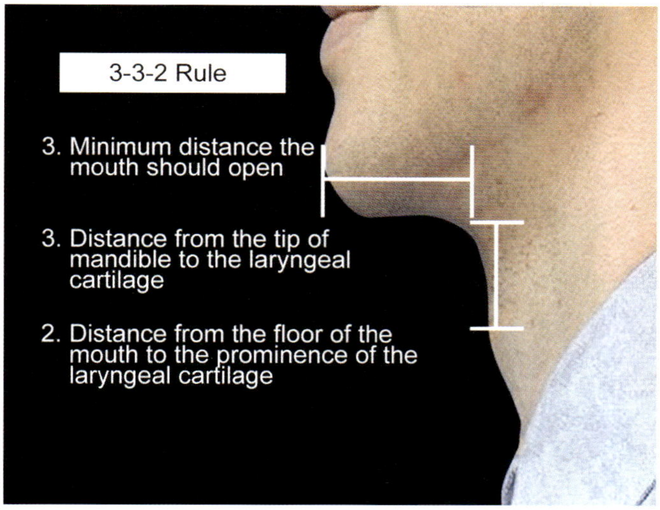

Figure 3 Evaluation method

- Burns
- Facial trauma
- Stridor
- Macroglossia **(Figure 2B)**.

E: Evaluate the 3-3-2 Rule (Figure 3)

- 3 fingers fit in mouth
- 3 fingers fit from mentum to hyoid cartilage
- 2 fingers fit from the floor of the mouth to the top of the thyroid cartilage.

M: Mallampati Classification (Figure 4)

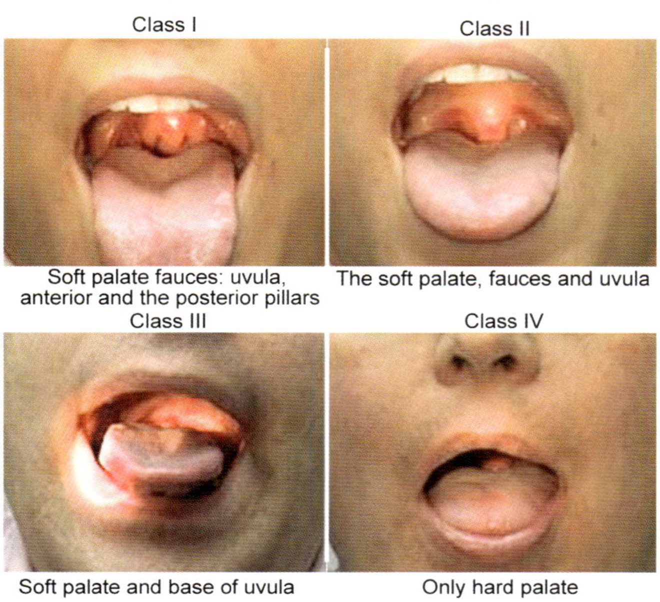

Figure 4 Classes of mallampati classification

O: Obstruction?

- Blood
- Vomitus
- Teeth
- Epiglottis
- Dentures
- Tumors
- Impacted objects.

N: Neck Mobility—Measurement of Atlanto-occipital Angle

Figure 5 shows neck mobility—measurement of atlanto-occipital angle.

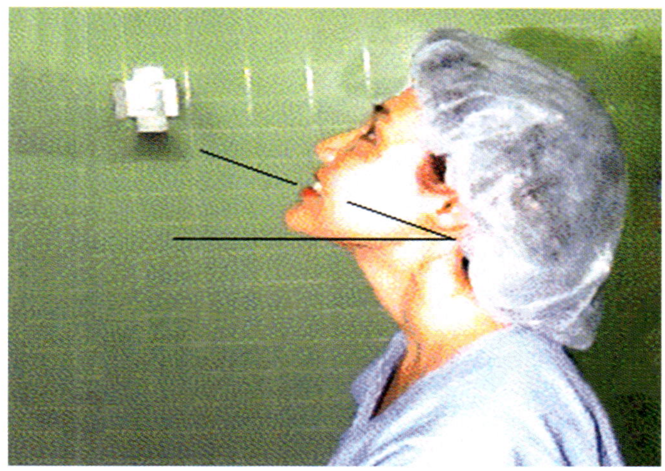

Figure 5 Neck mobility—measurement of atlanto-occipital angle

MANAGEMENT PLAN OF ANTICIPATED DIFFICULT AIRWAY

Is Laryngeal Visualization Going to be Difficult?

Cannot intubate—defined by 4 Ds

1. *Disproportion*: Acromegaly; prognathism
2. *Distortion*: Contracture, fibrosis
3. *Dysmobility*: TM joint ankylosis
4. *Dentition*: Edentulous; buck teeth.

Alternate Technique (Figures 6 and 7)

Alternative methods for difficult airway detection and alternate technique plan are shown in **Figures 6 and 7**.

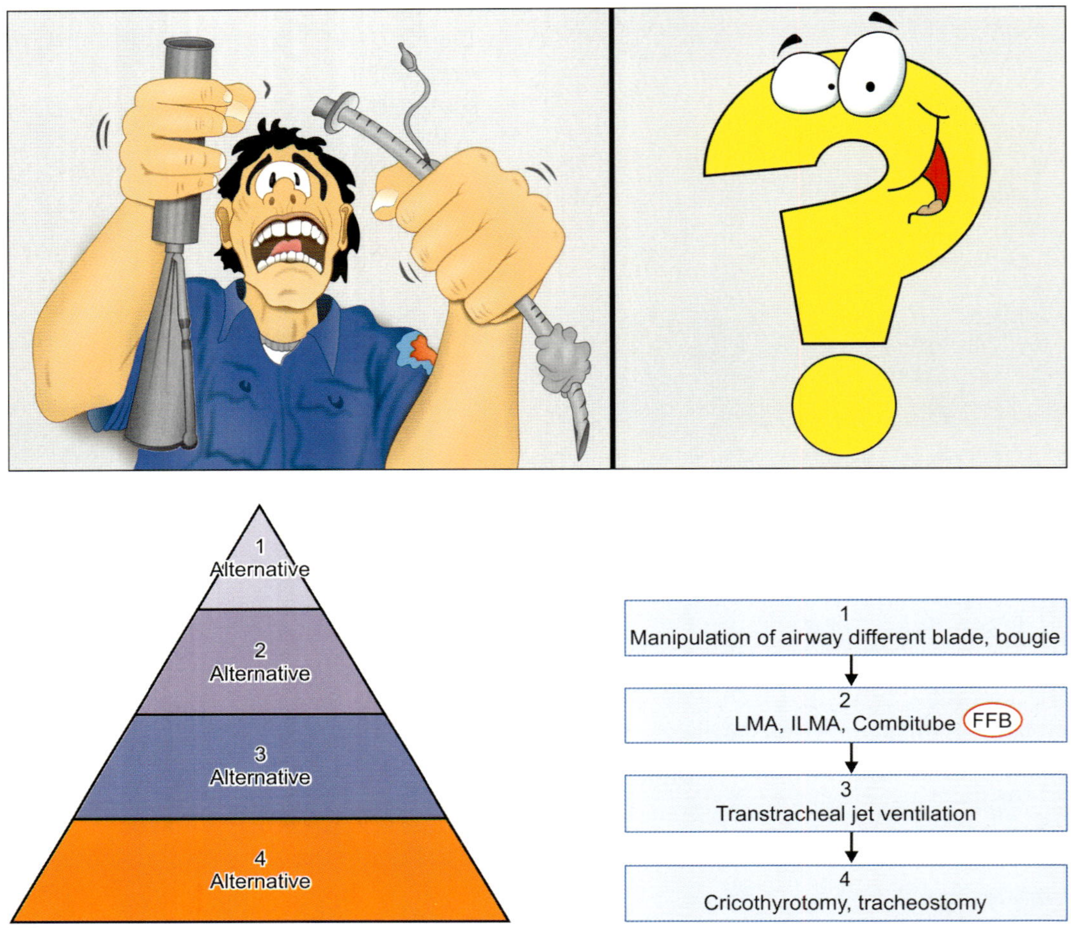

Figure 6 Alternative methods for difficult airway detection

INDICATIONS OF FFB: INTUBATION ELECTIVE

Diagnosed difficult airway:

- Morbid obesity, trismus, facial trauma, pharynx and larynx injury
- Limited flexion and extension of the neck, craniofacial disorders, jaw malformations
- Temporomandibular joint ankylosis, macroglossia, larynx tumors, laryngotracheobronchitis
- Glottic edema and epiglottitis.

REQUIREMENTS FOR THE PROCEDURE

- Ensure that you are familiar with using the fiberoptic scope, and have reviewed manufacturer's guidance on its use, including handling, cleaning and storage.
- Make sure that you have all the appropriate resuscitation equipment to hand.
- The patient should be fully monitored throughout the procedure (blood pressure, pulse oximetry, ECG). Ideally, capnography should be available.

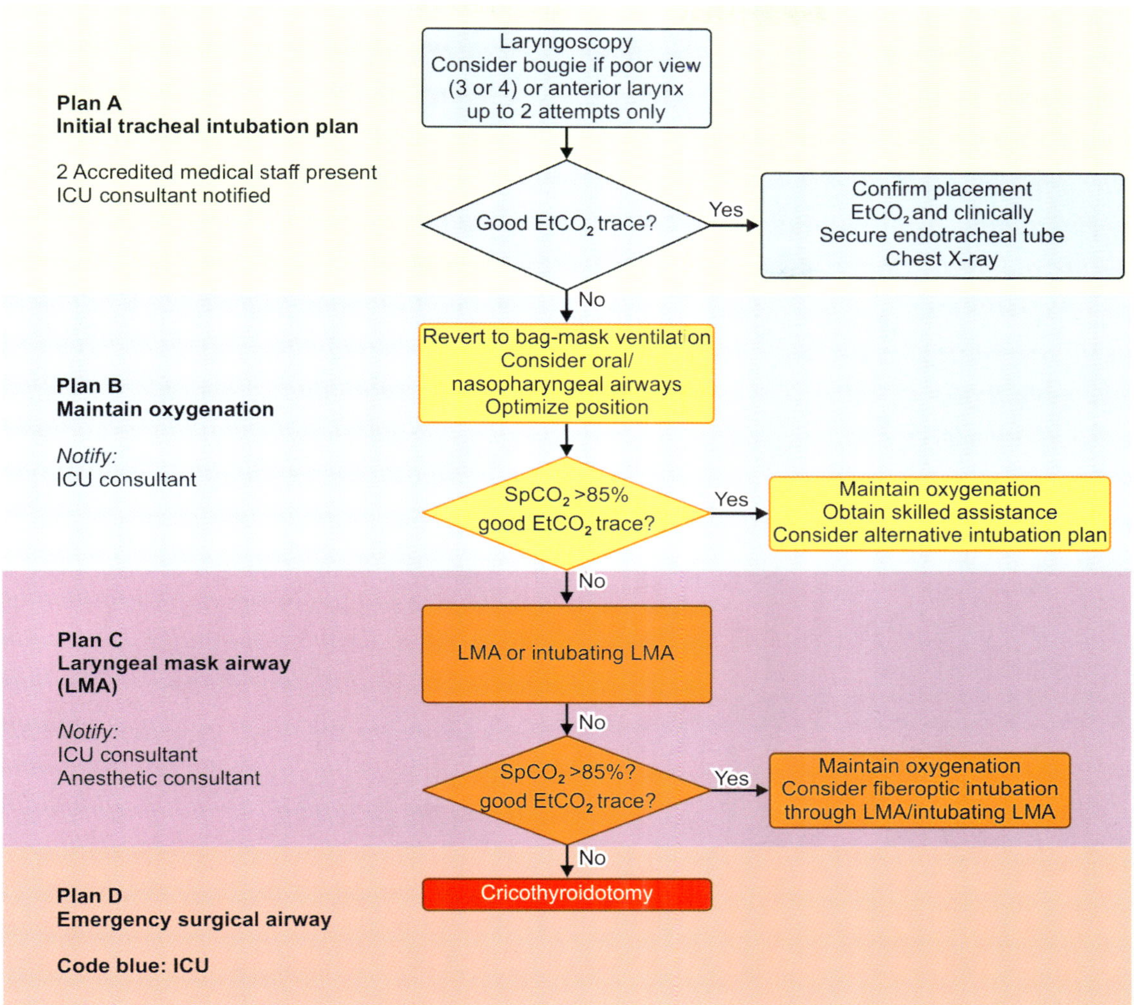

Figure 7 Alternate technique plan A, B, C, D

BASIC EQUIPMENT: BRONCHOSCOPE (FIGURE 8)

- Excellent optics
- Suction channel for LA/Oxygen
- Sufficient length (60 cm).

Accommodate Endotracheal Tube

Adequate distal segment maneurability

- ET threaded over distal tip → fed proximally → fixed in position near control handle.

WHAT SIZE TO CHOOSE? (TABLE 1)

- Intubation—snug fit between the endotracheal tube and bronchsocope

TABLE 1 Size of fiberoptic bronchoscope

Number	Bronchoscope (OD)	ET (ID)	Patient
1	5.9 mm	≥6.5	Adult
2	3.5 mm	≥4.5	Pediatric
3	2.7 mm	≥3.0	Infant

- Diagnostic or therapeutic bronchoscopy—concentric airway remaining should be adequate to provide ventilation.

ANESTHETIZING THE AIRWAY (TABLE 2)

- Lidocaine spray (10 mg/spray)
- Gargling lidocaine liquid (2–4%)—30 mL

CHAPTER 27

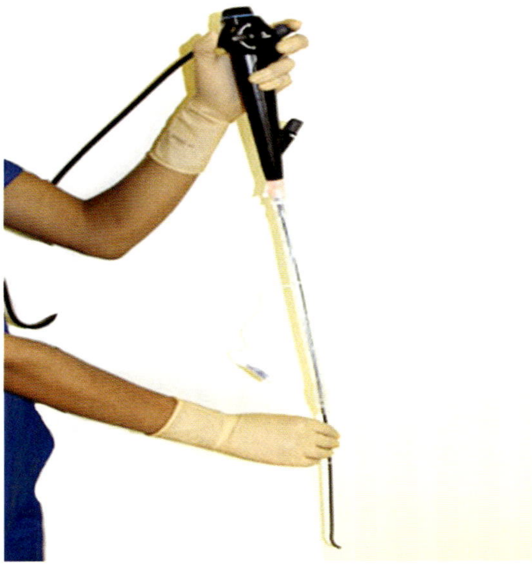

Figure 8 The bronchoscope

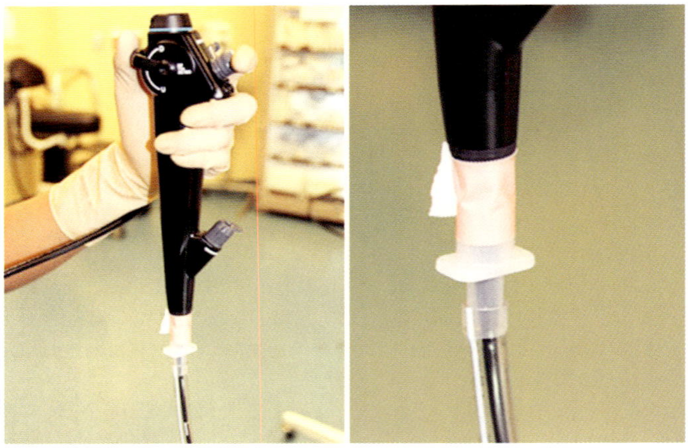

Figure 9 Loading endotracheal tube onto the bronchoscope

TABLE 2 Anesthetizing the airway

Anesthetic	*Conc.*	*Peak effect (min)*	*Safe dosage*
Lignocaine	2–4%	2–5	3–4 mg/kg
Tetracaine	0.45–2%	3–8	50–80 mg
Cocaine	4–10%	Immediate	1–3 mg/kg

- Nebulization (10 mL 2% lidocaine)
- Superior laryngeal nerve block
- For nasal intubation—vasoconstrictors (Oxymetazoline or xylometazoline 0.05–0.1%)
- Sedation—personal preference.

PROCEDURE STEPS

Loading the endotracheal tube over the scope.

Loading the Endotracheal Tube

Steps ...rotating the tube (Figures 9 and 10)

CAUTION POINTS

- Do not force the tube, but withdraw slightly, rotate 90 degrees anticlockwise, and readvance
- **Keep the carina in the field of vision**.
- Remove the fiberscope whilst visualizing, and maintaining the ETT in place, with the tip at 3–5 cm above the carina.

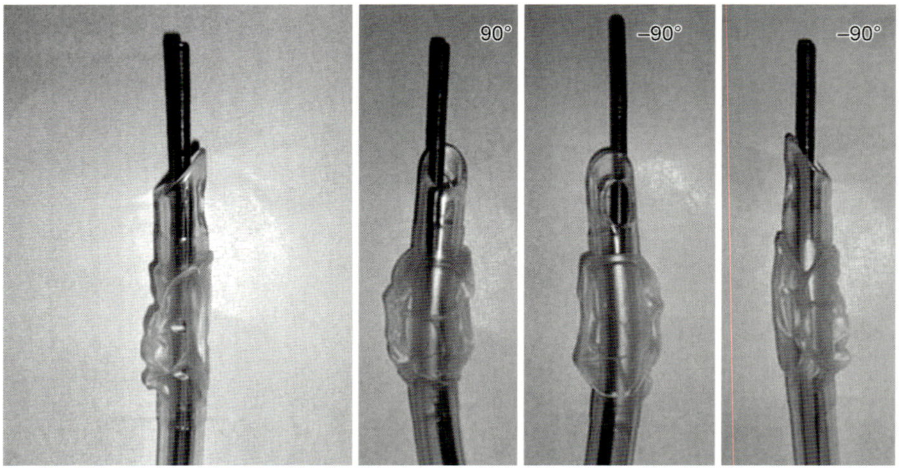

Figure 10 Rotating the tube

TABLE 3 Steps for FFB intubation

1. Selecting flexible fiberoptic bronchoscope and endotracheal tube.
2. Insertion of the FFB into tht lumen of the tracheal tube (lubrication is essential).
3. Introduction of the FFB through the nose or oral cavity with a mouthguard.
4. Advane of the FFB until the glottis is visible.
5. Introduction of the FFB into the trachea.
6. Slide the tube until reaching the distal tip of the FFB.
7. Introduction of the FFB and the tube until reaching the middle-third of the trachea.
8. Extraction of the FFB, retaining the tube within the trachea.
9. Fixation of the tube to the face, avoiding unplanned extubation.
10. Finally, tracheal tube is immediately connected to the oxygen source.

- Confirm the ETT position by capnography, auscultation, observation of chest movement and misting of the tube, and feeling air movement at the tip of the tube **(Table 3)**.

Postprocedure: Before Extubation

- Oxygenate with 100% for 3–5 min
- Any muscle relaxants adequately reversed
- The upper airway is free of all secretions—the airway may still be anesthetized, and hence, laryngeal reflexes are not intact. Pulmonary aspiration is therefore possible
- The patient is breathing spontaneously with adequate tidal volumes
- The patient is awake.

Contraindications to Flexible Fiberoptic Bronchoscope

- Lack of airway skills
- Difficult airway with impending airway obstruction
- Allergy to local anesthetic agents
- Infection/contamination of the upper airway—blood, friable tumor, open abscess
- Grossly distorted anatomy
- Fractured base of skull (CI to nasal route)
- Patient refusal or uncooperative patient.

Complications of Flexible Fiberoptic Bronchoscope

- Epistaxis
- Upper airway/vocal cord injury
- Tube block
- Laryngospasm, bronchospasm
- Tachycardia.

Problems in Bronchoscopic Intubation

- *During step 1*: Negotiating scope into trachea
  - Jaw thrust
  - Neck extension
  - Tongue protrusion
- *Step 2*: Passing endotracheal tube over scope into trachea
  - Apnea
  - Damage to upper airway

Sites which hamper insertion of tube over scope into trachea is a problem (Figures 11A and B)

- Anatomical factors, narrowed rasal passage, enlarged tongue, epiglottis, arytenoid cartilage,

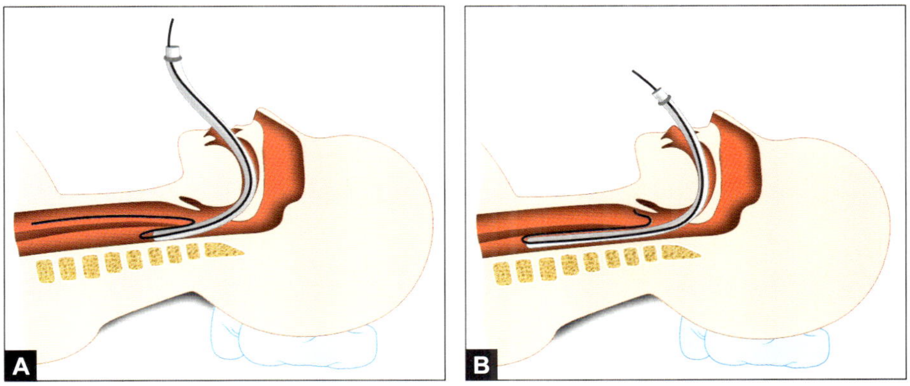

Figures 11A and B Sites of hamper insertion of tube over scope

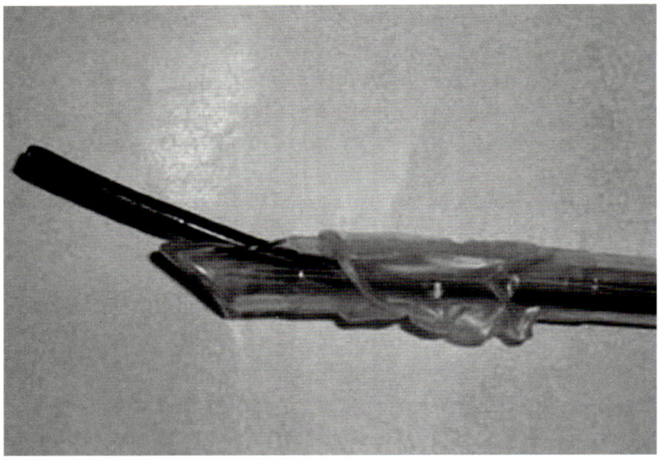

Figure 12 The bronchoscope should not protrude at an angle to the endotracheal tube tip

pyriform fossae, esophagus, device or procedure factors, Murphy eye of a tracheal tube, airway intubator, cricoid pressure, jaw thrusting.

- Main problems in oral insertion of tube over scope **(Figure 12)**:
  - Posterior migration onto arytenoids or esophagus
- Nasal intubation:
  - Nasal cavity obstruction
  - Epiglottis
- Accidental esophageal intubation—Incidence: up to 40–62%
- The Murphy eye...should be kept in mind, always

Solutions to the Problems Cited Above

- Reduction of the gap between bronchoscope and the tracheal tube
  - Use of a thick scope and a thin tracheal tube
  - Use a tapered tracheal tube
  - Use of gap fillers

FLEXI-TIP TUBES

Figures 13A and B show flexi-tip tubes.

FLEXI-TIP TUBES/ILM TUBES

Solutions... (Figures 14A and B)

- Release of jaw thrust
- Cricoid pressure

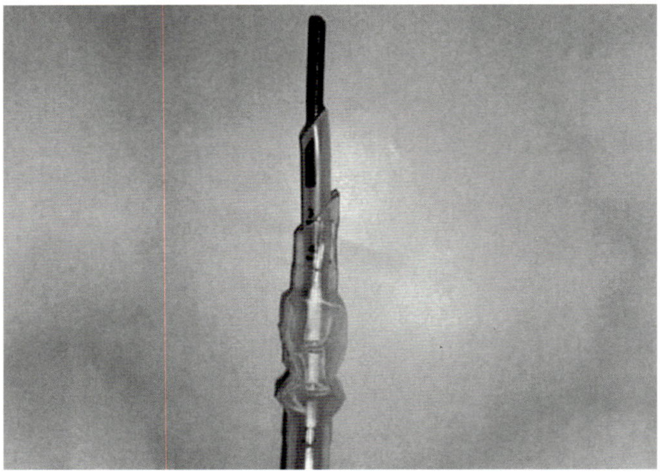

Figure 13A Flexi tip tube

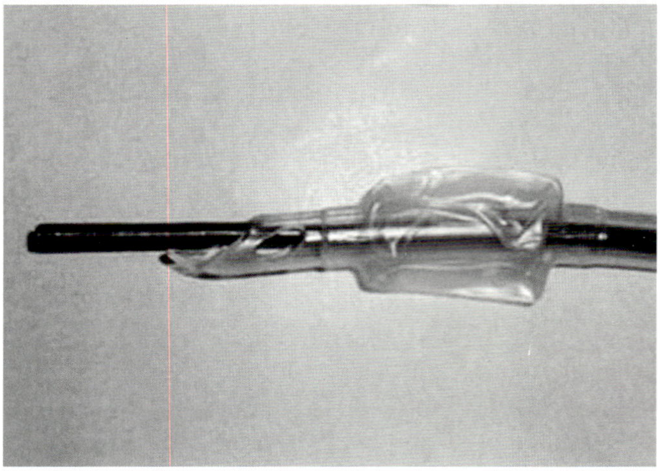

Figure 13B Flexi tip tube

- Use a laryngoscope
- Digital aid
- View scope movements.

SUMMARY OF PROCEDURE OF BRONCHOSCOPIC INTUBATION IN A DIFFICULT AIRWAY

- Use snug fitting tube over the scope
- Use flexible tracheal tube, if available
- Preload the scope and fix
- Use laryngeal mask airway (LMA)
- Try rotation movements
- Adjust head, neck positions, cricoid pressure.

SECTION 6

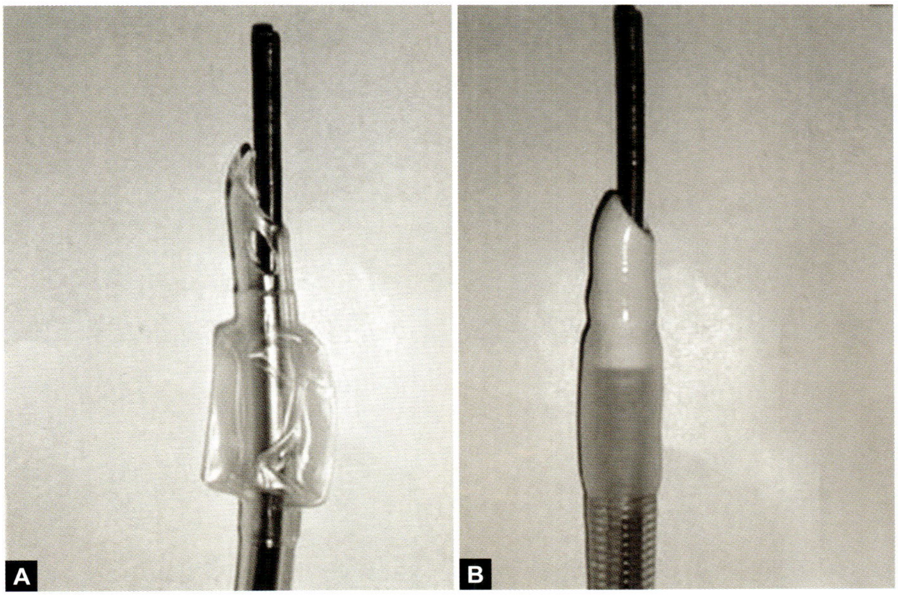

Figures 14A and B Flexi tip ILM tubes

CONCLUSION

- Difficult airways for intubation are common
- All patients classified as having a difficult airway as well as patients with failed intubation must be considered as potential candidates for endotracheal intubation with flexible fiberoptic bronchoscope
- Bronchoscopy must be performed by an experienced and skilled endoscopist
- There is a high rate of success using this technique.
- Complications are rare.

Chapter 28

Bronchoscopic Simulation: Role in Training of Pulmonary Physicians

JC Suri, D Bhattacharya

Chapter Outline

- Simulation Tools and Approaches
- Evolution of Simulation in Bronchoscopy
- Low Fidelity Bronchoscopy Simulation
- High Fidelity Bronchoscopy Simulation
- Bronchoscopy Simulator: The Equipment
- Bronchoscopy Simulators: Current Evidence

INTRODUCTION

Flexible bronchoscopy was first performed in early 70's. A sea change has taken place in the field of pulmonary endoscopy in general and interventional pulmonology in particular since then. Presently bronchoscopies are routinely performed in nearly every unit practicing pulmonary medicine. Training in bronchoscopy includes understanding the indications and contraindications, risks and benefits of the procedure in a given patient, sedation and local anesthesia, dexterity in handling and maneuvering the bronchoscope in the anatomically complex bronchial tree. It also mandates the knowledge of normal bronchial tree, interpretation of abnormal lesions, and the skill to perform endobronchial and bronchoscopic lung biopsies, transbronchial needle aspiration, and bronchoalveolar lavage. Other important issues are the art of communication with staff and patients, informed consent and care of the sedated patient. Traditionally learning the art of bronchoscopy follows the Halsted's approach or the 'apprenticeship model' based on " see one, do one, teach one" policy whereby trainees first learn the theory related to the procedure, then observe it first-hand. Once reasonable confidence is there in the teacher and student, the trainee initially performs the procedure in low risk patients under close supervision of the mentor and gradually progress to cases that are more complex and with progressive degree of independence. However, this approach has several limitations. Learning the complex procedural skills in the clinical scenario on a real patient can be stressful for the trainee and increases the potential for patient discomfort, procedure-related complications, and risk of wrong diagnosis. This method of training is also associated with significant variability in the acquisition of knowledge, skills, and competence. In order to overcome these deficiencies, bronchoscopic training at many centers is now being increasingly imparted in a structured manner with the help of low and high fidelity simulators which facilitate safe, cost-effective, and uniform training. Simulators help the trainee to learn the new procedures and hone their skills to the level of competence or mastery before the procedure is performed on live patients. Simulators also help the health professionals in fulfilling obligation to provide optimal care without compromising patient safety and wellbeing. Virtual reality bronchoscopic simulator with computerized module may also standardize the assessment of bronchoscopic competence, that otherwise is based on the number of procedures conducted and subjective evaluation of the trainer by direct observation for knowledge and procedural skills.

SIMULATION TOOLS AND APPROACHES

Simulation tools have been in use since several centuries as an aid for medical education. Probably, the first among such "simulators" or mannequins (also often referred to as phantoms) developed were those for teaching obstetrical skills, which, resulted in a fall in the maternal and infant mortality rates. Learning the art of giving an injection or suturing is undertaken on an orange and piece of cloth respectively to develop competence and confidence. Modern technology can go further in this direction imparting realistic feel and environment with the provision for feedback. Studies undertaken have verified the efficacy of screen based realistic simulators for improved technical and behavioral skills.

The modern day concept of simulation was first introduced in the aviation industry as a means to provide cost effective training to trainee pilots and to reduce errors and prevent disastrous accidents.

EVOLUTION OF SIMULATION IN BRONCHOSCOPY

Simulators expectedly have not evolved as a pulmonology educational tool overnight. Bronchology has evolved since the introduction of the rigid endoscope by Gustav Killian in 1897. Further developments in the rigid bronchoscopy instruments were made by Chevalier Jackson and H H Hopkins. However, it was only after the introduction of the flexible bronchoscope by Ikeda in 1970 along with rapid developments in fiberoptics, engineering and various instrumentation modalities that this discipline has evolved into its present state.

Traditionally, bronchoscopy training begins with didactic lectures of the bronchial anatomy, study of texts and atlases. The indications, contraindications, anesthesia, analgesia and sedation protocols must also be mastered before one can proceed to perform bronchoscopies. The knowledge that was attained from lectures, books and atlases can now be gained through videos, 'you tube' and from dedicated web based e-learning modules available on the internet. Inclusion of these readily available modes has significantly hastened the learning process. Once, one is armed with this background knowledge, it is essential to develop the mental to hand eye coordination for using the bronchoscope adeptly without missing out on important steps or comprehending subtle findings.

Simulation adds to the visual perception, analytical ability and develops the art of rapid decision making essential for impromptu actions required for a successful diagnostic or therapeutic bronchoscopic procedure. Simulation bronchoscopy training can be delivered either using low fidelity or high fidelity simulation depending on the complexity of the technology employed. Low fidelity simulation includes the use of live animal models, resected and preserved animal lungs or wet tissue models, and inanimate models of upper airways and bronchial tree made of various materials, whereas high fidelity simulation uses a computer based bronchoscopic simulators which are intended to provide a realistic bronchoscopic experience and feedback to trainee regarding the procedural skills.

LOW FIDELITY BRONCHOSCOPY SIMULATION

Low fidelity simulators for bronchoscopy are of various types and include animal models or inanimate models that may be used to develop bronchoscopic skills related to diagnostic and therapeutic procedures. Animal models have the limitations of anatomical variations besides being fraught with ethical issues. The commonly used inanimate models of upper airway and bronchial tree are made of wood, rubber, plastic or silicone. Each of these has their advantages and disadvantages. The wooden model with the "choose-the-hole" box comprises of three to five wooden panels drilled with holes through which the bronchoscope is required to be maneuvered. The synthetic models of plastic or rubber reproduced the branching pattern of

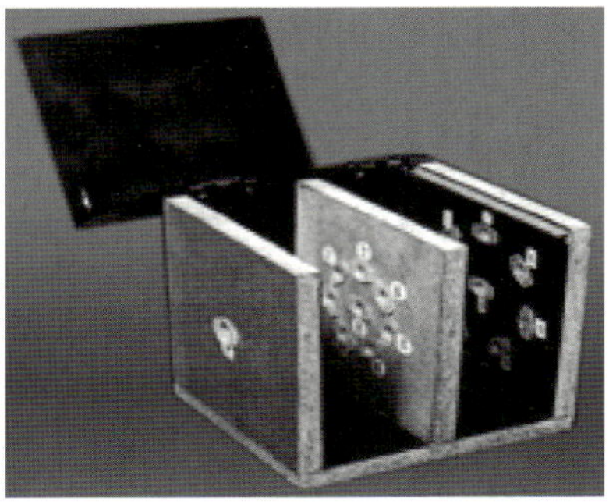

Figure 1 Choose-the-hole model
(*Source*: *http://ijaweb.org/articles/2011/55/5/images/IndianJAnaesth_2011_55_5_451_89866_f2.jpg*)

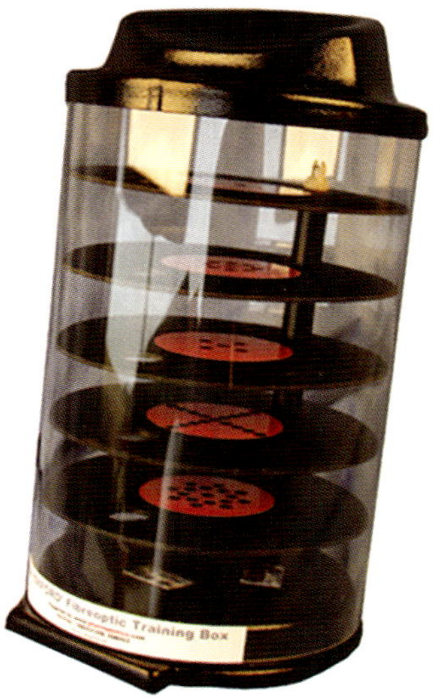

Figure 2 Oxford fiberoptic teaching box
(*Source*: *http://www.pharmabotics.com/files/eshoppics/oxford.jpg*)

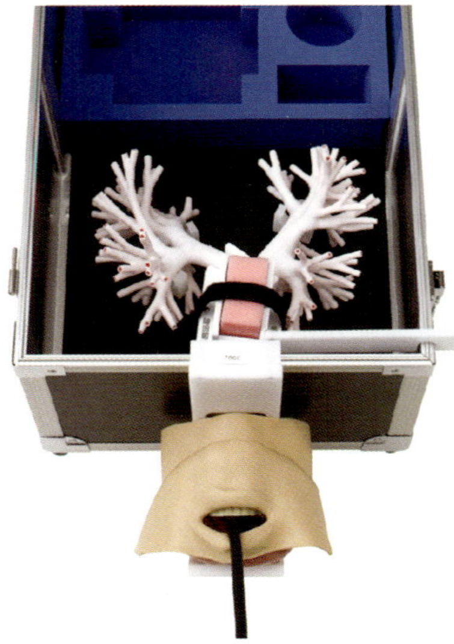

Figure 3 Ultrasonic bronchoscopy simulator
(*Source*: *http://www.erler-zimmer.de/media/catalog/product/cache/2/image/9df78eab33525d08d6e5fb8d27136e95/l/m/lm99.jpg*)

the bronchial tree better (**Figures 1 to 3**). In a recent study a, comparison was made between low- and high-fidelity bronchoscopy simulations for training in conventional transbronchial needle aspiration (TBNA) including the user preference. Based on the learner and trainer perceptions the low fidelity model of rubber trachea attached to the laryngotracheal airway was found to be superior to the high-fidelity virtual reality simulator for training in the three methods of conventional TBNA. Low fidelity models are usually disadvantaged by artificial appearance and feel, lack of adaption and experience with pathological lesions, and most importantly the absence of realism. This can be improved by use of real bronchoscopes or combination of two or more low-fidelity models to create a customized hybrid model. However, feedback from trainees suggests that low fidelity models provide an enjoyable learning experience especially as several of the hybrid models use a real bronchoscope. Therefore, though high-fidelity simulators may have their advantages low-fidelity models have a definite role in providing training in certain bronchoscopic techniques such as TBNA (**Table 1**).

HIGH FIDELITY BRONCHOSCOPY SIMULATION

High fidelity bronchoscopy simulation models find an ever-increasing role base as a learning tool to hone skills before performing the procedure on live patients. To some extent, this is because of the effect related to the preconceived knowledge of novelty and high technological sophistication producing the "halo" effect. On the positive aspect, the incorporation of physiological effects of cough, breathing, bleeding and the side effects of local anesthesia, etc. makes the experience more realistic. Further, incorporation of objective assessment modules along with work outcome

TABLE 1 Simulation tools used for bronchoscopy training

Tools	*Description*
Low fidelity simulators	Live animal models, extracted and preserved animal lungs wet lab model), inanimate models of bronchial tree (wood, rubber, plastic and silicone)
Computerized simulator	Preloaded programs to assess clinical knowledge and train aspects related to decision making in medical fields requiring critical and rapid decision making (e.g. critical care)
High fidelity computerized simulators	Highly complex instruments with visual, audio, touch and additional tools integrated with computers thereby creating a reality simulated device that replicate a clinical setting, e.g. bronchoscopy, arthroscopy, laparoscopic surgery, cardiology interventions, ultrasound, etc. surgery, cardiology interventions, ultrasound, etc.

assessment and direct observation of procedure skills make the high fidelity simulators more exciting. Finally, the liberty to practice till subjective and objective satisfaction is attained with the knowledge that there is no fear of harm caused to patients due to acts of omission or commission on the part of the trainee greatly helps in raising their confidence till satisfactory 'competence' is achieved.

BRONCHOSCOPY SIMULATOR: THE EQUIPMENT

There are currently about four to five bronchoscopy simulators models manufactured worldwide that are commercially available. They are expensive equipment costing between $25,000 to $1,00,000 depending on their complexity. It consists of a proxy flexible bronchoscope (FB), a robotic interphase device, a computer with a monitor loaded with the specific authorized simulation software and a graphics card to give a realistic feel to the experience. Used together it creates a realistic training environment for learning and practicing flexible bronchoscopy along with interventional procedures **(Figure 4)**.

The user is required to insert the proxy FB into the robotic interphase device which is shaped like a human face with the entry point being one of the 'nasal apertures'. The robotic interphase device tracks the motions of the proxy FB and gives the feel of an actual bronchoscopy. The proxy FB tracks the manipulations made on the tip control lever, suction button and video buttons. The device also keeps a track of manipulations of accessories within the instruments channel, thereby

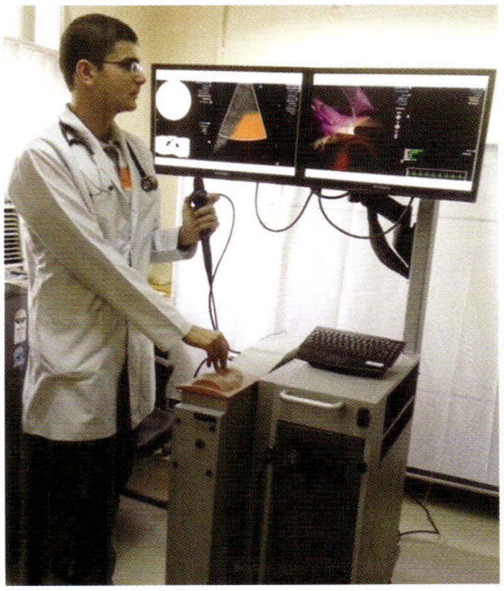

Figure 4 Virtual reality bronchoscopy simulator [with permission from: M/s Endo VR CAE Healthcare (Sarasota, FL, USA)]

enabling study of interventions (endobronchial biopsy, transbronchial biopsy, transbronchial needle aspiration, etc.) performed in the simulator.

The monitor of the simulator displays, computer generated images of the airway at the point where the tip of the FB is positioned as the FB is navigated in the robotic interphase. The images seen on the monitor are preloaded on the computer from 1 mm or thinner computed tomography and magnetic resonance imaging (MRI) images from a data bank. Further, in order to give a realistic look to the bronchial mucosa texture maps based on videotapes from actual bronchoscopy images are added. In addition common airway variations are loaded to give the user a feel of undertaking the procedure in a new case each time. In addition not only are the video pictures correct anatomically but also various physiologic functions like effect of breathing, coughing, bleeding (spontaneous or following an intervention) with or without changes in the 'patients' physiological parameters are also integrated in the software giving a life like feel to the experience. Also the 'virtual case' on the simulator is programmed to need lignocaine for local anesthesia as in normal bronchoscopy and overdose of which may result in 'seizures', 'cardiac arrhythmias' or even 'death'.

The bronchoscopy simulator is loaded with software to train novices the correct techniques of performing bronchoscopy, identifying the various segments and diagnosing common pathologies. The simulator is also programmed to train the user common interventions like bronchial sampling, bronchoalveolar lavage, transbronchial needle aspiration, difficult pediatric airways and performance of radial endobronchial ultrasound guided transbronchial needle aspiration of various lymph node stations **(Table 2)**.

The software is also programmed to record all the actions of the user in its database and at the end of the procedure give a report on the 'performance' of the procedure in the form of time taken for examination, times of 'red outs', i.e. the number of times the tip of the scope collides with the bronchial wall, percent of bronchial segments entered, use of help to verify location, amount of lignocaine used, unnecessary use of suction, etc. **(Table 3)**. The hardware specifications of the computer are continuously upgraded in order to produce the most realistic real time images.

Duration of Training

A certain level of training and practice man hours is essential to develop a level of competence in a task. This could be planned as time on the simulator or minimum number of cases performed for an accepted level of competence. As per the current evidence a minimum of 50 procedures were considered necessary for an individual to attain competency and majority

TABLE 2 Learning points of bronchoscopy simulation

On completion of the module, the trainee should know:
1. The indications, contraindications, and complications of flexible bronchoscopy.
2. Describe the correct technique for holding and manipulating the bronchoscope.
3. Should be competent with the procedural steps necessary to perform a bronchoscopic examination of the upper and lower airways.
4. Know about the common mistakes committed by a trainee.
5. Visualize and correctly identify the structures of the tracheobronchial tree.
6. Understand the anatomy of the upper and lower airway as viewed through a bronchoscope.
7. Be conversant with the anatomic structures external to the lungs that are relevant for bronchoscopists, especially those intending to undertake interventional procedures.
8. Know the special relationship of the tracheobronchial tree to adjacent anatomic structures.
9. Identify common endoscopic lesions (pathological/normal anatomic variations).
10. Should be able to appreciate the difference in airway anatomy of patients of different age groups and should be able to negotiate the bronchoscope in difficult pediatric airways.
11. Should be conversant with the indications and the steps to perform a bronchoalveolar lavage.
12. Should be conversant with the various bronchoscopic accessories (forceps, needles, brushes) required for endobronchial sampling. Know the correct procedural steps for obtaining the samples and should be able to diagnose and manage any complications that may occur during such a procedure.
13. Should know the correct indications, contraindications and complications of transbronchial needle aspiration (TBNA). Must identify correctly the locations of the various lymph node stations. Should master the correct technique of performing bronchoscopic TBNA.
14. Should be conversant with the indications, contraindications, and complications of EBUS-TBNA. Have knowledge of the anatomy of the lymph node stations and be able to negotiate the bronchoscope correctly and identify the different lymph node stations on endoscopic ultrasound. Should know the correct usage of the EBUS-TBNA sampling needle.

TABLE 3 Summary report of bronchoscopy competence assessment of trainee

1. Overall	
Description	*Result*
Time of procedure	5.16 minutes
Percent of bronchial segments entered	90%
Number of scope collisions with airway walls—"Red outs"	30%
Time in "Red outs"	50 seconds
Suction button used	0.09
2. Instilled fluids	
Fluid	*Amount used*
Lignocaine	6 Aliquots of 1 mL (2%–20 mg/mL)
Saline	2 Aliquots of 3 mL
Adrenaline	2 Aliquots of 1 mL (1/20,000)
3. Educational features	
Features	*Number of times used*
External view	0
Road signs	0

of the trainees would be deemed competent after 100 procedures. The use of bronchoscopy simulation can speed up the initial learning curve and master bronchoscopic skills that are highly dependent on hand eye coordination, which can then successfully be transferred to patient care. It is essential to understand that thereafter a minimum number of the said procedures must be performed regularly to maintain the level of competence.

Assessment of Bronchoscopy Training

Assessment in endoscopy is largely subjective. Performance outcome studies could vary from subjective or objective assessment by observers or computer generated estimates of performance outcomes. These could be evaluated for (a) process—technique and completeness (b) procedural time (c) procedural success, e.g. biopsy, needle aspiration, etc. (d) knowledge of user and (e) satisfaction of trainee and trainer.

The above assessments could be made as single group assessment or randomized controlled group assessment for content, quality, satisfaction or reliability.

Rationale for use of Simulators in Bronchoscopy Training

Having looked at the levels of simulation and the technical features of the bronchoscopy simulators it is pertinent to understand the rationale behind their use.

The primary responsibility of the health professional is towards the patient. Every patient who submits him/herself into the hands of a health professional deserves the right for the best medical care. Though it is understood that trainee health professionals, especially in teaching hospitals would partake in their care, albeit under supervision; it should not be at the risk of the patient's wellbeing. In these situations use of simulators can hone the competence of trainees before encountering an actual patient, thereby minimizing risks.

It is also essential that the future tier of health care providers be trained so that health professionals continue to have the same high standards of competence and the standard of medical education continue to be maintained. Use of simulators can help in a large way in furthering this end by preparing the trainees for different clinical situations. It allows trainees to spend as much time necessary to attain proficiency and confidence.

The simulators are also currently programmed to judge the competence levels of trainees by inbuilt scoring systems which would be improved on further in the future with technical improvements to simulate near live situations. Simulators could therefore prepare trainees to encounter real patients with greater level of confidence at the same time avoid several preventable medical 'accidents'.

However, despite all precautions taken the chances of a trainee making errors is higher and depending on whether damage control measures are effective or not the implications for the patient could be far reaching. Use of simulators could go a long way in preparing a trainee so as to prevent such injuries without compromising on the learning experience of trainees. Simulators could also prepare a trainee for the handling of situations that resulted in 'death' due to misplaced judgment of medical novices.

The final right to choose their caregiver, refuse certain treatments, or disagree to partake in research rests on the patient or their family. However, as often the risks related to a treatment are partly withheld or consents taken in a casual manner, patients may give their consent without the realization that they may be subjected to potentially risky procedures by a trainee. Moreover, often patients are sick, in pain, sedated, and under the influence of anesthetics and therefore unable to fully comprehend the 'implications of various procedures'. In such situations, simulators could substitute for patients without denying the opportunity for trainees to learn from an array of experiences.

In principle the responsibility for medical education, research and innovations must be borne by health professionals, administrators, and citizens alike, unfortunately this does not happen. Most centers of medical education are located in government run urban health institutions. Therefore, it is usually the poor who not being in a position to afford treatment in corporate hospitals face the risk of treatment related mishaps in the hands of trainees. As the use of animals and cadavers are not allowed for several teaching activities because of animal rights and social activism movements, simulators could substitute these and prevent health management related complications among the socially deprived group.

BRONCHOSCOPY SIMULATORS: CURRENT EVIDENCE

Current evidence on the role/benefits of bronchial simulation is varied and sparse. Trials which studied the role of simulators in bronchoscopy aided difficult intubations found that simulator training improved outcomes and procedure time in difficult intubations. Studies including one meta-analysis including animal models, mannequins, artificial models, endoscopic ultrasound training and virtual simulation concluded benefit for the use of simulation for bronchoscopy training. Based on the limited available studies the meta-analysis conducted also concluded that simulation-based bronchoscopy was more effective when compared to no intervention.

Results of simulation bronchoscopy studies depends on study design, duration, technology used and number of subjects included in the study. Measurement of parameters such as duration of procedure, identification of bronchial segments and 'red outs' showed that repetitive practice on the simulator increases muscle memory, hand eye co-ordination and outcomes. This was seen in both one off sessions as well as training over time. It was shown that with short periods of training novices compared with experienced endoscopists were able to perform thorough examination with high accuracy in both inanimate and VRS models. By assessing these outcomes, some investigators even claimed to distinguish between the levels of experience of different bronchoscopists. Unfortunately, most of the studies were handicapped because of small number of subjects, variation in study designs and use of different VR simulators. However, the small number of subjects in each study and varying study designs makes it difficult to reach at a consensus on the results.

A review of 17 studies comprising simulation based bronchoscopy training with no intervention or alternate instruction; simulation-based training was consistently associated with better learning outcomes. It was further noted from comparison of different training approaches, that training sessions that was longer and more structured were more effective and there was improvement in skills when authentic clinical context was included.

Unfortunately most outcomes on the role of simulation are limited by quantity and quality of original studies; it was found that simulation moderately favored process outcome and highly favored time outcomes and nearly all studies favored simulation based training in comparison to no intervention.

Reviews of simulation-based bronchoscopy training also showed that simulation-based bronchoscopy training is effective for a variety of tasks including inspection, rigid bronchoscopy, endobronchial ultrasound, transbronchial needle aspiration, therapeutic interventions such as foreign body removal as well as transfer of this learning to patient care. Therefore, uses of simulators are recommended for educational purposes barring resource constraints. Further, simulation-based training is complemented by simulation-based assessment tools that enhance competency based educational systems and help in mastering different procedural skills.

Use of simulators in health care lags behind because of high cost involved, lack of conclusive evidence of its usefulness and resistance to change. Keeping in mind Hippocrates's oath of "First do no harm" there is justification in introducing alternative modes of medical education like simulators to avoid treatment related patient injuries. Therefore, there is a pressing need for a change in the method of imparting education, clinical practice, and be open to the use of technology, backed by rigorous scientific evidence thereby breaking the inherent resistance among medical educators from a strong professional culture.

CONCLUSION

Therefore, from the current evidence base available one can safely conclude that simulation-based training is clearly effective. Evidence further suggests that longer and more structured training add greater value to the training. Although high fidelity simulation methods hold great promise, various low fidelity tools have also been found to be very useful and cost effective. High fidelity simulators have added advantages of planning the course curriculum as per choice include automated scoring systems, feedbacks and have the added advantage of unrestricted availability. Virtual reality bronchoscopy simulation clearly has a definitive role in the training and education of budding pulmonologists.

BIBLIOGRAPHY

1. Colt HG, Crawford SW, Galbraith O III. Virtual reality bronchoscopy simulation: a revolution in procedural training. Chest. 2001:120(4):1333-9.
2. Davoudi M, Colt HG. Bronchoscopy Simulation: A Brief Review, Advances in Health Science Education: Theory and Practice. 2009;14(2):287-96.
3. Davoudi M, Osann K, Colt HG. Validation of two instruments to assess technical bronchoscopic skill using virtual reality simulation. Respiration. 2008; 76(1):92-101.
4. Davoudi M, Wahidi MM, Zamanian Rohani N, et al. Comparative effectiveness of low and high-fidelity bronchoscopy simulation for training in conventional transbronchial needle aspiration and user preferences. Respiration. 2010;80(4):327-34.
5. Kastelik JA, Chowdhdhury F, Pathmanathan S, et al. Developments in simulation bronchoscopy training. Open Journal of Respiratory Diseases. 2013;3:154-63.
6. Kennedy CC, Maldonado F, Cook DA. Simulation-based bronchoscopy training: systematic review and meta-analysis. Chest. 2013;144(1):183-92.
7. Ost D, DeRosiers A, Britt EJ, et al. Assessment of a bronchoscopy simulator. Am J Respir Crit Care Med. 2001;164(12):2248-55.
8. Stather DR, Lamb CR, Tremblay A. Simulation in flexible bronchoscopy and endobronchial ultrasound: a review. J Bronchology Interv Pulmonol. 2011:18(3):247-56.
9. Weinberger SE, Pereira AG, Lobst WF, et al. Alliance for Academic Internal Medicine Education Redesign Task Force II. Competency-based education and training in internal medicine. Ann Intern Med. 2010;153(11):751-6.
10. Ziv A, Wolpe PR, Small SD, et al. Simulation-based medical education: an ethical imperative. Acad Med. 2003;78(8):783-8.

Chapter 29

Simulation for Airway Management

Kumar Belani

Chapter Outline

INTRODUCTION

One of the main thrusts of education in anesthesiology is training candidates to be professional world-class experts in airway care. The training for proper airway care begins in medical school and escalates to higher levels during medical internship with even more advanced training occurring during residency in anesthesiology. Anesthesia practitioners continue to improve their skills during the daily care of their patients. The maintenance of certification in anesthesiology requires anesthesia care providers to remain skilled in the provision of anesthesia services and an important component is being prepared to not only recognize but also be competent in newer technologies that become available for patient safety. The technologies for airway care are constantly improving and this has helped reduce airway related morbidity during the care of patients. Anesthesia care providers need to be aware of the practice guidelines that have been suggested by the American Society of Anesthesiologists (Apfelbaum, Hagberg et al. 2013). The **Figure 1** provided by this source is important for all practitioners involved in airway care for patients:

Nonanesthesiologists providing sedation or emergency room care also need to undergo training for the skills required for upper airway assistance namely, mask ventilation and endotracheal intubation. The same holds true for those obtaining certification for Advanced Cardiac Life Support.

AIRWAY ASSESSMENT

Proper assessment of the upper airway is a basic requirement before airway intervention or the use of drugs that may necessitate airway intervention. This is an important step during anesthesia care.

American Society of
Anesthesiologists

DIFFICULT AIRWAY ALGORITHM

1. Assess the likelihood and clinical impact of basic management problems:
   - Difficulty with patient cooperation or consent
   - Difficult mask ventilation
   - Difficult supraglottic airway placement
   - Difficult laryngoscopy
   - Difficult intubation
   - Difficult surgical airway access
2. Actively pursue opportunities to deliver supplemental oxygen throughout the process of difficult airway management
3. Consider the relative merits and feasibility of basic management choices:
   - Awake intubation vs. intubation after induction of general anesthesia
   - Noninvasive technique vs. invasive techniques for the initial approach to intubation
   - Video-assisted laryngoscopy as an initial approach to intubation
   - Preservation vs. ablation of spontaneous ventilation
4. Develop primary and alternative strategies

Figure 1 The difficult airway algorithm for all practitioners involved in airway care

Prior history of airway care, difficulty with mask ventilation, endotracheal intubation or extubation will be important to explore. Presence of anatomic deformities either congenital or acquired that result in airway distortion will suggest the presence of a difficult upper airway. The goal of airway assessment is to determine if there is adequate mouth opening, there is enough space in the oral cavity, that neck mobility is normal, that the lower jaw is anatomically normal in size and structure with a satisfactory submandibular distance and there is enough compliance in the submandibular area so as to allow proper alignment of the visual, oropharyngeal and laryngeal axes for easy oral endotracheal intubation. Normal intraoral structures combined with the described normal anatomy will allow for easy mask ventilation.

ENDOTRACHEAL INTUBATION

If the airway assessment indicates that the upper airway is feasible, then oral endotracheal intubation should be successful with traditional laryngoscopy. Proper mouth opening and technique with the appropriate sized curved (Macintosh) or straight (Miller) blades will allow for direct visualization of the larynx.

INABILITY TO SECURE THE AIRWAY

To minimize the chance of being unable to secure the airway especially during anesthesia care, there are various modalities and options. Practitioners need to be aware of these options as discussed in the difficult airway algorithm **(Figure 2)**. To obtain basic training in these options, difficult airway simulation workshops (Kennedy, Cannon et al. 2014, Mileder and Schmolzer 2014) have been a great resource. Pregnancy, multiple trauma and obesity are examples where airway establishment could be challenging leave alone other congenital and hereditary disorders.

As discussed earlier, the American Society of Anesthesiologists has established a difficult airway algorithm for practitioners to consider during a difficult upper airway situation. This requires preparedness and for effective implementation simulation training is helpful.[1-3]

At our own institution we have been conducting difficult airway workshops using biological (live animal, frozen then thawed tracheal lung, human cadaver) and manikin models including computer simulated full manikins. The value of using simulation technologies have been shown to be effective educational tools

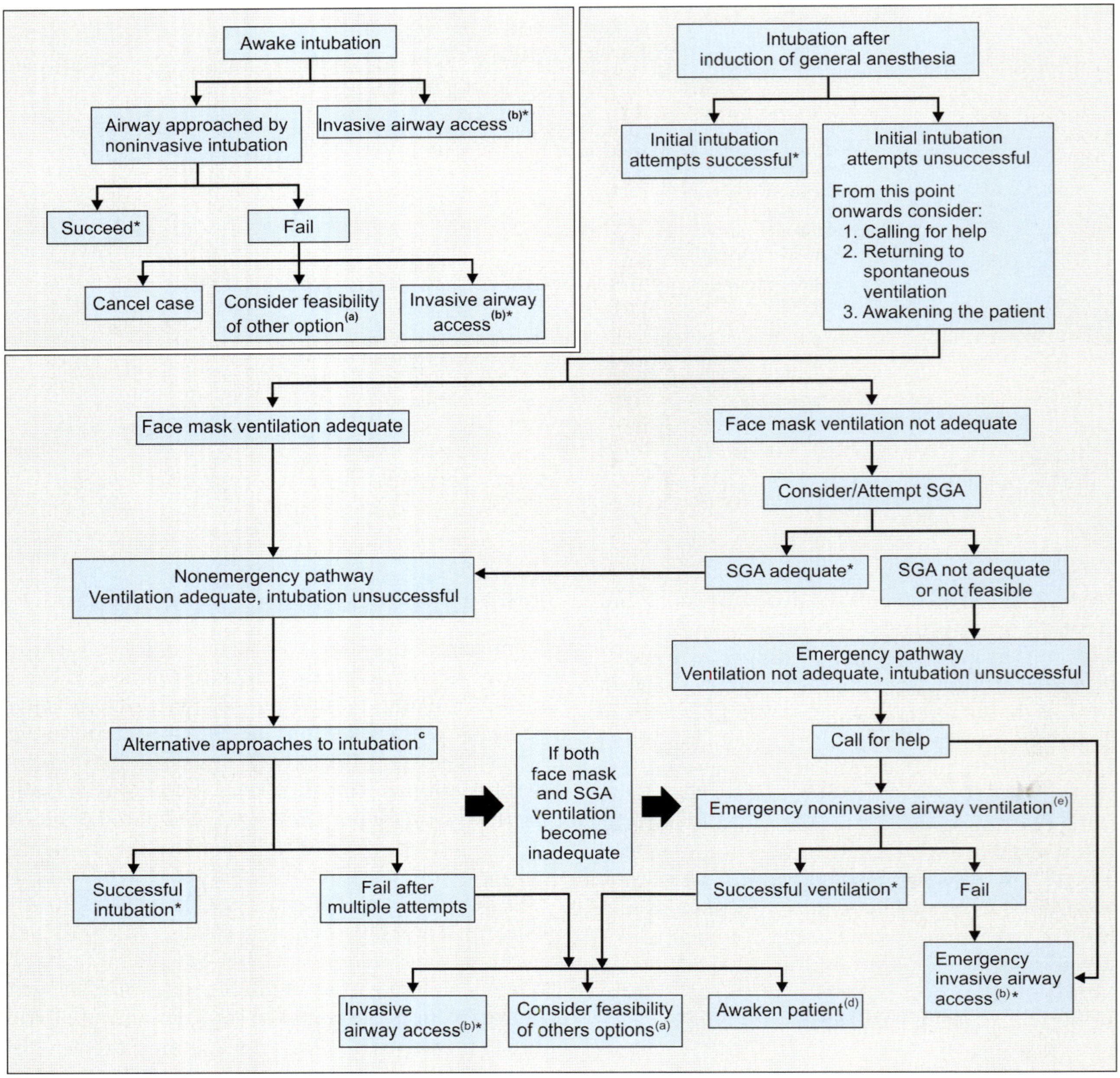

*** Confirm ventilation, tracheal intubation, or SGA placement with exhaled CO_2**

[a] Other options include (but are not limited to): Surgery utilizing face mask or supraglottic airway (SGA) anesthesia (e.g. LMA, ILMA, laryngeal tube), local anesthesia infiltration or regional nerve blockade. Pursuit of these options usually implies that mask ventilation will not be problematic. Therefore, these options may be of limited value it this step in the algorithm has been reached via the Emergency Pathway.

[b] Invasive airway access includes surgical or percutaneous airway, jet ventilation, and retrograde intubation.

[c] Alternative difficult intubation approaches include (but are not limited to): video-assisted laryngoscopy, alternative laryngoscope blades, SGA (e.g. LMA or ILMA) as an intubation conduit (with or without fiberoptic guidance), fiberoptic intubation, intubating stylet or tube changer, light wand, and blind oral or nasal intubation.

[d] Consider re-preparation of the patient for awake intubation or canceling surgery.

[e] Emergency noninvasive airway ventilation consists of a SGA.

Figure 2 The difficult airway algorithm for practitioners

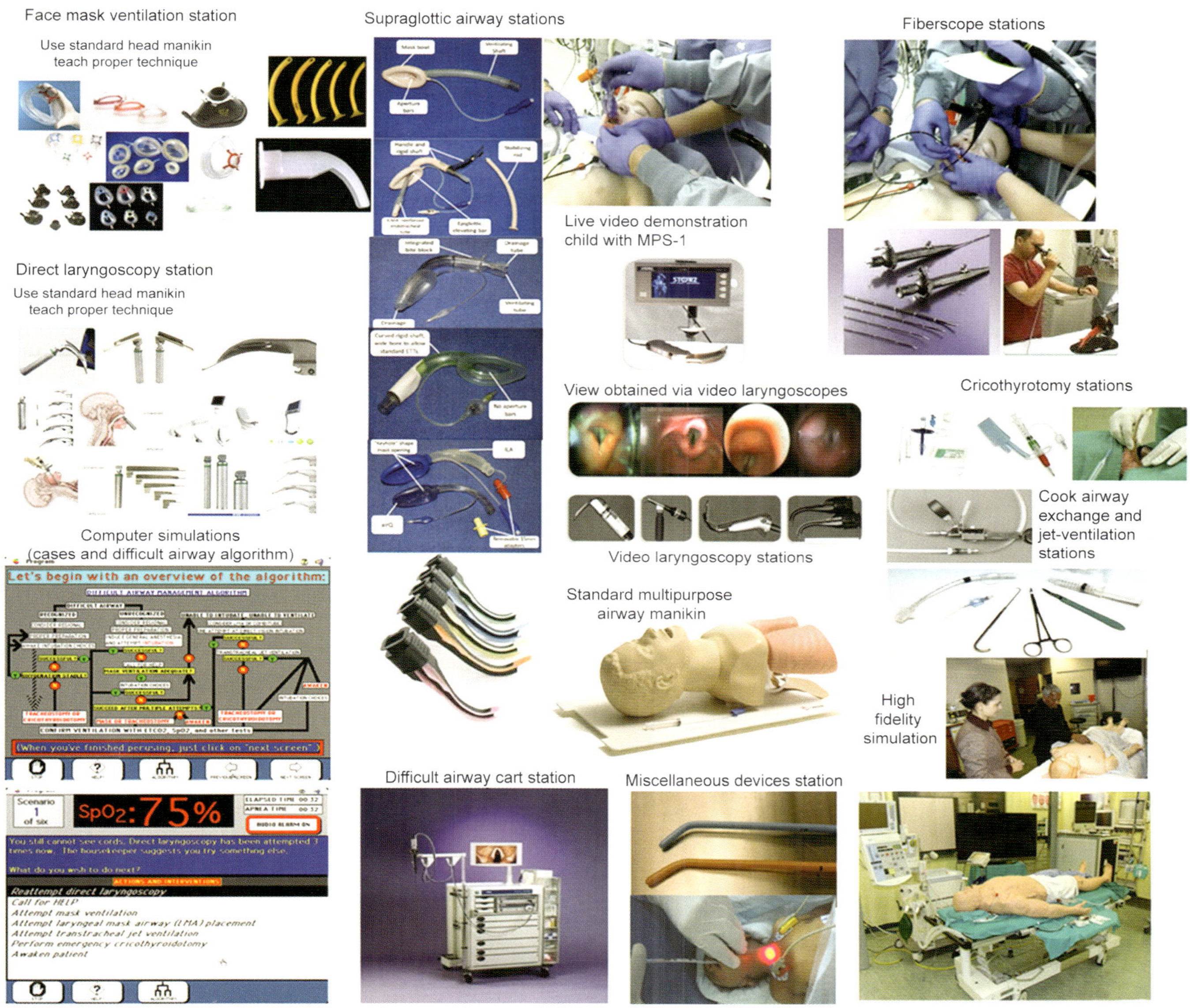

Figure 3 Components of the difficult airway workshop. The workshop detailed above is for those interested in advanced airway care. Other practitioners may also participate to learn different aspects of airway care

(Kennedy, Cannon et al. 2014, Mileder and Schmolzer 2014).

See the **Figure 3**, below for the different stations that are used during the basic and advanced airway training simulation.

SUMMARY

To reduce morbidity and mortality related to difficult upper airways, practitioners need to be aware of current technologies and options. These options can be easily learnt in difficult airway workshops. Experience in humans may be obtained in clinical facilities that offer such training.

REFERENCES

1. Apfelbaum JL, Hagberg CA, Caplan RA, Blitt CD, Connis RT, Nickinovich DG, Hagberg CA, Caplan RA, Benumof JL, et al. American Society of Anesthesiologists Task Force on Management of the Difficult. "Practice guidelines for management of the difficult airway: an updated report by the American Society of Anesthesiologists Task Force on Management of the Difficult Airway." Anesthesiology. 2013;118(2): 251-70.
2. Kennedy CC, Cannon EK, Warner DO, Cook DA. "Advanced airway management simulation training in medical education: a systematic review and meta-analysis." Crit Care Med. 2014;42(1):169-78.
3. Mileder LP, Schmolzer GM. "Simulation and its role in airway management training." Crit Care Med. 2014; 42(7):e541-42.

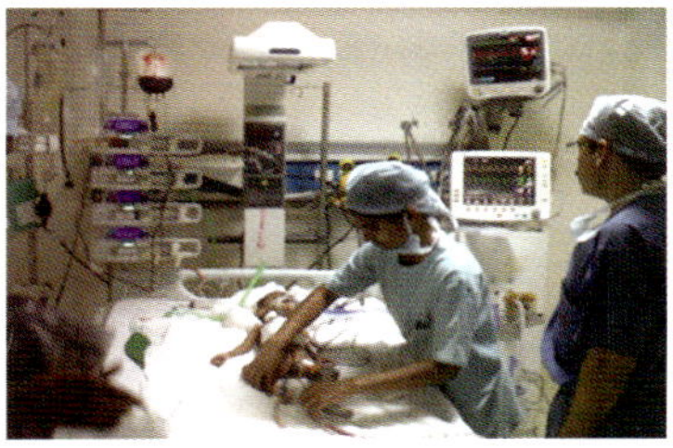

Section 7

Pediatric Simulation

Section Outline

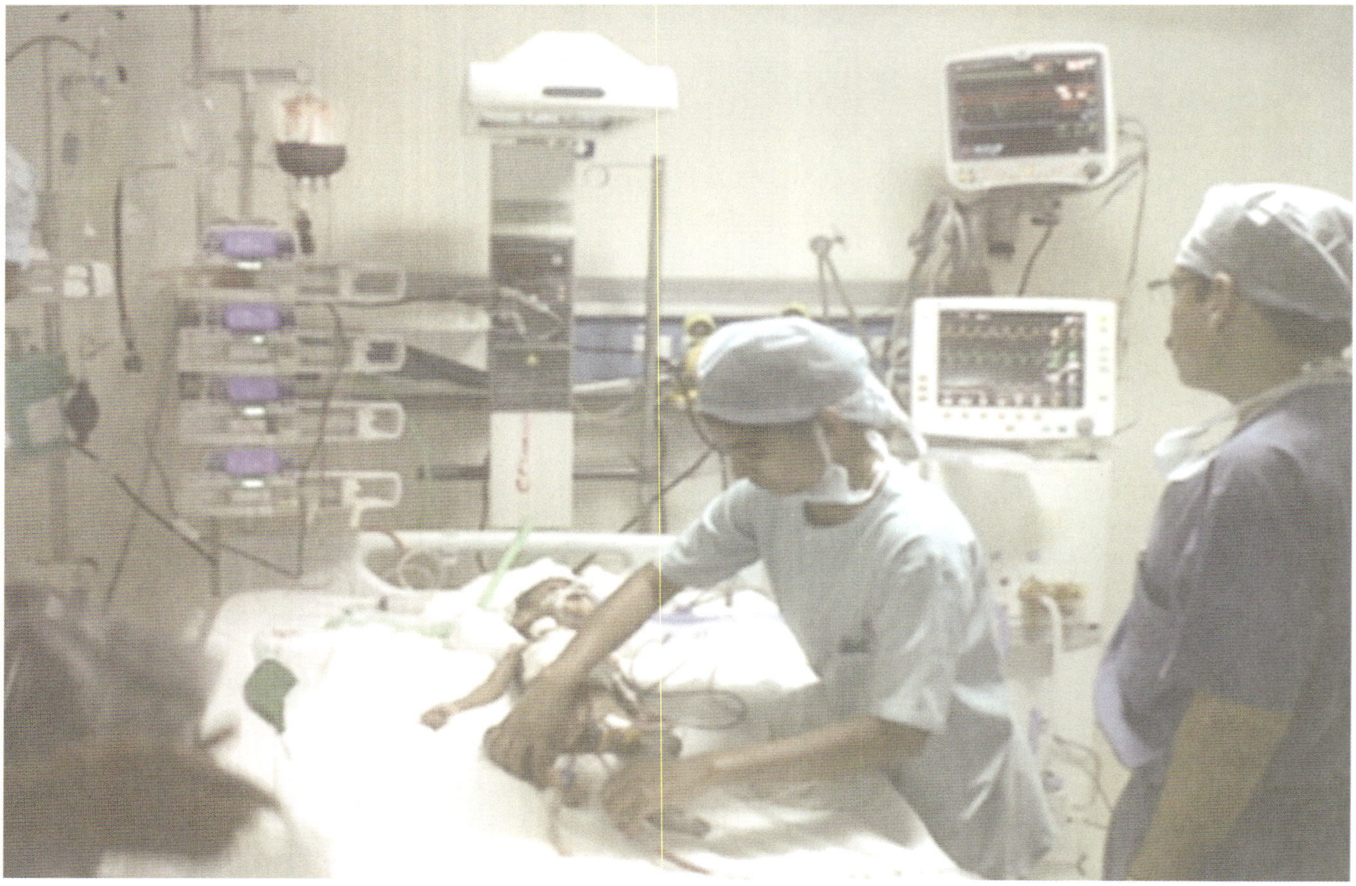

Chapter 30

Role of Simulation in Pediatrics

Sunit Singhi, Rakshay Shetty, Sujatha Thyagarajan

Chapter Outline

- Scope of Simulation-based Learning in Pediatrics
- Pediatric Emergency Medicine
- Pediatric and Neonatal Intensive Care
- Pediatric Anesthesia and Surgery
- Types of Simulation-based Education
- Part-task Trainers
- Role-play
- Standardized Patients
- Computer-based Simulators
- Scope of Simulation in Pediatric Acute Care Areas
- Fallacies
- The Indian Scenario
- Challenges and Future

Pediatrics is a challenging field where "Time is Essence" and the interplay of time-bound dynamics has a huge influence on the outcomes, particularly in an acutely ill child. In this context, simulation-based training appears to play a major role in training young pediatricians to develop critical decision making skills and learning in a risk-free environment.

SCOPE OF SIMULATION-BASED LEARNING IN PEDIATRICS

The scope of simulation-based training finds it vastly applicable in the care of acutely ill children. Pediatric cardiac arrests are infrequent and the survival in-hospital or out of hospital is poor. The focus hence is to prevent cardiac arrest through early detection and time based interventions to prevent the occurrence of arrest. This requires a good balance of theoretical knowledge, clinical experience, dexterity and critical time-bound decision making skills and leadership skills; a team approach is effective in managing crisis. Simulation based training has deviated from the traditional teaching on real patients to ensure patient safety and suitability to learners pace. Various sub-specialties in pediatrics have designed curricula based on the specific skill set required for completion of training in a safe environment and at the pace of the learner.

PEDIATRIC EMERGENCY MEDICINE

Specific curricula are designed to prepare the modern pediatric emergency trainees in majority of the institutions. Such training has been well rated too.

Skills based training such as insertion of intraosseous needles, umbilical line insertion, intubation, etc. team leading during resuscitation, revising the algorithms of commonly seen emergencies either at induction of training, during the fellowship training in the form of modules or through regular workshops have been highly valuable. Such curricula based training via simulation has been highly rated by trainees although the reflection on patient outcomes are yet to be clearly defined. Trauma team training, implementation of new protocols, mock codes on a regular basis have reinforced the learner's abilities and perceived confidence and performance.

PEDIATRIC AND NEONATAL INTENSIVE CARE

The scope of simulation in pediatric and neonatal critical care settings are manifold. The focus has been to inculcate team-training to hone in essential intensivist attributes such as leadership, team work, communication, resource utilisation and behavioural skills. In-situ simulation has been extremely productive in determining latent system errors in a safe environment. Team training has shown to identify and improve the communication failures and build the interprofessional relationships. Debriefing has a major role in enhancing the learner's experience. Procedural skills such as central line insertion and other rarely performed procedures such as emergency thoracotomy can be learnt well on simulated part-task trainers. The learners ability to reflect and retain based on the experience in a risk free environment appears to have added value compared to traditional teaching on a sick patient. Application of simulation in high risk areas where low volume and high risk seem a challenge, such as pediatric extracoporeal membrane oxygenation (ECMO), continuous renal replacement therapy (CRRT), and transport have found simulation based learning a valuable tool. There is some experience of utilizing high fidelity simulators for credentialing and certification of exams for specialists.

PEDIATRIC ANESTHESIA AND SURGERY

This is a high risk environment. Anesthetists and surgeons have specific task and team oriented simulation based curricula to engage and prepare them to deal with all crisis. Various simulation models are available for learning bronchoscopy, foreign body removal, laparoscopy, cleft lip repair, nerve blocks, lumbar puncture and other procedures so that the trainee can learn these skills including dexterity at their pace without compromising patient safety.

TABLE 1 Types of simulation-based tools

• *Task driven:* Specific task trainers (e.g. central line, arterial line, chest drain models)
• *Event driven* – Standardized patient/care actor – Hybrid simulation, e.g. standardized patient and part task trainer – *Computer-based*—low, medium and high fidelity.

TYPES OF SIMULATION-BASED EDUCATION

Types of simulation based education are summarised in **Table 1**.[1-5]

PART-TASK TRAINERS

Training of specific skills such as airway management, arterial line, central line, intraosseous line and chest drain placements can be taught using part task trainers. Commonly available as manikins or animal models and is useful for novice trainees to understand the techniques and practice in a low-risk situation without any patient-harm. Part-task trainers are widely utilized in various skills based workshops and life support courses.

ROLE-PLAY

This is an excellent way to train and assess communication skills. Role-play may be as child actors, parents, trauma victims, pregnant mothers, etc. Role-play sessions are particularly applicable for teaching breaking the bad news, explaining a procedure, taking consent, etc.

STANDARDIZED PATIENTS

It is used to demonstrate specific clinical skills and elicit signs, discuss approach and practical management. This is part of the traditional examination popular amongst various undergraduate and postgraduate curriculum assessments.

COMPUTER-BASED SIMULATORS

It is categorized on the basis of fidelity. Fidelity is the common industry term used in simulation to describe

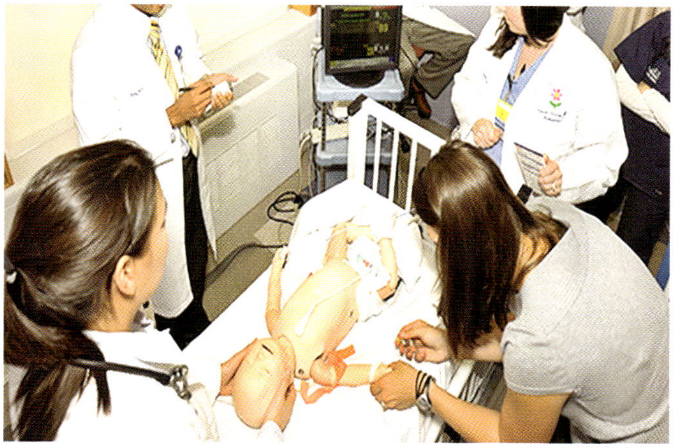

Figure 1 High fidelity simulator

the degree of realism and technical complexity of models. This is dictated by the needs of the application; more complex is the task, more is the fidelity of the model. Low fidelity models can be developed and updated rapidly while high-fidelity models cost more to engineer and maintain but are more flexible when applied to different uses. However, not everything needs to be taught in a high-fidelity simulation. A screen text simulator and static mannequins are examples for low fidelity simulators. Examples of medium fidelity simulators include virtual simulators like videogames and mannequins with mechanical movements like AMBU Man. A high fidelity simulator **(Figure 1)** is a full body computerized manikin that have realistic features, such as blinking eyes with reacting pupils, chests that rise and fall with respirations, palpable pulses, various heart and lung sounds, and the ability to cry, drool and bleed. They can respond physiologically to interventions, such as medication administration, intravenous fluid infusions and application of oxygen. They have procedural features to allow chest tube and tracheotomy management, defibrillation and urinary catheter insertion. Laerdal, METI and Gaumard are the most popular companies involved in pediatric simulation. Laedral as of now has a larger presence in India.

SCOPE OF SIMULATION IN PEDIATRIC ACUTE CARE AREAS

- Improving patient outcomes
- Discovering system errors
- Improving the quality of education
- Credentialing and exams.

Improving Patient Outcomes

Crisis resource management (CRM) is a method of team training that focuses on behavioral skills, resource utilization, communication, leadership, and teamwork. These skills are essential for effective clinical care, yet few medical personnel are exposed to formal training in these areas. Team training has been found to decrease medical errors.[6] Simulation offers an ideal setting to practice methods of CRM in a safe learning environment. A systematic review of team training studies found that 85% of the studies utilized simulation.[7] A 2007 study evaluating the effectiveness of a mock code-based educational intervention on the leadership skills of pediatric residents[8] displayed significantly improved leadership skills compared with residents who did not undergo training. Andreatta et al.[9] showed that conducting simulation-based mock codes significantly correlated with improved pediatric patient cardiopulmonary arrest survival rates.

Discovering System Errors

Communication failures account for many of the issues in patient safety. Simulation can be used to improve communication among team members and theoretically reduce patient errors. Interdisciplinary simulation can be used to identify institutional policies and practices that may be detrimental to patient care. For example, it can be used to improve the transition between emergency room and Pediatric Intensive Care Unit (PICU) or between anesthetists and intensivists. Running such kind of simulation can find out situation readiness and the adequacy of handover. Over a 6-month period, the Andreatta et al. implemented an interdisciplinary team training and simulation program to improve the management of obstetric emergencies.[10] Transcripts from the debriefing sessions identified five main types of system-level and specialty-specific practices, policies, and procedures that could potentially cause conflict within the clinical team or adversely affect patient care. These included institutional policies that were impossible carry out, policies between departments that contradicted one another, policies that participants did not realize existed, and a variety of communications barriers between different departments and specialties. This study showed how interdisciplinary communications simulation training can be used to identify critical systems-based obstacles and issues that despite being endemic, might otherwise have gone unaddressed.

Improving the Quality of Education

Curriculum based training in PICU is primarily driven by textbooks and clinical experience gained with real patients under supervision by trainers. Errors are inevitable and not without repercussions. The trainers and learners have little opportunity to facilitate training without the added pressure of time and patient safety. Procedural skills such as line insertions and the competency required with dexterity and slickness for high risk situations commonly encountered in PICU such as a patient in shock get undermined more frequently than not for novice trainees and hence more missed opportunities. Procedural skills may be learnt on simulated models or part-task trainers at the learner's pace with enough practice without causing patient harm. Learning in a non-risk environment facilitates better reflection and retention. Infact, simulation offers a unique advantage for learning rarely performed procedures. Studies looking into the skill retention showed that a skill learnt in skill laboratories can sustain upto 1 year.[11] McGaghie et al.[12] looked into a specific question of whether simulation with deliberate practice yields better results than traditional education. They screened over 3000 articles published between 1990 and 2010 and demonstrated an improvement in the simulation with deliberate practice group over traditional education. Largest metanalysis on simulation education was published by Cook et al. in JAMA,[13] also supported its superiority.

Credentialing and Exams

One more potential use of simulation is as a tool to evaluate competency and credentialing. It is a relatively new concept. Though computer based scenario oriented exams are being conducted, there is not much experience using scenarios based on high fidelity simulators. Results of the Israeli study[14] looking into usage simulation for board certification for anesthesiologists are promising. It might find more application in this regard as more studies look into their validity.

Advantages of Simulation-based Learning

Simulated practice environments are useful for reflection upon experience in clinical areas because it draws out learning points, develops clinical reasoning and integrates theory with practice. Mistakes may be made and learning can occur without risk to patients. Practical skills can be developed in a systematic supported manner. Furthermore, discussion of theoretical and ethical matters that are normally inappropriate in the presence of a patient can occur in parallel with the developing of practical skills. One significant advantage of simulation is that it permits both the trainer and the learner to study patient treatment processes in ways that nature prohibits. The simulation can be run many times with the values of the parameters being modified between runs and the changes in outputs observed. It also offers unique advantage of learning procedural skills or management of clinical situations that are of rare incidence.

FALLACIES

For simulation-based education to be effective, instructor needs to have a considerable experience in designing a realistic scenario. Instructor should be able to deliver an effective debriefing session tailoring to the needs of the trainee. As discussed above, if all the components of cycles of learning are not elicited during the simulation exercise, it might be underwhelming and might not lead to a desired learning experience.

THE INDIAN SCENARIO

The vision of Medical Council of India states that every medical college must make provisions for simulation equipment/labs. To date, we have about 24 simulation centers in the country but only half of them have Paediatric high fidelity simulation mannequins and supportive equipment. Even more challenging has been the availability of formally trained Paediatric trainers in simulation. In a web-based survey of all training institutes for PICU in India, conducted by Pedi STARS India in 2012, only 2 of the 20 institutions had pediatric simulation facilities available locally and only 3 of the 28 teaching faculty had some exposure to paediatric simulation.

There have been various 1–2 day workshops held in various parts of the country over the last 4 years with the assistance of international faculty and the technical support and high fidelity mannequins offered by simulation equipment companies based in India. The target audience have been specifically Paediatricians and paediatric critical care or acute care Paediatricians. These workshops have been highly rated indicating the inherent demand locally.

A web-based survey conducted via Pedi STARS India amongst all paediatricians practising in India showed that more than 90% favoured simulation based education.

CHALLENGES AND FUTURE

As we stride forward this century in India, we epitomise as one of the cost-effective models of healthcare. Simulation tools such as the high-fidelity simulators are very expensive and require trained personnel and specifically designed simulation labs equipped with the gadgets and technical support to facilitate simulation training. Few training institutions have already taken a leap in this direction and have set up state of the art simulation laboratory. However, there is a gross under-utilisation of these facilities due to lack of availability of simulation instructors. We need to create a bank of simulation instructors who can then inculcate effective training in our institutions. Point of care or in-situ simulation is a viable and more topical alternative to the expensive simulation labs in our set-up. We need to look at cost-effective models that can still work on the same principles of training and learning. We need a wider acceptance of a culture of quality and patient safety as a mandatory responsibility in our acute Pediatric areas such as PICU/NICU/Emergency Departments, transport and operating theaters and are prepared to evaluate ourselves periodically of how well we can improve based on the regular simulation exercises. The investment in resources that improve quality of care will eventually improve patient outcomes and hence become cost-effective. There is a felt need to promote networking and intelligence sharing across the international borders and within the country to create a pool of leaders and trainers/experts in paediatric simulation within India. One such initiative has been Pedi STARS India, which is now affiliated to Society of Simulation in Healthcare and International Paediatric Simulation Society.

CONCLUSION

Simulation offers tremendous promise to improve the quality of care and education in acute pediatrics. There is now a growing body of high-quality literature and evidence to support its growth. In the future, it can be expected that simulation will be used by practically every healthcare provider at some or multiple points in the training and certification process.

REFERENCES

1. Paul B. The history of simulation in medical education and possible future directions. Medical Education. 2006;40:254-62.
2. Goudar SS, Kotur PF. Trends in medical education. Indian J Anaesthesia. 2003;47:25-27.
3. Uth HJ, Wiese N. Central collecting and evaluating of major accidents and near-miss-events in the Federal Republic of Germany—results, experiences, perspectives. J Hazardous Mat. 2004;111:139-45.
4. Vozenilek J, Huff S, Reznek M, Gordon JA. See one, do one, teach one: advanced technology in medical education. Acad Emerg Med. 2004;11:1149-54.
5. Malone HR, Syed ON, Downes MS, D'Ambrosio AL, Quest DO,Kaiser MG. Simulation in neurosurgery: a review of computer based simulation environments and their surgical applications. Neurosurgery. 2010;67:1105-16.
6. Morey JC, Simon R, JayGD, et al. Error reduction and performance improvement in the emergency department through formal teamwork training: evaluation results of the MedTeams project. Health Serv Res. 2002;37:1553-81.
7. Salas E, DiazGranados D, Weaver SJ, et al. Does team training work? Principles for healthcare. Acad Emerg Med. 2008;15:1002-9.
8. Gilfoyle E, Gottesman R, Razack S. Development of a leadership skills workshop in paediatric advanced resuscitation. Med Teach. 2007;29:e276-83.
9. Andreatta P, Saxton E, Thompson M, et al. Simulation-based mock codes significantly correlate with improved pediatric patient cardiopulmonary arrest survival rates. Pediatr Crit Care Med. 2011;12:33-8.
10. Andreatta P, Frankel J, Boblick SS, et al. Interdisciplinary team training identifies discrepancies in institutional policies and practices. Am J Obstet Gynecol. 2011; 205:298-301.
11. Boet S, Borges BC, Naik VN, et al. Complex procedural skills are retained for a minimum of 1 year after a single high-fidelity simulation training session. Br J Anaesth. 2011;107:533-9.
12. McGaghie WC, Issenberg SB, Cohen ER, et al. Does simulation-based medical education with deliberate practice yield better results than traditional clinical education? A meta-analytic comparative review of the evidence. Acad Med. 2011;86:706-11.
13. Cook DA, Hatala R, Brydges R, et al. Technology-enhanced simulation for health professions education: a systematic review and meta-analysis. JAMA. 2011; 306:978-88.
14. Ben-Menachem E, Ezri T, Ziv A, et al. Objective structured clinical examination based assessment of regional anesthesia skills: the Israeli National Board Examination in Anesthesiology experience. Anesth Analg. 2011;112:242-5.

Chapter 31

Simulation and Crisis Resource Management in Pediatric Learning

Rakshay Shetty, Geethanjali Ramachandra

Chapter Outline

- Why Simulation?
- How do Adults Learn?
- Crisis Resource Management
- Lessons Learn from Aviation Industry
- Stages of Medical Simulation
- Factors Associated with Crisis
- Leadership
- Debriefing
- Focus of Debrief
- Barriers Associated with the Delivery of Simulation Training in India

WHY SIMULATION?

Traditional way of pouring information through lectures focus on improving the knowledge. This may not be the best way to improve outcome and safety of the patient in intensive care unit (ICU) environment. In the ICU, there is much emphasis on technical skills and not on communication, teamwork and leadership, resulting in clinicians being unprepared to meet the demands of the complex ICU environment.

Intensive care frequently results in unintentional harm to patients. The ICU environment is unforgiving for mistakes due to the multidisciplinary, time-critical nature of care and vulnerability of the patients. Human factors account for the majority of adverse events and a sound safety climate is therefore essential.

Simulation training is a powerful educational tool to help facilitate learning and change the practice to improve patient outcomes. Simulation allows the health professionals to practice and gain experience in a safe and structured environment without risk to patients. Simulation training with crisis resource management (CRM) focuses on teamwork, error management and blame free discussion of human mistakes.

Health care simulation prepares the physicians and nurses to face real patients. It offers a controlled, safe and reproducible environment to practice clinical skills. Simulation creates a zero-risk environment that allows medical teams to practice high-risk; low frequency events without endangering patients. Manikins used for simulation can come back alive despite errors, but not real patients!

Types of Simulation Training

- Simulation laboratory-environment with high fidelity computer controlled manikins.
- "In situ"-training, which is conducted on actual patient care units involving actual health care team members and actual organization processes.
- Role play.

HOW DO ADULTS LEARN?

Adult learning is different from that of children. Past experience allows adults to form mental models, which guide their practice. In health care, mental models form the basis for clinical decision-making.

Unlike lecture-based learning, simulation requires learners to apply their current mental models. Simulation provides a great opportunity for individuals refine their mental models. Educators can design simulations that stress existing mental models, helping the individual to identify areas where they need to learn and refine the mental models.

Experiences, either real or simulated, are simply catalysts for learning. The actual learning does not occur during the experience itself, but rather during the debriefing that follows. Experiences provide an opportunity for the reflection during debriefing. Learner can evaluate, refine and enhance the mental models. The learner must then "test," or experiment with revised mental models created by this reflection, leading to permanent change. The process of having an experience (concrete experience), reflecting on that experience (reflective observation), developing mental models (abstract conceptualization) and then testing that mental model (active experimentation) is based on Kolb's experiential learning cycle **(Figure 1)**.

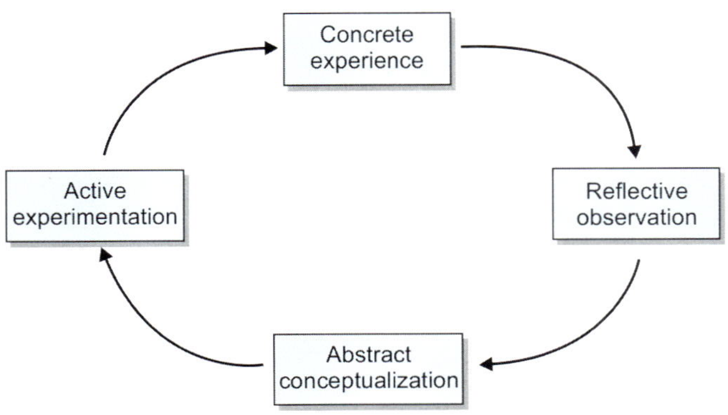

Figure 1 Kolb's experiential learning cycle

Circle of Adult Learning

Adult learning is a continuing process of attaining, maintaining, and enhancing clinical competence. Simulation adheres to the most important aspects of experiential adult learning by allowing hands-on experience in a safe environment, and subsequently providing guided reflection.

Adult learners develop new skills through repeated experience with simulation, allowing repeated exposure to both common and rare clinical scenarios. If conducted well and accompanied by constructive feedback simulation has been shown to improve trainee performance when faced with a similar situation again.

Unlike learning through lectures, confidentiality is a unique requirement for simulation based learning because all levels of individual performance are observed by the whole group.

CRISIS RESOURCE MANAGEMENT

What is Crisis?

A crisis can be defined as follows:

"A time of difficulty or danger which involves nonroutine circumstances, leading to an increase in workload, speed and complexity".[1]

It is the turning point of a disease when important changes take place, indicting either recovery or death.

What Happens in Crisis?

As a result of a crisis, such as a cardiac arrest, tasks get neglected and there could be a loss of situational awareness. Situational awareness allows one to predict what might happen next or to see the "big picture". The increased speed and complexity seen in a crisis may lead to confusion and lack of coordination and errors. These are often errors of fixation and omission.[2] For example, a blood pressure cuff not able to record blood pressure (BP) might actually represent hypotension, not malfunction.

What is Resource Management?

Management of the medical crisis often requires effective performance of multiple simultaneous tasks. It requires pooling of cognitive resources of multiple people, from several disciplines than an individual. The optimal team possesses a shared awareness of the situation and a shared decision-making process to prevent errors related to the time-critical environment.

CHAPTER 31

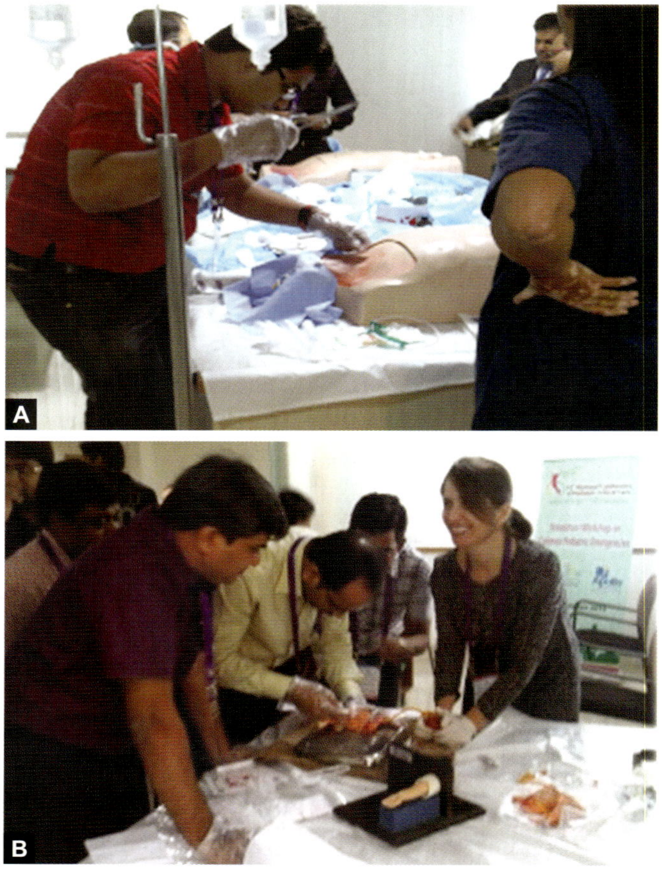

Figures 2A and B Task oriented simulation
(*Courtesy:* PediSTARS India)

Traditional medical education has focussed on individual learning and has not focussed on importance of team work and development of safe systems. Most medical errors occur due to system failure than individual error. Behaviors and actions result in under performance.

The evidences show that ICUs with a "team-oriented culture" have shorter lengths of stay **(Figures 2A and B)**, lower nursing turnover and higher quality of care and can better meet family members needs".[3]

LESSONS LEARN FROM AVIATION INDUSTRY

The concept of CRM-based culture change by the use of team training exercises from scenario is derived from aviation simulation expertise. Up to 1977 aviation industry could be classified as a professional-centered, hierarchic working environment. This all changed with the Tenerife disaster. A KLM Boeing 747 crash-later revealed that human factors contributed to the deadliest mishap in aviation history that claimed 583 lives. As part of the solution to prevent this from happening ever again, a compulsory human factor training for all aircrew personnel was developed in 1979 in a workshop (CRM) sponsored by NASA.

In aviation, nontechnical skills, a blame-free environment and team situational awareness (SA) are considered CRM core competencies. Team SA is defined as the ability to identify, process, and comprehend the critical elements of information about what is happening to the team with regards to the mission.

What are Nontechnical Skills?

Nontechnical skills (NTS) or human factors are the cognitive, social and personal resource skills that complement technical skills and contribute to safe and efficient task performance. NTS tell us how it should be done than what should be done!

Human factors (rather than equipment failure) were found to be the most common cause of serious accidents in aviation industries. Suboptimal performance among highly trained pilots was not always the result of lack of knowledge or deficiency in technical ability, but often due to short comings in communication, leadership, situational awareness, decision making and teamwork.

These so called "nontechnical skills" became a key component of pilot training and everyday operations with the introduction of "Cockpit resource management" (CRM). Training in NTS was subsequently introduced into numerous other industries, and the word "cockpit" in CRM was replaced with "crisis" (crisis resource management).

The importance of NTS in health care was recognized by anesthetists, who developed the first formal medical NTS training course piloted in 1990. The NTS model has subsequently been adapted to emergency situations in other branches of health care.

STAGES OF MEDICAL SIMULATION (TABLE 1)

First level of medical simulation training mainly focuses on technical skills, and level 2 of simulation training focuses on CRM. CRM helps the participants develop greater awareness of importance of effective communication, team work, situation awareness and

TABLE 1 Taxonomy for nontechnical skills used in crisis resource management

Categories	*Elements*
Task management	Planning and preparing Prioritizing Providing and maintaining standards Identifying and utilizing resources
Team working	Coordinating activities with team members Exchanging information Using authority and assertiveness Assessing capabilities Supporting others
Situation awareness	Gathering information Recognizing and understanding Anticipating
Decision making	Identifying options Balancing risk and selecting options Re-evaluating

management of resources during crisis. It is found to be both beneficial and enjoyable by participants and allows the opportunity for team building.

To be able to provide the best care to patients, there must be effective interdisciplinary team work between nurses, doctors and other healthcare providers. This teamwork must be maximized during a crisis situation, for the patient to receive the best care.

To successfully manage a crisis, several things need to happen simultaneously. We need to make a timely diagnosis, declare a crisis, mobilize resources and initiate appropriate medical management.

FACTORS ASSOCIATED WITH CRISIS[4,5]

Factors that cannot be changed include:

- Patient issues
- Disease process
- Circumstances of the crisis situation.

Factors that can be changed with effective communication and interdisciplinary training are:

- Leadership and role clarity for everyone in the team
- Communication and crosscheck techniques
- Situational awareness and recognition of adverse situation[6]
- Effective use of resources (personnel, equipment)
- Ongoing global assessment and feed back.

These are the five major principles in CRM.

CRM training focuses on risk management and decision-making, the effective use of checklists, identifying team roles, effective communication and performance feedback. Team members are taught how to communicate without creating conflict or in the face of apparent conflict **(Figures 3A and B)**.

LEADERSHIP

It is vital for the team leader to be:

- Be clear
- Organize team

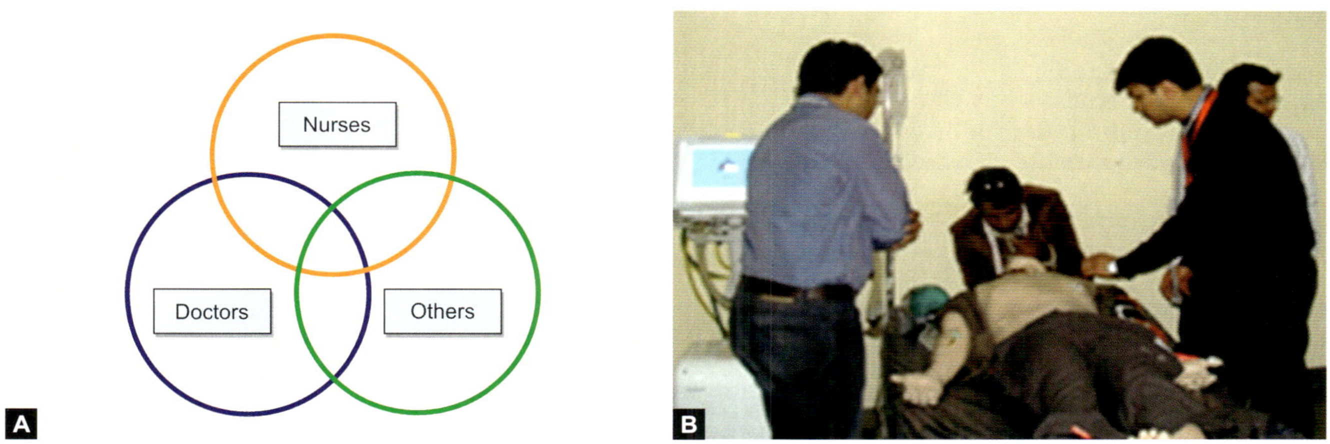

Figures 3A and B CRM training (*Courtesy:* PediSTARS India)

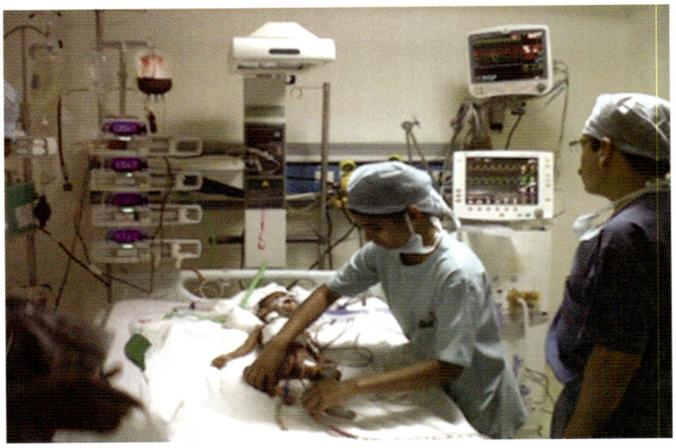

Figure 4 Global assessment during CRM-"20,000 meters view"

- Control communication
- Verbalize clear goals
- Transmit plans with frequent updates
- Maintain 20,000 meters view to avoid tasks and fixation **(Figure 4)**.

Why Communication is Important?

Communication is the glue that holds crisis management together. During a crisis, members of the team may have information and different ideas. This information may be critical to the patient's survival. It is important to create a respectful environment where information is shared. This creates situational awareness and equal distribution of work load.

Three Cs of communication–(1) Clarity, (2) Cite name, (3) Close the loop.

DEBRIEFING

The actual learning does not occur during the simulation experience itself, but rather during the debriefing that follows. A debriefing is a discussion that occurs immediately following the simulation. Educators and learners reflect together to analyze individual and group performance.

Debriefing provides an opportunity for learners to reflect on the simulation and their own performance. This reflective process allows the learner to identify gaps in mental models and to prepare for learning. Experience and reflection allow the learner to make sense of what happened, facilitates bridging to future experiences.

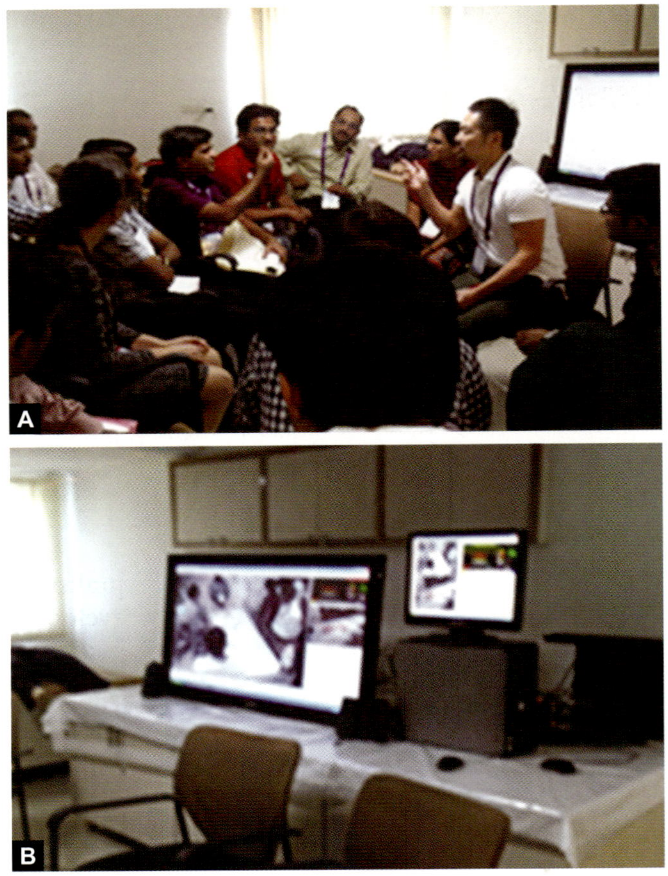

Figures 5A and B Debriefing with video recording (*Courtesy:* PediSTARS India)

After reflection, the learner is ready to adapt their mental model. Active experimentation promotes "cementing" of new knowledge and long-term changes in practice **(Figures 5A and B)**.

FOCUS OF DEBRIEF

- Individual performance (Competency management)
- Team performance (CRM).

The participants are guided through the events in a sequential order, accompanied by questions. The facilitators encourage a dialogue and an exchange of opinions regarding management, teamwork and communication skills. Video clips can be used to illustrate crucial points.

BARRIERS ASSOCIATED WITH THE DELIVERY OF SIMULATION TRAINING IN INDIA

- *Costs of training:* Especially for high-end immersive simulation, which requires medical equipment, manikins, personnel, simulation programming and facilities
- Lack of trainers.

The only solution to overcome this barrier lies within us; by motivating ourselves to achieve the best. Sharing the simulation equipment, encouragement of more *in situ* simulation in the hospital setting and training the trainers (TOT) are the way forward to see much wider use of simulation learning in our country.[5]

SUMMARY

Simulation has been shown to improve quality of patient care and increase patient safety, by developing new training methods for health care professionals.

Effective education must be delivered along a continuum, from simulation to the bedside, where each experience is seen as a problem to be solved or an opportunity to learn. Simulations should not only provide an opportunity for experience, but also one for reflection and refinement of mental models.

REFERENCES

1. CRM training. Children's Hospital Boston-International Quality Improvement Collaborative for Congenital Heart Surgery, 15th learning module of 2012.
2. Zigmont JJ, Kappus JJ, et al. Theoretical foundations of learning through simulation. Semin Perinatol. 2011;35:47-51.
3. Kolb DA. Experiential learning. Upper Saddle River, NJ, Prentice Hall, 1984.
4. Gillon S, Radford S, Chalwin R, et al. Crisis resource management, simulation training and the Medical emergency team. Crit Care Resusc. 2012;14:227-35.
5. Grant DJ, Marriage SC. Training using medical simulation ADC. Sept 15, 2011.
6. Marck HTM, Haerkens, Jenkins DH, et al. Crew resource management in the ICU: the need for culture change. Annals of Intensive Care. 2012;2:39.

Section 8

Simulation for ECMO and Pain Medicine

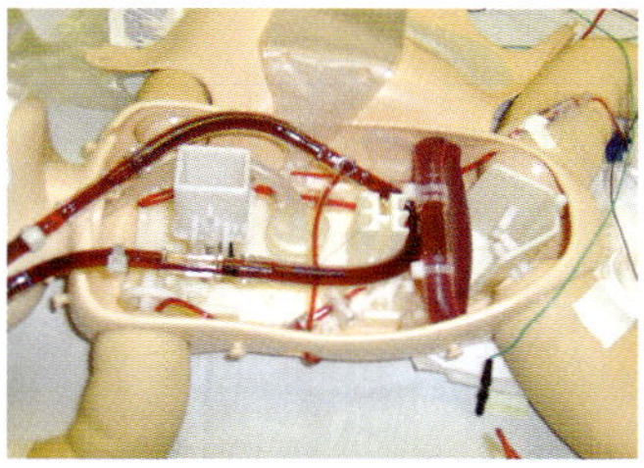

Section Outline

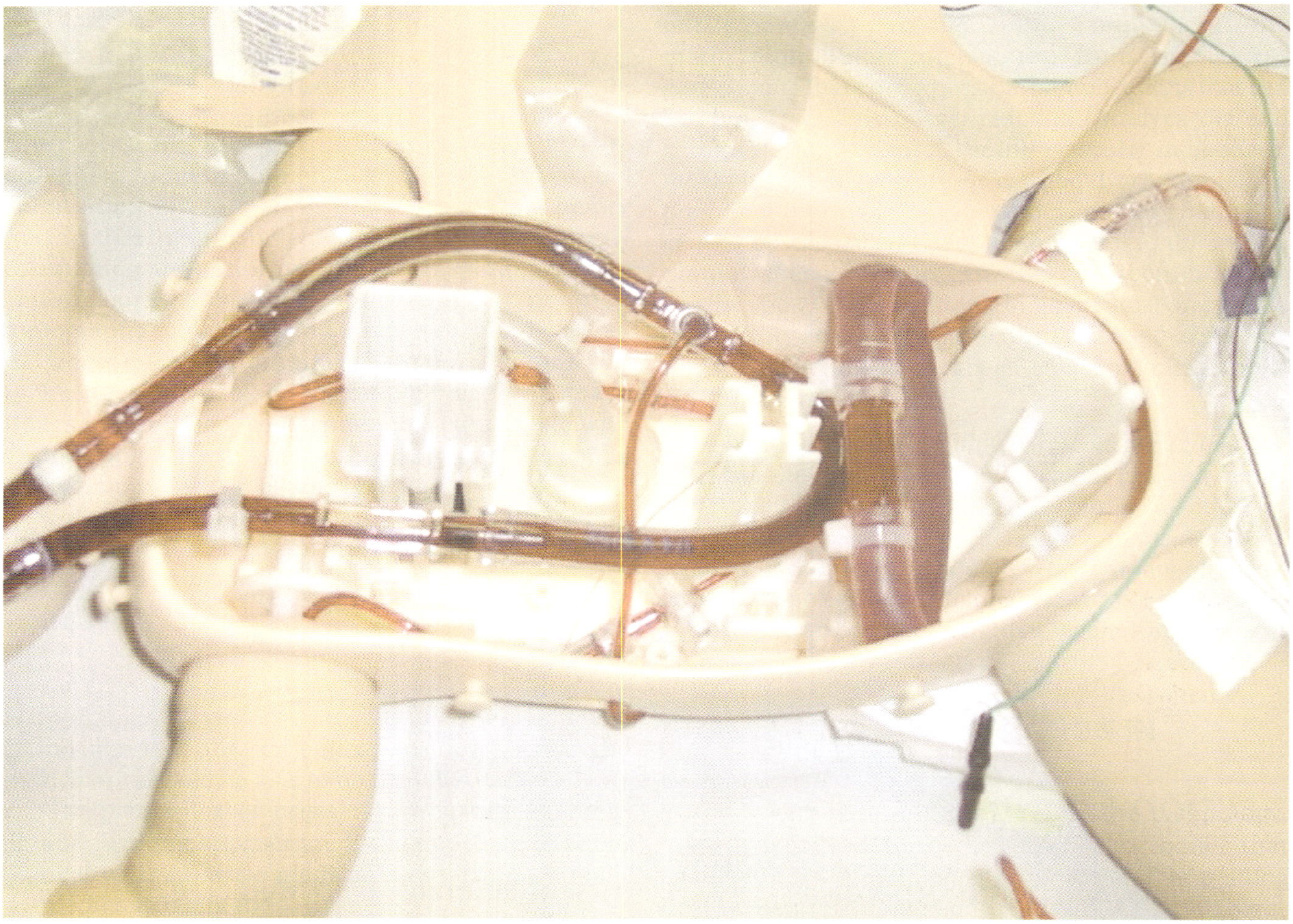

Chapter 32

Simulation for Extracorporeal Membrane Oxygenation

Pranay Oza, Venkat Goyal

Chapter Outline

- ECMO Training
- Traditional ECMO Training
- Advanced ECMO Training
- Impact of Simulation Training
- Methodology
- Scenario Design
- ECMO Simulation Systems
- Qualities of Simulation System
- Circulation Simulator
- ECMO Simulator
- ECMOjo
- MSE System

INTRODUCTION

The extracorporeal membrane oxygenation (ECMO) is a highly technical, advanced life support therapy and is used for critically ill newborns, children and adults, as a temporary means of cardiac and pulmonary support. A mechanical circuit allows the heart and lungs to rest and recover for patients with potentially reversible conditions. Patients who are potential candidates for ECMO support have complex cardiac, respiratory or mixed pathologies requiring significant support and often intensive therapy for recovery.

The ECMO supported patient has unique care requirements due to the complex interaction between the pathophysiology of the patient and the mechanical components of the ECMO circuit. The ECMO patient is managed by a group of ICU physicians collaboratively with both bedside nurses and technically trained ECMO specialists. Although unique to each centre that offers ECMO support, ECMO teams are large, multidisciplinary groups that can include physicians, fellows, residents, physician assistants, nurse practitioners, perfusionists, registered nurses and respiratory therapists.

ECMO TRAINING

While ECMO is not a new treatment modality, it is complex and requires a high level of training to acquire and maintain proficiency. The numbers of ECMO cases are very less and it involves lots of catastrophic, life-threatening complications which need to be diagnosed early and tackled immediately. This highly critical situation with high workload and stressful environment makes it more vulnerable for human

TABLE 1 Challenges of ECMO training

• Complexity
• Dynamism
• Major time pressure
• Rapidly evolving and changing information load
• High information ambiguity
• High workload and risks
• Criticality of conditions
• Stressful
• High tech environment

errors. A multidisciplinary team is needed to manage the patient. It is very essential that this team should have proper theoretical and practical training. Opportunities to develop teamwork skills and expertise to mitigate risks are very few. It is important to maintain cognitive, technical and behavioral skills in these cases and that can be acquired by an active learning environment **(Table 1)**.

Currently, training for ECMO primarily uses didactic education and occasionally includes various hands-on training modules. Simulation courses with mannequins are available at a few centers as supplemental training.

In Indian scenario, there is a big difference in ECMO-training programs between the ECMO-centres. In most of the centres, the ECMO training is mainly by water drills. Video-assisted real-time simulation and structured debriefing is not commonly used. No suitable ECMO-simulator on the market at this time. Only ECMO simulation available in India is web-based ECMOjo and MSE Simulator (personal version).

TRADITIONAL ECMO TRAINING

The traditional ECMO training involves the wet drills and animal lab which has its own advantages and disadvantages. But none of this can create the exact scenario of an ECMO runs and also it just helps us to develop only technical skills.

Wet Drills

It can be done easily and it helps us to have hands on circuit management and circuit-related complications **(Table 2)**.

TABLE 2 Advantages and disadvantages of wet drill

Advantages	*Disadvantages*
Cheap	No realism
Easy to set up for different shifts	Limited ability to test circuit emergencies
Gives a good hands on for circuit management	No testing of the team and its communication

TABLE 3 Advantages and disadvantages of animal labs

Advantages	*Disadvantages*
More realism than wet drills	Costly
Ability to see circuit and patient responses in real time	Labor-intensive
? Cannulation practice	Difficult to maintain for longer periods of time
	Difficult to test serious circuit emergencies without prematurely ending the session
	Limited testing of team roles and interactions
	Usually starting with healthy subject
	Sacrifice animal so difficult in Indian scenario

Animal Labs

Here the live animal is cannulated and connected to ECMO circuit **(Table 3)**. It is like a live case on ECMO, and then different mechanical as well as physiological scenarios are being created to demonstrate the hemodynamic response. It gives the realistic scenario and one can have patient responses to the different situations during an ECMO run. One can also have live demonstration of and hands on for cannulation.

ADVANCED ECMO TRAINING

ECMO training requires real-time decision making and diagnosis coupled with action to improve the clinical situation. As we know ECMO is a multidisciplinary team work, appropriate team behaviors and clear communication are of utmost importance in caring for ECMO patients. Traditional training methods do not adequately address these skills.

Medical simulation is a branch of simulation technology related to education and training in medical fields of various industries. Its main purpose is to train medical professionals to reduce accidents during surgery, prescription, and general practice. It is very useful tool in training multidisciplinary team especially in low volume cases with high-risk scenarios. It is a methodology for learning in which trainees:

- Are immersed in an environment filled with realistic visual, auditory and tactile clues
- Must integrate cognitive, technical and behavioral skills under often intense time pressure[1]
- Are provided the opportunity to reflect on their performance

ECMO simulation system is realistic training and mimics the real environment of pump, team and patient. It helps us to improve acquisition of cognitive, behavioral and technical skills. It sharpens our reflexes and can be used for frequent retraining and thereby train to weaknesses. One can plan rehearsal of the management of unusual or infrequent problems, particularly when multiple individuals are involved in the team.[2,3] ECMO simulation allows teams to incorporate a variety of learning objectives into each scenario, including medical knowledge, technical skills, team behaviors and communication. It also allows for the development of a standardized experience for all staff members.

IMPACT OF SIMULATION TRAINING

Simulation-based training is an effective method to improve safety, knowledge, attitudes, and teamwork surrounding ECMO emergencies.[4]

Anderson JM, et al. *Simulation in Healthcare*, 2006, conducted a study to evaluate the efficacy of a simulation-based approach to ECMO crisis training. It was a Prospective, randomized, controlled trial. They enrolled nine ECMO nurse specialists and each participated in two sequential, randomly assigned, simulated ECMO emergencies. All simulations were video-taped and key technical and behavioral skills were scored by reviewers blinded to the sequence of scenarios. They concluded that ECMO Sim was preferred by the study subjects, trainees felt more intellectually engaged and felt that ECMO Sim better developed their cognitive, technical and behavioral skills. It helps in reduction in response time and technical skills performed correctly more often in second simulation.[5] Behavioral skills were rated more highly in second simulation by masked reviewers. There was more trainee led discussion on ECMO Sim group than the traditional group.

TABLE 4 Why simulate?

• Zero-risk environment
• Allowance to practice high-risk, low-frequency events without endangering patients!
• Realistic clinical setting
• Reactions close to physiological responses in real life
• Active participation (immersion)
• Real-time: Time pressure

Another two studies conducted by researchers at Le Bonheur Children's aim to better prepare caregivers for high-risk emergencies in the Cardiovascular Intensive Care Unit (CVICU). The first study's findings suggest that simulation based training is an effective method for improving the knowledge, ability and confidence levels of novice ECMO specialists and physician trainees. A second study proves that simulation-based team training is effective in increasing teamwork and collaboration among multidisciplinary teams in the CVICU during an emergency.[6] The study's training course simulated a post-pediatric surgery cardiac arrest, a high-risk clinical situation with high morbidity and mortality. Findings show that participation in the simulation based training improves teamwork, confidence and communication during these high-risk events. The only disadvantage is the anxiety levels of trainees are high and is stressful.[7]

Repeated exposure to simulation is most beneficial to crisis resource management training and single, isolated exposure may not be sufficient **(Table 4)**.[8]

METHODOLOGY

The pre-requisite for the simulation system is the trainee should have a basic knowledge of perfusion and ECMO system. Here the trainee takes an active participation and responds to realistic cues in real-time. This is followed by objective and constructive debriefing by the instructors. The trainees will think, talk and do. He or she will be challenged to raise their performance to a higher level by being forced out of their comfort zone. They will make mistakes and will learn from them. The emphasis will be made to train to weaknesses at personnel and system level. The ideal simulation system has the virtual ECMO circuits which depict all circuit components, allows visualization of data and allows manipulation of the circuit.

SCENARIO DESIGN

Simulation scenario should be designed on real events and on a hierarchy of teaching strategies, i.e. clinical observation, diagnose the abnormality, treat the abnormality (With or without time pressure) and interaction with the team. The scenarios should be designed to meet important needs, with increasing complexity introduced in a controlled way. Scenarios should be practiced and repeated until the trainee passes, and if required to be modified to individual needs. The scenarios to be designed in following steps:

- Objectives
- Scenario
- Instruction to simulator and equipment
- Debriefing.

Objectives

First step to design the scenario is to determine primary learning objectivesand the assessment tools and methods. Create learning and assessment objectives as per the needs of learners. Always incorporate learners background in determining the learning objectives.

Scenario

The next step is to construct a set of norm-scenarios depending on learning objectives. One should focus on one or two learning objectives at a given time and make simplified scenario. The scenario should be realistic and have scientific and clinical merit (written procedures and references). The scenario should be integral to a clinical procedure guideline and include practitioner behaviors and skills that are measurable. The scenario should be from routine management issues to low frequency, high-risk emergencies. This can be used to create a standardized learning experience for all staff, and allow for exposure to very rare events that happen infrequently in clinical practice, but where prompt and correct actions are vital.

It should include scenario from:

- Normal ECMO-run
- Non-acute, non-critical complications during ECMO
- Critical technical events on ECMO
- Critical patient-related events on ECMO.

Normal ECMO-run

For the beginners, initially scenario of normal ECMO-run should be created to acclimatize them with ECMO circuit and parameters. They should learn to interpret patients vital parameter, ECMO-parameters (e.g. pressures in ECMO-system), anti-coagulation status. They should learn to perform basic actions like ACT-measurement, adjustments of ECMO-flow, FiO_2 and sweep gas flow and blood sampling. They should learn to deliver routine care on the ECMO-system like complete check of ECMO-system. These scenario should also make them learn the effect of various actions taken like increasing or decreasing the blood flow, FiO_2, sweep gas and heparin dose. They should also learn circulatory and ventilatory management on VV and VA-ECMO.

Non-acute, Non-critical Complications during ECMO

This includes routine ECMO management decisions, such as decreased venous return or management of a weaning and trial-off for VV and VA ECMO, or identification and management of recirculation. It should also include scenario on team behavior and communication focus, such as during cannulation or intra-hospital patient transport and imaging while on ECMO. This can also include the scenario of cardiac stunning, circuit-induced DIC (Blood clots in ECMO-system), etc.

Critical Technical Events on ECMO

This includes creating different scenarios of mechanical complications or circuit-related complications like oxygenator failure, air in circuit, pump or power failure, Cannula dislocation/malposition—arterial or venous, Tube leakage, etc. they should able to diagnose and treat it accurately. It should also be made with time pressure so as to be more realistic.

Critical Patient-related Events on ECMO

This includes the different scenarios of patient-related complications like bleeding, hypertension, hypotension, desaturation, cardiac arrhythmias and convulsions.

Introduction to Simulator and Equipment

In order to achieve the realism of the scenario experience, equipment and documentation (e.g. case notes, laboratory results, and patient records) potentially required for each scenario needs to be available and believable. These props are crucial. Faculty staff checks equipment and set-up the next scenario during debriefing of the previous scenario by other faculty members. A functioning ECMO system includes an ECMO trolley, gas blender, three pressure transducers (pre-pump, pre-oxygenator, and post-oxygenator), ECMO circuit of variable size according to patient age, oxygenator, heat exchanger and ECMO cannula placed through the neck into the mannequin's chest cavity **(Figure 1)**. The circuit is primed with artificially colored saline to simulate blood. Treatment including oxygen, ventilation, drugs, fluids and blood products are all given realistically, and investigations such as blood gases (patient and ECMO circuit), activated clotting time (ACT) are drawn and results reported in real time. SvO_2 monitoring should also be included in VA ECMO scenario as this is standard on ECMO support.

Trainees are then brought into the simulation room. They are oriented to the ECMO simulator and its capabilities, the equipment available (ventilator, defibrillator, etc.), documentation for patient vital signs, labs, ECMO flow sheets, and imaging studies, and the mechanism for requesting additional information or equipment. An instructor typically serves as a confederate during the scenarios to allow for efficient scenario flow.

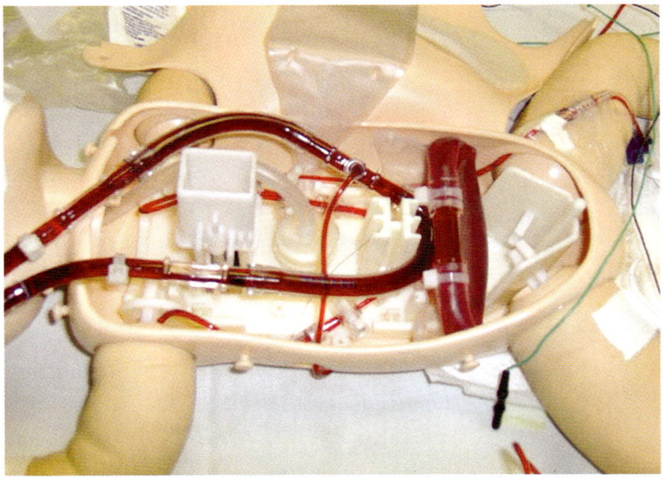

Figure 1 Mannequin's chest cavity with neck cannula

The scenario is then described, including the case history, present status and issues, IV access, and medications. Bedside vital sign flow sheets, ECMO flow sheets, laboratory studies and relevant imaging studies are available for review. Staff members are given the opportunity to ask questions, after which point the simulation takes place. Scenarios are videotaped and then reviewed by trainee and colleagues during debriefing session.

Debriefing

After the simulation is complete, participants move into a separate conference room for debriefing. In the "pre-briefing" period, confidentiality is again discussed, along with a timeframe and plan for the debriefing. All learners are expected to actively participate in the discussion, and the facilitator serves as a guide for the discussion, rather than a "lecturer." During debriefing, mislearning opportunities are being discussed and recommendations provided for improvement of technical and behavioral skills.

Reflection on scenario is very important as it gives impact of the experience. It should be guided by experienced facilitators, should be supportive, safe and with environment of trust. Video-assisted debriefing is strongly recommended as it allows participants to see how they performed rather than how they think they performed. Few centres even utilize 3D Model of Debriefing.[9] This strategy provides learners the opportunity to first "Diffuse" emotions elicited from the simulation.

Summary

The simulation ends with the completion of two simple, written evaluation instruments that give the facilitator and the learner the opportunity to evaluate the learning scenario. Finally, the entire session is analyzed. Here the scenario is tested on the basis of equipment, learner responses, timing, assessment tools, and methods through extensive pilot testing. Here a reflective observation of performance and identification of performance gaps that can be enhanced by facilitator's observations, participants' recalled experiences, and video review. Participants in this phase should ideally acquire new information to build or enhance their own mental model. At the last, facilitator provides a summary of lessons learned and is then carried into clinical practice.

ECMO SIMULATION SYSTEMS

The different type of ECMO simulation system is available which has either mechanical based, computer based or on virtual reality. Many of them have Mannequin human patient simulators. Many centers use custom-made simulators. Commercially, available simulators are:

- Orpheus cardiac perfusion simulator by ULCO technologies.
- *Virtual simulators:*
  - ECMOjo (Mark Ogino et al. University of Hawaii)
  - ECMO simulator from MSE.

The ECMO simulators are classified in to 3 categories depending their functions and computerizations. They are Low fidelity system, Medium Fidelity system and high fidelity system. The one which are easily available are:

- Low fidelity system:
  - *In situ* sim
  - Circulation simulator
- Medium fidelity system:
  - ECMO simulator
- High fidelity system like ECMO Sim
  - Virtual simulator, e.g. ECMOjo
  - Electronic simulator, e.g. MSE

QUALITIES OF SIMULATION SYSTEM

As there are many simulation systems available and many of the centres have their custom-made simulation system, one should have clear idea of what should be the minimum quality of their custom made simulation system.

- *Motive:* Simulation system should either be goal-driven or event driven. Initially, the simulation system should be goal driven and try to focus on what you want to simulate. This can later be modified into event driven and lastly the virtual (a complete artificial patient and ECMO-system).
- *Easy to operate:* It should be easy to operate as doctors are (in general) no computer or electronics geeks.
- *Inexpensive in use:* Budget cuts are common in all fields of medicine.
- *Use original ECMO-console:* This will help to get the realism in training. Candidates are used to the ECMO-console, so modifying or tampering with will distract the candidates and influence the learning experience.
- *Use video- and audiorecording:* Team training and non-technical skill training is very difficult to do without video- and audio-recording.
- *Use a manikin and patient monitor:* This will greatly enhance the sense of realism. Ideally, a manikin which provides feedback of the vital parameters

CIRCULATION SIMULATOR

Circulation simulator is a custom-made low fidelity simulator designed by ECMO physician and ECMO specialist from British Columbia Children's Hospital, Vancouver, BC, Canada.[10] It is a mechanical simulator which may be used in conjunction with any type of computer driven patient simulator, and to which may be attached any type of ECLS circuit: centrifugal or roller pump ECMO circuit, VAD, CRRT or plasmapheresis.

Basic Principle

It is a circulation simulator which has two components of preload (CVP) and afterload (MAP). Preload and afterload can be changed by adjusting the height of the reservoir tank. All the scenarios are created by changing the CVP and MAP of simulator and changing the patient parameters on computer-driven patient simulator **(Figure 2)**.

Scenario Design

The circulation simulator consists of two fluid reservoirs, the "CVP" or pre-load and the "MAP" or after load which connects to the venous and arterial ends of the ECLS circuit respectively. The height, in cm of water, of those columns can be adjusted by means of a height adjustable reservoir drain: that drain empties into a large holding tank. The two reservoirs are in turn filled by a pump submerged in that holding tank.

The ECLS circuit connects to the reservoirs and is turned on, with circuit flow as per scenario to be tested. The circuit "sees" the CVP and MAP reservoirs at the set heights and continuous circuit flow is enabled by the MAP reservoir draining to the holding tank. Fluid is pumped from the holding tank back to the CVP reservoir to the height determined by the adjustable drain.

A variable clamp, remotely controlled, is placed on both the arterial and venous limb of the circuit close to

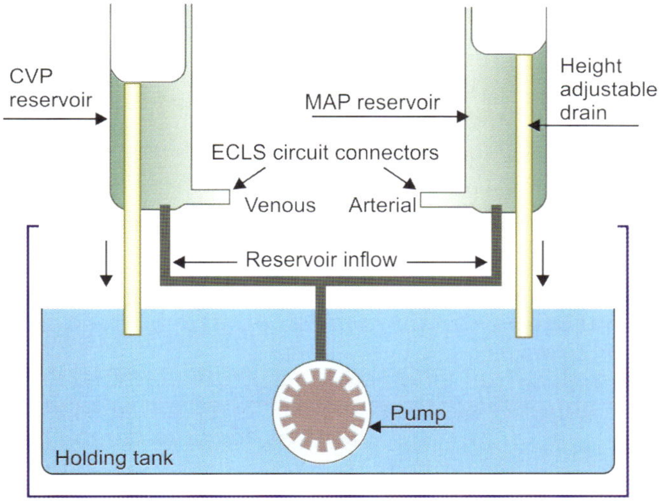

Figure 2 Circulation simulator

TABLE 5 Scenario created with circulatory simulator

Mechanical	*Patient related*
Cannula displacement	Hypovolemia
Cannula kinking	Hypervolemia
Cannula clotting	Temponade
	Tension pneumothorax
	Recirculation on VV-ECMO
	Inadequate sedation
	Hyperthermia
	Hypothermia
	Sepsis/decreased SVR
	Hypertension/increased SVR
	Seizures
	Surgical bleeding

the connection with the simulator, so that resistance to flow in one or both lumens may be applied. A wide range of scenarios may be tested by varying combinations of CVP, MAP and resistance to flow on either the venous or arterial limb of the circuit **(Table 5)**.

Advantages

- Simple in design and construction and could be easily completed by most hospitals, biomedical engineering departments at very modest cost
- Portable and small enough to be used in a typical PICU bed space for "mock code" type training exercises
- Works with the different computer-driven simulator manikins available in the hospital and with all of the different ECLS circuits used in the institution including ECMO, VAD, CRRT, hemodialysis and plasmapheresis.

ECMO SIMULATOR

It is medium-fidelity simulators which can create a complete ECMO simulation environment and is designed by group of people from Radboud University Medical Centre, Nijmegen, Netherlands **(Figures 3A and B)**.[11]

Basic Principle

It is basically a portable ECMO mechanical simulator which is connected with regular ICU simulation system.

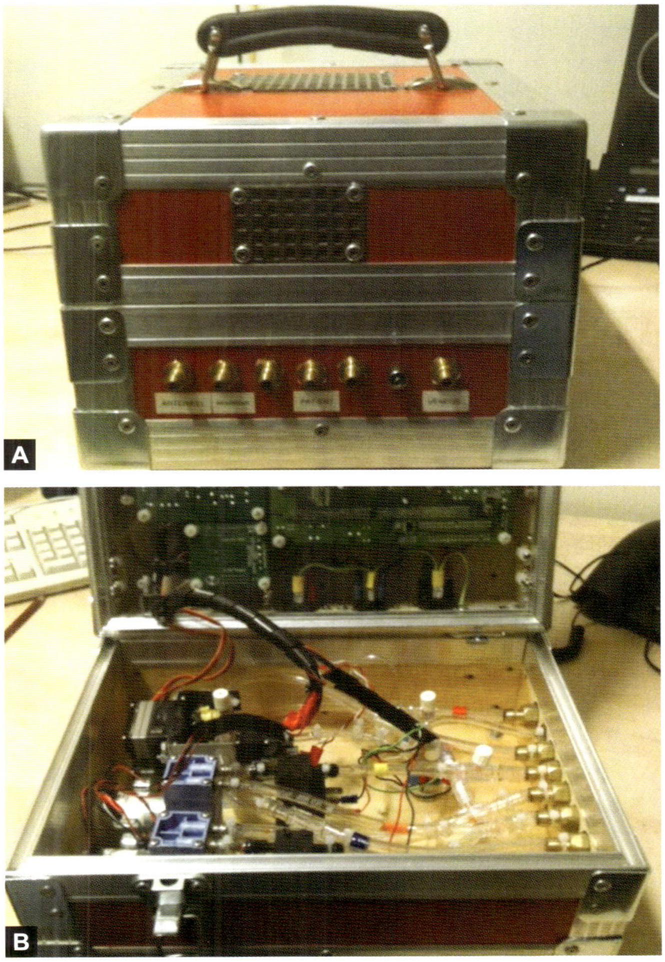

Figures 3A and B ECMO simulator

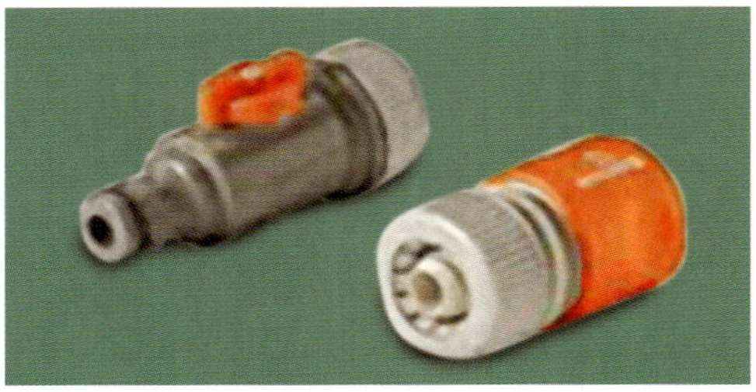

Figure 4 Garden hose

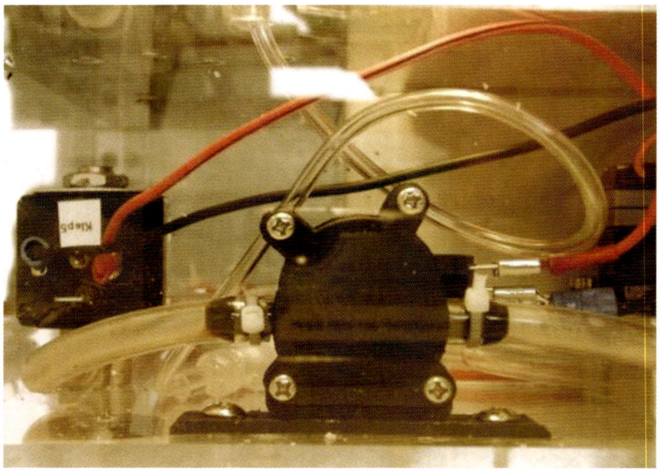

Figure 5 Windshield wiper pump

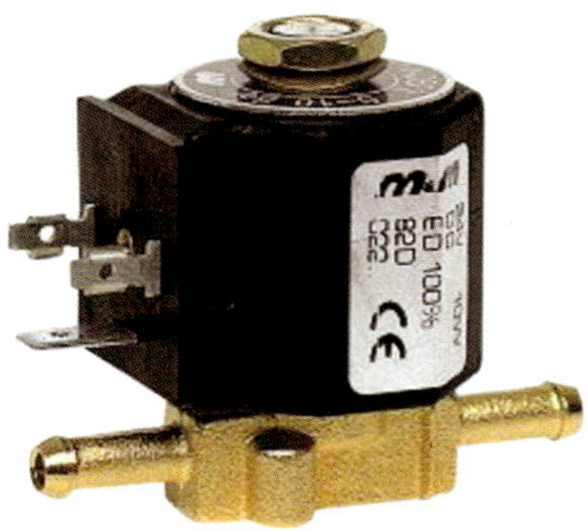

Figure 6 Magnetic valves

ECMO-related scenarios are created by regulating the flow, preload and afterload through the mechanical simulator. This can be achieved by controlling the diameter of servoregulated garden hose **(Figure 4)** and wind-shield wiper pump **(Figure 5)**. Pre- and postoxygenator pressures are controlled by magnetic valves **(Figure 6)**. Hemodynamic changes can be demonstrated by ICU simulators.

Scenario Design

Most of the ECMO-related complications both mechanical as well as patient-related complications can effectively created and even few procedures can be performed by this simulator **(Table 6)**.

Advantages

- Complete real-time wireless control.
- Simulates all common ECMO-related technical emergencies.
- Connection to any ECMO system (roller pump or centrifugal systems).
- Portable system.
- Easy to operate.
- Manikin is connected to the ECMO system which can mimic Heart- and breath sounds, spontaneous breathing movements
- Various procedures like functional intravascular access (umbilical lines, CVP and arterial lines), chest

TABLE 6 Scenarios created with ECMO simulator

Normal ECMO-run
Non-acute, non-critical complications during ECMO:
• Blood gas interpretation on ECMO
• Circulation and ventilation on VV and VA-ECMO
• Anticoagulation therapy
• Imaging on ECMO
• Cardiac stun
• Blood clots in ECMO system
Critical technical events on ECMO:
• Artificial lung failure
• Tubing leakage
• Power failure
• Arterial and venous air embolus
• Cannula dislocation/malposition
• Bladder box alarm
Critical patient-related events on EMO:
• Cardiac temponade
• Hemothorax
• Intracranial bleeding
• Pneumothorax
• Hypertension
• Hypotension
• Desaturation

tube or needle decompression, pericardiocentesis on Manikin is possible.

- Detection of fluid status
- Complete control of venous and arterial side of the ECMO circuit
- Complete patient monitor simulation including arterial and venous curves and real-time ECG.
- Can displays laboratory results, X-ray, ECG or other imaging.

ECMOjo

ECMOjo is a simulator and trainer for extracorporeal membrane oxygenation. ECMOjo is a computer application implemented in Java. ECMOjo is available for all major operating systems including Windows, Macintosh, Linux and Unix.[12] The application consists of a graphical user interface to teach physicians, nurses and students the basics of extracorporeal membrane oxygenation. ECMOjo has been developed by the Telehealth Research Institute (TRI), John A Burns School of Medicine (JABSOM) of the University of Hawaii.

Basic Principle

ECMOjo is a computerized simulator system in which there are pre-set tutorials and scenarios. The tutorial is basically an introduction to the ECLS components and the simulation system. The different scenarios are created with time limit of 5 minutes in which the trainee has to identify problems and correct it. The scenario is being made realistic by online changing values of patient's parameters and constant alarm. Here the tutorials and scenarios are already pre-set and new one cannot be created by the operators.

Scenario Design

All the scenarios are pre-existing **(Figure 7)**. It is divided into three categories—tutorials, scenarios and simulations. Tutorials give a basic introduction to ECMO system and simulation. Then there are various scenarios of ECMO- related complications followed by test simulation in which realistic event of ECMO-related complication is being created and trainee has to diagnose the problem and treat it within the span of 5 minutes **(Table 7)**.

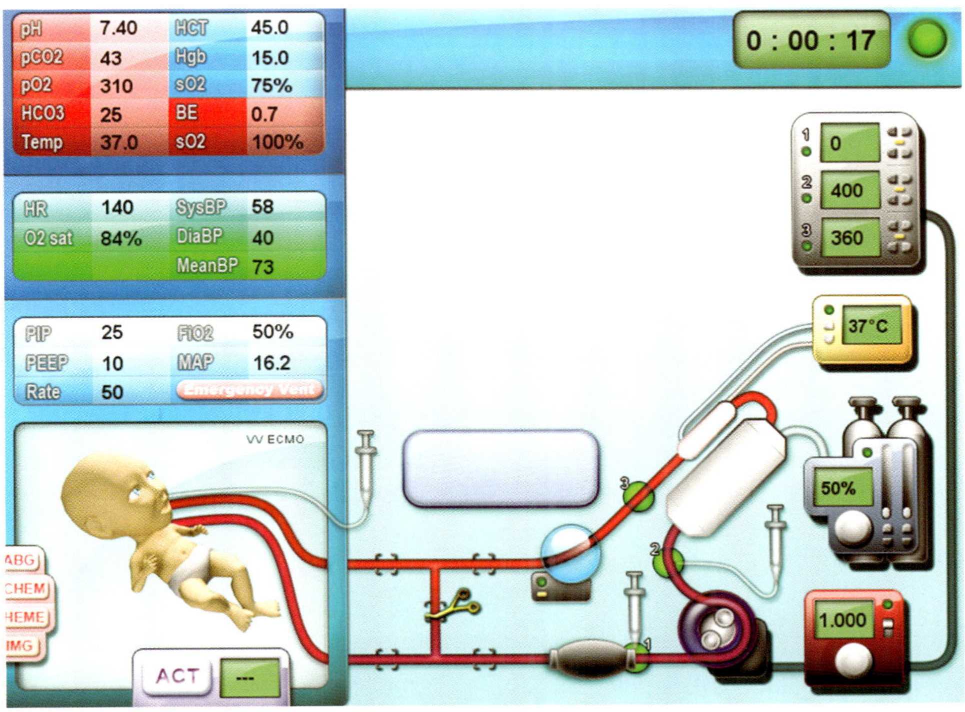

Figure 7 ECMOjo virtual circuit

TABLE 7 Scenarios existing in ECMOjo

Tutorials	*Scenarios*	*Simulations*
Tutorials—overview	Coming off roller pump	Continuous Simulation
Tutorials—introduction	Coming off centrifugal pump	Simulation 1
Tutorials—detail	Large blood loss from circuit	Simulation 2
Tutorials—advanced	Air in arterial limb	Simulation 3
Circuit check	Accidental arterial decannulation	Simulation 4
Temperature control	Pump failure	
Sweep gas 1	Air in venous limb	
Sweep gas 2	VA ECMO pump flow	
	VV ECMO pump flow	
	Oxygenator failure	
	Oxygenator rupture	
	Circuit failure	
	High preoxygenator pressure	
	High postoxygenator pressure	
	Negative venous pressure	
	ECMOism	

Advantages

It has a virtual circuits **(Figure 7)** and patient with different patient parameters and treatment options. One can see the real time effect of treatment given in a simplified form. Few scenarios are with time pressure and have to be solved in that particular time. This helps in realistic feeling and also helps to sharpens reflexes. At the end of the scenario, there is a session of debriefing which helps the trainee to understand their mistakes.

MSE SYSTEM

The MSE ECMO simulator is a screen-based implementation of a high-fidelity, medical simulation system—The Modular Simulation Environment (MSE).[13] It is being developed by Dr DA Pybus from Sydney, Australia. The simulator can be installed on computers running under the 32 or 64 bit versions of the Microsoft 'Windows XP', 'Vista' or 'Windows 7' operating systems. It has been designed for use by single users or small groups in a 'tutorial' setting and is intended to run on a 'Full HD' television display or a computer which has a screen resolution of at least 1920 × 1080 pixels. It is available in 3 version—evaluation version, personal version and Institutional version **(Figure 8)**.

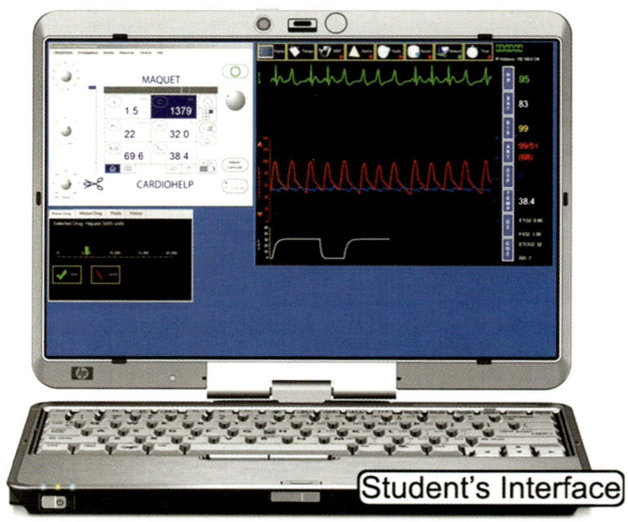

Figure 8 MSE system—trainee screen

Basic Principle

It is basically a software program which consists of the unsupervised mode and supervised mode. The ECLS circuit is not present in this system. Unsupervised mode is basically a demonstration of different complication and management of ECMO. The supervised mode consists of two computers one for the trainee and other for supervisor or instructor. In this, the instructor creates different situation on computer by altering different parameters and trainee has to identify problem and can try the various treatment modality available on it. One can even see the effect of treatment given by them. This system helps one to understand the complete case scenario of ECMO right from initiation of ECMO till weaning along with all possible ups and down of the ECMO run. The patient consists of about 20 real-time models, which can be adjusted by a supervisor to reproduce a wide variety of clinical states. The trainee can then treat the patient using any of the available devices or drugs.

Scenario Design

The simulator incorporates various MSE components which include a 'Virtual' patient, Centrifugal pump-based ECMO system Hollow-fibre oxygenator, Physiological monitor, Ventilator and Defibrillator.[14] It has the compendium of drugs and fluids which can be used to treat the 'virtual' patient. It also has data recording system in which the digital data can be saved in terms of some photos, videos, power point slides, PDF formats, etc. This 'Scenario' database can be used to provide a large variety of relevant clinical data to the trainee. This can be used to make virtual case more lively and realistic. It also has Series of VV and VA ECMO tutorials **(Table 8)**.

TABLE 8 Scenarios created with MSE

• Variation in blood flow through the oxygenator
• Variation in gas flow through the oxygenator
• Heating or cooling of the patient
• Changing the position of the drainage cannula
• Insertion of a second drainage cannula
• Changing the size of the return cannula
• Changes in central venous pressure on venous drainage
• The impact of VA ECMO on systemic blood flow
• Differential hypoxemia (circulation)
• Back flow through the system
• Oxygenator failure
• Inlet obstruction
• Outlet obstruction
• Fresh gas disconnection
• Massive blood loss
• Changes in lung function
• Changes in cardiac function

Advantages

It is software-based virtual program so one can create the scenario by themselves and can have actual ECMO run starting from initiation to weaning and trial off. No ECMO circuit so circuit-related issues cannot be taken care like air in circuit clots in circuit, etc.

Summary

Thus ECMO simulation system is more interesting, more intellectually engaged and helps to develop cognitive, technical and behavioral skills. It also helps in reducing the response time. ECMO simulation is a new learning tool which is 10% science, 10% programming and 80% fun. High-fidelity simulation with well-staged and realistic scenarios followed by a debriefing session appears to be the most promising educational tool for health-care team members.[15-18] With the use of high fidelity simulators, ECMO can be simulated in a laboratory environment, and the care team can practice high-risk situations without fear of adverse outcome to a real patient.[19]

The ECMO simulation program has been used to identify systems issues and change practice to improve patient safety. Issues identified during ECMO simulations helped to streamline the process of medication administration. Team training has been widely recognized as a method by which to improve patient safety and decrease rates of medical errors. Development of an institutional ECMO simulation program confers many benefits for all members of the multidisciplinary ECMO team. Working with perfusionists and simulation specialists, a wide variety of clinical experiences can be recreated, including routine management decisions as well as emergency situations. Combining these clinical experiences with effective debriefing allows adult learners to enhance their understanding of the clinical situations and improve their skills. These sessions can be used to guide quality improvement efforts, and further enhance patient safety initiatives.

REFERENCES

1. Halamek LP, et al. *http://www.pediatrics.org/cgi/content/full/106/4/e45.* [Online]
2. Rogalski J, Plat M, Antolinn-Glenn P. Training for collective competence in rare and unpredictable situations. R Samurcay, M Fischer N Boreham (Eds). Work Process Knowledge. London: Routledge : S.N., 2004.
3. Bosseau MW, Foster PA. Crisis resource management amongst strangers: principles of organising a multidisciplinary group for crisis resource management. J Clin Anaes. 2000;12:633-8.
4. Burton KS, Pendergrass TL, Byczkowski TL, Taylor RG, Moyer MR, Falcone RA, Geis GL. Impact of simulation-based extracorporeal membrane oxygenation training in the simulation laboratory and clinical environment. Simul Health Care. 2011;6:284-91.
5. Anderson JM, Murphy AA, Boyle BB, Yaeger KA, Halamek LP. Simulating extracorporeal membrane oxygenation (ECMO) emergencies, Part II: Qualitative and Quantitative assessment and validation. Simulation in Healthcare. 2006;1:228-32.
6. Figueroa, Mayte, Shah, Samir, et al. Studies-show-benefit-of-ECMO-simulation. *http://www.lebonheur.org/articles.* [Online] 2013.
7. GR Nimmo, G Wylie, J Scarth, J Simpson, E Gracie, I Torrance, M Liddell, C Davies. Critical events simulation for neonatal and paediatric extracorporeal membrane oxygenation. Journal of Intensive Care Society. 2008;9:1:20-2.
8. Stocker M, Allen M, Pool N, Costa KD, et al. Impact of an embedded simulation team training programme in a paediatric intensive care unit: a prospective, single-centre, longitudinal study. Journal of Intensive Care Medicine. 2011;10:2371-5.
9. Zigmont JJ, Kappus LJ, Sudikoff SN. Seminars in Perinatology. 2011;35:52-8.
10. Cogswell A, Pitfield S, Chalmers M, Mintak R, Salt D, Singh AJ. Use of a circulation simulator for teaching and skills maintenance in an ECLS Program. Vancouver, BC, Canada: British Columbia Children's Hospital.
11. Timothy Antonius. Workshop ECMO Simulation challenges and lessons learned. [prod.] Radboud University Medical Centre. Nijmegen, Netherlands : S.N.
12. ECMOjo. *http://ecmojo.sourceforge.net/.* [Online] Telehealth Research Institute (TRI), John A Burns School of Medicine (JABSOM) of the University of Hawaii, 2009.
13. Pybus DA. Adult ECMO simulator. *www.ecmosimulation.com.* [Online] MSE (Australia) PL, 2009.
14. ECMO Simulation User Manual v 5.4. *www.ecmosimulation.com.* [Online] MSE (Australia) PL, 2010.
15. Sahu S, Lata I. Simulation in resuscitation teaching and training: an evidence based practice review. J Emerg Trauma Shock. 2010;3:378-84.
16. Schroder T, van Heymann CH, Ortwein H, Ran J, Wernecke KD, Spies C. Simulation-based anaesthesia crisis resource management training. Results of a survey on learning success. Anaesthesist. 2009;58:992-1004.
17. VanSchaik SM, von Kohorn I, O'Sullivan P. Pediatric resident confidence in resuscitation skills relates to mock code experience. Clin Pediatr. 2008;47:777-83.
18. Dine CJ, Gersk RE, Leary M, Rigby BS, Bellini LM, Abella BS. Improving cardiopulmonary resuscitation quality and resuscitation training by combining audiovisual feed back and debriefing. Crit Care Med. 2008;36(10):2817-22.
19. Anderson JM, Murphy AA, Boyle BB, Yaeger KA, Halamek LP. Simulating extracorporeal membrane oxygenation (ECMO) emergencies to improve human performance, Part I: Methodologic and Technologic Innovations. Simulation in Healthcare. 2006;1:220-7.

Chapter 33

Simulation in Pain Medicine

GP Dureja, Dhruv Bibra

Chapter Outline

- Need for Simulation in Pain Medicine
- Techniques of Simulation in Pain Medicine
- Case Scenarios
- Challenges of Simulation in Pain Medicine

INTRODUCTION

A training simulation is a virtual medium through which various types of skills can be acquired. Training simulations has been used in a wide variety of genres; however, they are commonly used in corporate situations to improve business awareness and management skills, aviation industries, fire departments, disaster management, etc.

Primum non-nocere 'above all, do no harm' is considered a fundamental of medical practice. Medicine has traditionally relied on a '**see one, do one**' approach to learning and experience. This inevitably exposes patients to inexperienced healthcare practitioners, and the dangers and harm associated with this are increasingly unacceptable. The term 'learning curve' has repeatedly been used to account for higher complication and mortalities, as well as longer procedure times, among inexperienced practitioners and teams. Climbing the steep learning curve can no longer be done by trial and error.

Medical schools and residencies are currently facing a shift in their teaching paradigm. The increasing amount of medical information and research makes it difficult for medical education to stay current in its curriculum. As patients become increasingly concerned that students and residents are "practicing" on them, clinical medicine is becoming focused more on patient safety and quality than on bedside teaching and education. Educators have faced these challenges by restructuring curricula, developing small-group sessions, and increasing self-directed learning and independent research. Nevertheless, a disconnect still exists between the classroom and the clinical environment. Many students feel that they are inadequately trained in history taking, physical examination, diagnosis, and management.

Medical simulation has been proposed as a technique to bridge this educational gap. In medical training, simulation has been demonstrated to lead to improvements in medical knowledge, comfort in procedures, and improvements in performance during retesting in simulated scenarios. Simulation has also been shown to be a reliable tool for assessing learners and for teaching topics such as teamwork and communication. Multiple studies have demonstrated the effectiveness of simulation in the teaching of basic science and clinical knowledge, procedural skills, teamwork, and communication as well as assessment at the undergraduate and graduate medical education level.[1]

NEED FOR SIMULATION IN PAIN MEDICINE

Pain medicine services, both hospital- and freestanding clinic–based, provide diagnosis and treatment for patients with a wide range of pain complaints. These include those associated with perioperative pain control, cancer-related pain, and chronic pain due to a variety of underlying causes. Providers of these services come from multiple primary specialties, including anesthesiology, neurology, physiatry, internal and oncologic medicine, rheumatology, surgery, and nursing. The treatment of pain, chronic and cancer related often requires a multidisciplinary approach, involving pharmacologic management, invasive procedures, psychological or psychiatric evaluation, and physical therapy. Although serious adverse treatment-related events rarely occur, the potential for acute life-threatening complications is inherent to the medications and procedures that are routinely used in pain medicine. In addition, the practice of pain medicine regularly generates ethical and interpersonal challenges for healthcare providers. The management of critical events requires practiced skillful action and teamwork. The wide range of training backgrounds and experience of pain practitioners at any acute medical complication adds to this general need for practiced teamwork.[2]

The role of simulation in training programs is variable; however, in technical specialties such as surgery and anesthesiology it is quickly becoming standard. Pain fellowship programs are relatively short in duration, and must teach clinical diagnostic skills, pharmacology, pathophysiology, and interventional skills to fellows with varying residency backgrounds and skill sets. However, observing these skills and offering feedback for improvement is challenging in a short duration of fellowship. Simulation offers fellows increased opportunities to safely develop skills in emergency scenarios, and in communication and professionalism.

Simulation provides active learning as fellows experience challenging patient scenarios, stressful peri-procedural events, and cases that require emergency algorithm recall and action. An example is the simulation of total spinal anesthesia requiring airway and hemodynamic support during a stellate ganglion block, followed by the challenging conversation discussing the complication with the patient's family. Learners take turns participating as the physician, and participate in additional roles to gain team situation awareness. Faculty members participate as moderators and lead the postsimulation discussion and debriefing. Simulation ensures fellows' exposure to rare but potentially devastating crisis situations and allows opportunities for observed fellow-driven patient interactions and self-reflection. It is unknown how performance in these simulations correlates to clinical skills, however, prior meta-analysis has shown improved outcomes after simulation training across many medical specialties.

TECHNIQUES OF SIMULATION IN PAIN MEDICINE

Clinical Simulation

The specialty of pain medicine is a discipline within the field of medicine that is concerned with the prevention of pain, and the evaluation, treatment, and rehabilitation of persons in pain. Some conditions may have pain and associated symptoms arising from a discrete cause, such as postoperative pain or pain associated with a malignancy, or may be conditions in which pain constitutes the primary problem, such as neuropathic pains or headaches **(Figure 1)**.[2]

Pain medicine specialists use a broad-based approach to treat all pain disorders, ranging from pain as a symptom of disease to pain as the primary disease. The pain physician serves as a consultant to other physicians but is often the principal treating physician (as distinguished from the primary care physician) and may provide care at various levels, such as treating the patient directly, prescribing medication, prescribing rehabilitative services, performing pain relieving procedures, counseling patients and families, directing a multidisciplinary team, coordinating care with other healthcare providers and providing consultative

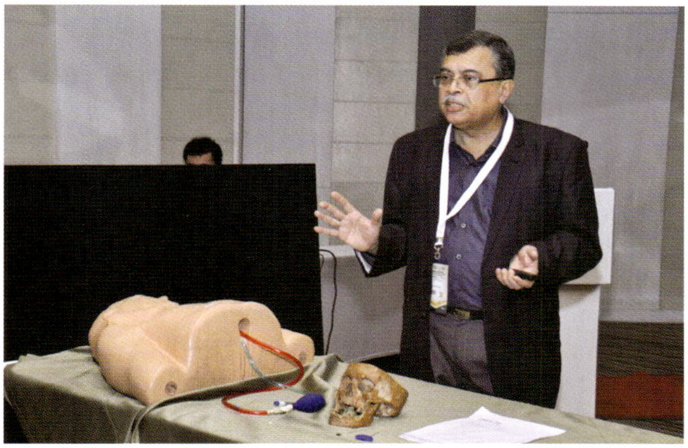

Figure 1 Simulation for Pain—teaching pain blocks with hands-on training on the simulator limbs and body is best practice for perfecting the art

services to public and private agencies pursuant to optimal health care delivery to the patient suffering from pain. The objective of the pain physician is to provide quality care to the patient suffering from pain. The pain physician may work in a variety of settings and is competent to treat the entire range of pain encountered in delivery of quality health care.

Pain medicine specialists typically formulate comprehensive treatment plans, which consider the patients' cultural contexts, as well as the special needs of the pediatric and geriatric populations. Evaluation techniques include interpretation of historical data; review of previous laboratory, imaging, and electrodiagnostic studies; assessment of behavioral, social, occupational, and avocational issues; and interview and examination of the patient by the pain specialist.

The cornerstone of pain medicine is history taking and detailed clinical examination of the patient. Keeping these principles in mind lot of emphasis needs to be given on this aspect. Hence clinical simulation can be further divided into:

- Clinical history
- Examination
- Making a diagnosis and then management plan.

Clinical History

Taking a relevant history goes a long way in diagnosing and treating painful conditions. Hence lot of emphasis needs to be given on this aspect. The bases of good clinical history taking can be taught as well as tested by means of simulating good clinical scenarios. All these scenarios need to be under the hawk of a good moderator who can really guide the trainee in improving his clinical skills **(Table 1)**. The skills can be assessed on the grounds of confidence, ability to connect with the patient, extraction of relevant medical history, etc. depending on the module design and level of the clinician being assessed.

TABLE 1 Critical skills that can be taught and evaluated in simulation sessions

• Critical event recognition
• Teamwork
• Communication skills
• Patient care handsoff
• Group dynamics
• Empathetic listening
• Crisis management

Examination

A thorough medical examination needs to be done based on the medical history of the patient. This aspect requires greatest amount of learning as a mistake can influence the management of the patient greatly. An error at this level can land the physician in a legal soup, e.g an absence of ankle jerk is a contraindication for any interventional procedure. Hence, a patient or a computer generated simulation is preferred.

Making a Diagnosis and Management Plan

Based on the clinical history and examination the pain physician should be able to make a provisional diagnosis.

We investigate the patient to come to the final diagnosis. These investigations must be discussed with the patient and his relatives to explain the importance of the investigation in the management of the patient. After proper evaluation of the investigations we come to the final diagnosis. The management plan is made for the patient depending on the final diagnosis. The management protocols developed by the institutes based on evidence based data needs to be followed.

Patient or computer based simulation algorithms based on the combination of history, examination and specific investigation can be created and the competence of the pain physician needs to be tested. This apart from testing the basic skill of the person can be used as a tool for constant evaluation and quality control among pain relief providers.

Procedural Simulation

Interventions are an important tool in the armamentarium of pain physicians. A pain physician should be fully trained in these procedures before performing them on real patients. Interventional techniques are performed under imaging guidance {fluoroscopy, ultrasonography (USG), computed tomography (CT) Scan} and very rarely blindly based on anatomical landmarks. Therefore simulation techniques have to be developed keeping these things into perspective. Mannequins compatible with fluoroscope are used for performing intricate spinal interventions under real time imaging.

Kohman injection Phantom is another simulation devise used for learning interventions techniques employed in pain medicine.

Crisis Simulation (Emergency Situation Simulation)

In the simulation-based educational experience, the participant should be able to do the following:

- Use principles of crisis resource management and institute appropriate life support measures to deal with an acute medical complication of pain medicine treatment;
- Implement a team process for ethical decision making in an acute pain medicine-related situation;
- Understand the principles of pain medicine-related medical error evolution, prevention, and treatment and be able to appropriately disclose and apologize to patients and their families for medical errors when they occur.

Because of the rare and essentially unpredictable nature of critical events in pain medicine practice, the educational program should ideally include all the aspects of crisis management.

CASE SCENARIOS

Case 1: *Esponding to catastrophic decompensation during Stellate Ganglion Block*

A middle-aged patient receives a local anesthetic block of the stellate ganglia performed by a junior trainee (actor) under the supervision of the course participant. The trainee impulsively injects the medication before instruction from the course participant. There are 4 possible complications that can be simulated: a vasovagal reaction (bradycardia and cardiovascular collapse), an intravascular injection of local anesthetic (seizure or cardiac dysrhythmias), a pneumothorax (hypotension and respiratory difficulty) caused by misplacement of the needle into the nearby pleural space, and an intrathecal injection in the nearby spinal canal resulting in high spinal anesthesia (respiratory arrest). The participant will need to manage the acute physiologic derangements depending on the complication depicted.

Case 2: *Resuscitating anaphylaxis in the pain clinic*

A middle-aged paraplegic inpatient presents to the pain clinic requiring an epidural steroid injection for severe back pain. During the procedure, the patient, while in the prone position, develops an anaphylactic reaction to an antibiotic that was previously started. The simulation can proceed to mild or severe consequences of anaphylaxis.

CHALLENGES OF SIMULATION IN PAIN MEDICINE

There have been rapid advances in the technology, augmented availability and a growing belief that simulation is a useful and appropriate tool for training healthcare practitioners of the future. Although high-tech simulators are exciting, to date most advances in simulation have been made through low-fidelity, low-cost approaches. This is important because simulation has tremendous potential to be used globally, removing the patient from the healthcare practitioner's learning curve and improving patient safety.

Nonetheless, simulation-based medical education should not be viewed as a panacea or silver bullet to solve current challenges within the healthcare system: working hour's restrictions, patient safety, quality and service targets and the emergence of new technologies.

Although simulation-based training can certainly extinguish the early part of the learning curve, instill the adoption of safe practices and reduce patient harm, it is unlikely that simulation will replace the importance of key clinical experiences, and learning from them. Furthermore, the road to expertise might only be achieved through clinical practice rather than repeated exposure within the simulation laboratory.

Ultimately, the major challenge to adopting simulation-based training is to show that a difference is being made on real clinical outcomes.

In the macro environment, it is likely that simulation-based training will become the norm. Practicing in an environment where it is permissible to make mistakes and being able to do so repetitively and deliberately, will improve training outcomes.

It is necessary for simulation-based training to be fully integrated and funded within training programs for clinicians at all stages. It is also necessary to train the trainers through the development of a skilled faculty of expert clinical facilitators, supported by adjunctive support staff in dedicated simulation suites. Further research is needed to extend the use of simulation to serve as a tool in identifying suboptimal performers, credentialing, revalidation and learning new technologies. There must also be a move away from using experience as a proxy for competence and, on a continuous basis, to analyze a practitioner's skills. Simulation, therefore, has an immense capacity to become an integral part of the drive to build a safer healthcare system for patients everywhere.

REFERENCES

1. American Board of Anesthesiologists. Simulation Education: American Society of Anesthesiologists. 2012 Park Ridge, IL American Society of Anesthesiologist.
2. Brenner, Gary J Nemark, Jordan L, Raemer, Daniel. Curriculum and Cases for Pain Medicine Crisis Resource Management Education Anesthesia and Analgesia. 2013;116(1):107-10.

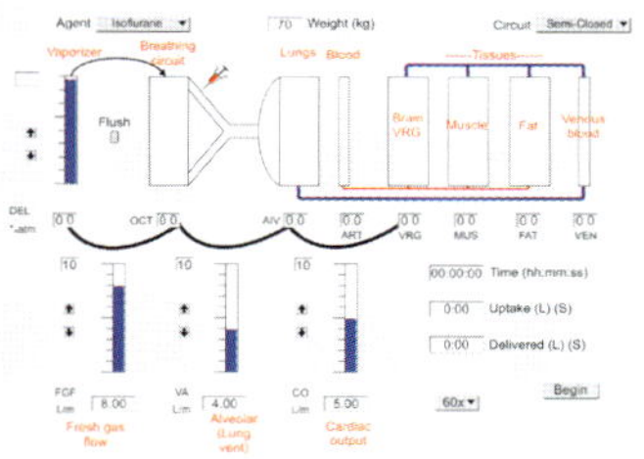

Section 9

Simulation, Cardiac Critical Care and Resources

Section Outline

- Analysis of Inhalation Agents: Using Simulated Gas Man® Model
- Simulation Resources
- Simulation in Cardiac Critical Care Medicine

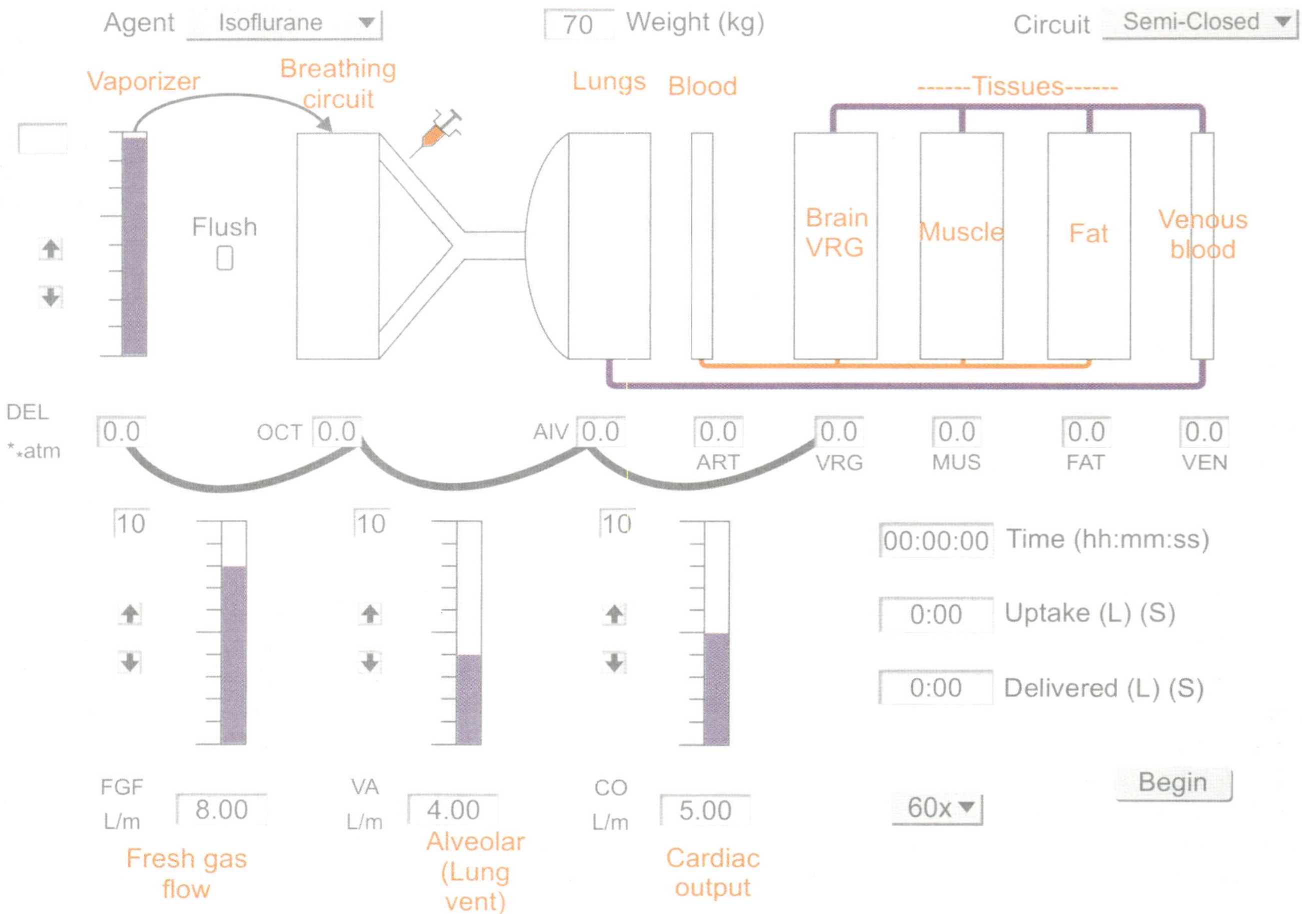
Agent
Isoflurane
70
Weight (kg)
Circuit
Semi-Closed
Vaporizer
Breathing circuit
Lungs
Blood
------Tissues------
Flush
Brain VRG
Muscle
Fat
Venous blood
DEL
*atm
0.0
OCT
0.0
AIV
0.0
0.0
ART
0.0
VRG
0.0
MUS
0.0
FAT
0.0
VEN
10
10
10
00:00:00
Time (hh:mm:ss)
0:00
Uptake (L) (S)
0:00
Delivered (L) (S)
FGF
L/m
8.00
VA
L/m
4.00
CO
L/m
5.00
60x
Begin
Fresh gas flow
Alveolar (Lung vent)
Cardiac output

Chapter 34

Analysis of Inhalation Agents: Using Simulated Gas Man® Model

Rakesh Garg

Chapter Outline

INTRODUCTION

The understanding of pharmacokinetics of inhaled anesthetic agents has been well described. It is described in terms of various physiological models based on tissue partition coefficients, tissue perfusion and different tissue compartments. In spite of this knowledge, its applicability and its understanding for a specific patient or in other words, its clinical application for a particular patient remains complex. Also, as teacher, explaining these concepts to novice or at times, even trained anesthesiologists becomes difficult because of various models, concepts, mathematics and its relation to clinical application. The understanding of few concepts related to volatile anesthetics like use of low flow to an experience anesthesiologists (not using low flow), becomes difficult in the absence of its demonstration. Experimenting or learning on patient model may not always be acceptable.

NEED OF SIMULATION

The pharmacokinetics of inhalational agents has been reported in the literature with extensive evaluation leading to development of complex compartmental models to understand the distribution of volatile inhalational agents in humans.[1] The kinetics of inhalational agents is difficult to understand or to teach. The present understanding is based on these theoretical backgrounds. Its extrapolation to clinical application is difficult. These difficulties entail the need of an easy to understand simulator. With the evolving concepts of multi-compartment model, understanding kinetics and distribution of the drugs including inhalational agents becomes more complex and difficult to interpret using mathematical models in real time scenarios.

Simulation has come a big way in medical sciences for understanding various medical aspects without compromising the safety of patient. Its repeatability, standardization, "stop and go" technique, practice at ease, recording, storing and rewinding are the various advantages of simulation. Valid and reliable simulated clinical scenarios based on learning objective may be prepared for teaching and learning.

The use of simulators in anesthesia practice is evolving rapidly. Several types of simulators are available starting from simple mannequins to advanced high fidelity mannequin.[2] The fidelity is related to its extent of mimicking to real time clinical scenario. These may be associated with computer based software to understand complex situation in graphical representation or related to clinical end point.

SIMULATION FOR VOLATILE ANESTHETICS

Computer based simulations were developed to understand the complex models for understanding and teaching purpose.[3-6] The impact of variables affecting the inhalational agent kinetics like ventilation parameters, cardiac output has been incorporated in these models to analyze their impact. Such tools are necessary as inhaled anesthetics are used round the world for millions of patients and its increasing use mandates its thorough understanding by its user anesthesiologists.

GAS MAN® MODEL SIMULATION FOR VOLATILE ANESTHETICS

The Gas Man® is computer based software simulator and is considered a low fidelity simulator.[5] The Gas Man® model has been updated frequently to incorporate variables to match the real time situations. These simulators are an easy tool for understanding and teaching various aspects including pharmacokinetics of inhalational agents. These are also considered as excellent tool for changing the behaviors of anesthesiologists like explaining the benefits of using low flow anesthesia, etc.

The pharmacokinetics of inhalational agents is usually considered by the physiological model. The Gas Man® simulation uses physiological model and thus relevant variables have been incorporated to mimic real time clinical scenario. This simulator uses Euler's method for the simultaneous differential equations. The Gas Man® model is based on four compartments distribution including the lung, vessel-rich group, muscle, and fat in addition to a breathing circuit as an additional compartment. This is based on understanding of the tissue partition coefficients, tissue volumes and organ blood flows.[7]

Gas Man® simulation is based on Euler integration with linear coefficients that govern the five compartment system to represent breath-by-breath kinetics of inhalational agents.[8] The Gas Man® utilizes standard values for organ volumes, anesthetic solubility and regional blood flows.

This tool has been used for various purposes:[5,8,9]

- To learn inhalational anesthesia concepts
- To teach inhalational anesthesia principles and kinetics
- To experiment various inhalational anesthesia options
- To plan an anesthesia with different clinical scenarios
- To understand and interpret the anesthetic monitors
- To design inhalational agents experiments.

The different concepts that could be understood by Gas Man® simulation are:[5,8-11]

- One compartment model and its step response or wash- in
- Two sequential compartments
- Alveolar tension curve
- Plateau height determined by blood/gas solubility
- Overpressure and optimal anesthesia course for clinical anesthesia
- Concentration effect
- Low flow anesthesia
- Closed circuit anesthesia with liquid injection
- Second gas effect
- Emergence
- Effect of patient weight on inhalational kinetics
- Analyzing cost of agents and techniques **(Figure 1)**.

Gas Man® simulation is a computer simulation (screen based simulation program and runs on Microsoft and Apple operating systems) for simulation to understand pharmacokinetics, i.e. uptake and distribution of the inhalational agents.[4,5,8,11] It utilizes mathematical model for kinetics of inhalational agents and displays in pictorial and graphical representation of the volatile agent and vapor tension for better understanding and capture **(Figure 2)**.

The agents include desflurane, enflurane, ether, halothane, isoflurane, nitrogen, nitrous oxide,

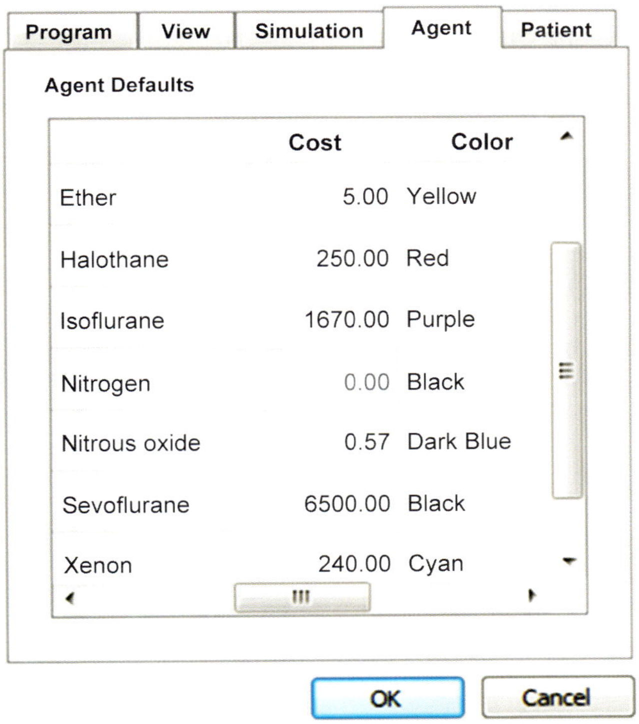

Figure 1 The Inhalational agents and their costs in Gas Man® model

sevoflurane, and xenon **(Figure 1)**. The vaporizer concentration and fresh gas flow will be as per user setting[8] **(Figure 2)**. Other parameters that can be set include volatile agent(s), circuit type, alveolar ventilation, cardiac output, weight of the patient[8] **(Figure 3)**.

The interactive graphics displays the inhalational volatile agent concentration in various tissue compartments at various time periods. The Gas Man® simulation displays the tension of volatile agents in various compartments like breathing circuit, lungs, arterial blood, vessel rich group (including brain), muscle, fat, and venous blood.[8] **(Figures 4 and 5)**.

The Gas Man® simulation has interestingly refute certain clinical practice like changing from isoflurane to desflurane toward the end of anesthesia accelerate recovery, hyperventilation speeds emergence etc.[12] Other important clinical practice confirmed by Gas Man® model includes use of vital capacity induction for loss of consciousness, simulated context-sensitive decrement times explain recovery profiles, usefulness of low gas flow over high fresh gas flow, advantage of reducing fresh gas flow and not the vaporizer setting during intubation procedure, re-anesthetization with hypoventilation after extubation etc.[8] This highlights the usefulness of this simulation model in clinical practice. It allows practicing impact of various techniques related to inhalational anesthesia like overpressure, impact of high and low flow of gases, the type of circuits used (open, closed, semi close) and its impact, and helps in exploring various tissue solubility and various alveolar inhalational concentrations and its extrapolation to clinical parameters. It allows understanding of routine and advanced clinical techniques related to the use of inhalational agents. The understanding of simple single-compartment wash-in to more complex multi-compartment model is easier with Gas Man® simulations. The interaction of multiple agents may also be mimicked here and can be compared using an overylay graph[8] **(Figure 6)**.

The financial implication of various inhalational techniques can be assessed **(Figure 6)**. This model also allows comparing various techniques for inhalational agents and this may help in better understanding to the extent of acceptance of better technique. This simulator is a good tool for understanding concepts related to induction techniques like vital capacity breath, three minute tidal volume breath with regards to inhalational agents. It explains in easier representation the concept of vaporizer overpressure and brief high fresh gas flow for altering the faster anesthetic depth alterations. The understanding of second gas effect and concentration effect can be represented using this model. The interaction of ventilation changes (hyperventilation, hypoventilation, normoventilation) and cardiac output changes (reduced or increased) and its impact on inhalational agent uptake and changes in anesthetic depth may be understood using the Gas Man® simulation **(Figure 3)**. The implication of hypoventilation after emergence and reanesthetization if muscle tissue has achieved 1 MAC anesthetic tension may also be understood. The impact of various parameters like breathing circuit, venous return, anesthetic uptake, and liquid vaporization can be altered to clarify concepts of kinetics in the Gas Man® simulation.[8] The second gas effect can be mimicked by including or removing the effect of uptake on ventilation.[8] The uptake characteristics of various inhalational agents in different clinical scenarios can be run on the simulation models. The volatile agent effect changes with change in cardiac output. The cardiac output varied intraoperatively due to various

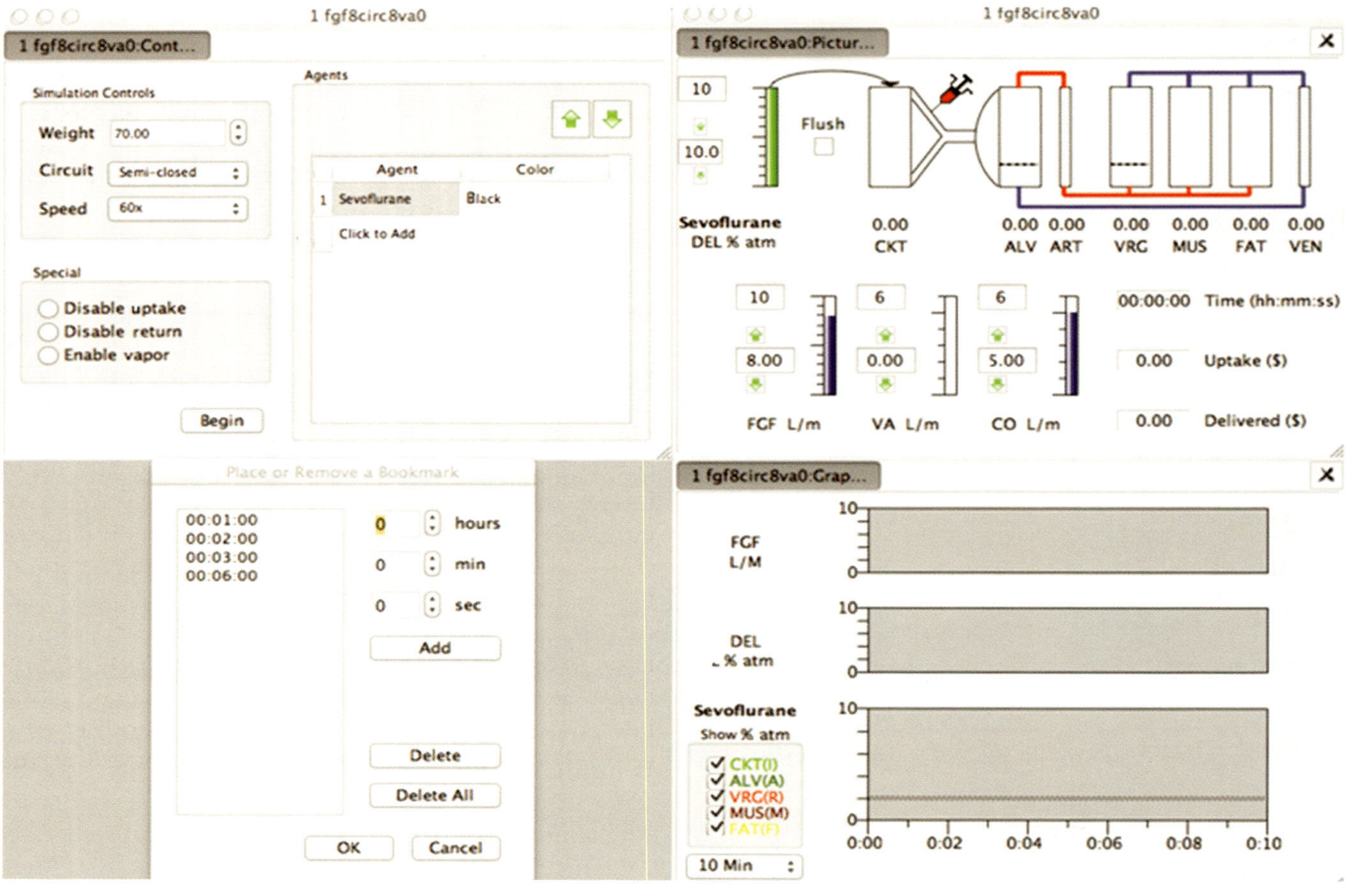

Figure 2 Screen of Gas Man® simulation showing settings, pictorial and graphical representation of various parameters

reasons like drugs, stress, regional blocks, volume status, etc. this at times mandates use of cardiac output monitor. The Gas Man® model can predict the impact of inhalational agents based on change in cardiac output. By entering the cardiac output parameters, the Gas Man® simulation will automatically show the changes on the inhalational agent. The discrepancy between the vaporizer dial concentration and gas analyzer inspired agent concentration is seen especially with low flows and in a rebreathing circuit. The understanding of dilution effect of rebreathing can be simulated in the Gas Man® model.

The awakening after the stoppage of an inhalational agent would depend on many factors including volatile agent tissue solubility and duration of its use. The solubility varies among tissues as well. Some tissues equilibrate faster like brain, heart, liver, kidney, while other tissue compartments like muscle and skin are slower and further tissues like fat are the slowest. It is well known fact the agents like desflurane and sevoflurane will have faster awakening as compared to agents like isoflurane or halothane due to differences in solubility. However, based on duration of its usage in a patient, the prediction of awakening time may be done using Gas Man® model.[13]

It was evaluated whether kinetics of different anesthetic agents generated by a physiological uptake model of Gas Man® are comparable to human compartmental model and found to be comparable.[7] It was reported that pretest and post-test scores of residents improved with regard to understanding of various aspects of uptake and distribution of inhalational agents when they were made to understand kinetics using Gas Man® model.[14]

The prediction of the outcomes with a set of settings for the use of inhalational agent in a particular patient

SECTION 9

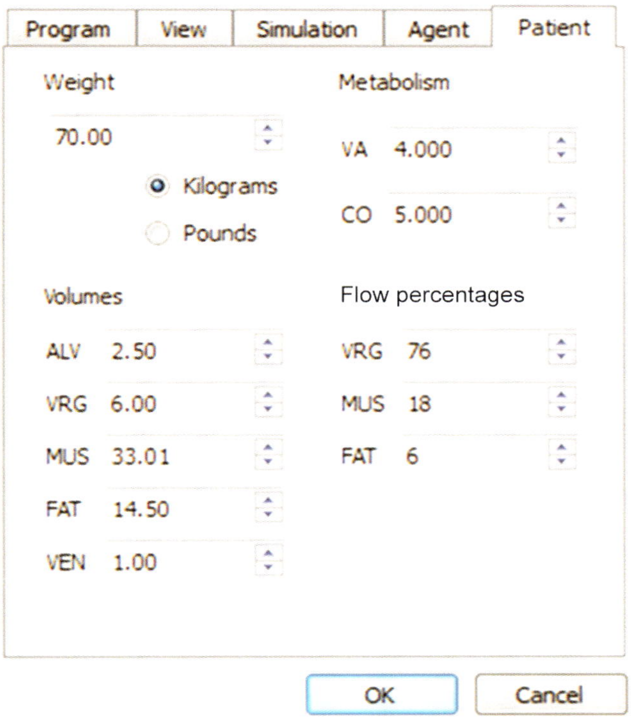

Figure 3 The Gas Man® simulation: The basic parameters

may satisfactorily be done using Gas Man® simulator.[15] The authors compared the real time end tidal sevoflurane concentration with alveolar sevoflurane concentration from Gas Man® software program at various phase of anesthesia and reported to be comparable.[15] Gas Man® software was compared with real time measured end tidal isoflurane concentrations with a semi closed circle system in anesthetised patients.[1] The authors reported that end-tidal isoflurane concentration was comparable to those predicted by Gas Man® software. This would help in predicting the end tidal concentration where end tidal monitoring for volatile agents may not be available or not functional for monitoring. The concept of minimum alveolar concentration (MAC) and MAC awake is usually linked to end tidal concentration of inhalational agents and with clinical endpoints of immobility and consciousness respectively.[7] Both these clinical endpoints are important and depend on various factors. Predicting time for these clinical endpoints also carries with the patient. Simulation or using kinetic models like Gas Man® computer software, prediction of the end points becomes clearer. Not only prediction becomes predictable but also its understanding as to why this will occur becomes clear with understanding

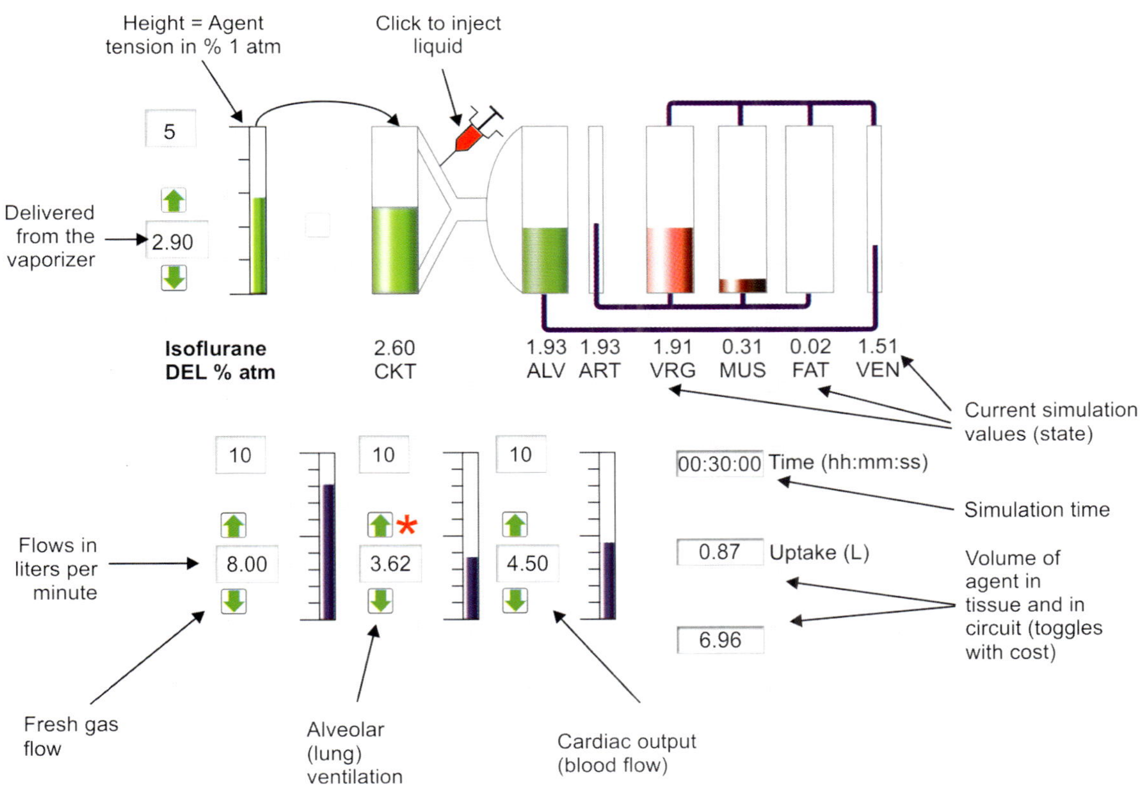

Figure 4 The Gas Man® components and compartments

Abbreviations: CKT, breathing circuit; ALV, alveoli (lungs); ART, arterial blood; VRG, vessel rich group (including brain); MUS, muscle; FAT, fat; VEN, venous blood

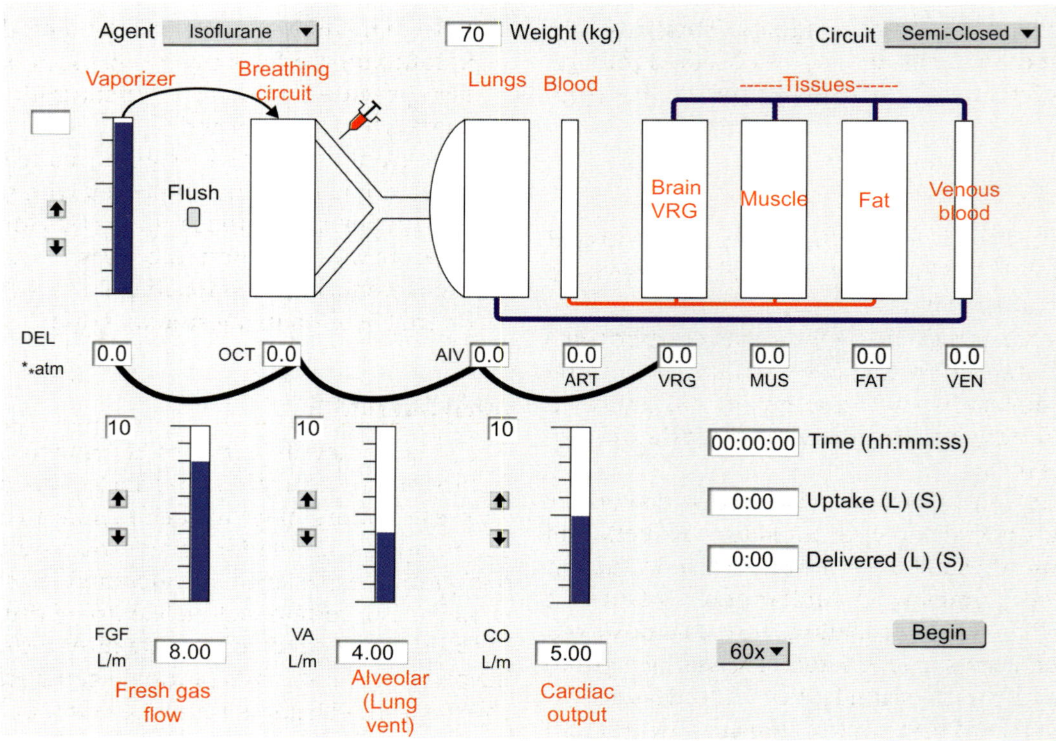

Figure 5 The Gas Man® simulation—compartments and flows

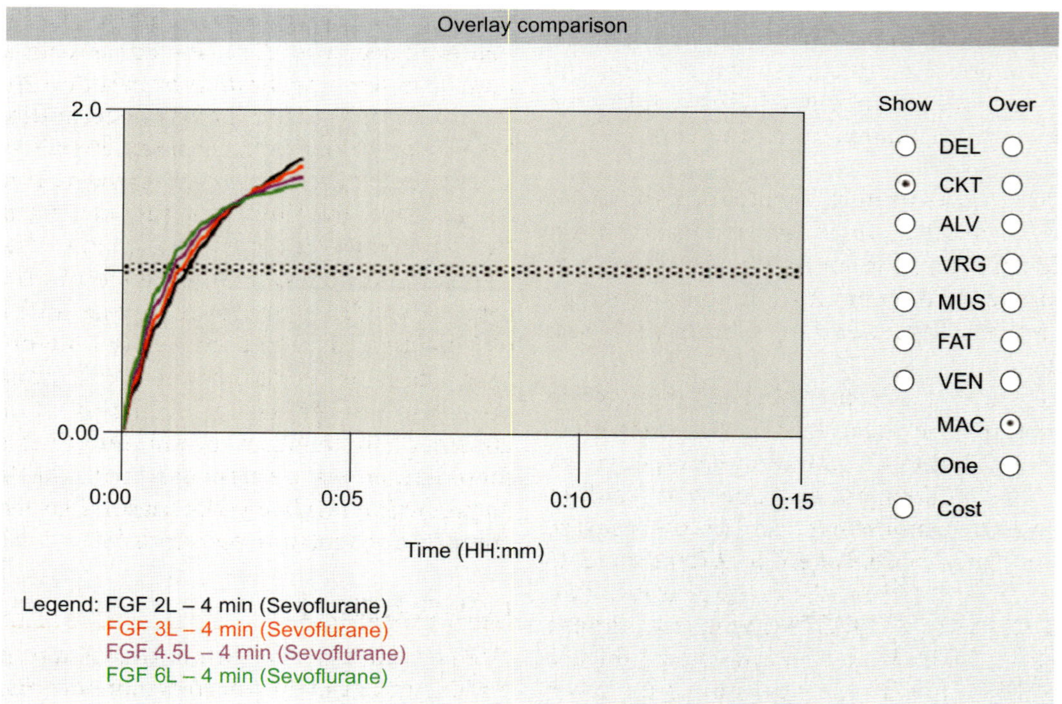

Figure 6 The Gas Man®: The over lay comparison (comparison of different fresh gas flows and anesthetic concentration in breathing circuit)

of the kinetics of inhalational agents. Their wash in and wash out characteristics may be observed through these simulation models and can be applied directly to patient care.[7]

Clinical Impact

The usefulness of Gas Man® has been well demonstrated in the literature.[8,9,10,16] The Gas Man® tool has been used to elucidate various clinical situations:

- Switchover of anesthetic agents for faster emergence was evaluated using Gas Man® simulation.[17] The authors observed that change of isoflurane to desflurane toward the end of anesthesia did not accelerate recovery.
- Gas Man® was used to compare intravenous induction vs. vital capacity inhalation induction of general anesthesia.[18] They observed that induction and recovery times were similar and explained it based on Gas Man® simulation. They also observed that use of nitrous oxide increases vessel rich group inhalational agent tension faster by about 5 secs.
- The authors explored context-sensitive decrement times across anesthetic agents for variable duration.[13] This allows selection of appropriate anesthetic agent in various clinical scenarios.
- The use of Gas Man® simulation would avoid patient exposure fro evaluating some newer protocols related to inhalational agents.[19] This would save resources and any harm to human or animal subjects.
- The Gas Man® was used to evaluate the utility of end-tidal anesthetic concentration vs. inspired anesthetic concentration for depth of anesthesia.[20] The authors reported that end-tidal concentration as target was better for attaining clinically relevant end point.
- The impact of ventilation strategy at emergence was evaluated suing Gas Man®.[21] They observed that hyperventilation do speed up emergence for an insoluble volatile agent and does not result in re-anesthetization unless hypoventilation is severe or unless a highly soluble agent (e.g. isoflurane) is used. Also, sever hypoventilation after extubation may lead to re-anesthetization with all modern agents due to accumulated agent in skeletal muscle especially when anesthetic exposure if for more than 2 hours.[22]
- Low flow anesthesia and its implications have been demonstrated using Gas Man®. The concerns related to keeping flows on and switching off the vaporizer at intubation affects operating room pollution and also provide inadequate concentration of volatile agent when reconnected.[23]
- The hazard with high inspired concentration for inhalational induction in patient with risk of airway obstruction was emphasized by Gas Man® model.[24] After airway obstruction occurs, redistribution of inhalational agents is insufficient to reduce alveolar, arterial, and brain anesthetic tension.

LIMITATIONS

The volatile agents' kinetics is impacted by varying factors and some vary from patient to patient. Mimicking all these factors may not be feasible in simulations. So, it appears simulation should be used with clinical background experience of concerned anesthesiologists as well. Also, certain factors like use of drugs including opioids, benzodiazepines, dexmedetomidine may have impact on the inhalational agents effect and this effect may not be adjusted on the Gas Man® Simulation model as such. The Gas Man® model uses mathematical calculation for an exponential change in the inhalational agents' tension in various compartments. However, it appears same change may not occur in real time scenario. Also, the anesthesia workstations may have some calibration or baseline discrepancy in measurements of flows and concentration while Gas Man® is error free for these parameters. So the outcome in Gas Man® may not truly reflect the real time in day-to-day practice. The simulation models may be limited by the fact of many assumptions made in the simulation. The simulation assumes absence of an arterial-end expired gradient, uniform uptake and distribution of inhalational agents and instantaneous.[7] The Gas Man® does not have provision for compensation for correcting inter-tissue diffusion of anesthetics, anesthetic metabolism, or pulmonary shunt.[8] Though these limitations are associated with Gas Man® model, its prediction has been with reasonable accuracy when compared in real time scenarios.[1]

CONCLUSION

The simulation for inhalational agents helps in understanding of the pharmacokinetics and thus would improve patient care. The Gas Man® simulation mimics several real time scenarios and can be used for patient management by better understanding in an individual patient. Such simulation would help in optimizing the use of these unique drug and concerns related to impact on patient and environment.

REFERENCES

1. Athiraman U, Ravishankar M, Jahagirdhar S. Performance of computer simulated inhalational anesthetic uptake model in comparison with real time isoflurane concentration. J Clin Monit Comput. 2015; DOI 10.1007/s10877-015-9776-6.
2. Schwid HA. Anesthesia simulators-technology and applications. IMAJ. 2000;2:949-53.
3. Rietbrock S, Wissing H, Kuhn I, Fuhr U. Pharamcokinetics of inhaled anesthetics in a clinical setting: description of a novel model based on routine monitoring data. Br J Anaesth. 2000;84:437-42.
4. Bouillon T, Shafer SL. Hot air or full steam ahaed? An empirical pharamacokinetic model of potent inhalational agents. Br J Anaesth. 2000;84:429-31.
5. Dean JM. Gas Man®. MD Comput. 1986;3:537.
6. Kennedy RR, French RA. The development of a system to guide volatile anesthetic administration. Anaesth Intensive Care. 2011;39:182-90.
7. Hendrickx JFA, Lemmens HJM, Shafer SL. Do distribution volumes and clearances relate to tissue volumes and blood flows? A computer simulation. BMC Anesthesiology. 2006;6:7 doi:10.1186/1471-2253-6-7.
8. Philip JH. Using screen based simulation of inhaled anesthetic delivery to improve patient care. Br J Anaesth. 2015;S2:ii89-ii94.
9. Garfield JM, Paskin S, Philip JH. An evaluation of the effectiveness of a computer simulation of anesthetic uptake and distribution as a teaching tool. Med Educ. 1989;23:457-62.
10. Bouillon T, Shafer S. Editorial–Hot air or full steam ahead? An empirical pharmacokinetic model of potent inhaled agents. Br J Anaesth. 2000;84:429-31.
11. Philip JH. Gas Man®—An example of goal oriented computer-assisted teaching which results in learning. Int J Clin Mon. 1986;3:165-71.
12. Lawson D. Gas Man®, Understanding Uptake and Distribution. Book Reviews. Anesth Analg. 1991;73: 240-2.
13. Eger II EI, Shafer SL. Tutorial: context sensitive decrements times for inhaled anesthetics. Anesth Analg. 2005;101:688-96.
14. Garfield JM, Paskin S, Philip JH. An evaluation of the effectiveness of a computer simulation of anesthetic uptake and distribution as a teaching tool. Med Edu. 1989;23:457-62.
15. Panchal NN, Swadia VN, Patel MG. National Journal of Medical Practice. 2014;40:156-60.
16. Hendrickx JFA, Shafer SL. The Kinetics of Gas-Man®- I. Model Derivation. Anesthesiology. 2005;103:A764.
17. Neumann MA, Weiskopf RB, Gong DH, Eger EI, Ionescu P. Changing from isoflurane to desflurane toward the end of anesthesia does not accelerate recovery in humans. Anesthesiology. 1998;88:914-21.
18. Philip BK, Lombard LL, Roaf ER, Drager LR, Calalang I, Philip JH. Comparison of vital capacity induction with sevoflurane to intravenous induction with propofol for adult ambulatory anesthesia. Anesth Analg. 1999;89: 623-27.
19. Pott LM. Simulation saves resources. J Clin Anesth. 2009; 21:539-40.
20. van Zundert T, Hendrickx J, Brebels A, de Cooman S, Gatt S. Effect of the mode of administration of inhaled anesthetics on the interpretation of the FA/FI curve—a Gas Man® simulation. Anaesth Intensive Care. 2010;38: 76-81.
21. De Wolf A, van Zundert TC, De Cooman S, Hendrickx JF. Theoretical effect of hyperventilation on speed of recovery and risk of rehypnotization following recovery—a Gas Man® simulation. BMC Anesthesiol. 2012;12:22.
22. Leeson S, Roberson RS, Philip JH. Hypoventilation after inhaled anesthesia results in reanesthetization. Anesth Analg. 2014;119:829-35.
23. Feldman JM. A simple strategy for faster induction and more cost-effective use of anesthetic vapor. J Clin Monit Comput. 1999;15:17-21.
24. Vijjeswarapu MA, Kuo AS, Philip JH. Incomplete spontaneous recovery from airway obstruction during inhaled anesthesia induction: a computational simulation. Anesth Analg. 2016;122:698-705.

Chapter 35

Simulation Resources

Poonam Malhotra Kapoor, R Gopinath, Manju Mani

Chapter Outline

SIMULATION SOCIETIES ACROSS THE WORLD

- Society for simulation in healthcare
- World Simulation Society (WSS)
- *ABRASSIM:* Brazilian Association of Simulation in Healthcare
- *ASPiH:* Association for simulated practice in healthcare
- The Center for Medical Simulation in Poznan
- Association of Standardized Patient Educators (ASPE)
- The International Nursing Association for Clinical Simulation and Learning
- The International Pediatric Simulation Society (IPSS)
- Simulation Network
- Swiss Conference on Standardized Patients and Simulations (SPSIM)
- *SESAM:* Society in Europe for Simulation applied to Medicine.

SIMULATION WEBSITES

- *http://www.feinberg.northwestern.edu/sites/dme/simulation*
- *http://www.ucc.ie/en/assert*
- *http://www.gcrme.miami.edu*
- *http://hscj.ufl.edu/csesar*
- *http://www.med.umich.edu/umcsc*
- *http://www.upmc.com/about/why-upmc/quality/pages/wiser.aspx*
- *http://inspiresim.com*
- *http://www.nursingsimulation.org*
- *www.ssih.org*
- Simulation on the web.

BOOKS FOR SIMULATION STUDIES

- **The Comprehensive Textbook of Healthcare Simulation**
  Levine AI, DeMaria Jr S, Schwartz AD, Sim AJ (Eds.)
  ISBN 978-1-4614-5993-4

- **Simulation-Based Case Studies in Logistics**
  Education and Applied Research
  Merkuryev Y, Merkuryeva G, Piera MA, Guasch Petit A (Eds.) 2009, XXIV, 232 p.
  ISBN 978-1-84882-187-3
- **Advanced Research on Computer Education, Simulation and Modeling**
  International Conference, CESM 2011, Wuhan, China, June 18-19, 2011. Proceedings, Part I
  Editors: Song Lin, Xiong Huang
  ISBN: 978-3-642-21782-1 (Print) 978-3-642-21783-8 (Online)
- **Patient Safety and Quality: An Evidence-Based Handbook for Nurses.**
  Hughes RG, editor. Rockville (MD): Agency for Healthcare Research and Quality (US); 2008 Apr.
- **Simulation-Based Case Studies in Logistics: Education and Applied Research Hardcover–2009**
  Yuri Merkuryev (Editor), Galina Merkuryeva (Editor), Miquel ANgel Piera (Editor), Antoni Guasch Petit (Editor)
  ISBN-13: 978-0195177664
- **Clinical Simulation in Nursing**
  Suzie Kardong-Edgren, PhD, RN, ANEF
  Vol. 10 Issue 9, September 2014
- **Simulation in Healthcare Education: A Best Evidence Practical Guide.**
  October 2013, Vol. 35, No. 10, Pages e1511-e1530 (doi:10.3109/0142159X.2013.818632)
  Ivette Motola[1*], Luke A Devine[2], Hyun Soo Chung[3], John E Sullivan[1], S Barry Issenberg

JOURNALS FOR SIMULATION

- *Education and research*: Nursing Plus - Editorial
- *Simulation and gaming*: An Interdisciplinary Journal of Theory, Practice and Research
- *Journal of surgical simulation (JSS)*: The international peer-reviewed journal for surgeons using simulation to enhance practice and patient safety.
- The online journal of issues in nursing practice: Simulation in Nursing Practice—The Impact on Patient Care.
- The Medical Journal of Australia
- International Journal of Gaming and Computer-Mediated Simulations (IJGCMS).

Chapter 36

Simulation in Cardiac Critical Care Medicine

Kalpana Irpachi, Poonam Malhotra Kapoor, Rohan Magoon

Chapter Outline

- Computer-based Simulation
- Whole Body Simulation
- Simulation Scenarios in the Intensive Care Unit
- Simulation in Hemodynamic Monitoring
- Simulation in Extracorporeal Membrane Oxygenation
- Simulation in Resuscitation Training
- Crisis Resource Management
- Role of Simulation in Pediatrics
- Simulation for Procedural Training
- Future of Critical Care Simulation

ABSTRACT

Simulation is educational tool, it improves trainees' knowledge and skills in cardiac critical care such as invasive procedures, management of medical and surgical emergencies and communication skills. A growing body of literature supports the use and effectiveness of low-fidelity and high-fidelity simulators for procedural training. This review highlights simulation-based training in cardiac critical care medicine tools to provide realistic simulated critical care events without placing patients at undue risk to improve patient safety and outcome.

INTRODUCTION

Patient care is complex in postoperative cardiac intensive care unit (ICU) following cardiac surgery which is comprised of critically ill patients, high emotionality, and fatiguing work schedules represents a particularly high stakes environment for human error and system failures, this is compounded by the need for simulation training on team function.[1,2]

Simulation is a "computer-based realistic training device that duplicates artificially the conditions likely to be encountered in critical care set-up". Even after successful surgical repair, patients may have complications of depressed myocardial contractility, bleeding, hypo- or hypertension, hypo- or hypervolemia, hypo- or hyperthermia, heart block, tamponade, and anemia. Hence, simulation offers a controlled, safe and reproducible environment to practice clinical skills, in solving healthcare challenges as well as it is an excellent educational tool to help facilitate learning and change the practice to improve patient outcomes.[3]

Based on work done on aviation industry, medical simulation pioneered in 1980s developed simulation environment in which clinician could interact with patient simulator and the clinical environment, allowing the trainees to engage in real-time clinical scenarios.[4]

There is a wide diversity of training methods, utilizing equipment ranging from low-fidelity manikins for skills practice to the high-fidelity models used for scenario-based learning in simulation centers. Scenarios can be tailored to reflect local and critical incidents, and site-specific system errors may be identified. In this article, we review simulation-based training in cardiac critical care medicine requires procedural competence in many technical domains, including vascular access, airway management, basic and advanced bronchoscopy, pleural procedures, and critical care ultrasonography.

It is a teaching strategy for nursing education and orientation skills in critical care medicine.[5] Simulation-based medical education is an educational tool for healthcare professionals while individuals achieve a high level of technical competency which is a strong signal that improves the patients outcome. Several simulation programs have been set-up in ICUs around the world simulation-based interventions are required to promote resident confidence and skills across many competency domains.

OBJECTIVES

- To develop the approach to simulation in critical care training
- Help to improve clinician response in highly stressful, life-threatening situations
- To develop the use and effectiveness of low-fidelity and high-fidelity simulators for procedural training and assessment
- Clinical rehearsal
- Simulation as a teaching tool
- Promote simulation-based education through research and collaboration
- Performance assessment.

COMPUTER-BASED SIMULATION

Computer-based simulation prior to mannequin-based simulation improves the participants' skills confidence and satisfaction with the activity during the more real-life setting achieved in the mannequin-based simulation.[6]

Computer-based simulation training also improves high-level and lower-level the learning outcomes in mannequin-based simulation exercises. The simulator has some type of physical representation with sensing instruments that inform the computer of the user's movements. The program that computes the changes that should take place within the model and projects the correct response onto the screen. Systems may include some sort of three-dimensional (3D) imaging to make the environment more realistic.

WHOLE BODY SIMULATION

Whole body simulation is an efficient means of training a large group of trainees, allows a trainees to experience rare, life-threatening conditions, to make medical errors without harmful consequences to patients, enables faculty to provide feedback, permits trainees to repeat performances until educational objectives are achieved.

Use of high-fidelity human simulators is poised to take on a greater role for the training of residents, medical students and critical care nurses within the specialties of pulmonary and critical care medicine. High-fidelity simulator training led to more rapid acquisition of skills compared with conventional training. Objective assessment for rapid acquisition of technical skills consists of endotracheal intubation, advanced cardiac life support protocols, central venous catheter insertion, bronchoscopy, and complex case-based simulation skills such as respiratory distress, pulseless rhythms, stable and unstable supraventricular arrhythmias, septic shock, anaphylaxis, status epilepticus and hypertensive crisis.

SIMULATION SCENARIOS IN THE INTENSIVE CARE UNIT

Airway Scenarios

Emergency intubation of a patient with a dilated cardiomyopathy and cardiogenic shock, severe asthma, septic shock and severe metabolic acidosis, recognition of endotracheal tube dislodgement.

Cardiothoracic Surgery Scenarios

Pericardial tamponade postcardiac surgery, end of life and organ donation scenarios, hemodynamics/

shock and vasopressors scenarios, hypotension due to disconnected inotropes, hypertension due to measurement error.

Renal Scenarios

Hyperkalemia and cardiac arrest due to acute kidney injury (AKI), VF arrest (unexpected cardiac arrest due to ventricular fibrillation), sedation and delirium scenarios.

Application of Simulation in Cardiac Critical Care Medicine

To accomplish the goal, different types of simulation technologies relevant to critical care environment are discussed here.

SIMULATION IN HEMODYNAMIC MONITORING

The critical care and hemodynamic monitoring simulation training system consists of a personal computer, software, and human torso designed to enable to practice insertion of a hemodynamic monitoring catheter; the cardiac monitor displays feeding the catheter through the heart into the pulmonary artery, inflating the balloon at the tip of the catheter, and interpreting the measured pressure and other information obtained.[7] There is further evidence that simulation-based training can reduce catheter-related bloodstream infections as well as the major implications for ICU outcomes.[8] Special screen calculators in the program may be used to determine hemodynamic, respiratory, ventilatory, and renal function indices. The computer also displays patient histories, laboratory results, treatment options, patient responses, and a real-time cardiac monitor.

Hemodynamic monitoring simulations incorporate the Laerdal SimMan and SimMan 3G software partnered to Edwards' life sciences provide a range of hemodynamic monitoring solutions. This simulation toolkit includes 19 preprogrammed scenarios to interpret and prudently act upon hemodynamic data developed specifically to challenge cardiac critical care staff or students.

AQAI SIS models are a growing technology continuously develops new applications to make all relevant hemodynamic values (e.g. Global End diastolic volume, extravascular lung water) more realistic on the basis of the actual patient findings. AQAI SIS is a flexible software system which synchronizes the heart rate of the cardiac simulator with the heart rate of the patient which is a physiological model in cath lab simulations. AQAI SIS combines with TestChest is a high end artificial lung simulator with its own models on lung mechanics, gas exchange and heart lung interactions properties. The SIS model analyses all relevant drugs for anesthesia, calculates drug interactions and generates a simulated bispectral (BIS) index. This module includes several scenarios, e.g. volume loss, severe sepsis, acute respiratory distress syndrome (ARDS) which is combined with appropriate learning modules.

PiCCO is a tool for advanced hemodynamic monitoring. It uses transpulmonary thermodilution and pulse contour analysis to derive various parameters of the cardiovascular system. Communication to the PiCCO monitor allows all regular user interactions on the monitor. Finally the hemodynamic situation can be analyzed and treated by the trainee.

SIMULATION IN EXTRACORPOREAL MEMBRANE OXYGENATION

Anderson et al. were the first to publish the simulation for extracorporeal membrane oxygenation (ECMO), showed a decreased number of errors in ECMO emergencies in those individuals receiving simulation training.[9] ECMO system consists of two components, neonatal mannequin and a standard neonatal ECMO circuit primed with an artificial blood, which is adjusted to reflect the particular clinical scenario. Both venoarterial (VA) and venovenous (VV) ECMO can be simulated, and the cannulae are changed to reflect the appropriate scenario **(Figure 1)**. Simulation specialists adjust the circuit pressures, patient monitoring equipment, and vital signs in real-time of a wide variety of clinical scenarios and ECMO emergencies, thereby enhancing the overall realism of the setting.

SIMULATION IN RESUSCITATION TRAINING

The quality of education, CPR guidelines and the chain of survival all contribute to patient outcome following cardiac arrest. Gavin discussed the role of task trainers,

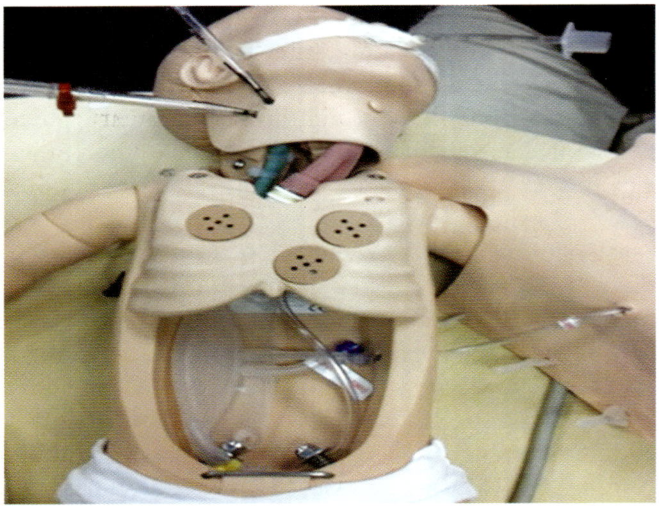

Figure 1 ECMO Mannequin's chest cavity with neck cannula

high- and low-fidelity patient simulators and computer-assisted simulation as teaching tools. Skill-based training offers a simulation-based skills and team work training program such as BLS and ACLS.[10]

SimMan™ 3G is a very high-fidelity recent version virtual reality wireless device widely used for cardiopulmonary resuscitation (CPR). During CPR scenarios can be preprogrammed or actively programmed. Monitors record chest compression rate, depth of compression, time without compression (hands off time), palpable pulses, respiratory rate, arterial blood gases, ECG waveforms, ECG artifacts, critical event recognition (e.g. cardiac arrhythmia) and responses to various drug injections. SimMan™ 3G mannequin provides realistic patient experiences for deliberate practice of teamwork, leadership, and communication skills in high-risk, low frequency emergency scenarios.

CRISIS RESOURCE MANAGEMENT

Crisis resource management (CRM) is the new way of teaching including the application of realistic simulation exercises, to improve the patient safety in acute care domains. Crisis resource management principles forms the foundation for efficient team functioning and subsequent error reduction in high-stakes environments such as acute care pediatrics setting. Principles of CRM provided the tools necessary to help build the simulation-based CRM teaching into pediatric training programs.[11]

ROLE OF SIMULATION IN PEDIATRICS

A high-fidelity simulator is a full body computerized manikin that have realistic features, such as blinking eyes with reacting pupils, chest that rise and fall with respiration, palpable pulses, various heart and lung sounds and ability to cry, drool and bleed. They can respond physiologically to interventions, such as medication administration, intravascular fluid infusions and application of oxygen. They have a procedural features to allow chest tube and tracheotomy management, defibrillation and urinary catheter insertion. Laerdal, METI and Gaumard are the most popular companies involved in pediatric simulation.

SIMULATION FOR PROCEDURAL TRAINING

Simulation enhances the resident confidence in critical care and procedural skills.[12] It is an effective and efficient way for the trainees to acquire bronchoscopy skills. Simulator training in flexible bronchoscopy include low-fidelity simulation which incorporates a live animal models, resected and preserved animal lungs or wet tissue models, and inanimate models of upper airways and bronchial tree made up of various materials, whereas high-fidelity simulation uses a computer- based bronchoscopic simulators which are intended to provide a realistic bronchoscopic experience and allows the operator to navigate through computer-generated airway images which gives the feedback to trainee regarding the procedural skills.

SimMan is a full size, portable patient simulator designed for practising resuscitation skills and scenarios. The manikin can be used for training in airway management with the facility to induce trismus, glottic swelling and cannot ventilate/cannot intubate scenarios and invasive procedures such as needle and surgical cricothyroidotomy, chest drain insertion and intravenous cannulation. It also generates realistic heart rate, breathing, blood pressure and bowel sounds. An online survey performed across the UK regarding complications and airway management in the ICU. Twenty-seven patients were died of adverse airway events. Upon survey found that a majority of junior trainees inexperienced with tracheotomy care and emergencies and felt low confidence levels with airway management in critical care. Hence, Cook et al created a multidisciplinary airway training program at the point of care to practice critical incident drills.[13]

Simulation using high-fidelity simulators in image acquisition for transesophageal echocardiography should be relevant to all three aspects image acquisition, image interpretation, and clinical applications. Limitation of performing ultrasonography and echocardiography include cost, logistics, and lack of pathology in normal models. Advanced critical care echocardiography is also a tool to monitor hemodynamics in the ICU, but requires acquisition of technical skills in transesophageal echocardiography (TEE). Gwénaël demonstrated the addition of virtual reality simulator sessions to a standardized 6-month curriculum improves the acquisition of practical and technical skills for the hemodynamic evaluation of ventilated ICU patients.[14] The use of computerized echocardiographic simulation improves the learning curve for transesophageal hemodynamic assessment in critically ill patients **(Figure 2)**.

EchoCom simulator was the first to publish as a simple 'Windows' interface based on the concept of augmented reality in training of echocardiographic simulation. Augmented reality couples virtual with real data (in particular, 3D image data) **(Figure 3)**. It supported the spatial orientation and hand-eye coordination. The advantage of this application is that trainees can tailor their course according to their own timetable and needs. Difficult procedures can be trained without setting patients at risk.[15]

Vimedix simulation is the most sophisticated versatile ultrasound simulator that supports on one platform: transthoracic echocardiography (TTE), transesophageal echocardiography (TEE) and abdominal/pelvic scanning, including focused assessment with sonography for trauma (FAST). It provides a realistic method of image acquisition and improves the spatial relationship **(Figures 4 and 5)**.

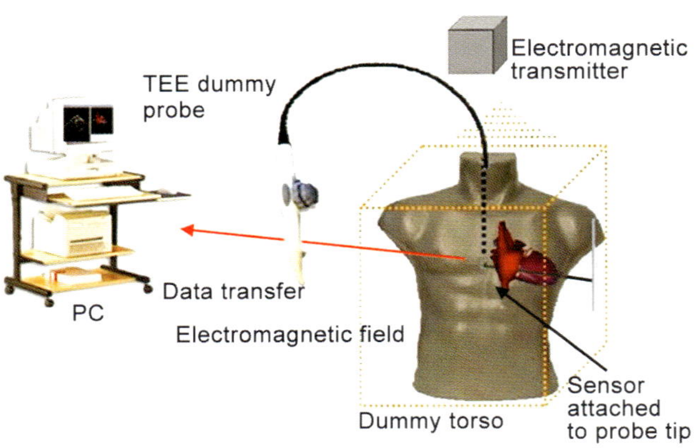

Figure 2 Parts of a transesophageal echocardiography (TEE) simulator

Cost

The costs involved with simulation-based medical education technology requires complete reporting and accounting of cost. A systematic review conducted to evaluate the economic analysis of simulation-based medical education for the financial implications of the educational intervention.[16] The cost of simulation typically increases as the fidelity increases. More recently, several studies demonstrated the comparison

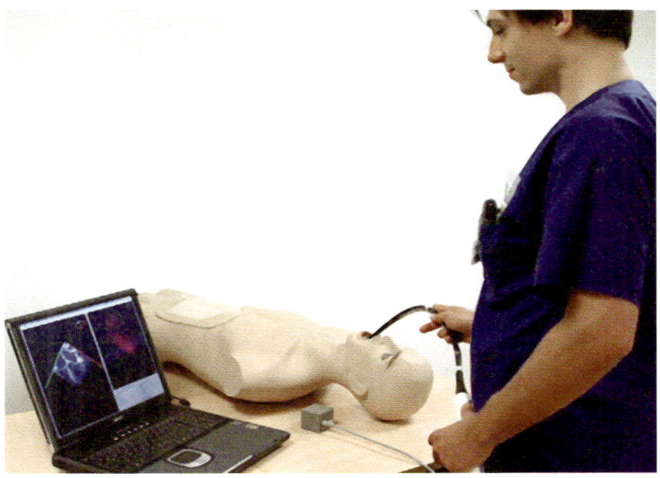

Figure 3 EchoCom simulation system shows virtual heart model depicting transthoracic/transesophageal echocardiographic probe, and EchoCom software installed on a computer

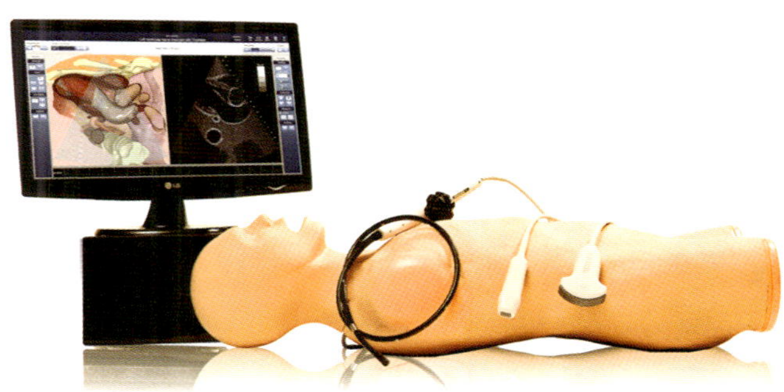

Figure 4 Vimedix simulation

CHAPTER 36

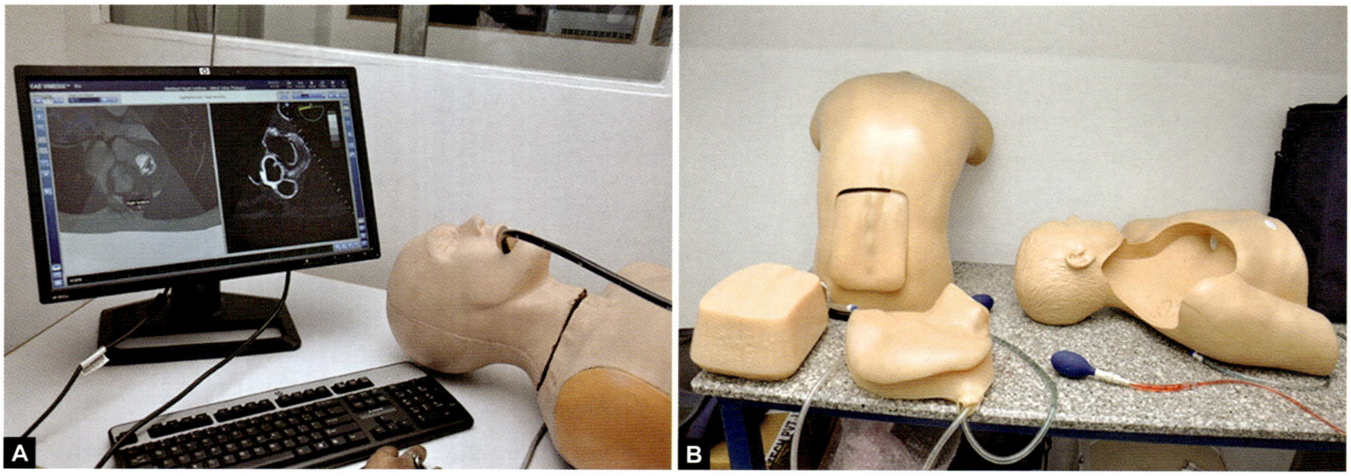

Figures 5A and B Vimedix simulator mannequin system consists of a full-sized mannequin, transthoracic echocardiographic, transesophageal echocardiographic, abdominal scanning probes, and a dedicated computer

of low versus high-fidelity models, and consistently found that low-fidelity models can be similarly effective and less expensive compared with their high-fidelity counterparts. Weinstock developed a low-space mobile cart with a reduced-cost to provide an actual clinical environment to hospital teams as a model for cost-effective, transportable, widespread simulation-based education internationally.[17]

FUTURE OF CRITICAL CARE SIMULATION

Simulation has proved to study human factors and failure modes during critical care, in the developmental research of new treatment concepts (e.g. checklist use and telemedicine), and in the support of bioengineering system development (e.g. device beta-testing, educating the manufacturers' workforce).[18] Future research should continue to assess the efficacy of traditional teaching methods for performance assessment versus computer simulations. In the near future, medical simulation could serve the impact or benefit of simulation-based training across the various dimensions.

CONCLUSION

Simulation is a well-accepted teaching method for critical care and procedural skills and improves resident confidence. Simulation has been used effectively in a growing number of critical care domain as a standard of training and certification. Teamwork conducted in the simulated environment offer traditional didactic instruction, enhance performance, and possibly also reduce errors in clinical/procedural skills, as well as robust quality improvement tool to identify deficiencies of practice. Hence, the expanded role of simulation training reduces procedural errors, mortality rates, and malpractice claims.

REFERENCES

1. Frengley RW1, Weller JM, Torrie J, Dzendrowskyj P, Yee B, Paul AM, Shulruf B, Henderson KM. The effect of a simulation-based training intervention on the performance of established critical care unit teams. Crit Care Med. 2011;39(12):2605-11.
2. Rosen MA1, Salas E, Wu TS, Silvestri S, Lazzara EH, Lyons R, Weaver SJ, King HB. Promoting teamwork: an event-based approach to simulation-based teamwork training for emergency medicine residents. Acad Emerg Med. 2008;15(11):1190-8.
3. Datta R, Upadhyay K, Jaideep C. Simulation and its role in medical education. Med J Armed Forces India. 2012; 68(2):167-72.
4. Chang CH. Medical simulation is needed in anesthesia training to achieve patient's safety. Korean J Anesthesiol. 2013;64:204-11.
5. Rauen CA. Simulation as a teaching strategy for nursing education and orientation in cardiac surgery. Crit Care Nurse. 2004;24(3):46-51.
6. Curtin LB, Finn LA, Czosnowski QA, Whitman CB, Cawley MJ. Computer-based simulation training to

improve learning outcomes in mannequin-based simulation exercises. Am J Pharm Educ. 2011;75(6):113.
7. McSparron JI, Michaud GC, Gordan PL, Channick CL, Wahidi MM, Yarmus LB, Feller-Kopman DJ, Makani SS, Koenig SJ, Mayo PH, Kovitz KL, Thomson CC. Skills-based Working Group of the American Thoracic Society Education Committee. Simulation for Skills-based Education in Pulmonary and Critical Care Medicine. Ann Am Thorac Soc. 2015;12(4):579-86.
8. Cohen ER, Feinglass J, Barsuk JH, et al. Cost savings from reduced catheter-related bloodstream infection after simulation-based education for residents in a medical intensive care unit. Simul Healthc. 2010;5(2):98-102.
9. Anderson JM, Murphy AA, Boyle KB, Yaeger KA, Halamek LP. Simulating extracorporeal membrane oxygenation emergencies to improve human performance. Part II:assessment of technical and behavioral skills. Simul Healthc. 2006;1(4):228-32.
10. Perkins GD. Simulation in resuscitation training. Resuscitation. 2007;73(2):202-11.
11. Cheng A, Donoghue A, Gilfoyle E, Eppich W. Simulation-based crisis resource management training for pediatric critical care medicine: A review for instructors. Pediatr Crit Care Med. 2012;13:2.
12. James M. Cooke, Janet Larsen, Stanley J. Hamstra, Pamela B. Andreatta. Simulation Enhances Resident Confidence in Critical Care and Procedural Skills. Fam Med. 2008;40(3):165-7.
13. SC Cook, JJ Gatward, FE Kelly, J Bell, FM O'Higgins and MJ Thomas. Simulation training at the point of care to decrease the incidence of airway complications on the intensive care unit. Critical Care. 2010;14(Suppl 1):P463.
14. Prat G, Charron C, Repesse X, Coriat P, Bailly P, L'her E, Vieillard-Baron A. The use of computerized echocardiographic simulation improves the learning curve for transoesophageal hemodynamic assessment in critically ill patients. Ann Intensive Care. 2016;6:27.
15. Weidenbach M, Drachsler H, Wild F, Kreutter S, Razek V, Grunst G, Ender J, Berlage T, Janousek J. EchoComTEE—a simulator for transoesophageal echocardiography. Anaesthesia. 2007;62(4):347-53.
16. Zendejas B, Wang AT, Brydges R, Hamstra SJ, Cook DA. Cost: the missing outcome in simulation-based medical education research: a systematic review. Surgery. 2013;153(2):160-76.
17. Weinstock PH1, Kappus LJ, Garden A, Burns JP. Simulation at the point of care: reduced-cost, in situ training via a mobile cart. Pediatr Crit Care Med. 2009; 10(2):176-81.
18. Marcus Rall, David M. Gaba, Peter Dieckmann, christophbernhardeich. Patient Simulation. In Miller's Anesthesia, 2-Volume Set, 8th Edition, Year 2014, Chapter 8, p. 167-209

INDEX

Page numbers followed by *f* refer to figure and *t* refer to table.